Summary of Catecholamine Receptor Activity

Receptor Subtype	Action When Stimulated	Stimulating Drugs	Action When Blocked	Blocking Drugs
Alpha (α)				
α₁ Postsynaptic areas of neurons, blood vessels α₂ Presynaptic and post-synaptic areas of neurons, blood vessels	Vasoconstriction ↑ BP ↑ SVR ↑ CO	Phenylephrine* Methoxamine* Epinephrine Norepinephrine Dopamine Ephedrine	Vasodilation ↓ BP ↓ SVR ↕ CO	Prazosin Labetalol Clonidine Methyldopa Phentolamine
Beta (β)				
β₁ Myocardial surface	↑ Contractility ↑ HR ↑ BP ↑ CO	Dobutamine Dopamine Epinephrine Isoproterenol Norepinephrine	↓ Force of contraction ↓ HR ↓ BP ↓ CO	At_ Es_ M_ La_ N_ Pr_ Ti_
β₂ Blood vessels, bronchial and GI smooth muscle	Vasodilation ↓ BP Bronchodilation ↑ Blood glucose	Dobutamine Epinephrine Isoproterenol	Slight vasoconstriction Slight ↑ BP Bronchospasm	La_ N_ Pr_ Ti_
Dopaminergic				
Renal and mesenteric blood vessels	Renal vasodilation Mesenteric vasodilation ↑ UO ↑ GI motility	Dopamine† (<7 μg/kg/min)	Renal vasoconstriction Mesenteric vasoconstriction ↓ Urine output ↓ GI motility	D_ (_)_ N_ Pt_ M_ Ej_ Ej_

↑ = Increase; ↓ = decrease; ↕ = may increase or decrease   *Alpha, stimulation only.   †Pure dopaminergic effects ≤ 2 μg/kg/min

Mosby's Critical Care and Emergency Drug Reference

Mosby's
Critical Care
and
Emergency
Drug Reference

Janet Hicks Keen, RN, MS, CCRN, CEN

Staff Nurse, Level II
Saint Joseph's Hospital of Atlanta
Atlanta, Georgia
Clinical Instructor
Gordon College
Barnsville, Georgia
Consultant in Emergency, Trauma, and Critical Care

Marianne Saunorus Baird
RN, MN, CCRN

Clinical Nurse Specialist
Critical Care
Saint Joseph's Hospital of Atlanta
Atlanta, Georgia

Jody H. Allen
PharmD

Assistant Clinical Professor
Virginia Commonwealth University
Richmond, Virginia

CONTRIBUTOR **Bob Aucker,** PharmD

Consultant in Critical Care
   Pharmacology
Clinical Pharmacist
Saint Joseph's Hospital of Atlanta
Atlanta, Georgia

ⅤⅤ Mosby

St. Louis   Baltimore   Boston

Carlsbad   Chicago   Naples   New York   Philadelphia   Portland

London   Madrid   Mexico City   Singapore   Sydney   Tokyo   Toronto   Wiesbaden

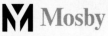
Mosby

Dedicated to Publishing Excellence

A Times Mirror
Company

Vice President and Publisher: Nancy Coon
Editor: Robin Carter
Developmental Editor: Elizabeth Fathman
Project Manager: Mark Spann
Production Editor: Jenny Doll
Designer: Judi Lang
Manufacturing Supervisor: Tony McAllister

A NOTE TO THE READER

The authors and publisher have made every attempt to check dosages and nursing content for accuracy. Because the science of pharmacology is continually advancing, our knowledge base continues to expand. Therefore we recommend that the reader always check product information for changes in dosage or administration before administering any medication. This is particularly important with new or rarely used drugs.

Printed in the United States of America
Composition by TSI Graphics
Printing/binding by R.R. Donnelley & Sons Company

Mosby-Year Book, Inc.
11830 Westline Industrial Drive
St. Louis, Missouri 63146

ISBN 0-8151-5054-7

96   97   98   99   00   /   9   8   7   6   5   4   3   2   1

To
Jean Snyder Hicks, RPh
who taught me respect for the power of medications
supported my aspirations
and without whose help and encouragement
this endeavor would not have been possible.

J.H.K.

Foreword

Cindy Brown, RN, MN, CEN
1984-1985 President, ENA
Atlanta, Georgia

It is not easy being a nurse in today's world, if, indeed, it has ever
been "easy" to be a nurse. With mergers, consolidations, hospital
closings, downsizing, work redesign, cross-training, decreased cen-
sus and increased acuity, increased regulation, and fear of legal ram-
ifications, change is the *only* constant; and the resultant chaos is
barely manageable. How does today's nurse survive the whirlwind,
and more important, how will that nurse and the ones to come, survive the future?

In addition, nurses face an ever-expanding array of treatment modalities, technologies, and drug therapies with each year that passes.
Information assaults us at a truly awesome pace. How is it possible
to keep up? Is it possible to remember everything?

The answer to the above questions are, "No, it is not possible, nor
even desirable, to try to remember all the bits of data required of
us." The ability to function effectively lies in knowledge. Knowledge is the only way to keep one's head above water, and the only
way to remain knowledgeable is to marshall all available resources—
books, journals, manuals, guides—and keep them at hand, ready at a
moment's notice for reference.

Mosby's Critical Care and Emergency Drug Reference is just
such a resource. There are many drug guides on the market, but this
one is unique in that it was written specifically by and for critical
care and emergency nurses, who have a clear understanding of the
information necessary to function as one must in these milieus.

Critical information is presented first: generic name, trade name,
classification(s), usual dose, actions, and pharmacokinetics. This is
followed by precautions and contraindications, including not only
the warning, but why that particular caution is important. For example, one is warned to use adenosine cautiously in the asthmatic
patient because it may cause bronchoconstriction.

Additional pertinent data include pediatric doses, interactions/
compatibilities, therapeutic levels, symptoms of toxicity/overdose,
patient care implications, monitoring/hemodynamic guidelines,
physical assessment guidelines, and patient/family teaching. Appendixes include such topics as how to manage toxicity due to overdose, ACLS guidelines, management of acute allergic reactions, infusion rate guidelines, relative activity of pressor agents, and how to

ix

manage extravasation of pressor agents. Serious warnings are in bold print, capturing immediate attention. The prose is written in simple, commonly used language. No pseudosophistication here!

I am proud to introduce *Mosby's Critical Care and Emergency Drug Reference,* the definitive answer to the need for quickly accessible information for critical care and emergency nurses. I think you will find it an indispensable part of your armamentarium for practice.

Foreword

Sandra B. Dunbar, RN, DSN
1986-1987 President, AACN
Associate Professor and Coordinator of Critical Care Nursing
Nell Hodgson Woodruff School of Nursing
Emory University
Atlanta, Georgia

Critical care nurses have experienced a remarkable evolution of knowledge and responsibility over the past three decades. As new modalities and technologies have been developed to treat the patient with life-threatening illness, the nurse's responsibility and account-ability for implementing therapy have increased concomitantly. In-dependent and collaborative assessment and management of human response to life-threatening illness and its treatment are hallmarks of critical care nursing practice.

Complex pharmacologic regimens are commonplace in critical care. The combined vulnerability of the critically ill patient and po-tency of the drugs require the critical care nurse to administer multi-ple agents with expert knowledge of their compatibilities and side effects. Complex decision-making is involved in the process of al-tering or titrating drugs on the basis of rapidly changing patient re-sponses. Constant vigilance for side effects and prompt intervention when adverse responses occur are inherent in this role.

Current knowledge of pharmacology, pharmacokinetics, and drug administration particulars is essential to safely implement this role. Critical care nurses must have ready access to information that sup-ports their decisions. With *Mosby's Critical Care and Emergency Drug Reference,* the authors have met an important challenge by creating a reference with knowledge about drugs that is highly spe-cific for critical care. Attention to pharmacologic effects on hemo-dynamic changes and special circulatory systems is an important extension not available in most drug guides. Implications for elders and children are welcome additions to the set of references of criti-cal care nurses.

Points for consideration in patient teaching and management of side effects or adverse responses are well described. This extensive compilation of information is a valuable reference for nurses who provide care for the critically ill in many types of settings.

Preface

As an active critical care and emergency caregiver, I identified a need for an easy-to-use, portable reference with up-to-date, specific drug information. *Mosby's Critical Care and Emergency Drug Reference* was conceived in response to this need. It is designed for busy practitioners who require an exceptionally reliable and thorough, yet quick, reference for everyday use in the care of patients with critical or emergent illnesses or injuries.

The most frequently used critical care and emergency medications, together with important hemodynamic effects and implications for critical care monitoring, have been included in the book. Essential information is provided concisely, yet in greater detail than usually provided in general drug references. This compendium enables the critical care practitioner to apply the information to our uniquely complex patient care situations.

Mosby's Critical Care and Emergency Drug Reference is intended to augment the user's basic understanding of pharmacology and critical care. Each drug description and all supporting material have been carefully written to emphasize information most useful in critical and emergency care. For example, since so many seriously ill patients are receiving multiple medications, comprehensive information is provided on drug interactions and physical compatibility.

Because this is a quick reference, some information is limited. For example, pediatric applications are briefly addressed for drugs commonly used for children. The highly specialized area of neonatal pharmacology has not been included. Specialized references should be consulted for neonates or for complex pediatric situations. Dosage adjustments for patients with renal or hepatic insufficiency are briefly summarized, but the prescribing practitioner is encouraged to consult specialized references for complete information when prescribing medications for patients with functional impairment of any major organ.

Medication administration under any condition is a tremendous responsibility. This responsibility is extreme during emergencies or when the patient's physiologic status is critical. The user of this, or any drug reference, must consider the unique characteristics of each patient and use the information accordingly.

Mosby's Critical Care and Emergency Drug Reference is written by, and uniquely for, critical care and emergency caregivers. In keeping with a commitment to provide the most relevant and accurate information in this rapidly changing field, the authors welcome and value suggestions from users.

Janet Hicks Keen

Acknowledgments

We are grateful to the many individuals who supported us during the writing of this manuscript. We offer our thanks to:

Our families, especially Raymond, Laura, Glenna, Thom, Rachel, Michael, Kathryn, John, Elizabeth, and Margaret, whose patience and neverending love helped us endure many difficult moments.

Pam Swearingen, RN, whose wisdom and encouragement led to the concept of this project.

Bob Aucker, Pharm D, whose expertise is valued by all of the authors.

All of the exceptional individuals at Mosby, especially Robin Carter.

REVIEWERS

We would like to extend our gratitude to the reviewers of *Mosby's Critical Care and Emergency Drug Reference.* Their careful examination of the enclosed contents resulted in a wealth of informed, insightful recommendations. We appreciate their dedication, knowledge, and good efforts.

Elisabeth Buck, RN, CCRN, LT, NC, USN
Naval Medical Center
Portsmouth, VA
and
Acute Care Department
Branch Medical Clinic Norfolk
Norfolk, VA

Roberta Secrest, PhD, PharmD, RPh
Senior Associate Scientist
Marion Merrell Dow Research
    Institute
Cincinnati, OH

Elizabeth Warmke, RN, MS
Pediatric/PICU Clinical Nurse
    Specialist
Christ Hospital and Medical Center
Oak Lawn, IL

Contents

About this book: How to use *Mosby's Critical Care and Emergency Drug Reference*

Mosby's Critical Care and Emergency Drug Reference is carefully arranged for rapid retrieval of essential content. Medications are listed alphabetically by the most commonly used generic name. Infusion tables for vasoactive agents, Advanced Cardiac Life Support recommendations, and many other helpful tables and charts are located in the Appendixes. Frequently used information is located inside the front and back covers. A comprehensive, screened index lists medications by generic and trade names.

Name

The common generic name is followed by any alternate generic name(s) and then by commonly used trade names, which are capitalized. Icons indicate Canadian trade names ✤, if they are different from the standard United States trade name. Frequently used combination products (e.g., Tylenol No. 3) are listed after the single product. The drug monograph applies to the agent listed first and generally does not include information on combination products.

Classifications

Major functional and chemical classifications are listed.

Controlled substances schedule

The Drug Enforcement Administration (DEA) controlled substance schedule is listed. Appendix E explains the meaning of each category.

Usual dose

The usual dose or dosage range is given. Dosage variations for special populations (e.g., children or older adults) are listed separately, as applicable. Icons **P** for pediatric considerations and **G** for geriatric considerations facilitate immediate identification of these unique dosages. Indication for use or preexisting medical conditions (e.g., renal insufficiency) often influences dosage, and these changes are noted.

IV, Direct

The term *IV, direct* is used to indicate a bolus or direct injection of the medication. It refers to medications that are injected directly into a vein, via capped intermittent infusion device (e.g., heparin lock, INT), or through the tubing of a freely flowing IV solution. Direct IVs are generally given in a brief period (e.g., less than 5 minutes).

IV, intermit inf

The term *intermit inf* is used to indicate IV medications that are infused over a given length of time, generally 10 to 60 minutes. This heading includes Y-site or piggyback infusion, as well as infusion through capped intermittent infusion devices.

IV, cont inf

The term *continuous infusion* is used to indicate IV medications that are infused on an ongoing basis over a long or an indefinite period.

---

italic = common side effects   **bold** = life-threatening reactions

Administration

Special instructions for administration by various routes are noted. Recommendations regarding timing of direct IVs and infusions are listed. A triangular symbol **V** allows immediate identification of minimal administration times for direct IV dosages during emergency situations. IV tubing is included in this section. Atypical routes of administration are briefly explained as applicable. When administration technique or route varies according to age group, this is noted. If not noted otherwise, the medication may be administered similarly in all age groups. Compatibilities with commonly used infusion solutions (usually included under "Preparation"), are included here if the medication comes premixed or if there are no special recommendations for preparation.

Preparation

This section includes brief instructions for preparation of IV admixtures and other routes of administration that require special preparation. Compatibilities with commonly used infusion fluids are listed. As indicated, special instructions on storage or stability of admixtures are noted.

Actions

Pharmacologic effects are described with an emphasis on cellular effects, when known. Special attention is given to effects that are relevant to critical care, particularly hemodynamic activity. Generally, explanations of the pharmacologic activity are followed by a brief statement of therapeutic effect, unless otherwise obvious by pharmacologic action.

Pharmacokinetics

Times given for onset, duration, peak, and half-life are approximate and vary according to individual patient factors. The percentage of agent bound to protein (when known) is listed under distribution. This information is especially relevant to the many hypoproteinemic critically ill patients.

Indications

Major indications are listed, with particular emphasis on emergency and critical care applications. Investigational or non–FDA-approved uses are listed if they are relevant to critically ill or injured patients. Specific institutional guidelines should be followed during investigational or unlabeled use of any medication.

Precautions/contraindications

Major precautions are listed. Contraindications follow. Recommendations for pregnancy, lactation, or use in children are briefly explained in this section, as applicable. A bold capital letter in the margin indicates the pregnancy category, which is explained in Appendix D.

Adverse effects

Common and serious side effects are listed according to the body system affected. Common side effects are *italicized;* serious or life-threatening ones are **bold.** Generally, the most frequent side effects are listed first. Extremely rare side effects (i.e., those with isolated reports in the literature) or side effects with questionable relationship to a specific agent are omitted unless there are overriding critical care implications.

P pediatric   **G** geriatric   **V** Direct IV

Toxicity/overdose

A brief listing of symptoms of toxicity and recommendations for management is included. The emphasis is placed on acute toxicity and initial stabilization. Appendix I outlines the general management for a patient with drug overdosage.

Interactions

Drug interactions are listed alphabetically, with a brief description of the specific interaction. The list of agents is generally limited to those commonly used in critical care or emergency settings. Specialized references are available for more detailed information (see References).

Compatibilities/Incompatibilities

Compatibilities and incompatibilities with IV agents commonly used in critical care or emergency settings are listed. Compatibility refers to physical compatibility; not all solutions were tested for loss of drug potency. Specialized references (see References) should be consulted for more detailed information.

Patient care implications

Specific recommendations for each medication are outlined in simple language. When the medication is commonly prescribed for use outside of the hospital setting, an "Outpatient" section is included. The following recommendations apply to any agent prescribed for use outside the hospital, and the patient or family member should be instructed accordingly:
• Take medications exactly as prescribed. Call the prescriber before discontinuing or changing dose.

• Never take prescription medicine that was not prescribed specifically for you.
• Keep all medications away from children. Safely dispose of outdated medication and used transdermal units.
• Follow-up appointments are important for safe and effective long-term therapy.

Available forms

Available forms commonly used in critical or emergency care are listed. The availability of specific preparations changes frequently. In addition, the hospital pharmacy may not stock all available preparations. Any special instructions on storage of the product in the original container are included here.

---

italic = common side effects   **bold** = life-threatening reactions

Medication use in Critical and Emergency Care

Medication administration is an awesome responsibility, particularly in critical and emergency care, wherein complex patients are very ill, decisions are made rapidly, and potent agents are used, often intravenously. The following guidelines are recommended to facilitate safe medication administration.

IV administration

Inspect all solutions for discoloration or particulate matter before administration. Do not use solutions that are discolored or cloudy or that contain visible particles. If uncertain of usual appearance, consult specialized reference.

Y-site/piggyback infusion

This technique calls for intermittent infusion through the Y-site or stopcock of an existing IV solution. Special care is required to prevent complications such as physical or chemical incompatibility and uneven or unsafe infusion rates. Ascertain compatibility with the primary solution before hanging the secondary solution. If the solutions are not compatible or information is not available, the following measures are recommended: discontinue the primary solution, flush the primary IV tubing with compatible solution, and then initiate secondary infusion. With simultaneous infusion, be certain to control the flow rate of both the primary and secondary solutions. Simultaneous infusion of agents with potent vasoactive or respiratory depressant effects is not recommended. After completing the secondary infusion, flush the secondary tubing with compatible solution to ensure complete delivery of all medication and to prevent incompatibility with subsequent agents.

Intermittent injection/ infusion

When administering medications intermittently, be certain to flush the IV tubing or catheter plug with compatible solution before and after each injection/infusion. Significant loss of therapeutic action and/or incompatibility with subsequent agents may occur if flushing is omitted. In addition, if flushing is omitted, up to one third of the total daily dose of medication may be unknowingly discarded with routine tubing changes. Verify compatibility if heparin is used in the flush solution because heparin is physically incompatible with many agents.

Potent vasoactive agents

Y-site infusion of titrated vasoactive agents (e.g., nitroglycerin, nitroprusside, dopamine, and epinephrine) or respiratory depressant agents (e.g., propofol and midazolam) should be avoided. In unusual circumstances such as cardiac arrest, simultaneous administration of potent vasoactive agents is occasionally necessary until additional IV access can be obtained.

IV filters

Standard 0.22 µm in-line IV filters are often used to reduce the complications of IV therapy. Notable exceptions include agents administered in very low concentrations and slowly in-

---

italic = common side effects   **bold** = life-threatening reactions

fused or agents that are absorbed or neutralized by filters (e.g., nitroglycerin). In some instances, specially designed filters may be indicated. Follow institutional guidelines and specific manufacturers' recommendations. See Appendix M for additional information on filtering.

Distribution

Binding to serum proteins affects the activity of many agents commonly used in critical care (e.g., phenytoin, digoxin, warfarin). Low serum protein (reflected by serum albumin level) results in increased activity of free or unbound drug. An increased incidence of adverse effects or toxicity may occur at usual doses when highly protein-bound medications are used in hypoalbuminemic patients. In addition, the concurrent administration of two highly bound agents may cause displacement, thus interfering with therapeutic effects of either agent.

Pregnancy and lactation

Avoid using any drug that is not clearly necessary during pregnancy and lactation. The woman should be informed of any potential risks when medications with unknown or questionable safety are used.

MEDICATION ADJUSTMENTS FOR SPECIAL POPULATIONS

Medication dosage and administration must be individualized according to the unique characteristics of the individual for whom the medication is prescribed. Failure to adjust the "usual" dosage to individual requirements could result in serious consequences, including toxicity or ineffectiveness. This section describes situations for which dose adjustments are often required.

Special age groups

P Children: Size is the most obvious factor influencing the child's response to medications; however, age and developmental stage also influence response to drug therapy.

Medication dosage is adjusted to body size using a number of different approaches. One simple and common method is to adjust the dosage according to the child's body weight. In very small children and infants, this method may result in inadequate doses. An alternate method is to use body surface area for estimating dosages in children. This method more accurately approximates dosage requirements over a wide range of body sizes.

Pediatric pharmacokinetics vary according to developmental stage. For example, preadolescent children typically eliminate certain medications (e.g., theophylline, phenytoin) more rapidly and require more frequent dosing to maintain a steady-state level. Reduced protein binding of certain agents (e.g., phenytoin, lidocaine, furosemide, propranolol, diazepam) in infants and young children affects therapeutic levels and drug efficacy. The reader who frequently cares for children is encouraged to consult specialized references (see References) for additional information on pediatric pharmacokinetics.

Drug administration in children requires special expertise. Oral medications may need to be crushed and mixed in juice or other foods. Care should be taken to administer these and

---

other extemporaneous preparations promptly, since the stability of such mixtures is often unknown. IM and SC injection sites should be carefully selected to avoid nerve or tissue damage. IV catheters should be carefully placed and secured to prevent inadvertent dislodgement. Intraosseous administration is an alternative to IV therapy in emergency situations (see Appendix C).

Whenever medications are administered to children, care should be taken to explain the procedure and expected sensations to the child and parents. All explanations must be adjusted to the child's developmental level.

G **Older adults:** Many critically ill and emergency patients are older than age 65. Changes caused by physiologic aging affect drug pharmacokinetics. For example, increased gastric pH and reduced intestinal blood flow may affect absorption of some medications (e.g., prazosin, levodopa, controlled-release preparations). Drug distribution may be affected by a decrease in total body water or an increase in body fat. The administration of "usual" doses of digoxin, which is primarily distributed in body water, may result in excessive blood levels. Lipid-soluble drugs, such as diazepam, may accumulate, resulting in undesired prolonged effects. Debilitated older adults with decreased albumin levels may be expected to have elevated free concentrations of highly protein-bound drugs (e.g., diazepam, warfarin, phenytoin) and are at a greater risk for toxicity.

Decreased hepatic blood flow and reduced hepatic metabolism may delay excretion of some drugs. This is particularly relevant for drugs with high hepatic extraction ratios, such as barbiturates, lidocaine, and propranolol. Impaired renal elimination in older adults is the result of a multitude of factors, including loss of functional renal cells, arteriosclerotic changes, diminished cardiac output, and a decrease in the ability to concentrate urine. Important drugs that are highly dependent on renal elimination include aminoglycosides, atenolol, cephalosporins, digoxin, furosemide, metoclopramide, procainamide, ticarcillin, and vancomycin. Many older adults receive a number of prescription drugs and frequently medicate themselves with over-the-counter products. The simultaneous use of a number of different medications increases the risk of drug interactions and errors in administration. Impaired vision or hearing may interfere with safe use of medication, and adjustments should be made for patients with sensory deficits. Medication use should be minimized whenever possible, and alternatives to drug therapy are to be encouraged when available.

Alterations associated with organ impairment

Hepatic failure: The liver metabolizes most drugs, usually to an inactive state. Hepatic function in the critically ill may be adversely affected by chronic alcohol ingestion, viral disease, trauma, or diminished cardiac output. Renal hemodynamics are altered in patients with

---

italic = common side effects   **bold** = life-threatening reactions

chronic hepatic failure (e.g., cirrhosis) and pose additional problems for this population. Finally, certain drugs affect the metabolism of other drugs by induction or inhibition of metabolic enzymes. It is difficult to predict the effect of hepatic impairment on drug disposition, in part because readily available measures of hepatic function are not in widespread use. "Liver function" tests (e.g., albumin, prothrombin time, bilirubin, AST, ALT, and alkaline phosphatase) reflect liver damage but do not measure hepatic function. According to the degree of hepatic impairment and the pharmacokinetic characteristics of the specific drug, a 25% to 50% reduction in dose may be necessary. When possible, drug use should be minimized in patients with known or suspected hepatic impairment. When medications are necessary, blood level monitoring and careful assessment for signs of toxicity are essential.

Renal failure: Critically ill patients often have some degree of renal impairment as a result of impaired renal blood flow, multiple organ system dysfunction, or age-related decreases in renal function. Whenever there is impaired glomerular filtration rate and other derangements associated with renal failure, dosing adjustments and careful monitoring of medications are necessary. Generally the dose is reduced and/or the dosing interval lengthened to compensate for reduced renal clearance and prolonged half-life. The degree of renal function is estimated, usually by creatinine clearance, and dosage adjustments are made

accordingly. When available, drug levels are an additional method used to monitor dosage requirements for a given patient. Levels of aminoglycosides, digoxin, vancomycin, digoxin, lidocaine, quinidine, procainamide, and other agents are used to optimize dosing.

Congestive heart failure: Right-sided heart failure results in increased venous pressure and passive congestion of the liver and digestive organs. Drug absorption and metabolism are slowed. Left-sided heart failure results in diminished cardiac output with reduced renal blood flow and impaired renal elimination of many medications. Other factors associated with heart failure, such as altered acid-base balance and increased extravascular volume, also affect drug distribution and clearance.

The precise effects of many drugs in patients with heart failure are unknown. In general, medications tend to be metabolized erratically, and the half-life may be prolonged. Drugs should be used cautiously, and in many instances in reduced doses, in patients with heart failure. Drugs with short half-lives are advantageous, particularly in patients whose hemodynamic status is unstable. Drug levels should be followed closely and the patient monitored for concurrent hepatic and/or renal failure. Dose adjustments are necessary with any change in the patient's hemodynamic status.

Summary
Numerous factors influence medication effects in critically and emergently ill patients.

P pediatric   **G** geriatric   **V** Direct IV

Whenever multiple medications are prescribed for a patient with functional impairment of any major organ, a pharmacist review of the drug profile is recommended. Careful assessment and cautious use of any medication is necessary in seriously ill patients.

abciximab
(ab-sis'i-mab)
ReoPro, c7E3 Fab

Classifications: Biological anti-coagulant, monoclonal antibody Fab fragment

USUAL DOSE

Direct IV, adults: 0.25 mg/kg or 0.125 ml/kg initial dose given 10-60 min before angio-plasty; followed by IV, continuous. For example, 20-mg or 10-ml initial dose used for 80-kg patient.

IV, cont inf, adults: 10 µg/min (17 ml/hr) for 12 hr after angioplasty, unless discontinued because of complications • If percutaneous transluminal coronary angioplasty (PTCA) fails, stop infusion.

Abciximab intended for use along with the following medications: aspirin, 325 mg, PO 2 hr before procedure and once daily thereafter; heparin, initial bolus of 10,000-12,000 U, IV, then additional boluses up to 3,000 U during PTCA. Continue heparin infusion for 12 hr after procedure; adjust to maintain APTT of 1.5-2.5 times normal.

ADMINISTRATION

▼**Direct IV:** Inject initial bolus over 5 min.

IV, cont inf: Infuse at rate of 10 µg/min, which is 17 ml/hr, using concentration of 9 mg/250 ml. • Use volumetric infusion pump and 0.22-µm, low protein-binding filter. • Use separate IV line; do not infuse with other medications. • Stop infusion for serious/uncontrolled bleeding.

PREPARATION

Direct IV: Use 0.22-µm filter needle to withdraw into syringe. Do not dilute or mix with other medications.

IV, cont inf: For recommended concentration of 9 mg/250 ml, withdraw 4.5 ml abciximab and add to 250 ml compatible solution.

Compatible solutions: D₅W, 0.9% NaCl

Stability: Mixed solution stable for 12 hr when refrigerated. Discard unused portion after 12 hr.

ACTIONS

Binds to platelet protein receptors that mediate platelet aggregation; inhibits aggregation/adhesion by preventing final common pathway of aggregation. Extensive platelet inhibitory effects reduce risk of acute closure after angioplasty and may shorten time to reperfusion. • Antiplatelet effects much greater than those of aspirin. • Derived from mouse-human sources, but has a low likelihood of triggering hypersensitivity reactions; has not been associated with anaphylaxis.

PHARMACOKINETICS

ROUTE	ONSET	PEAK	DURATION
IV	Immed	Approx 2 hr	Approx 48 hr

DISTRIBUTION
Platelet-bound; throughout circulation
ELIMINATION
Half-life 10-30 min. Low levels may remain for 10 days.

INDICATIONS

Prevention of acute myocardial ischemic complications in coronary angioplasty or atherectomy

---

italic = common side effects   **bold** = life-threatening reactions

patients at high risk for acute closure of the affected coronary artery. Risk factors to be considered include unstable angina or non-Q wave MI, acute Q wave MI within 12 hr of symptom onset, and other American College of Cardiology/American Heart Association defined risk factors related to coronary arterial morphology and clinical features. Intended for concurrent use with aspirin and heparin.

PRECAUTIONS/ CONTRAINDICATIONS

Precautions: Major bleeding complications possible: arterial access site bleeding; internal retroperitoneal or spontaneous GI/ GU bleeding; during coronary artery bypass graft (CABG). Major bleeding reported in 14% of patients in one study. • Increased risk of bleeding complications associated with body **G** weight <75 kg, age >65 years, history of GI disease, recent thrombolytic therapy. • Risk of bleeding complications may be increased with PTCA within 12 hr of symptom onset, PTCA lasting >70 min, failed PTCA. **Use caution with:** Readministration of abciximab; data not available; may cause hypersensitivity reaction, thrombocytopenia, or reduce benefit • Concomitant heparin, aspirin, thrombolytic, oral anticoagulant, NSAID, dipyridamole, ticlopidine therapy; increased bleeding risk
c Pregnancy category: Use only if safer alternative not available
Contraindications: Hypersensitivity to abciximab or murine (mouse) proteins. • Active internal bleeding • Recent (within 6 wk) significant GI/GU bleeding • CVA within 2 yr or with significant neurologic deficit • Bleeding diathesis • Oral anticoagulant therapy within 7 days unless PT is ≤1.2 times control • Platelet count <100,000 cells/ μl • Recent (within 6 wk) major surgery or trauma • Intracranial neoplasm, atrioventricular (AV) malformation, aneurysm • Severe uncontrolled hypertension • History of vasculitis • Use of IV dextran before or during PTCA • Safe and effective use **P** in children has not been established.

ADVERSE EFFECTS
CNS: Intracranial hemorrhage
CV: *Hypotension,* bradycardia
GI: *Nausea,* vomiting, hematemesis, other bleeding
GU: Hematuria
MS: Pain, altered sensation of extremities
Hema: *Bleeding,* thrombocytopenia, decreased hgb, hct
Misc: Hypersensitivity, positive human anti-chimeric antibody (HACA) titers

TOXICITY/OVERDOSE
Experience with overdosage in humans has not been reported.
• For acute allergic reaction, see Appendix N.

INTERACTIONS
anticoagulants, incl. heparin, thrombolytics, warfarin: ↑ risk of bleeding
Antiplatelet agents (NSAIDs, dipyridamole, ticlopidine): ↑ risk of bleeding

COMPATIBILITIES

Do not mix or infuse through same line with other medications.

PATIENT CARE IMPLICATIONS

• Review history for contraindications.
• Hypersensitivity reactions to protein content of abciximab are possible. Have emergency resuscitation equipment, incl. epinephrine, dopamine, theophylline, antihistamines, corticosteroids, immediately available.
• Risk of bleeding complications is great; early detection is essential; physicians and equipment must be readily available to manage hemorrhage. If unable to control serious bleeding with direct pressure, stop abciximab and any heparin therapy.
• Avoid unnecessary arterial and venous punctures, IM injections. If possible, use saline or heparin lock for drawing blood. If venipuncture necessary, hold manual pressure over site for 20 min or until bleeding stops.
• Avoid arteriovenous invasive procedures in areas where direct pressure is difficult to apply: subclavian, jugular veins. Document and monitor all IV sites/attempts and other puncture sites. Apply pressure dressings to unsuccessful venipuncture attempts.
• Minimize risk of bleeding at sheath insertion site by maintaining complete bed rest, limiting head of bed elevation to ≤30°, restraining affected limb in a straight position, providing adequate sedation/analgesia. Discontinue heparin for at least 4 hr before sheath removal. After removal, hold manual or mechanical pressure for at least 30 min. Apply pressure dressing and maintain bed rest for 6-8 hr after sheath removal or cessation of abciximab therapy, whichever is later.
• As possible, avoid use of urinary catheters, NG tubes, nasotracheal intubation, and other catheters that may cause tissue irritation/trauma and bleeding.

Vital signs/hemodynamics:
• Monitor VS at frequent intervals according to patient condition. Avoid or minimize use of automatic blood pressure cuffs.
• Immediately notify physician of severe or uncontrolled hypertension: SBP >180 or DBP >110 mm Hg. Prepare to initiate hypotensive therapy.
• Monitor ECG for ST depression/elevation, inverted T waves, Q wave >0.04, other indicators of injury/infarction.

Physical assessment: Assess chest pain intensity, character, location, radiation, duration. Note any associated symptoms.
• Frequently assess potential bleeding sites: femoral artery sheath placement site, other catheter insertion sites, arterial/venous punctures, cutdowns, needle punctures. • Frequently check insertion site and distal pulses of affected leg while sheath is in place and for at least 6 hr after removal. Observe insertion site for hematoma; measure and monitor for enlargement. • Assess for intracranial hemorrhage, evaluate baseline neurologic status, and reassess for signs of neurologic dysfunction or ↑ intracranial pressure. Immediately notify physician of changes. • Assess for other bleeding: retroperito-

neal (bluish discoloration of flank), GI (nausea, blood in emesis/stools), GU (pink/bloody urine).

Laboratory tests: Monitor: platelet count, ACT, PT, APTT, cardiac enzymes • **May cause:** Development of human antichimeric antibody (HACA) and increase likelihood of hypersensitivity reaction to diagnostic/therapeutic monoclonal antibodies • If platelet count <100,000 or decreases by 25% from baseline, repeat platelet count using ethylenediaminetetraacetic acid (EDTA), citrate, or heparin-containing tubes. If thrombocytopenia confirmed, discontinue therapy and continue to monitor platelets until normal.

PATIENT/FAMILY TEACHING

Purpose of medication is to help prevent abrupt closure of blocked coronary arteries treated by PTCA. • Frequent monitoring is necessary because of many side effects. • Report chest pain or discomfort; unusual bleeding from IV sites, nose, mouth, or in urine or feces. • Remain on bed rest throughout therapy. • Avoid possible tissue damage from shaving, toothbrushing, excessive activity for 24 hr after therapy.

AVAILABLE FORMS

Parenteral for IV injection/infusion

---

acebutolol
(ase-bute'oh-lole)
Sectral, Monitan ✹,
Rhotral ✹, Sectral ✹

Classifications: Class II antidysrhythmic, cardioselective beta-adrenergic blocker, antihypertensive

USUAL DOSE

PO, adults: 200-800 mg/day, given in one or two daily doses. Up to 1,200 mg/day has been used. • **Older adults:** Use lower dose range; monitor carefully. Do not exceed 800 mg/24 hr.

ACTIONS

Selective blockade of beta-1-adrenergic receptors of myocardium, decreasing HR, BP, force of contraction • Little effect on beta-2 receptors of vasculature, bronchial smooth muscle unless dose exceeds 800 mg/day • Mild sympathetic stimulation limits negative inotropic effects, resulting in larger CO, smaller reduction in HR than with other beta-blockers. • Membrane-stabilizing properties (similar to quinidine) present at higher doses.

PHARMACOKINETICS

ROUTE	ONSET	PEAK	DURATION
PO	<1 hr	2-8 hr	24-30 hr

DISTRIBUTION
Wide; does not cross blood-brain barrier
ELIMINATION
Eliminated by liver, kidneys; half-life 13 hr, longer in older adults

INDICATIONS

Control of hypertension alone, or with diuretics or other antihypertensive agents • Control of ventricular dysrhythmias, including PVCs, couplets, R on T phenomenon, especially in patients with COPD, type I diabetes mellitus, peripheral vascular disease • Useful when other beta-blockers are not tolerated because of excessive bradycardia

Unlabeled/investigational: SVTs, chronic stable angina, acute MI

PRECAUTIONS/ CONTRAINDICATIONS

Precautions: Symptomatic bradycardia, hypotension • Abrupt cessation of therapy may induce angina, ventricular dysrhythmias, acute MI.
Use caution with: Heart failure, valvular heart disease; may precipitate severe failure • Raynaud's syndrome, peripheral/mesenteric vascular disease; may worsen arterial insufficiency • Asthma, COPD; use low dose, monitor for bronchospasm. • General anesthesia; additive impairment of cardiac contractility; consider withdrawal before elective surgery. • Diabetes; beta-blocking effects mask hypoglycemic symptoms. • Hyperthyroidism; beta-blocking effects mask symptoms. • Renal/hepatic impairment; reduce dose. • Mental depression; may worsen
symptoms. • Children: Safety, efficacy not established
B Pregnancy category: Safety not clearly established
Contraindications: Hypersensitivity to acebutolol • Severe bradycardia, 2nd, 3rd degree heart block • CHF (unless resulting from tachycardia) • Cardiogenic shock

ADVERSE EFFECTS

CNS: *Fatigue, dizziness, headache,* insomnia, depression, lethargy, paresthesias
Resp: Dyspnea, rhinitis, **asthma, bronchospasm**
CV: Bradycardia, **hypotension, CHF, edema, angina**
GI: Diarrhea, constipation, flatulence, abdominal pain, elevated liver enzymes
GU: Urinary frequency, dysuria, nocturia, decreased libido
Endo: Blocked symptoms of hypoglycemia/hyperthyroidism
Syst: Arthralgia, myalgia, positive ANA, lupus-type syndrome

TOXICITY/OVERDOSE

Symptoms: Symptomatic bradycardia, HR < 45, profound hypotension, loss of consciousness, heart failure, advanced heart block, bronchospasms, hypoglycemia, possible seizures
Management: After recent ingestion, implement guidelines for management of acute overdose (Appendix I). • **Symptomatic bradycardia, heart block:** Atropine, isoproterenol according to ACLS guidelines (Appendix P) • **Bronchospasm:** Isoproterenol, aminophylline • **Heart failure:** Inotropic agents (e.g., dobutamine, dopamine), diuretics, digoxin • **Hypotension:** Elevate legs, administer IV fluids; use vasopressors (e.g., norepinephrine) if severe and refractory to inotropes. • Implement seizure precautions; administer diazepam, phenytoin as needed. • Hemodialysis may be helpful.

---

italic = common side effects   **bold** = life-threatening reactions

INTERACTIONS

amiodarone Severe bradycardia; ventricular dysrhythmias

antidiabetics (insulin, oral agents) Prolonged recovery from hypoglycemic episodes; hyperglycemia

barbiturates ↓ effectiveness of acebutolol

diltiazem Extreme bradycardia; hypotension

disopyramide Additive negative inotropy; reduced CO

epinephrine, other α-adrenergic stimulants, including cold, allergy remedies Unopposed alpha stimulation with hypertension, dysrhythmias; ↓ epinephrine effectiveness in anaphylaxis

isoproterenol ↓ isoproterenol effectiveness

lidocaine ↑ risk of lidocaine toxicity; ↓ CO

nicardipine Hypotension

nifedipine Hypotension

NSAIDs ↓ acebutolol effectiveness

phenothiazines Hypotension; synergistic effects

prazosin Hypotension

quinidine Additive cardiac depression

rifampin ↑ beta-blocker metabolism; higher acebutolol doses required

theophylline ↓ bronchodilation

verapamil Extreme bradycardia; hypotension

PATIENT CARE IMPLICATIONS

• Use lowest possible dose for dysrhythmia control.
• Administer with food if possible, or administer consistently with regard to meals to minimize variation in absorption.

• Monitor closely if other antidysrhythmics or hypotensive agents used.
• Gradually withdraw therapy to avoid rebound hypertension, angina, possible acute MI.
• **COPD, asthma:** Monitor closely; avoid high-dose therapy (>800 mg/day), which may precipitate bronchospasm. Have bronchodilator such as aminophylline or β$_2$-stimulant readily available.
• **Hyperthyroidism, diabetes, heart disease, vascular disease:** Special precautions necessary; see Precautions.

Vital signs/hemodynamics: Assess BP, HR, RR frequently when initiating therapy and adjusting dose. Consult physician for hypotension, symptomatic bradycardia, tachypnea. • As available, observe ECG for heart block, severe bradycardia, prolongation of PR interval, widening of QRS complex. If present, consult physician.
• Measure CVP, PAP, CO as available. Consult physician if ↓ CO/ ↑ PCWP or other symptoms of heart failure.

Physical assessment: Assess for perfusion/oxygenation deficit: ↓ level of consciousness, activity intolerance, hypotension, chest discomfort, dizziness.
• Assess for evidence of pulmonary edema: ↑ respiratory rate, bibasilar crackles, frothy sputum; especially important in patients with preexisting heart disease. • Assess patients with diabetes for sweating, because tachycardia and tremors associated with hypoglycemia may be blocked by therapy.

Laboratory tests: Monitor: Blood glucose, liver enzymes, ANA titers, CBC regularly

---

throughout therapy • Blood glucose frequently in patients with diabetes.

PATIENT/FAMILY TEACHING

Purpose of medication is to lower BP or regulate abnormal heartbeats. • May cause drowsiness, dizziness, low BP; change positions slowly, particularly when getting out of bed. • Report breathing difficulty, palpitations, dizziness, chest pain, extreme fatigue. • Avoid excessive amounts of coffee, tea, or caffeinated soft drinks, which may counteract drug's BP-lowering effects.

Outpatient: Take medication exactly as prescribed. Do not stop taking medicine, even if you feel better. If medication is abruptly discontinued, you may develop dangerously high BP, serious heartbeat irregularities, and angina. • Check and record resting pulse each day and BP each week. Contact health care provider if pulse < 50 bpm or BP significantly different. • Medication is not a cure for high BP, and other therapies, including life-style modifications, must be continued. • Avoid driving and other activities requiring mental alertness until individuals response to drug known. • Drinking alcohol may cause extreme dizziness, drowsiness, impaired mental alertness. • Consult health care provider before taking over-the-counter preparations, particularly cold or allergy preparations. • Carry medical identification card identifying drug, dosage, specific indication. • Notify physicians and dentists of therapy before any treatment. • Therapy blocks elevated HR and BP, so hyperthyroid and diabetic patients must be aware of other symptoms of crisis.

AVAILABLE FORMS

Capsules

acetaminophen
(a-seat-a-mee'noe-fen)
APAP, paracetamol
Acephen, Aceta, Datril, Feverall, Liquiprin, Panadol, Tempra, Tylenol, Abenol ✦
acetaminophen with codeine phosphate
Phenaphen No. 1-4, Tylenol No. 1-4
acetaminophen with oxycodone
Oxycet, Percocet, Roxicet, Roxilox, Tylox

Many formulations available alone and in combination with aspirin, caffeine, codeine, diphenhydramine, oxycodone, propoxyphene, pseudoephedrine, other agents
Classifications: Nonnarcotic analgesic, antipyretic

USUAL DOSE

Ⓟ **PO/rectal, adults/children >11 yr:** 325-650 mg q4h as needed; up to 1 g may be used as single dose. • Do not exceed 4 g/day or 2.6 g/day if used chronically • Do not exceed 2 g/day if history of chronic alcohol use.
Ⓟ **PO/rectal, children <12 yr:** Dose according to weight (see following page) q4h. • Do not exceed 5 doses/day.

---

italic = common side effects   **bold** = life-threatening reactions

P Approx PO/rectal doses for children ≤11 yr:

AGE	DOSE (mg)
Newborn-3 mo	40
4-11 mo	80
12-24 mo	120
2-3 yr	160
4-5 yr	240
6-8 yr	320
9-10 yr	400
11 yr	480

ACTIONS

Reduces pain and fever • Analgesia primarily caused by peripheral effects, probably prostaglandin inhibition • Temperature-lowering effects caused by direct effect on heat-regulating center of hypothalamus

PHARMACOKINETICS

ROUTE	ONSET	PEAK	DURATION
PO	10 min; food delays absorption	10-60 min	4-8 hr

DISTRIBUTION

Rapid; into most body tissues

ELIMINATION

Metabolized in liver, excreted in urine; half-life 1.25-3 hr. prolonged with cirrhosis, acetaminophen overdose

INDICATIONS

Relief of mild to moderate pain • Fever reduction • Used with opiate-agonist analgesics (e.g., codeine, oxycodone) for greater analgesia

PRECAUTIONS/ CONTRAINDICATIONS

Precautions: Excessive doses hepatotoxic; do not exceed recommended dosage. • Some PO formulations contain aspartame (NutraSweet); avoid use with phenylketonuria. • Some commercial preparations contain sulfites, which can cause serious allergic reactions.

Use caution with: Impaired hepatic function • Chronic alcohol use • Malnutrition

B Pregnancy category: Safety not clearly established

Contraindications: Hypersensitivity to acetaminophen • Chronic use in individuals with anemia or cardiac, pulmonary, renal, hepatic disease

ADVERSE EFFECTS

Hema: Hemolytic anemia, leukopenia, pancytopenia, neutropenia, thrombocytopenia, agranulocytosis (rare)
Derm: Rash, urticaria

TOXICITY/OVERDOSE

Symptoms: Chronic: Anemia, renal damage, GI disturbances • **Acute:** Initially, nausea, vomiting, abdominal pain, diaphoresis, followed by right upper quadrant pain, with elevations in liver enzymes, bilirubin, PT; later, serious hepatotoxicity with jaundice, hypoglycemia, encephalopathy; possible renal failure; CNS stimulation followed by depression, coma; respiratory/circulatory failure possible with large overdose; minimum toxic dose, 10 g in adults

Management: After recent ingestion, implement guidelines for management of acute overdose (Appendix I). • Administer PO loading dose of acetylcysteine (Mucomyst); 140 mg/kg, then 70 mg/kg q4h for 17 doses. If charcoal has been administered, lavage stomach before administering acetylcysteine. • Administer O_2/support ventilation as needed. • Monitor UO; rehydrate as necessary. Avoid diuretics, forced diuresis.

• Monitor glucose; treat hypo-glycemia with IV glucose. • For prolonged PT, administer vita-min K, fresh-frozen plasma.

INTERACTIONS

alcohol Acetaminophen toxicity with doses as low as 2 g/day.
barbiturates ↓ Acetaminophen effectiveness; ↑ risk of toxicity
cholestyramine ↓ Acetamino-phen effectiveness
phenothiazines Severe hypo-thermia

PATIENT CARE IMPLICATIONS

Assess for history of chronic alcohol use/malnutrition, which increase likelihood of hepato-toxicity.
Vital signs/hemodynamics: **Antipyretic use:** Monitor tem-perature before and 1-2 hr after administration. • **Analgesic use:** Recognize antipyretic ac-tivity and possibility that fever associated with infection could be masked.
Physical assessment: Assess level of pain before and at in-tervals after administration.

PATIENT/FAMILY TEACHING

Purpose of medication is to re-lieve pain or reduce fever. • Do not exceed recommended dos-age. • Consult physician if pain continues for longer than 10 days in adults or 5 days in children or if fever persists for more than 3 days or recurs.
• **Infants/children:** For home use, make sure parents under-stand correct dosage according to child's body weight.

AVAILABLE FORMS

Tablets, capsules • Chewable tablets • Oral solution • Rectal suppositories

acetazolamide
(a-set-a-zole'a-mide)
Diamox, AK-Zol

acetazolamide sodium
Diamox

Classifications: Carbonic anhy-drase inhibitor, diuretic, anticon-vulsant

USUAL DOSE

PO/IM/IV adults: CHF, edema: 250-375 mg or 5 mg/kg given in AM, every other day, or 2 of 3 days; intermittent dosing required for maximal ef-fectiveness • **Epilepsy:** 8-30 mg/kg/day (usually 375-1,000 mg) given in 1-4 divided doses • **Glaucoma:** 250-1,000 mg/day given in 1-4 divided doses • **High-altitude sickness:** 500-1,000 mg/day given in 1-4 di-vided doses. Initiate therapy 24-48 hr before ascent and con-tinue for ≥ 48 hr while at high altitude • Do not exceed single dose of 250-500 mg.
PO/IV children: CHF, edema: 5 mg/kg or 300-900 mg/m²/day, given in AM, every day, or 2 of 3 days; intermittent dosing re-quired for maximal effective-ness • **Epilepsy:** 8-30 mg/kg/day (usually 375-1,000 mg) given in 1-4 divided doses • Do not exceed single dose of 250 mg or maximal dose of 1.5 g/day.

---

italic = common side effects   **bold** = life-threatening reactions

ADMINISTRATION

▼ Direct IV, adults/children:
Ⓟ Inject dilute solution at rate of 100-500 mg/min.
Ⓟ IV, adults/children: When added to IV solution, infuse over 4-8 hr.

PREPARATION

IV: Add 5 ml sterile water for injection to 500-mg vial for concentration of 100 mg/ml; may be further diluted in compatible fluid for IV infusion.
Compatible solutions: D_5W, 0.9% NaCl, LR, prepared combinations of these solutions

ACTIONS

Inhibits enzyme, carbonic anhydrase, thus reducing hydrogen ions in renal tubules • Increases excretion of bicarbonate, sodium, potassium • Decreases reabsorption of water, increases urine volume, alkalizes urine • Effects may result in metabolic acidosis. • Diuresis inhibited with metabolic acidosis; enhanced with metabolic alkalosis • Decreases formation of aqueous humor, thus lowering intraocular pressure (IOP) • Ocular effects independent of diuresis and acid-base variations • Decreases frequency of seizures; mechanism not clearly defined • Anticonvulsant effects independent of diuresis

PHARMACOKINETICS

ROUTE	ONSET	PEAK	DURATION
PO, tabs	1 hr	1-4 hr	8-12 hr
PO, ext rel	2 hr	3-6 hr	18-24 hr
IV	2 min	15 min	4-5 hr

DISTRIBUTION
Throughout body; high concentrations in RBCs, kidneys
ELIMINATION
Excreted unchanged by kidneys

INDICATIONS

Edema associated with CHF • With other anticonvulsants in epilepsy, particularly petit mal seizures • Open-angle glaucoma not controlled by miotics alone. • Short-term reduction of IOP before surgery • Promote altitude tolerance, lessen symptoms of high-altitude sickness
Unlabeled/investigational:
Prevention/treatment of alkalosis after open heart surgery; promote urinary excretion of lithium carbonate, other agents during acute toxicity

PRECAUTIONS/ CONTRAINDICATIONS

Precautions: Metabolic acidosis, which causes cessation of diuresis, typically occurs within 4 days of initial therapy. • Tolerance to anticonvulsant effects develops quickly, but effectiveness often restored after temporary cessation of therapy.
Use caution with: Respiratory acidosis, COPD, pulmonary infection/obstruction • Diabetes mellitus • Concurrent high-dose aspirin therapy • Sulfonamide sensitivity; serious allergic reactions possible
ⓒ Pregnancy category: Fetal damage possible; use only if risk explained to woman and benefits exceed risk.

Ⓟ pediatric   **Ⓖ** geriatric   **▼** Direct IV

Contraindications: Hypersensitivity to acetazolamide • Cirrhosis, hepatic failure • Renal insufficiency • Calcium-containing renal calculi • Hyponatremia, hypokalemia • Hyperchloremic acidosis • Adrenocortical insufficiency

ADVERSE EFFECTS

CNS: Drowsiness, hearing disturbances, headache, confusion, paresthesias, **seizures**
Resp: Alkalosis and associated **respiratory depression/ failure**
CV: Dysrhythmias
GI: Nausea, vomiting, anorexia, diarrhea, constipation, dry mouth, thirst, **hepatic coma** (preexisting liver disease)
GU: Dysuria, renal colic, renal calculi
Endo: Hyperglycemia, glycosuria
F&E: Hypokalemia, metabolic acidosis, hyponatremia, elevated ammonia
Hema: Bone marrow depression, aplastic anemia, thrombocytopenia, leukopenia
Misc: Elevated uric acid, gout, **anaphylaxis, Stevens-Johnson syndrome**

TOXICITY/OVERDOSE

Symptoms: Electrolyte imbalance, acidosis, CNS depression or excitation
Management: After recent ingestion, implement guidelines for management of acute overdose (Appendix I). • Support respiration as needed with O_2 and/or mechanical ventilation. • Administer IV fluids, replace electrolytes based on serum levels. Closely monitor potassium balance/acid-base status. Administer bicarbonate for acidosis.

• Hemodialysis may be effective.

INTERACTIONS

amphetamines Prolonged amphetamine effects
amphotericin B Severe hypokalemia
aspirin (high doses) Metabolic acidosis, tachypnea, lethargy, coma, death
corticosteroids Severe hypokalemia
digitalis glycosides Hypokalemia leading to toxicity
diuretics Synergistic enhancement of diuresis; severe hypokalemia
lithium ↑ Excretion; impaired lithium effectiveness
phenobarbital ↑ Excretion; impaired phenobarbital effectiveness
procainamide ↓ Excretion; prolonged procainamide effects
quinidine ↓ Excretion; prolonged quinidine effects
TCAs ↓ Excretion; prolonged TCA effects

COMPATIBILITIES

Cimetidine, ranitidine

INCOMPATIBILITIES

Diltiazem, multivitamins

PATIENT CARE IMPLICATIONS

• Loss of diuretic/anticonvulsive effectiveness may be avoided by giving drug intermittently.
• IV route preferred; IM injections painful and not recommended for children
• May induce metabolic acidosis, which impairs diuresis
• May diminish mental alertness; safety precautions indicated

---

Vital signs/hemodynamics:
Monitor VS, UO frequently, especially with parenteral therapy, pulmonary disease.
Physical assessment: Assess for CHF: dyspnea, bibasilar crackles, peripheral edema, weight gain, S₃ gallop, neck vein distention. • Assess for electrolyte imbalance: dysrhythmias, confusion, weakness, muscle cramps, paresthesias, thirst, vomiting. • Evaluate visual acuity, assess for ↑ ocular pressure: pain, loss of side vision, blurred vision, halos, other visual disturbances. • Weigh patient daily.
Laboratory tests: Monitor: Electrolytes, acid-base status, CBC, liver enzymes, uric acid before and at intervals throughout therapy • Blood glucose frequently in patients with diabetes. • **May cause:** False-positive urinary protein • Depression of iodine uptake by thyroid

PATIENT/FAMILY TEACHING

Purpose of drug is to eliminate excess body fluids, reduce pressure within the eye, or reduce frequency of seizures. • Report signs/symptoms of heart failure: breathing difficulty, activity intolerance, chest pain. • Report any changes in visual acuity, eye pain, visual disturbances.
Outpatient: Use caution in performing hazardous tasks requiring mental alertness or physical coordination. • Avoid frequent use of aspirin without consulting health care provider. • Report sore throat, unusual bleeding or bruising, fever, rash.
Glaucoma: Provide periodic ophthalmologic testing to detect worsening of glaucoma.

Diuresis: Weigh twice per wk: report weight gain or edema.
Patients with diabetes: Increased blood glucose levels possible; insulin dose may need adjustment.

AVAILABLE FORMS

Tablets • Sustained-release capsules • Parenteral for IV/IM use

acetylcysteine
(a-se-til-sis'tay-een),
N-acetylcysteine
Mucomyst, Mucosol

Classification: Mucolytic

USUAL DOSE
Nebulization, adults/
(P) children: 3-5 ml 20% solution or 6-10 ml 10% solution three to four times daily • Up to 10 ml 20% solution or 20 ml 10% solution may be used.
Intratracheal instillation,
(P) adults/children: 1-2 ml 10%-20% solution q1-4h
(P) PO, adults/children: For acetaminophen overdose only: Loading dose of 140 mg/kg, then 70 mg/kg q4h for 17 additional doses (see Appendix J for quick reference table with specific dosage guide) • Repeat if patient vomits within 1 hr of administration • Initiate therapy as soon as possible. • Continue full course of therapy unless acetaminophen levels fall well below predicted hepatotoxic range.

ADMINISTRATION
Nebulization: Schedule treatments 30-60 min before meals to minimize nausea. • Instruct patient to clear airway by deep

breathing/coughing before treatment. • 20% solution may be diluted with 0.9% NaCl. • Dilution of 10% solution unnecessary • Use conventional plastic or glass nebulizers.

PO: May administer chilled/use glass straw to ↑ palatability • May dilute 1:3 with carbonated soft drink, orange or grapefruit juice • Gastric or duodenal tube: dilute with water and administer within 1 hr of preparation. Flush tube with 30-50 ml water after administration.

ACTIONS

Inhal: Reduces viscosity of pulmonary secretions by breaking disulfide linkages of mucoproteins • Facilitates secretion removal by coughing, postural drainage, suctioning • No action on living tissue

PO: ↓ hepatotoxic effects of acetaminophen by increasing hepatic glutathione, which inactivates toxic metabolites associated with acetaminophen overdose

PHARMACOKINETICS

ROUTE	ONSET	PEAK	DURATION
Inhal	Immed	Rapid	Var
PO	Rapid	ND	Approx 4 hr

DISTRIBUTION

PO: absorbed from pulmonary epithelium; inhal: absorbed from GI tract

ELIMINATION

Metabolized by liver

INDICATIONS

Inhal: To reduce viscous pulmonary secretions associated with pneumonia, bronchitis, emphysema, tuberculosis, cystic fibrosis, other pulmonary disorders

Intratracheal instillation: To prevent ET crusting, reduce need for bronchoscopy

PO: Antidote in treatment of acetaminophen overdose

PRECAUTIONS/ CONTRAINDICATIONS

Precautions: ↑ volume of liquefied bronchial secretions may obstruct airway. • Bronchospasm possible, especially with asthma

Use caution with: Asthma, asthmatic bronchitis • Older adults, debilitated patients with respiratory insufficiency • Severe hepatic failure; nitrogen content may contribute to encephalopathy

Pregnancy category: Safe use not well-established

Contraindications: Hypersensitivity to acetylcysteine • Hepatic encephalopathy

ADVERSE EFFECTS

CNS: *Dizziness, drowsiness,* headache, fever, chills

Resp: *Rhinorrhea,* **bronchospasm,** chest tightness, bronchial irritation, hemoptysis

CV: Hypotension

GI: *Nausea,* stomatitis, vomiting, anorexia

Derm: Urticaria, rash

Misc: Clamminess, fever, chills

TOXICITY/OVERDOSE

Wide margin of safety; toxicity unlikely • Large PO doses have caused reversible elevations in liver enzymes.

COMPATIBILITIES

Aluminum, glass, plastic, stainless steel

INCOMPATIBILITIES

Copper, hydrogen peroxide, iron, rubber; do not mix in solution with antibiotics.

PATIENT CARE IMPLICATIONS

Inhal/instillation: Have equipment for ET suction immediately available.

Acetaminophen overdose:
• If unfamiliar with use of acetylcysteine as antidote to acetaminophen overdose, contact local poison control center or Rocky Mountain Poison Center (800-525-6115) for assistance.
• If activated charcoal has been administered, it must be completely removed by gastric lavage before initiating acetylcysteine therapy.
• Initiate therapy as soon as possible; optimal results obtained if administered within 8-16 hr of acetaminophen ingestion; useful within 24 hr after ingestion. Do not delay therapy to obtain acetaminophen levels.
• Repeat dose if patient vomits within 1 hr of administration. Dilution with soda or juice minimizes vomiting. Use duodenal tube if patient unable to retain PO doses.
• See Administration for additional recommendations.

Vital signs/hemodynamics: Monitor VS for hypotension, tachycardia, tachypnea, fever.
• Monitor ECG for tachycardia, dysrhythmias.

Physical assessment: Inhal/instillation: Assess respiratory status: coughing, breath sounds, respiratory rate and effort, quantity and character of bronchial secretions. • Assess for ↑ volume of liquefied bronchial secretions that may obstruct airway. Encourage coughing; use ET suctioning if necessary to remove secretions. • Assess for bronchospasm: wheezing, rhonchi, dyspnea, diminished breath sounds. Administer bronchodilator treatment if needed. Discontinue acetylcysteine for severe or progressive bronchospasm. • **Acetaminophen overdose:** Assess level of consciousness, neurologic status frequently.

Laboratory tests: Inhal/instillation: Monitor ABGs for improvement in oxygenation CO_2 retention. • **Acetaminophen overdose:** Monitor: Acetaminophen levels • Liver enzymes, bilirubin, PT • Electrolytes, serum glucose • Obtain acetaminophen levels as soon as possible after ingestion, but not sooner than 4 hr to ensure that peak concentrations measured; monitor levels at established intervals.

PATIENT/FAMILY TEACHING

Inhal/instillation: Purpose of medication is to liquefy secretions in lung and facilitate removal by coughing or suctioning. • Unpleasant odor is anticipated. • Adequate fluid intake helps liquefy secretions.
• Rinse mouth and wash face to remove irritating and sticky residue. • May cause drowsiness; do not drive or perform activities requiring mental alertness until individual effects of medication determined. • Avoid alcohol or other drugs that may cause sedation.

Acetaminophen overdose: Purpose of medication is to reduce levels of toxic substances that may cause serious liver

---

P pediatric   **G** geriatric   **V** Direct IV

damage. • Report breathing difficulty, chest pain, palpitations, activity intolerance, swelling of feet and ankles.

AVAILABLE FORMS

10%, 20% solutions
Storage: Store in refrigerator after opening. Slight purple discoloration does not affect potency.

acyclovir
(ay-sye'kloe-ver)
Zovirax

Classification: Antiviral

USUAL DOSE

PO, adults: 200-800 mg, q4h, 5 times daily for 5-10 days
PO, children: 20 mg/kg, 4 times daily for 5 days. Single dose not to exceed 800 mg.
IV, intermit inf, adults: 5-10 mg/kg, q8h for 7-10 days
• **Obesity:** Dose according to ideal body weight • **Renal insufficiency:** Reduce dose or adjust dosing intervals; give supplemental dose after hemodialysis
IV, intermit inf, children
<12 yr: 250-500 mg/m², q8h or 7.5-45 mg/kg/day given in evenly divided doses q8h for 7-10 days • Do not exceed maximal dose of 500 mg/m².

ADMINISTRATION

IV, intermit inf: Infusion pump necessary. Infuse prepared solution at constant rate over 1 hr; **do not infuse for <1 hr.** Rapid infusion results in crystalluria, renal tubular blockage, acute renal failure.

PREPARATION

IV: Dilute 500-mg vial with 10 ml sterile water for injection; use 20 ml for 1,000-mg vial. Resulting concentration is 50 mg/ml. Add to 50-125 ml compatible solution; dilute solution should not exceed concentration of 7 mg/ml to reduce risk of phlebitis. • **Do not dilute with bacteriostatic water,** which may contain benzyl alcohol or parabens and cause precipitation
Compatible fluids: D_5W, 0.9% NaCl, LR, prepared combinations of these solutions
Stability: Reconstituted solution stable for 12 hr; fully dilute solution stable for 24 hr at room temperature.

ACTIONS

Inhibits viral DNA synthesis; has selective activity against herpes simplex virus, varicella-zoster virus, Epstein-Barr virus, and cytomegalovirus

PHARMACOKINETICS

ROUTE	ONSET	PEAK	DURATION
IV	rapid	2 hr	Approx 8 hr

DISTRIBUTION
Wide; 9%-33% plasma protein bound.
ELIMINATION
Renal excretion of unchanged drug. Terminal half-life is 2.5 hr; prolonged with decreased creatinine clearance.

INDICATIONS

Initial and recurrent simplex viral (HSV) infection in immunocompromised and certain other patients • Severe initial herpes genitalis in nonimmunocompromised patients • HSV encephalitis in patients older than 6 months • Acute varicella-zoster infection (chickenpox) • Varicella-zoster infection

---

italic = common side effects   **bold** = life-threatening reactions

(shingles) in immunocompromised patients

Unlabeled/investigational:
Cytomegalovirus (CMV) infection in immunocompromised patients; disseminated primary eczema herpeticum; varicella pneumonia; certain severe herpes simplex infections

PRECAUTIONS/ CONTRAINDICATIONS

Precautions: Acyclovir powder for reconstitution and IV use only; do not administer by SC, IM, or other routes. • May cause renal impairment; ↑ risk with rapid or bolus administration, dehydration, presence of other nephrotoxic agents, preexisting renal insufficiency

Use caution with: Preexisting renal or hepatic insufficiency • Concurrent use of other nephrotoxic drugs • Neurologic abnormalities, seizure disorders, electrolyte disturbances, hypoxemia; may cause neurotoxicity/ seizures • Previous neurologic reaction to cytotoxic drug

c **Pregnancy category:** Use only if safer alternative not available

Contraindications: Hypersensitivity to acyclovir, ganciclovir

ADVERSE EFFECTS

CNS: *headache, dizziness,* confusion, **seizures, coma,** hallucinations
GI: elevated liver enzymes, nausea
GU: elevated BUN/creatinine, proteinuria, **renal failure,** *vaginitis, moniliasis*
Hema: **bone marrow depression, leukopenia, granulocytopenia, thrombocytopenia, megaloblastic anemia**
Derm: rash, urticaria, pruritus

Local: *pain, phlebitis* at IV site
Misc: fever, pain

TOXICITY/OVERDOSE

Symptoms: Elevated BUN/creatinine, renal failure • Lethargy, seizures, coma
Management: Discontinue drug if symptoms of toxicity. • After recent ingestion, implement guidelines for management of acute overdosage (Appendix I). • Treat symptomatically. • Hemodialysis may be helpful.

INTERACTIONS

interferon Synergism, neurotoxicity
ketoconazole Synergist
methotrexate, intrathecal Neurotoxicity
probenecid Reduced acyclovir excretion
zidovudine Neurotoxicity

COMPATIBILITIES

Allopurinol, amikacin, ampicillin, cefamandole, cefazolin, cefoperazone, cefotaxime, cefoxitin, ceftazidime, ceftizoxime, ceftriaxone, cefuroxime, cephapirin, chloramphenicol, cimetidine, clindamycin, dexamethasone, doxycycline, erythromycin, fluconazole, gentamicin, heparin, hydrocortisone, hydromorphone, imipenem-cilastatin, lorazepam, magnesium sulfate, methylprednisolone, metoclopramide, metronidazole, multivitamins, nafcillin, oxacillin, paclitaxel, penicillin, pentobarbital, perphenazine, piperacillin, potassium chloride, ranitidine, sodium bicarbonate, theophylline, ticarcillin, tobramycin, trimethoprim-sulfamethoxazole, vancomycin, zidovudine

---

INCOMPATIBILITIES

Diltiazem, diphenhydramine, dobutamine, dopamine, meperidine, morphine, odansetron, piperacillin-tazobactam

PATIENT CARE IMPLICATIONS

Initiate therapy as soon as possible after initial symptoms occur. Obtain C&S before initiating treatment; start treatment after specimen collected. • Maintain adequate hydration by encouraging fluid intake of 2-3 L/day throughout duration of therapy. • Assess for history of seizure or other neurologic disorders.

IV use: Rotate veins and confirm patency with each use because drug will cause thrombophlebitis. • Promote abundant urine flow during first 2 hr after each dose, which is time of maximal acyclovir concentration. • Optimal UO is ≥500 ml/g acyclovir. With encephalitis, benefits of hydration must be weighed against risk of cerebral edema.

Vital signs/hemodynamics: Monitor urine output/I&O ratio throughout therapy; consult prescriber for diminished UO or increased BUN/creatinine.

Physical assessment: Evaluate resolution of infection: diminished pain, itching, lesions. • Assess for neurologic abnormalities, including level of consciousness; consult prescriber at onset of neurologic changes. Neurotoxicity more likely with **advanced age** or debilitation. • Assess for signs of infection, anemia, and unusual bruising or bleeding.

Laboratory tests: Monitor: BUN, creatinine, CrCl, UA, urine protein • RBC, WBC, platelets, bleeding time • Liver enzymes • C&S

PATIENT/FAMILY TEACHING

Purpose of medication is to treat certain herpes viral infections. It controls symptoms, but does not cure the infection. • Be sure to drink plenty of fluids while taking this medicine. • Report mental changes, which could indicate toxicity. • Report sore throat, fever, fatigue, unusual bleeding or bruising, which could indicate infection or blood dyscrasias.

Outpatient: Start therapy at first sign of itching or pain, which is usually before skin eruptions. • Take acyclovir at evenly spaced intervals around the clock. • Virus remains dormant and can still spread to others. Inform sexual partners of history of herpes. Always use condoms.

AVAILABLE FORMS

Capsules, tablets, suspension • Powder to be reconstituted for IV use • Ointment

adenosine
(ah-den'oh-seen)
Adenocard

Classification: Antidysrhythmic

USUAL DOSE

Direct IV, adults: Initially 6 mg rapid bolus; if ineffective after 1-2 min, follow with 12 mg dose, which may be repeated once; doses >12 mg not recommended.

---

italic = common side effects   **bold** = life-threatening reactions

℗ Direct IV, children (unlabeled/investigational): 0.1-0.2 mg/kg rapid bolus; if ineffective after 1-2 min, may follow with additional doses for a total of three doses; doses >12 mg not recommended.

ADMINISTRATION

▼ Direct IV: Inject rapidly over 1-2 sec directly into a peripheral vein or very proximal IV injection site; follow with rapid saline flush of 10 ml or more to clear IV tubing completely. Central venous administration has been reported without untoward effects.

ACTIONS

Naturally occurring nucleoside that slows conduction time through AV node • Interrupts reentry pathways through AV node and restores normal sinus rhythm in patients with supraventricular tachycardia (SVT) including that associated with WPW • No systemic hemodynamic effects at usual dose; larger doses may decrease peripheral vascular resistance, BP • Effects not blocked by atropine • Effects antagonized by methylxanthines

PHARMACOKINETICS

ROUTE	ONSET	PEAK	DURATION
IV	Seconds	<10 sec	Seconds

DISTRIBUTION
Wide

ELIMINATION
Rapidly metabolized by erythrocytes, vascular endothelial cells

INDICATIONS

Conversion of SVT to sinus rhythm, including SVT associated with accessory bypass tracts (e.g., WPW) • Not effective in converting atrial fibrillation or flutter, ventricular tachycardia • Considered choice agent for SVT • Particularly useful for SVT that fails to respond to verapamil or when other conditions (e.g., CHF, beta blockade, hypotension, left ventricular dysfunction) limit verapamil use

PRECAUTIONS/CONTRAINDICATIONS

Precautions: May cause brief 1st, 2nd, or 3rd degree heart block; transient asystole; other dysrhythmias at time of conversion • Safe use in children has not been established; controlled studies have not been conducted.

Use caution with: Asthma; may cause bronchoconstriction

c Pregnancy category: Use only if clearly needed.

Contraindications: Hypersensitivity to adenosine • 2nd or 3rd degree AV block or sick sinus syndrome, except with functioning artificial pacemaker • High-level block after previous administration • Atrial flutter, atrial fibrillation, ventricular tachycardia; not effective in converting these rhythms

ADVERSE EFFECTS

CNS: Lightheadedness, dizziness, paresthesias
Resp: *Shortness of breath, dyspnea,* hyperventilation
CV: *Conversion dysrhythmias* (e.g., *PVC, PAC, sinus bradycardia, sinus tachycardia*), heart block, **asystole,** *flushing,* sweating, palpitations, chest pain/pressure, hypotension
GI: Nausea, metallic taste, tightness in throat

TOXICITY/OVERDOSE

Symptoms are usually brief and self-limiting because of short half-life (<10 sec). Treat life-threatening dysrhythmias in accordance with ACLS guidelines (Appendix P). Bradycardias may not respond to atropine.

INTERACTIONS

aminophylline ↓ adenosine effectiveness

caffeine ↓ adenosine effectiveness

carbamazepine ↑ heart block

dipyridamole Potentiates adenosine effects

INCOMPATIBILITIES

Because of specific use and administration, do not mix with any other drug or solution.

PATIENT CARE IMPLICATIONS

• Try vagal maneuvers to convert rhythm before administration.

• Confirm labeling to avoid confusion with adenosine phosphate, which is used IM for relief of varicose vein complications

• Entire dose must reach systemic circulation as bolus. Inject very rapidly; follow with rapid saline flush.

• Emergency resuscitation equipment, preferably including external pacemaker, and ACLS drugs must be immediately available.

• Other antidysrhythmics (e.g., beta-blockers, digoxin, quinidine, calcium channel blockers) are not likely to interfere with action. Follow-up antidysrhythmic may be initiated immediately after conversion with adenosine.

Vital signs/hemodynamics: Continuously monitor ECG. Observe for dysrhythmias, which are most prevalent at time of conversion and are usually self-limiting. Sinus pause of ≥3 sec may occur. Be prepared to manage prolonged dysrhythmias, including heart block. If high-level block occurs, do not administer additional doses.

• Monitor BP immediately before and frequently after each bolus dose.

PATIENT/FAMILY TEACHING

Purpose of drug is to restore regular heart rhythms. • Close monitoring is necessary during therapy.

AVAILABLE FORMS

Parenteral for IV use

Storage: Refrigeration may cause crystallization; if this occurs, dissolve by warming to room temperature.

albumin, normal serum, human 5%/25%
(al-byoo'min)
Albuminar, Albutein, Buminate, Plasbumin

Classifications: Blood derivative, plasma protein fraction, plasma volume expander

USUAL DOSE

IV, adults: 25-125 g/day. Do not exceed 2 g/kg/day or 250 g/48 hr. • **Shock:** 500 ml 5% solution q30min; repeat as necessary. • **Hypoproteinemia:** 1,000-2,000 ml 5% solution once daily • **Major burns:** Initially 5% solution as needed to restore/maintain plasma volume; after stabilization, 25% solution as necessary to maintain plasma albumin level of 2.5-4 g/dl

P IV, children: 0.5-1.5 g/kg/day in nonemergency situations.
• **Hypovolemic shock:** Initially 50 ml 5% albumin or 10-20 ml/kg for infants; repeat as necessary. • Maximum dose: 6 g/kg/day

ADMINISTRATION

IV, adults: Normovolemia: 5% solution at rate of 2-4 ml/min (250 ml over 1-2 hr); 25% albumin at rate of 1 ml/min (50 ml over 1 hr)
• **Shock:** 500 ml 5% albumin given rapidly over 15-30 min, as tolerated; rate slowed as plasma volume restored • Too rapid infusion may result in fluid volume overload, pulmonary edema.
P IV, children: Administer at ¼-½ adult rate.

PREPARATION

Remove seal, swab stopper top with antiseptic solution, puncture with administration set provided by manufacturer. • 20-gauge or larger needle/catheter required because of solution viscosity • Solution should be clear amber to orange-brown; do not use if turbid or contains deposit. Infuse within 4 hr of opening
• May be diluted (not recommended)
Compatible fluids: D_5W, $D_{10}W$, 0.45% and 0.9% NaCl, LR, prepared combinations of these solutions

ACTIONS

Sterile solution prepared from pooled donors • Regulates plasma volume and tissue fluid balance by colloidal oncotic pressure; encourages fluid shift from interstitial to intravascular spaces • In volume-depleted states, expands/maintains intravascular volume for many hours • Reduces edema caused by low serum protein levels • 5% solution osmotically equivalent to plasma • 50 ml of 25% solution will draw 175 ml of additional fluid into intravascular space within 15 min (unless patient is dehydrated). • Does not contain major antibodies; may be given without matching blood type or Rh factor • Processing removes risk of hepatitis, HIV transmission • Does not contain clotting factors

PHARMACOKINETICS

ROUTE	ONSET	PEAK	DURATION
IV	Immed	Rapid	Many hours if volume depleted

DISTRIBUTION
Intravascular, except with impaired capillary permeability

ELIMINATION
Variable depending on clinical state

INDICATIONS

Plasma volume expansion/maintenance of CO in serious hypovolemia resulting from burns, hemorrhage, trauma, surgery, other conditions • Hypoproteinemia related to acute nephrosis, acute hepatic cirrhosis, toxemia of pregnancy, anuria, hypercatabolic states, other conditions • 5% solution used for hypovolemic conditions, acute hypoproteinemia, initial burn injury • 25% solution used for hypoproteinemic conditions, cerebral edema, adult respiratory distress syndrome (with diuretics), hyperbilirubinemia, erythroblastosis fetalis as adjunct to exchange transfusions, and during hemodialysis.

PRECAUTIONS/CONTRAINDICATIONS

Precautions: Rapid infusion may cause circulatory overload • Not to replace transfusion therapy
Use caution with: Sodium-restricted patients (contains 130-160 mEq Na/L) • Pulmonary capillary membrane impairment (e.g., ARDS); may worsen pulmonary edema • Renal impairment (may contain aluminum, which could accumulate)
c **Pregnancy category:** Use only if clearly needed.
Contraindications: Hypersensitivity to albumin • Severe anemia • Cardiac failure • Increased intravascular volume

ADVERSE EFFECTS

CV: **Circulatory overload;** elevated CVP, PCWP; hypotension with rapid administration (rare)
Resp: Dyspnea, **pulmonary edema** (particularly if pulmonary capillary membrane impairment)
Misc: Allergic-like response with chills, fever, nausea, vomiting, urticaria

TOXICITY/OVERDOSE

Symptoms: Circulatory overload, ↑ CVP, ↑ PCWP, dyspnea, pulmonary edema
Management: Stop infusion and consult physician. Use diuretics cautiously if necessary.

INCOMPATIBILITIES

Avoid infusion with other agents. Addition of more than 25 g/L to parenteral nutrition solutions may occlude filters. Separate administration is recommended.

PATIENT CARE IMPLICATIONS

• Dose, rate, type of solution (5%, 25%) vary according to clinical condition, 5% solution osmotically equivalent to plasma, generally used in hypovolemic states. 25% solution equal to 5 times osmotic value of plasma, generally used for hypoproteinemia. Carefully evaluate fluid volume status, confirm labeling before administration.
• Infuse through 20-gauge or larger needle/catheter.
• Not replacement for transfusion therapy. For actively bleeding or anemic patients, use as adjunct to transfusions.
Vital signs/hemodynamics: Monitor BP, HR q1-2h depending on indication, rate of administration. Monitor q5-15min in unstable patients or with rapid administration. • Monitor CVP, PCWP, CO as available. Titrate rate, dosage to restore intravascular fluid volume and avoid overload. For CVP >6 mm Hg or PCWP > 12 mm Hg or elevated above desired range for patient, slow/stop infusion and consult physician. • Monitor hourly UO
Physical assessment: Assess for symptoms of circulatory overload: crackles (rales), S_3 gallop, dyspnea, jugular venous distention, elevated PAPs/CVP.
• As indicated, assess for improvement in edema, ascites, sequestrated fluid. • Restoration of volume in patients with surgery, trauma, other bleeding increases

---

italic = common side effects

bold = life-threatening reactions

intravascular pressure and may result in renewed or increased bleeding. Assess for indicators of bleeding. • Assess for allergic-type reactions, such as chills, fever, nausea, vomiting, urticaria.

Laboratory tests: Monitor: • Hgb/Hct, albumin, protein, electrolytes • Albumin levels >4 g/dl may increase catabolism in patients with burns, other hypercatabolic states.

PATIENT/FAMILY TEACHING

Purpose of drug is to provide necessary blood proteins. • Frequent monitoring may be necessary. • Immediately report chills, fever, nausea, vomiting, rash, itching, difficulty breathing

AVAILABLE FORMS

5%, 25% solutions with IV infusion sets

---

albuterol
(al-byoo'ter-ole)
Proventil, salbutamol ✦
Ventolin

Classification: Beta-2-adrenergic agonist

USUAL DOSE

Metered-dose inhaler,
ⓟ adults/children >4 yr: 1-2 puffs q4-6h
Nebulizer/IPPB, adults/
ⓟ children >12 yr: 2.5 mg three to four times daily • Up to 10 mg has been used in adults.
ⓟ Nebulizer/IPPB, children
<12 yr: 1.25-2.5 mg three to four times daily
ⓟ PO, adults/children >12 yr: 2-4 mg three to four times daily; do not exceed single dose

of 8 mg or total dose of 32 mg/
ⓖ day. Older adults may be more sensitive to sympathomimetic effects; lower dose range must be used. • **Extended-release tablets:** 4-8 mg q12h • Maximum dose 16 mg q12h
ⓟ PO, children 6-12 yr: 2 mg three to four times daily • Maximum dose 24 mg/day

ADMINISTRATION

Nebulizer/IPPB: Dilute desired dose with 0.9% NaCl for final volume of 3 ml. • Adjust flow rate of nebulizer to deliver albuterol over 5-15 min.

ACTIONS

Stimulates beta-adrenergic receptors; predominant effects on beta-2 (bronchial, uterine, vascular smooth muscle) receptors; minimal beta-1 (cardiac) effects • Results in bronchodilation, mild vasodilation, slight decreases in BP • May cause reflex tachycardia, especially at higher doses • Little or no effect on alpha-adrenergic receptors • Promotes intracellular shift of potassium from serum, thus decreasing elevated/normal potassium levels.

PHARMACOKINETICS

ROUTE	ONSET	PEAK	DURATION
Inhal	5-15 min	30-120 min	3-6 hr
PO, std	30 min	2 hr	4-6 hr

DISTRIBUTION
Does not cross blood-brain barrier
ELIMINATION
Metabolized in liver, rapidly excreted in urine, feces

INDICATIONS

Relief of bronchospasm in asthma, chronic bronchitis, emphysema, cystic fibrosis • Prevention of exercise-induced

---

ⓟ pediatric   ⓖ geriatric   ▼ Direct IV

asthma and bronchospasm
• Longer duration and less likely to cause cardiac stimulation than isoproterenol

PRECAUTIONS/CONTRAINDICATIONS

Precautions: Tolerance may develop with prolonged use.
• Repeated or excessive use may lead to paradoxical bronchoconstriction.
Use caution with: Cardiac disorders • Hypertension • Hyperthyroidism • Diabetes mellitus • Children <5 yr • Older adults
Pregnancy category: Use only if safer alternative unavailable.
Contraindications: Hypersensitivity to albuterol

ADVERSE EFFECTS

CNS: *Tremors, nervousness,* insomnia, headache, dizziness, restlessness, hallucinations, irritability
EENT: Dry or irritated nose/throat, dilated pupils
Resp: Bronchospasm, cough
CV: Palpitations, tachycardia, hypo/hypertension
GI: Nausea, vomiting
Misc: Tolerance

TOXICITY/OVERDOSE

Symptoms: Similar to adverse effects • Angina, hypertension, tachycardia, hypokalemia
Management: After recent ingestion, implement guidelines for management of acute overdose (Appendix I). • If necessary, administer selective beta-1-adrenergic blocker (e.g., metoprolol tartrate); use extreme caution because severe bronchospasm may occur. • Hemodialysis not recommended

INTERACTIONS

beta blockers ↓ Albuterol effectiveness
Digoxin ↓ Digoxin levels
sympathomimetics (epinephrine, isoproterenol) Tachycardia, dysrhythmias, hypertension, angina; avoid concurrent use

PATIENT CARE IMPLICATIONS

• For optimal benefits in controlling bronchospasm, schedule doses at regular intervals.
• Administer PO doses with meals.
Vital signs/hemodynamics: Monitor ECG for tachycardia, dysrhythmias. • Monitor VS for hypo/hypertension, improved RR. • Use pulse oximeter to evaluate O_2 saturation before and after administration.
Physical assessment: Assess work of breathing, ventilatory excursion, breath sounds.
• Evaluate peak flow, forced expiratory volume, other pulmonary function measurements before and after treatment.
Laboratory tests: Monitor: ABGs, potassium

PATIENT/FAMILY TEACHING

Purpose of medication is to relieve bronchospasm, improve breathing. • Report increased breathing difficulty, chest pain, palpitations. • Sips of water or sugarless gum may help dry mouth. • Take oral doses with meals to decrease stomach irritation. • Check with health care provider before taking cold or cough preparations. • Use metered-dose inhaler as demonstrated. Be certain to exhale completely before use, close lips firmly around mouthpiece,

---

italic = common side effects   **bold** = life-threatening reactions

and inhale deeply while activating inhaler. Hold breath for as long as possible and exhale slowly. • Use exactly as directed. If ineffective, do not increase dose or frequency of use; consult health care provider.

AVAILABLE FORMS

Solution for PO inhal therapy • Metered-dose inhaler • Tablets, ext. rel. tablets • PO syrup

---

alcohol, ethyl
ethanol

Classification: Antidote

USUAL DOSE

IV, cont inf, adults: Antidote, 10% solution: Loading dose of 7.6-10 ml/kg or 0.6-0.8 g/kg given over 30-60 min; use lower dose with concurrent ethanol ingestion. Maintenance dose according to body weight, drinking history (see below); for example, 111 ml/hr is usual amount required in 80-kg average drinker. Individualize maintenance dose to maintain ethyl alcohol levels of approx 100-200 mg/dl. Increase maintenance dose during hemodialysis.

Approx volume of 10% ethanol required to maintain blood ethanol level of 100 mg/dl

PREVIOUS DRINKING HISTORY	APPROXIMATE VOLUME REQUIRED (ml/kg/hr)
Nondrinker	0.83
Average drinker	1.39
Chronic drinker	1.95

Sedative, 5% solution: 1 ml/min

ADMINISTRATION

Administer 10% solution via large vein. If use of small vein unavoidable, more dilute (e.g., 5% ethanol) solution may be necessary. However, large volumes may be required to maintain desired blood levels.

ACTIONS

Limits toxicity from methanol (wood alcohol) or ethylene glycol (antifreeze) by preventing metabolism to by-products that cause metabolic acidosis, tissue destruction. Ethanol has greater affinity for enzyme that converts methanol and ethylene glycol to toxic by-products. • Relieves delirium associated with acute alcohol withdrawal states • May cause hypoglycemia, especially ❶ in children

PHARMACOKINETICS

ROUTE	ONSET	PEAK	DURATION
IV	Immed	Rapid, rate dependent	Metabolized at rate of 10-20 ml/hr

DISTRIBUTION
Wide; crosses placenta, blood-brain barrier

ELIMINATION
90% metabolized by liver; remainder excreted unchanged via kidneys, lungs; half-life dose dependent

INDICATIONS

Antidote for methanol/ethylene glycol poisonings • Sedative for acute alcohol withdrawal states (use is controversial)

PRECAUTIONS/ CONTRAINDICATIONS

Precautions: Hypoglycemia ❶ possible, especially in children • Crosses placenta, enters fetal circulation, may cause CNS de- ❶ pression of newborn • Use as antidote may result in disulfiram (Antabuse)-type reaction: flushing, sweating, severe hypotension, cardiac dysrhythmias.

• Large volumes (100-200 ml/hr) typically required to maintain desired ethanol levels may result in fluid volume overload.
• May precipitate acute gout
• Direct toxin to liver/brain

Use caution with: Chronic alcohol abuse • Diabetes (may cause hypoglycemia) • Hepatic/renal impairment • Shock, hemorrhage (risk of hypotension) • Recent cranial surgery, other CNS depression • Simultaneous blood administration; may cause pseudoagglutination

c Pregnancy category: Fetal damage possible; use only if safer alternative unavailable.

Contraindications: Epilepsy, active infection, diabetic coma

P • Children: Safety not established

ADVERSE EFFECTS

CNS: *Intoxication, sedation,* vertigo, disorientation, restlessness
CV: **Hypotension,** hypervolemia
Local: Pain/irritation at infusion site, venous thrombosis or phlebitis
Misc: **Hypoglycemia,** flushing, fever

TOXICITY/OVERDOSE

Symptoms: Alcohol intoxication with vertigo, flushing, disorientation, excessive sedation
Management: Slow or stop infusion

INTERACTIONS

antidiabetics (e.g., insulin, sulfonylureas) Hypoglycemia
antihypertensives Hypotension
barbiturates Additive CNS depression
benzodiazepines Additive CNS depression

cephalosporins (e.g., cefamandole, cefoperazone, cefotetan) Flushing, tachycardia, vomiting
chloral hydrate Additive CNS depression
disulfiram (Antabuse) Flushing, tachycardia, vomiting
diuretics Hypotension
meprobamate Additive CNS depression
metoclopramide Additive CNS depression
metronidazole Flushing, tachycardia, vomiting
narcotic analgesics Additive CNS depression
nitrates Hypotension
phenothiazines Additive CNS depression

PATIENT CARE IMPLICATIONS

• Infuse via large peripheral vein using small-bore needle or catheter. Check infusion site frequently.
• Do not administer simultaneously with blood.
• Ethanol infusions generally inappropriate in managing acute alcohol withdrawal, particularly in critically ill patients; benzodiazepines (e.g., diazepam, lorazepam) safer, more effective

Methanol or ethylene glycol poisoning: Use 10% alcohol solution. Use of 5% solution would require administration of excessive volumes to maintain desired alcohol level. • Observe for disulfiram (Antabuse)-type reaction (e.g., flushing, sweating, hypotension, cardiac dysrhythmias). If present, slow or stop infusion and consult physician. Treat hypotension with fluids/vasopressors as necessary.

Vital signs/hemodynamics: Monitor BP, HR, RR frequently.

• Measure/record all I&O.

Methanol or ethylene glycol poisoning: Continuously monitor ECG for cardiac dysrhythmias during initial loading dose and until VS stable. • Monitor BP at 5-15–min intervals during initial loading dose and at 15-min intervals until stable.

Physical assessment: Assess for changes in neurologic status: restlessness, excessive sedation, intoxication. Reduce infusion rate as necessary. • Assess for fluid volume overload: dyspnea, crackles (rales), hypertension, S_3 gallop, neck vein distention. • Assess for hypoglycemia (e.g., tachycardia, sweating, tremors, **P** hypotension), especially in children, patients with diabetes.

Laboratory tests: Monitor: Electrolytes, blood glucose, acid-base balance • Blood ethanol levels hourly and less frequently as patient stabilizes • Maintain ethyl alcohol blood levels of approx 100-200 mg/dl (approx 100 ml/hr of 10% solution). • Continue alcohol infusion until ethylene glycol or methanol levels <20 mg/dl.

PATIENT/FAMILY TEACHING

Purpose of drug is to limit damage caused by certain toxins. • Frequent blood samples, close monitoring are required. • Inform health care provider immediately of feelings of vertigo, intoxication, sedation, pain at infusion site. • Alcoholic odor on breath is anticipated side effect.

AVAILABLE FORMS

5% or 10% ethanol and D_5W for IV use

---

alprazolam
(al-pra′zoe-lam)
Xanax, Apo-Alpraz ✦,
Nu-Alpraz ✦

Classifications: Benzodiazepine, sedative/hypnotic, antianxiety (anxiolytic) agent
Schedule IV Controlled Substance

USUAL DOSE

PO, adults: 0.25-0.5 mg bid-tid
G • Older adults: 0.25 mg bid-tid • Use smallest effective dose, increase if needed every 3-4 days • maximum dose, 10 mg/day

ACTIONS

Facilitates action of gamma-aminobutyric acid (GABA, major inhibitory neurotransmitter), producing CNS depression; anxiety reduced, mild sedation occurs • No respiratory depressant effects at usual dose • No analgesic effects

PHARMACOKINETICS

ROUTE	ONSET	PEAK	DURATION
PO	<1 hr	1-2 hr	6-12 hr

DISTRIBUTION
Widely distributed, highly protein bound
ELIMINATION
Metabolized by liver, eliminated by kidneys; half-life 11 hr, 16 hr in older adults

INDICATIONS

Management of anxiety disorders, anxiety associated with depression; short-term relief of anxiety symptoms • Treatment of panic disorder, agoraphobia • Not for long-term use

---

PRECAUTIONS/ CONTRAINDICATIONS

Precautions: Risk of dependence; short-term use only • Abrupt cessation of therapy may lead to withdrawal

G Use caution with: Older adults; excessive sedation, hypotension possible; use reduced dose • COPD, hepatic/renal insufficiency, debilitation, opiate analgesics, alcohol, phenothiazines, other CNS depressants, low serum albumin; pronounced CNS depression possible; use reduced dose.

D Pregnancy category: Risk of congenital malformations, prolonged CNS depression, withdrawal symptoms in newborn; use only if risk explained to woman and safer alternative unavailable.

Contraindications: Hypersensitivity to alprazolam • Acute angle-closure glaucoma • Myasthenia gravis • Severe pulmonary disease • Children: Safety/ effectiveness not established

ADVERSE EFFECTS

NOTE: Most likely during initial therapy

CNS: *Drowsiness,* dizziness, fatigue, impaired coordination, memory impairment, confusion, headache, paradoxical excitement, especially in psychiatric patients

CV: Hypotension, tachycardia

GI: Constipation, dry mouth, diarrhea, nausea, vomiting

GU: Difficulty voiding, menstrual disorders

Misc: Dependence/withdrawal symptoms, including seizures

TOXICITY/OVERDOSE

Symptoms (acute toxicity): Somnolence, impaired coordination, confusion, coma, diminished reflexes • Hypotension, tachycardia, shock • Respiratory depression/serious toxicity more likely with ingestion of alcohol, other CNS depressants

Management: After recent ingestion, implement guidelines for management of acute overdose (Appendix I). • Maintain airway/support ventilation as necessary. • Use flumazenil to reverse effects • Hypotension: Elevate legs, administer IV fluids; use vasopressors (e.g., dopamine, norepinephrine) if not responsive to fluids • Do not use barbiturates for paradoxical excitation. • Hemodialysis not generally useful

INTERACTIONS

alcohol, ethyl ↑ Sedation

antacids Altered alprazolam absorption

antihistamines ↑ Sedation

barbiturates ↑ Sedation

beta blockers ↑ Sedation

cimetidine ↓ Alprazolam clearance; ↑ sedation

digoxin ↑ Serum concentration; risk of toxicity; monitor digoxin levels

disulfiram ↑ Sedation

flumazenil ↓ Sedation

isoniazid ↑ Sedation

ketoconazole ↑ Sedation

opiate analgesics ↑ Sedation

probenecid ↑ Sedation

propoxyphene ↑ Sedation

rifampin ↓ Sedation

theophylline ↓ Sedation

---

italic = common side effects   **bold** = life-threatening reactions

PATIENT CARE IMPLICATIONS

• Individualize dosage, increase cautiously. Always use smallest effective dose.
• Administer with food to reduce gastric irritation.
• Avoid sudden cessation of therapy, especially with long-term (>2-3 mo) therapy; may cause withdrawal symptoms and seizures. Manage seizures with diazepam, phenytoin, and/or barbiturates.
• Limit quantity prescribed for patients with severe depression, suicidal tendencies, history suggesting likelihood of substance abuse.
G • Older adults, debilitated patients, low serum albumin: Use lower dose, increase cautiously, monitor closely for adverse effects
• Periodically assess/document need for continued therapy.
Physical assessment: Assess for excessive sedation, impaired physical coordination. Reduce dose as necessary.
Laboratory tests: Monitor: Liver enzymes, CBC regularly throughout therapy

PATIENT/FAMILY TEACHING

Purpose of drug is to reduce anxiety. • May cause drowsiness or dizziness, especially during first few days of therapy; use caution with activity until individual effects recognized.
• Avoid concurrent use of alcohol or other drugs that cause sedation while taking this medication. • Cigarette smoking interferes with drug effectiveness. • Take with food to minimize upset stomach. • Report possible pregnancy. • May cause psychologic and physical dependence; seizures may develop if you suddenly stop taking this medication. Consult prescriber before increasing dose or discontinuing.

AVAILABLE FORMS

Tablets • Oral concentrate

---

alteplase
(al-teep′-lase)
rt-PA, t-PA, tissue-type plasminogen activator (recombinant)
Activase, Actilyse ✦

Classification: Thrombolytic agent

USUAL DOSE

IV, adults, coronary thrombolysis: 3-hr regimen: For patients ≥65 kg, administer total of 100 mg over 3 hr as follows: First hr—60 mg; give initial 6-10 mg as direct injection over 1-2 min; remainder of 60-mg dose infused over 1 hr. Second, third hr—40 mg remaining dose infused at rate of 20 mg/hr. For patients <65 kg, administer total of 1.25 mg/kg over 3 hr as follows: First hr—60% of total dose; initial 6%-10% of which is given as direct injection over 1-2 min; remainder of 60% infused over 1 hr. Second, third hr —40% remaining dose evenly infused over 2 hr. • **Accelerated regimen:** For patients >67 kg, administer total of 100 mg over 90 min as follows: Direct injection of 15 mg over 1-2 min; then 50-mg infusion over next 30 min; then 35-mg infusion over next 60 min. For patients ≤67 kg, administer total

---

P pediatric   **G** geriatric   **V** Direct IV

dose over 90 min as follows:
Direct injection of 15 mg over
1-2 min; then 0.75 mg/kg (but
not >50 mg) infusion over next
30 min; then 0.5 mg/kg (but not
>35 mg) infusion over next 60
min. Increased effectiveness
with prompt therapy (within 6
hr of symptom onset), concurrent heparin, aspirin therapy
• Other dosing regimens used
• Do not use ≥150-mg dose of
alteplase; ↑ Risk of intracranial
hemorrhage

**IV, intermit inf adults, acute
pulmonary embolism:** 100
mg IV over 2 hr • Followed by
heparin therapy • Other dosing
regimens used

ADMINISTRATION

IV, adults: Injection/infusion
rate varies according to indication (see above). Use volumetric
infusion pump. DO NOT FIL-
TER. Do not add other medication to solution. After infusion
complete, flush line with 25-30
ml saline.

PREPARATION

Prepare immediately before use.
• **20- or 50-mg vials:** Reconstitute using 1 ml/mg sterile water for injection WITHOUT
PRESERVATIVES (e.g., 20 ml
for 20-mg vial; 50 ml for 50-
mg vial). • Use 18-gauge or
larger needle and direct diluent
into powder. Roll or gently tilt
to mix; do not agitate. Foaming
settles if left undisturbed for 2-3
min. • Reconstituted solution
contains 1 mg/ml; may further
dilute in 0.9% NaCl or D_5W to
concentration of 0.5 mg/ml or
greater. Precipitation occurs
with more diluted solutions.
Gently invert or swirl to mix;
do not shake all solutions.

• **100-mg vials:** Reconstitute
using diluent and transfer device
provided by the manufacturer.
Pierce upright vial of diluent
with one end of transfer device.
Hold alteplase vial upside down
and pierce center of vial with
other end of transfer device.
Place alteplase vial upright and
hold diluent upside down to allow transfer of diluent into the
alteplase vial (does not contain
a vacuum). Transfer takes about
2 min, and a small amount of
diluent (0.5 ml) will remain in
diluent vial. Remove transfer
device from alteplase vial and
gently swirl to mix; do not
shake. May insert infusion device into existing puncture in
alteplase vial and hang by plastic ring on bottom of vial. • Inspect for particulate matter, discoloration before infusing.

Compatible fluids: After reconstitution compatible in 0.9%
NaCl, D_5W at concentrations
not <0.5 mg/ml

Stability: Reconstituted solution stable for 8 hr at room
temperature

ACTIONS

Promotes thrombolysis (clot dissolution) by binding to fibrin
within clot and activating plasminogen to form plasmin (enzyme that dissolves fibrin clots,
fibrinogen, some clotting factors) • Results in improved
blood flow through previously
obstructed vessel, usually within
1-2 hr • Prompt reperfusion
minimizes loss of myocardial
tissue due to ischema, common
promotes improved ventricular
function. • Reductions in circulating clotting factors may cause
significant bleeding complications.

---

italic = common side effects   **bold** = life-threatening reactions

PHARMACOKINETICS

ROUTE	ONSET	PEAK	DURATION
IV	Immed	20-120 min	5-10 min

DISTRIBUTION

Distribution to CNS, placenta, milk unknown

ELIMINATION

Rapid plasma clearance, primarily by liver; >80% cleared within 10 min. Some effects present for several hours.

INDICATIONS

Thrombolysis in evolving acute MI: Restoration of coronary perfusion to limit infarct size, improve ventricular function, reduce incidence of heart failure; indicated only during initial phase of acute MI, preferably within 6 hr of symptom onset. Concomitant anticoagulant therapy (e.g., heparin) and platelet-aggregation inhibitors (e.g., aspirin) reduces incidence of reocclusion. • **Lysis of acute pulmonary emboli:** Restores pulmonary blood flow in serious pulmonary embolic obstruction (entire lobe or multisegments involved, patient hemodynamically unstable); reduces pulmonary hypertension, reverses right ventricular dysfunction, improves hemodynamic stability; use concomitant anticoagulant therapy.
Unlabeled/investigational: Unstable angina pectoris. Pulmonary artery administration for lysis of acute pulmonary emboli. Lysis of peripheral arterial occlusions, occlusions in bypass grafts, other thromboembolic conditions.

PRECAUTIONS/ CONTRAINDICATIONS

Precautions: Bleeding, bruising, hematomas may occur, especially at vascular access sites, after invasive procedures, with IM injections. • Cerebral and other serious or fatal spontaneous bleeding may occur.
• Atrial/ventricular dysrhythmias may occur during coronary reperfusion.
G Use caution with: Older adults, history of cerebrovascular disease, doses >100 mg; ↑ risk of cerebral hemorrhage
c Pregnancy category: Safety not established; use only if safer alternative unavailable.
Minor relative contraindications: Recent (within 10 days) minor trauma, including CPR
• History of cerebrovascular disease • Pregnancy • Likelihood of left-sided heart thrombus (e.g., atrial fibrillation, severe left ventricular dyskinesia)
• Acute pericarditis • Subacute bacterial endocarditis • Hemostatic defects (including those associated with liver/renal dysfunction), anticoagulant therapy
• Diabetic hemorrhagic retinopathy, other hemorrhagic ophthalmic conditions • Age >75 yr
• Septic thrombophlebitis or occluded AV cannula at seriously infected site • Any condition in which serious bleeding likely or difficult to control
Major relative contraindications: Recent (within 10 days) major surgery, serious trauma, obstetric delivery, organ biopsy, puncture of noncompressible vessels • GI/GU bleeding within 10 days • Hypertension (SBP >180 or DBP >110 mm Hg)
Absolute contraindications: Hypersensitivity to alteplase
• Active internal bleeding • Recent CVA • Recent (within 2 mo) intracranial neoplasm, arteriovenous malformation/aneurysm • Recent (within 2 mo) in-

tracranial/intraspinal surgery, trauma • Bleeding diathesis • Severe, uncontrolled hypertension • Children: Safety not established

ADVERSE EFFECTS

CNS: **Cerebral hemorrhage**
EENT: Gingival bleeding, epistaxis
CV: *Reperfusion dysrhythmias* (e.g., accelerated idioventricular rhythm, PVCs, **ventricular tachycardia/fibrillation,** PACs, atrial fibrillation, junctional rhythm, sinus bradycardia), **hypotension**
GI: *Nausea/vomiting,* bleeding
GU: Hematuria
Misc: *Puncture site and soft tissue bleeding, bruising, ecchymosis/hematoma*

TOXICITY/OVERDOSE

Symptoms: Bleeding, bruising, hematomas; spontaneous bleeding from cerebral, retroperitoneal, GU, GI, soft tissue sources • Dose-dependent depletion of clotting proteins, production of fibrin degradation products
Management: Stop infusion. • Initiate local measures such as manual compression followed by pressure dressings. • Administer plasma volume expanders (avoid dextran), packed RBCs, fresh-frozen plasma, cryoprecipitate, as indicated by blood loss, clotting studies. • Antifibrinolytics (e.g., aminocaproic acid) have been used for life-threatening bleeding (e.g., intracranial hemorrhage).

INTERACTIONS

antifibrinolytic agents ↓ Fibrinolysis
anticoagulants (e.g., heparin, warfarin) ↑ Bleeding risk

antiplatelet agents (e.g. abciximal, dipyridamole, NSAIDs, ticlopidine) ↑ Bleeding risk
cefamandole, cefoperazone, cefotetan: cephalosporin may ↓ prothrombin/ ↑ bleeding risk

Y-SITE COMPATIBILITIES

Lidocaine, metoprolol, propranolol

Y-SITE INCOMPATIBILITIES

Dobutamine, dopamine, heparin, lidocaine, nitroglycerin

PATIENT CARE IMPLICATIONS

Before starting therapy:
• Obtain baseline 12-lead ECG.
• Review history for contraindications.
• Have emergency resuscitation equipment, including epinephrine, lidocaine, atropine, immediately available.
• Apply pressure dressings to unsuccessful venipuncture attempts.
• Place 2 or more 18-gauge or larger catheters for laboratory samples; medications, fluids, emergency use.
• Use volumetric or syringe infusion pump; do not use drop-counting infusion devices.
• Infuse through separate IV line; do NOT use IV filter.
During and immediately after therapy:
• Avoid unnecessary venipuncture, invasive procedures, IM injections.
• If venipuncture necessary, hold manual pressure over site for 20 min or until bleeding stops, then apply pressure dressing. Inspect frequently for bleeding.

---

italic = common side effects   **bold** = life-threatening reactions

- If arterial puncture necessary, avoid femoral site and hold manual pressure over puncture site for 30 min or until bleeding stops. Apply pressure dressing, inspect frequently for bleeding.
- Avoid arterial/venous invasive procedures in areas inaccessible to manual compression (e.g., internal jugular, subclavian).
- Transient dysrhythmias, reduced chest pain, reduction of ST segment elevation suggest successful thrombolysis, coronary reperfusion.
- Consult physician for significant dysrhythmias, unusual or excessive bleeding, change in neurologic status, unrelieved or recurrent chest pain, allergic reactions.

Vital signs/hemodynamics: Initially, monitor BP, HR 5-15 min; when stable, progress to q30-60min during and for several hr after infusion. Hypotension may result from reperfusion dysrhythmias, hemorrhage, impaired myocardial contractility; carefully evaluate each case.
- Immediately notify physician of severe or uncontrolled hypertension (SBP >180 or DBP >110 mm Hg). Prepare to initiate hypotensive therapy. • Continuously monitor ECG for dysrhythmias, changes in ST segment elevation. Anticipate reperfusion dysrhythmias; if symptomatic, manage dysrhythmias according to ACLS guidelines (Appendix P).

Physical assessment: Assess/document chest pain intensity, character, location, radiation, duration. Note any associated symptoms. • Monitor all vascular access sites; assess for bleeding q15min during and immediately after infusion, then q4h for 24 hr. If bleeding occurs, apply pressure, continue to monitor closely. Infusion may need to be discontinued if bleeding becomes excessive.
- Assess peripheral pulses for diminished intensity, especially those distal to arterial puncture or other invasive procedures.
- Assess neurologic status before initiating therapy and frequently thereafter. Immediately notify physician of changes.
- Assess for retroperitoneal bleeding (e.g., low back pain, flank ecchymosis). • Note blood in urine, other body fluids. Check emesis, stools for occult blood.

Laboratory tests: Monitor: CPK, CBC, PT, PTT, fibrinogen before and after therapy • Cardiac enzymes in coronary thrombolysis • *May cause:* unreliable results with coagulation studies; notify lab and consider use of aprotinin/aminocaproic acid

PATIENT/FAMILY TEACHING

Purpose of drug is to dissolve clots blocking blood flow to vital organs. • Frequent monitoring is necessary because of many side effects. • Inform health care provider immediately of chest pain or discomfort, unusual bleeding (e.g., from venipunctures, nose, mouth, urine), itching. • Remain on bed rest throughout therapy.
- Avoid potential trauma from shaving, toothbrushing, excessive activity for 24 hr after therapy.

AVAILABLE FORMS

Parenteral for IV injection/infusion

amikacin sulfate
(am-i-kay′ sin)
Amikin

Classification: Aminoglycoside antibiotic

USUAL DOSE

IV/IM, adults/children >1 mo: 15 mg/kg/24 hr in equally divided doses q8-12h • Dose for 70-kg adult is 500 mg q12h or 350 mg q8h. • Do not exceed 15 mg/kg/24 hr or 1.5 g/24hr.
• **Extensive burns:** Altered pharmacokinetics may cause reduced serum levels; adjust individually to therapeutic levels.
• **Renal insufficiency:** Reduce dose and/or frequency; adjust individually to creat. cl. and therapeutic levels.

ADMINISTRATION

IM injection: Inject deep into large muscle mass (e.g., gluteus maximus, lateral thigh)
IV, intermit inf: Infuse prepared solution over 30-60 min.

PREPARATION

IV, intermit inf: Dilute single dose in 100-200 ml (less for children) of compatible IV solution.
Compatible fluids: D_5W, 0.9% NaCl, LR, prepare combinations of these solutions
Stability: Reconstituted solution stable for 24 hr at room temperature

ACTIONS

Bactericidal effects; inhibits bacterial cell protein synthesis, causing cellular death • Active against many aerobic gram-negative bacteria, including *Pseudomonas aeruginosa, Aci-netobacter, Escherichia coli, Enterobacter, Klebsiella, Proteus, Serratia* • Active against some aerobic gram-positive bacteria, including *Staphylococcus aureus, S. epidermidis* • Generally reserved for strains resistant to other aminoglycosides

PHARMACOKINETICS

ROUTE	ONSET	PEAK	DURATION
IM	Rapid	45 min-2 hr	Approx 8-12 hr
IV	Immed	End of infusion	

DISTRIBUTION
Widely distributed; CSF levels unpredictable

ELIMINATION
Filtered through glomeruli and excreted; half-life = 2-3 hr ↑ with renal impairment, liver disease, cystic fibrosis advanced age, and in infants

Therapeutic levels: Peak levels of 15-30 µg/ml; trough levels of 5-10 µg/ml

INDICATIONS

Treatment of serious, gram-negative bacterial infections (e.g., skin infections in burn patients; septicemia; bone, respiratory tract, complicated urinary tract, or postop intraabdominal infections); particularly useful with strains of *Proteus, Serratia, Klebsiella, Pseudomonas* resistant to gentamicin, other aminoglycosides • Frequently combined with extended-spectrum penicillin (e.g., piperacillin, ticarcillin) for treatment of serious *Pseudomonas* infections, particularly in immunosuppressed patients • Not indicated for gram-positive bacterial infections if other, less toxic antibiotic could be used

---

italic = common side effects   **bold** = life-threatening reactions

PRECAUTIONS/ CONTRAINDICATIONS

Precautions: Bacterial or fungal overgrowth possible • Excessive serum levels associated with toxicity • Systemic absorption with toxicity possible when used in irrigating solutions or for intrapleural/peritoneal instillation • Some preparations contain sulfites, which can cause serious allergic reactions in susceptible individuals.

G P Use caution with: Renal impairment, advanced age, infants, preexisting hearing disorder, high-dose/prolonged therapy, dehydration; ototoxicity and/or nephrotoxicity more likely • Preexisting neuromuscular disease, hypocalcemia, massive transfusions of citrated blood, general anesthesia, NMBAs; neurotoxicity with paralysis more likely • Concurrent use of other ototoxic, neurotoxic, nephrotoxic agents, including other aminoglycosides

D Pregnancy category: Risk of fetal damage, avoid pregnancy; use only if safer alternative unavailable and risks explained to woman.

Contraindications: Hypersensitivity to amikacin, possibly other aminoglycosides

ADVERSE EFFECTS

CNS: *Ototoxicity*, dizziness, permanent hearing loss, peripheral numbness/twitching, weakness, neuromuscular blockade
GI: Nausea, vomiting, elevated liver enzymes
GU: *Nephrotoxicity*, tubular necrosis, **renal failure**
Local: Local irritation/pain

Misc: Hypersensitivity; superinfection, colonization

TOXICITY/OVERDOSE

Symptoms: Ototoxicity, nephrotoxicity • Neurotoxicity with neuromuscular blockade, possible respiratory paralysis, seizures
Management: Discontinue drug. • Initiate symptomatic/supportive measures, including airway management/ventilation. • Hemodialysis or peritoneal dialysis may be helpful.

INTERACTIONS

aminoglycosides Cumulative toxicity possible
amphotericin B ↑ Risk of nephrotoxicity
anticoagulants, oral Additive PT prolongation
cephalosporins (e.g., cephalothin) ↑ Risk of nephrotoxicity; synergistic antibacterial activity. Chemical inactivation of amikacin possible. Administer at separate sites; stagger schedules.
cyclosporine ↑ Risk of nephrotoxicity
diuretics ↑ Risk of oto nephrotoxicity
ethacrynic acid ↑ Risk of nephrotoxicity; extreme caution indicated
NSAIDs ↑ Risk of nephrotoxicity
penicillins Synergistic antibacterial activity; chemical inactivation of aminoglycoside, particularly with ticarcillin, carbenicillin. Administer at separate sites; stagger schedules

Y-SITE COMPATIBILITIES

Acyclovir, amiodarone, diltiazem, enalaprilat, esmolol, fluconazole, furosemide, labetalol,

---

P pediatric   **G** geriatric   **V** Direct IV

lincomycin, magnesium sulfate, morphine sulfate, ondansetron

Y-SITE INCOMPATIBILITIES

Amphotericin B, cephalosporins, heparin, hetastarch, penicillins, phenytoin

PATIENT CARE IMPLICATIONS

• Obtain specimens for culture and sensitivity before initiating antibiotic therapy. Therapy may be initiated before results received.
• IV route must be used for severe infections or when shock present.
• Contact with heparin may cause precipitation. Flush heparinized devices with 0.9% NaCl before and after administration.
Vital signs/hemodynamics: Monitor VS for indicators of infection • Carefully monitor UO, evaluate I&O ratio. Keep patient well hydrated with oral or parenteral fluids of sufficient volume to produce UO of O.5-1 ml/kg/hr. Older, debilitated, seriously ill, or renal impaired patients are at greater risk for toxicity. • As available, monitor CVP, PCWP, central hemodynamics to optimize fluid volume balance.
Physical assessment: Assess for improvement in primary infection or symptoms of super/suprainfection: appearance of sputum, urine, stool, wound drainage; presence of fever, candidiasis, vaginitis. • Assess for evidence of neuromuscular blockade: numbness, tingling, muscle twitching, weakness; possible progression to apnea; particular vigilance required for at-risk patients (see Precautions). • Assess hearing before

initiating therapy. Monitor at intervals for symptoms of ototoxicity: tinnitus, roaring in ears, hearing loss, dizziness, vertigo, nausea; particularly important with advanced age, preexisting hearing disorder, renal impairment, high-dose/proglonged therapy
Laboratory tests: Peak/ trough levels: Draw peak levels immediately after IV infusion complete or 30-60 min after IM injection. Draw trough levels just before next dose.
• Narrow therapeutic range requires close monitoring, particularly with advanced age, high-dose therapy, renal insufficiency. • **Monitor:** Electrolytes, liver enzymes, WBC • Urinalysis, BUN, creatinine, creat. cl. before and regularly during therapy; follow closely with older adults, renal impairment, high-dose/prolonged therapy. If signs of renal irritation (e.g., casts, proteinuria), increase hydration. Discontinue for renal dysfunction.

PATIENT/FAMILY TEACHING

Purpose of drug is to limit growth of infection-causing bacteria. • Report rash, itching, diarrhea, fever, vaginal itching or discharge, dizziness, hearing difficulties. • Report possible pregnancy.

AVAILABLE FORMS

Parenteral for IV/IM use

---

italic = common side effects   **bold** = life-threatening reactions

aminocaproic acid
(a-mee-noe-ka-proe'ik)

epsilon-aminocaproic acid, EACA
Amicar

Classifications: Hemostatic agent, antifibrinolytic

USUAL DOSE

PO, adults: Follow IV dosing regimen.

IV, adults: Priming dose, 4-5 g in 250 ml compatible solution given over 1 hr; follow with continuous infusion, 1-1.25 g/hr for 6-8 hr or until hemorrhage controlled • Do not exceed 30 g/24 hr.

P IV, children (investigational/ unlabeled): Priming dose, 100 mg/kg diluted in compatible solution given over 1 hr; follow with continuous infusion, 33.3 mg/kg/hr for 6-8 hr or until hemorrhage controlled. • Do not exceed 18 g/m^2/24 hr.

ADMINISTRATION

IV: Administer priming dose over 1 hr; follow with continuous infusion for 6-8 hr or until hemorrhage controlled. • Always dilute before administration. • Use infusion pump.
• Rapid administration or insufficient dilution may cause hypotension, bradycardia, other dysrhythmias.

PREPARATION

DILUTION	CONCENTRATION
5 g/250 ml	20 mg/ml
5 g/500 ml	10 mg/ml

Compatible fluids: D$_5$W, 0.9% sodium chloride, LR, sterile water for injection

ACTIONS

Promotes stabilization of clots by inhibiting fibrin breakdown. Primarily inhibits proteolytic activity of plasminogen but also inhibits plasmin at higher doses

PHARMACOKINETICS

ROUTE	ONSET	PEAK	DURATION
PO	Rapid	1 hr	ND
IV	Immed	Rapid	3 hr

DISTRIBUTION
Widely and rapidly distributed

ELIMINATION
40%-60% excreted unchanged in urine within 12 hr

Desired plasma level: 0.13 mg/ml

INDICATIONS

Acute, life-threatening bleeding associated with overactive fibrinolytic system, such as hyperfibrinolysis associated with heart surgery, portacaval shunts, hepatic cirrhosis, liver transplantation, abruptio placentae, aplastic anemia, certain carcinomas
• Urinary fibrinolysis associated with severe trauma, anoxia, shock, GU surgery/procedures
• Hematuria associated with polycystic/neoplastic renal disease
• Laboratory confirmation of hyperfibrinolysis required
Unlabeled/investigational:
Thrombolytic overdose; prevention of recurrent subarachnoid hemorrhage (efficacy not clearly established); amegakaryocytic thrombocytopenia to reduce need for platelet transfusion

PRECAUTIONS/ CONTRAINDICATIONS

Precautions: Confirm hyperfibrinolysis by checking platelet count (normal), protamine paracoagulation (negative), euglobu-

lin clot lysis (reduced) before initiating therapy. • Do not administer to patient with DIC unless concomitant heparin therapy.
Use caution with: Upper urinary tract hematuria; may cause obstruction via glomerular capillary or renal pelvic thrombosis • Cardiac, hepatic, renal disease; reduce dose.

c **Pregnancy category:** Use only if safer alternative unavailable.

Contraindications: Hypersensitivity to aminocaproic acid • Active intravascular clotting with fibrinolysis and bleeding • DIC • Thrombosis

ADVERSE EFFECTS

CNS: Dizziness, tinnitus, headache, **seizures** (rare)
CV: Thrombophlebitis, hypotension, bradycardia, cardiac dysrhythmias, cardiac muscle damage
GI: Nausea, cramping, diarrhea
GU: Diuresis, elevated serum potassium
MS: Weakness, fatigue, myopathy, acute rhabdomyolysis

TOXICITY/OVERDOSE

Symptoms: Thrombophlebitis, thromboembolic complications, elevated CPK, myopathy
Management: Stop infusion. Manage according to symptoms.

INTERACTIONS

estrogens ↑ Risk of thrombosis
oral contraceptives ↑ Risk of thrombosis
thrombolytics (e.g., alteplase, streptokinase) Inhibition of therapeutic effects

Y-SITE INCOMPATIBILITIES

Not determined; do not administer with other drugs.

PATIENT CARE IMPLICATIONS

Monitor IV site closely for signs of thrombophlebitis. Stabilize catheter/tubing to minimize movement.
Vital signs/hemodynamics: Monitor BP, HR frequently according to severity of bleeding • Monitor UO for decreasing amount or I&O imbalance.
Physical assessment: Assess for thromboembolic complications: positive Homan's sign, leg pain or edema, dyspnea, hemoptysis, chest pain. Consult physician for significant findings. • Monitor neurologic status frequently in patients with subarachnoid hemorrhage.
Laboratory tests: Confirm hyperfibrinolysis by checking platelet count (normal), protamine paracoagulation (negative), euglobulin clot lysis (reduced) before initiating therapy. Monitor platelet count, clotting factors throughout therapy. May type and screen for hemorrhaging. • **Monitor:** Electrolytes, particularly potassium, which may be elevated, especially with impaired renal function • CPK, AST (SGOT), for elevations associated with myopathy; discontinue therapy as necessary.

PATIENT/FAMILY TEACHING

Purpose of drug is to regulate clotting and prevent excessive bleeding. • Frequent monitoring is required with IV therapy. • Change position slowly to avoid orthostatic hypotension. • Inform healthcare provider im-

---

italic = common side effects   **bold** = life-threatening reactions

mediately of leg pain or swelling, chest pain, shortness of breath, recurrent bleeding.

AVAILABLE FORMS

Parenteral for IV infusion • Tablets • Oral solution

aminophylline
(am-in-off'-lin)

theophylline ethylenediamine
Aminophyllin,
Corophyllin,
Phyllocontin,
Somophyllin, Truphylline

Classifications: Bronchodilator, xanthine derivative

USUAL DOSE

P PO, adults/children >1 yr:
Loading dose, patient not receiving theophylline: 5 mg/kg
Dose requires individual adjustment to patient response, serum levels; excessive dosage results in serious toxicity; dosage based on lean body weight

P IV, adults/children >1 yr:
Loading dose, patient not receiving theophylline: 6 mg/kg
IV, maintenance dose:

ADULTS	DOSE (mg/kg/hr)
Nonsmoking	0.5
Smoking	0.8
Advanced Age	0.3
Cor pulmonale	0.3
CHF, hepatic failure	0.1-0.2
P CHILDREN	
1-9 yr	1.0
9-16 yr	0.8

Oral maintenance dose

ADULTS	DOSE
Nonsmoking	3 mg/kg q^{8h}
Smoking	3 mg/kg q^{6h}
Advanced Age	2 mg/kg q^{8h}
Cor pulmonale	2 mg/kg q^{8h}
CHF, hepatic failure	1-2 mg/kg q^{12h}
P CHILDREN	
1-9 yr	4 mg/kg q^{6h}
9-16 yr	3 mg/kg q^{6h}

ADMINISTRATION

IV, loading inf: Infuse loading dose over 20-30 min. • Do not exceed rate of 20 mg/min; rapid administration may cause ventricular fibrillation, cardiac arrest. • Infusion pump required. • Stop infusion for 5-10 min if tachycardia, dysrhythmias, hypotension, other adverse reactions.
IV, cont inf: Use infusion pump or other rate-controlling device.

PREPARATION

IV infusion: Dilute in 100-250 ml compatible solution. Aminophylline, 500 mg in 250 ml, yields concentration of 2 mg/ml. • More concentrated solutions may be used, but do not exceed concentration of 25 mg/ml. • Do not use crystallized solutions.

DILUTION	CONCENTRATION
250 mg/250 ml	1 mg/ml
500 mg/250 ml	2 mg/ml
1000 mg/250 ml	4 mg/ml

Compatible fluids: D$_5$W, 0.9% NaCl, LR, prepared combinations of these solutions

ACTIONS

Contains 89%-90% theophylline • **Respiratory:** Relaxes respiratory smooth muscle, relieves bronchospasm; increases flow rates, vital capacity; dilates pulmonary arterioles, reduces pulmonary hypertension, increases pulmonary blood flow; unlike sympathomimetic bronchodilators, tolerance rarely develops. • **CNS:** Stimulates vagal, vasomotor, vomiting centers, constricts cerebral vasculature, decreases cerebral blood flow; increases sensitivity of medulla to CO_2 and may increase rate and depth of ventilation. • **CV:** Direct arteriolar/venous dilation decreases peripheral vascular resistance preload; vasodilation usually offset by increased CO and vasomotor stimulation with vasoconstriction; slight BP increases seen with moderate doses; higher doses rapid IV injection cause vagal stimulation with bradycardia, reflex tachycardia, dysrhythmias, hypotension. • **Renal:** Mild diuresis caused by increased CO, slight renal arteriolar dilation

PHARMACOKINETICS

ROUTE	ONSET	PEAK	DURATION
PO, std	30 min	1-2 hr	
PO, ext rel		4-5 hr	
IV	Rapid	30 min	Var

DISTRIBUTION
Wide

ELIMINATION
Metabolized in liver, renal elimination; half-life 7-9 hr, shorter in children, smokers; half-life longer with CHF, COPD, liver disease, sustained fever, advanced age, and in infants

Therapeutic levels: 10-20 µg/ml

INDICATIONS

Reversible bronchospasm associated with chronic asthma, chronic bronchitis, emphysema

• IV route used with status asthmaticus refractory to epinephrine • To counteract bronchospasm associated with propranolol
Unlabeled/investigational:
IV route to relieve periodic apnea, in patients with Cheyne-Stokes breathing; adjunct in management of CHF to relieve dyspnea, decrease venous filling pressure, increase CO

PRECAUTIONS/ CONTRAINDICATIONS

Precautions: Rapid IV administration may cause profound bradycardia, PVCs, hypotension, cardiac arrest. • Stimultaneous administration by more than one route or with other xanthines increases risk of toxicity and should be avoided. • Some commercial preparations contain sulfites, which may cause serious allergic reactions.
Use caution with: Smokers (cigarettes, marijuana), young children; larger or more frequent doses may be necessary. •• Children: Adverse CNS effects more common • Sustained high fever, active influenza, older adults, heart failure, COPD, renal/hepatic impairment; use reduced dose and monitor closely • History of peptic ulcers • Hyperthyroidism • Glaucoma • Diabetes mellitus • Severe hypoxemia • Hypertension • CV disease • Seizure disorders
c **Pregnancy category:** Use only if safer alternative unavailable.
Contraindications: Hypersensitivity to theophyllines, caffeine, theobromine, ethylenediamine • Uncontrolled seizure disorder • Active peptic ulcers

---

italic = common side effects   **bold** = life-threatening reactions

ADVERSE REACTIONS

CNS: *Headache, irritability, restlessness,* nervousness, insomnia, muscle twitching, **seizures**

Resp: Tachypnea

CV: *Palpitations, tachycardia,* flushing, **ventricular dysrhythmias, hypotension, circulatory failure**

GI: *Nausea, vomiting, anorexia,* epigastric pain

GU: Diuresis

Misc: Dehydration, SIADH

TOXICITY/OVERDOSE

Symptoms: Nausea, vomiting, extreme thirst • Headache, irritability, agitation, maniacal behavior, delirium, seizures • Tachycardia, palpitations, dysrhythmias, diaphoresis, hypotension, ventricular fibrillation, cardiac standstill

Management: After recent ingestion, implement guidelines for management of acute overdose (Appendix I). • Charcoal may be administered q4h until aminophylline level ≤20 µg/ml. • **Seizures:** Establish airway; administer O_2, IV diazepam. • **Hypotension:** Elevate legs, administer IV fluids; use dopamine for severe hypotension. • **Extreme tachycardia:** Administer propranolol. • Consider charcoal hemoperfusion for levels >40 µg/ml.

Toxic levels: >20 µg/ml

INTERACTIONS

barbiturates ↓ Theophylline levels

benzodiazepines ↓ Sedation

beta blockers ↓ Bronchodilation

cabamazepine ↓ Theophylline levels

calcium channel blockers ↑ Theophylline levels

cimetidine ↑ Theophylline levels

ciprofloxin ↑ Theophylline levels

digoxin Cardiotoxicity

erythromycin ↑ Theophylline levels

lithium ↑ Lithium excretion

phenytoin ↓ Theophylline and phenytoin levels

propranolol ↑ Theophylline

quinolone antibiotics ↑ Theophylline levels

rantidine ↑ theophylline levels

rifampin ↓ Theophylline levels

sympathomimetics Dysrhythmias

Y-SITE COMPATIBILITIES

Amrinone, atracurium, cimetidine, enalaprilat, esmolol, famotidine, fluconazole, heparin, labetalol, morphine, netilmicin, pancuronium, piperacillin, potassium chloride, ranitidine, vecuronium

Y-SITE INCOMPATIBILITIES

Amiodarone, cefotaxime, ciprofloxacin, diltiazem, dobutamine, epinephrine, hydralazine, hydroxyzine, isoproterenol, norepinephrine, ondansetron, phenytoin, prochlorperazine, promethazine, vancomycin

PATIENT CARE IMPLICATIONS

• Toxic effects occur rapidly. Discontinue and consult physician for onset of any side effect.

• To reduce GI irritation, administer after meals, with full glass of liquid, or with antacids. For faster absorption with PO loading, administer with full glass of water 30-60 min before or 2 hr after meals.

• Extended-release preparations helpful in patients with continu-

ous asthmatic symptoms or rapid theophylline elimination (e.g., children, young smokers) • Do not crush or chew extended-release preparations.
• Beuzodiazepine anti-anxiety agent may be necessary to relieve aminophylline-associated agitation.
• Many drug interactions possible; pharmacist review of drug profile recommended

Vital signs/hemodynamics: As available, monitor ECG for tachycardia, dysrhythmias; continuous ECG monitoring necessary with IV loading, history of cardiac disorder. • Monitor VS for hypo/hypertension, improved RR. • Use pulse oximeter to evaluate O_2 saturation.

Physical assessment: Assess work of breathing, ventilatory excursion, breath sounds.
• Evaluate forced expiratory volume, other pulmonary function measurements. • Monitor I&O. Diuresis may lead to dehydration in susceptible individuals (e.g., older adults, young children)

Laboratory tests: Monitor: ABGs • Theophylline levels; therapeutic range, 10-20 µg/ml

PATIENT/FAMILY TEACHING

Purpose of medication is to relieve bronchospasm and improve breathing. • Report increased breathing difficulty, symptoms of toxicity: chest pain, palpitations, nausea, vomiting, twitching, convulsions.
Outpatient: Take exactly as prescribed at precise intervals. Do not skip or double doses.
• Dizziness is possible; avoid driving and hazardous activities until individual effects established. • Take with meals to de-

crease stomach irritation.
• Check with physician or pharmacist before taking cold or cough preparations. • Avoid excessive caffeine intake (e.g., coffee, tea, carbonated beverages). • Notify physician or prescriber of change in smoking habit; dosage adjustment may be necessary.

AVAILABLE FORMS

Solution for parenteral use
• Tablets, ext. rel. tablets • Oral solution • Rectal suppositories

---

amiodarone HCl
(a-mee'oh-da-rone)
Cordarone

Classifications: Antidysrhythmic, membrane-stabilizer, Vaughan-Williams Class III

USUAL DOSE

PO, adults: Initially 800-1,600 mg/24 hr in equally divided doses q6-12h for 1-3 wk or until dysrhythmia controlled • After initial stabilization, 200 mg q6-8h for 1 mo. then maintenance dose • Maintenance, 400 mg once daily or 200 mg q12h
• Initiate therapy only in critical care/telemetry unit with continuous ECG monitoring, capacity for electrophysiologic evaluation, close supervision by knowledgeable professionals
• Highly toxic; always use lowest effective dose.
PO, older adults: Use lower dose range because of increased susceptibility to bradycardia, conduction disturbances.
IV, adults: Initial dose of 75-150 mg administered over 10 min; up to 300 mg may be nec-

---

italic = common side effects   **bold** = life-threatening reactions

essary for dysrhythmia suppression. Follow by loading infusion of 1 mg/min for 6 hr; then infuse 0.5 mg/min until condition stabilized. Other dosing regimens are used. • Convert to oral therapy as soon as possible.

ADMINISTRATION

▼ **Direct IV:** Administer initial dose over 10 min • Too rapid administration may cause profound hypotension, bradycardia.
IV, cont inf: Infuse at rate of 0.5-1 mg/min; use lowest effective dose. • Must use infusion pump • Do not infuse in same line as other medications, solutions.

PREPARATION

Dilute to concentration of 2 mg/ml in D_5W; do not dilute in other solutions. Use glass container.
Compatible fluids: D_5W

ACTIONS

Delays repolarization; prolongs action potential duration, effective refractory period throughout normal/accessory conduction pathways • Inhibits alpha- and beta-adrenergic effects throughout myocardium • Relaxes vascular smooth muscle, causing vasodilation; has slight negative inotropic effects • Sinus node depression reduces heart rate by up to 20%.
• Membrane-stabilizing effects similar to those of procainamide, lidocaine • Prolongs PR and QT intervals, alters T wave contour: U waves develop

PHARMACOKINETICS

ROUTE	ONSET	PEAK	DURATION
PO	Slow, var 2-3 days to 3 wk	2-12 hr	≥1 mo after therapy ends

DISTRIBUTION
Wide, highly protein-bound

ELIMINATION
Metabolized in liver, eliminated in bile; half-life 25 days

Therapeutic level: 1.0-2.5 µg/ml

INDICATIONS

Suppression/prevention of refractory ventricular fibrillation and symptomatic, unstable, refractory ventricular tachycardia. IV form also used for refractory atrial fibrillation/flutter with rapid ventricular response • **Profound, life-threatening adverse effects;** generally used as last choice for dysrhythmia control • **Life-threatening toxicities possible;** prescribed only by physicians familiar with drug's complex pharmacokinetics
Unlabeled/investigational: Suppression/prevention of paroxysmal reentrant SVT (e.g., WPW), refractory atrial fibrillation

PRECAUTIONS/ CONTRAINDICATIONS

Precautions: Serious pulmonary toxicities occur often and include infiltrates, inflammation, and fibrosis; fatalities have been reported. • Adult respiratory distress syndrome (ARDS) has occurred after cardiothoracic, other surgery. • May cause new or worsened dysrhythmias, heart block, CHF • Potentially fatal hepatic toxicities occur infrequently. • Corneal microdeposits may cause significant visual disturbances. • Neuromuscular dysfunction, hyperthyroidism, hypothyroidism have been widely noted. • Hypokalemia, hypomagnesemia increase dysrhythmia occurrence

Use caution with: Pulmonary
G disease (e.g., COPD) • Older adults; toxicity more likely
D **Pregnancy category:** Use only if safer alternative unavailable and risk explained

Contraindications: Hypersensitivity to amiodarone • Preexisting severe sinus node dysfunction with marked bradycardia • 2nd, 3rd degree heart block unless functional ventricular pacemaker in place or readily available • Any bradycardia associated with syncope, except with artificial pacemaker

ADVERSE EFFECTS

CNS: *Fatigue, peripheral neuropathy, involuntary movements, itaxia,* headache, sleep disturbances

Resp: *Progressive cough and dyspnea,* **pulmonary inflammation or fibrosis**

CV: **Dysrhythmias, heart failure, hypotension, severe sinus bradycardia, sinus arrest with suppression of escape pacemakers**

GI: *Nausea, vomiting, anorexia, constipation,* elevated liver enzymes

Ophth: *Corneal microdeposits,* visual disturbances

Endo: *Hypothyroidism, hyperthyroidism,* hypo/hyperglycemia (rare)

Hema: Coagulation abnormalities

Derm: *Photosensitivity,* blue-gray skin discoloration

TOXICITY/OVERDOSE

Symptoms: Severe hypotension, severe sinus bradycardia, complete heart block, paroxysmal ventricular tachycardia, ventricular fibrillation, heart failure, respiratory failure, abdominal pain, hepatitis

Management: After recent ingestion, implement guidelines for management of acute overdose (Appendix I). • **Heart failure:** Administer inotropics (e.g., dobutamine, dopamine); use vasopressors (e.g., norepinephrine) if hypotension also present. • **Symptomatic bradycardia:** Use beta-adrenergic agonists (e.g., isoproterenol) or transvenous cardiac pacemaker; may not respond to atropine.
• **Ventricular dysrhythmias:** Use ACLS guidelines (Appendix P). • Dialysis is not useful.

INTERACTIONS

anticoagulants, oral (e.g., ***warfarin*)** Prolonged PT; excessive bleeding

antidysrhythmics Exacerbation of dysrhythmias; conduction disturbances

beta-blockers Symptomatic bradycardia, sinus arrest, AV block

calcium channel blockers Symptomatic bradycardia, sinus arrest, AV block

digoxin ↑ Digoxin levels, symptomatic bradycardia, toxicity possible

phenytoin ↑ Phenytoin levels; ↓ amiodarone levels

procainamide ↑ Procainamide levels

quinidine Exacerbation of dysrhythmias; conduction disturbances; elevated plasma levels; potential toxicity

---

italic = common side effects   **bold** = life-threatening reactions

theophylline ↑ Theophylline levels

Y-SITE INCOMPATIBILITIES

Aminophylline, cefazolin, heparin

PATIENT CARE IMPLICATIONS

• Serious adverse effects occur often in patients receiving >400 mg/day. Therapy usually is terminated if CHF, paroxysmal ventricular tachycardia, pulmonary fibrosis or infiltrates, persistent liver enzyme elevation, or hepatomegaly occurs.
• Baseline/periodic checks of pulmonary function and vision/ocular health should be performed.
• Initiate therapy in hospital using continuous ECG monitoring; electrophysiologic monitoring should be available. Expect days to weeks of monitoring because of long, irregular half-life and frequent, serious adverse effects.

Vital signs/hemodynamics: During initiation/adjustment of therapy (1-3 wk), continuously monitor ECG for dysrhythmias, ST segment changes. Use lowest effective dose. Notify physician of failure to resolve ventricular dysrhythmias, heart block, symptomatic bradycardia or sinus arrest, ST segment elevation/depression. • Monitor and evaluate VS for possible complications (e.g., hypotension, ARDS). • Monitor pulse oximetry if pulmonary complications suspected. • When available, measure for ↑ CO/ ↓ PCWP, which suggest onset of heart failure.

Physical assessment: Assess for perfusion/oxygenation defi-cit: decreased level of consciousness, chest pain, activity intolerance, hypotension, dizziness. Blue-gray skin discoloration is drug side effect and does not indicate perfusion/oxygenation deficit. • With prolonged therapy, be alert for development of dyspnea, cough, wheezes, crackles, which may indicate pulmonary complications. • With prolonged therapy, be alert for symptoms of hepatotoxicity: abdominal discomfort, distention, weight gain, jaundice, hepatomegaly. • Note abnormal bruising, prolonged or occult bleeding.

Laboratory tests: Monitor: Electrolytes; correct imbalances. • ABGs; correct hypoxia. • Liver enzymes • Thyroid function studies • Amiodarone plasma levels; therapeutic levels, 1-2.5 µg/ml • May cause: Elevated liver enzymes • Blood glucose disturbances

PATIENT/FAMILY TEACHING

Purpose of drug is to reduce frequency of dysrhythmias.
• Close monitoring is necessary because of possible dangerous adverse effects • Promptly report dyspnea, cough, activity intolerance, abdominal pain, edema, weight gain, chest pain, severe visual disturbances.
• Take with food to reduce stomach upset. • Use sunscreen, protective clothing to protect skin from sunlight.

AVAILABLE FORMS

• Tablets

amlodipine besylate
(am-lode'i-peen)
Istin, Norvasc

Classifications: Calcium channel blocker, antianginal, antihypertensive

USUAL DOSE
PO, adults: 5-10 mg, once daily • *Hepatic insufficiency*—start at 2.5 mg, once daily
G PO, older adults: 2.5-5 mg, once daily

ACTIONS
Inhibits movement of calcium ions across myocardium and vascular smooth muscle with greater effect on vascular smooth muscle • Dilates peripheral arteries, decreases peripheral vascular resistance, reduces BP • Inhibits coronary arterial vasospasm • Afterload reduction and decreased myocardial O_2 demand contribute to antianginal effectiveness • May slightly increase CO • SA or AV conduction unchanged • Serum calcium levels not affected

PHARMACOKINETICS

ROUTE	ONSET	PEAK	DURATION
PO	90 min	6-12 hr	≥24 hr

DISTRIBUTION
93% protein-bound
ELIMINATION
90% converted to inactive metabolite by liver; 10% excreted unchanged by kidneys. Terminal half-life 30-50 hr.

INDICATIONS
Hypertension • Chronic stable angina • Vasospastic angina
Unlabeled/investigational:
Congestive heart failure

PRECAUTIONS/ CONTRAINDICATIONS
Precautions: May cause hypotension 1-2 hr after dosing • Abrupt withdrawal may increase frequency, severity, duration of chest pain.
Use caution with: CHF, conduction disorders, artificial pacemakers, hepatic insufficiency
P • Children: safe use not established
C Pregnancy category: Use only if safer alternative not available.
Contraindications: Hypersensitivity to amlodipine • Sick sinus syndrome, 2nd or 3rd degree AV block except with functioning pacemaker

ADVERSE EFFECTS
CNS: *Headache, fatigue, dizziness,* somnolence, paresthesia
EENT: *Gingival hyperplasia*
Resp: Dyspnea
CV: Peripheral edema, flushing, palpitations, hypotension, chest pain, dysrhythmia
GI: *Nausea,* abdominal pain
Hema: Antiplatelet effects with bruising, petechiae, bleeding

TOXICITY/OVERDOSE
Symptoms: Hypotension, reflex tachycardia
Management: After recent ingestion, implement guidelines for management of acute overdosage (Appendix I). • Monitor HR, BP, RR at frequent intervals. • **Hypotension:** Elevate legs, administer IV fluids; consider dopamine, phenylephrine, or other vasopressors if necessary. • IV calcium gluconate may reverse hemodynamic effects of calcium channel block-

---

italic = common side effects   **bold** = life-threatening reactions

ade. • Hemodialysis is not likely to be helpful.

INTERACTIONS

Antihypertensives Profound hypotension

beta-blockers Profound hypotension

calcium Reduced amlodipine effectiveness

PATIENT CARE IMPLICATIONS

• Adjust dose to patient requirements; titrate over 7-14 days.
• Nitrates, O_2 can be used to manage chest pain while initiating therapy.
• Discontinue slowly to avoid increase in angina symptoms.
G • **Older adults** more likely to experience hypotension. Use lowest effective dose; monitor closely.

Vital signs/hemodynamics: Monitor BP to insure effective therapy; hypotension rare because of gradual onset of vasodilation.

Physical assessment: Monitor for frequency, duration, severity of chest pain. • Assess for perfusion/oxygenation deficit: decreased level of consciousness, hypotension, activity intolerance, chest discomfort. • Assess for dysrhythmias.

PATIENT/FAMILY TEACHING

Purpose of medication is to control high BP or relieve angina pain.

Outpatient: Take exactly as prescribed. Do not stop taking medicine even if you feel better. If medication is abruptly discontinued, you may develop dangerously high BP, chest pain.
• Medication is not a cure for high BP; other therapies, including life-style modifications, must be continued. • Consult health care provider before taking nonprescription preparations.

AVAILABLE FORMS

Tablets

amoxicillin
(a-mox-i-sill′in)
Amoxil, Polymox, Trimox, Wymox
Amoxican ✲
Apo-Amoxi ✲
Novamoxin ✲

Classifications: Penicillin antibiotic, aminopenicillin

USUAL DOSE

P **PO, adults/children >20 kg:** 250-500 mg q6-8h • Bacterial endocarditis prophylaxis: 3 g before procedure, followed by 1.5 g 6 hr after procedure • Single dose of 3 g sometimes used for acute genital/urethal infections caused by *Neisseria gonorrhoeae*

P **PO, children 1 mo-20 kg:** 20-40 mg/kg/24 hr in equally divided doses q8h

ACTIONS

Semisynthetic aminopenicillin with bactericidal action; interferes with bacterial cell wall synthesis/division • Greater activity against gram-negative bacteria than natural penicillins (e.g., penicillin G) and penicillinase-resistant penicillins (e.g., nafcillin, oxacillin) • Similar to ampicillin but requires less frequent dosing and less likely to cause diarrhea • Active against most gram-positive/gram-negative aerobic cocci (except penicillinase-producing strains), some gram-positive bacilli, some spirochetes • Notable activity against streptococci, pneumococci, enterococci, *Proteus mirabilis, Salmonella, Escherichia coli,* non–penicillinase-producing *Neisseria gonorrhoeae, Haemophilus influenzae, Corynebacterium diphtheriae, Listeria monocytogenes*

PHARMACOKINETICS

ROUTE	ONSET	PEAK	DURATION
PO	≤30 min	1-2 hr	Approx 6 hr; dose dependent

DISTRIBUTION
Widely distributed; CSF levels higher with probenecid administration

ELIMINATION
Primarily excreted in urine; half-life 1-1.5 hr, prolonged with renal impairment

INDICATIONS

Respiratory tract infections, sinusitis, otitis media • Urinary tract, skin, soft tissue infections • Ambulatory pelvic inflammatory disease, acute sexually transmitted epididymitis, along with probenecid, doxycycline administration • Bacterial endocarditis prophylaxis before specific procedures • Not to replace penicillin for treatment of streptococcal or staphylococcal infections
Unlabeled/investigational:
Helicobacter pylori infection associated with peptic ulcer disease

PRECAUTIONS/ CONTRAINDICATIONS

Precautions: Bacterial or fungal overgrowth may occur.
Use caution with: Hypersensitivity to cephalosporins or other drugs; risk of allergic re-

action • Renal insufficiency; lower dose/frequency
B Pregnancy category: Safety not clearly established
Contraindications: Hypersensitivity to any penicillin • Immediate hypersensitivity to cephalosporins or other beta-lactam antibiotic • Infectious mononucleosis

ADVERSE EFFECTS

CNS: Agitation, hyperactivity
GI: *Nausea, vomiting, diarrhea,* gastritis, elevated AST (SGOT)/ALT (SGPT), pseudomembranous colitis
Hema: Eosinophilia, hemolytic anemia, other blood dyscrasias
Derm: *Rash,* urticaria, pruritus
Misc: *Hypersensitivity,* including **anaphylaxis,** serum sickness; superinfection, colonization

TOXICITY/OVERDOSE

Symptoms: Neuromuscular excitability • Acute allergic reaction, including anaphylaxis
Management: Discontinue drug. Initiate symptomatic/supportive measures. • After recent ingestion, implement guidelines for management of acute overdose (Appendix I). • For acute allergic reaction, see Appendix O. • Hemodialysis may be effective.

INTERACTIONS

allopurinol ↑ Incidence of "ampicillin rash"
aminoglycosides (e.g., amikacin, gentamicin) ↑ Antibacterial activity
clavulanic acid ↑ Bactericidal activity
methotrexate (MTX) ↑ MTX levels

---

italic = common side effects   **bold** = life-threatening reactions

probenecid ↑ Amoxicillin blood levels

tetracycline ↓ Bactericidal activity

PATIENT CARE IMPLICATIONS

• Obtain specimens for culture and sensitivity before initiating antibiotic therapy. Therapy may be started before results received.

• Determine previous antibiotic use, including reactions to penicillins, cephalosporins. Cross-reactivity with cephalosporin allergies may occur.

• Have epinephrine, antihistamine, resuscitation equipment available for use with severe allergic reaction.

• May be administered without regard to meals

• Stagger doses if chloramphenicol or tetracycline also prescribed.

Vital signs/hemodynamics: Monitor VS at beginning and throughout therapy. • Monitor **[G]** I&O for imbalance; older, debilitated, seriously ill, or renal impaired patients at greater risk for nephrotoxicity

Physical assessment: Assess for improvement in primary infection or symptoms of super/suprainfection: appearance of sputum, urine, stool, wound drainage; presence of fever, candidiasis, vaginitis. • Observe for symptoms of hypersensitivity: rash, pruritus, wheezing, laryngeal edema, hypotension. • Observe for "ampicillin rash," a nonallergic, maculopapular rash generally appearing 3-14 days after initiation of therapy.

Laboratory tests: Monitor: Electrolytes, BUN, creatinine, CBC with differential with pro-

longed use; particularly important in patients with renal or **[G]** cardiac impairment and elderly or debilitated patients • May cause: Falsely elevated serum albumin • Positive direct antiglobulin (Coombs') test

PATIENT/FAMILY TEACHING

Purpose of drug is to limit growth of infection-causing bacteria. • Immediately report rash, swelling, intense itching, difficulty breathing. • Report diarrhea, fever, vaginal itching or discharge, furry growth on tongue. • Chewable tablets must be thoroughly chewed before swallowing.

Outpatient: Take at evenly spaced intervals over each 24-hr period. • Take all of medication exactly as prescribed. Do not stop taking medicine even if you feel better. Failure to take all of antibiotic may result in recurrence or additional infection. Do not save or share unused medicine.

AVAILABLE FORMS

Capsules • Chewable tablets • PO suspension • Pediatric drops

amoxicillin/clavulanate potassium
(a-mox-i-sill'in klav'u-lah-nate)
Augmentin, Clavulin ✣

Classifications: Penicillin antibiotic, aminopenicillin

USUAL DOSE

Dosage expressed as amoxicillin component

NOTE: Tablets contain different amounts of clavulanic acid and are not inerchangeable (e.g., 250-mg chewable tablets and 250-mg film-coated tablets are not equivalent; two 250-mg film-coated tablets are not equivalent to one 500-mg film-coated tablet).

P PO, adults/children >20 kg: 250-500 mg q8h

P PO, children 1 mo-20 kg: 20-40 mg/kg/24 hr in equally divided doses q8h; use chewable tablets or PO suspension.

ACTIONS

Semisynthetic aminopenicillin with bactericidal action; interferes with bacterial cell wall synthesis/division • Greater activity against gram-negative bacteria than natural penicillins (e.g., penicillin G) and penicillinase-resistant penicillins (e.g., nafcillin, oxacillin) • Clavulanic acid inhibits bacterial enzymes (beta-lactamases) responsible for inactivating amoxicillin and extends spectrum of activity to include many strains of bacteria resistant to amoxicillin alone.
• Notable activity against streptococci, pneumococci, enterococci, many enterobacteriaceae, including *Proteus mirabilis, Klebsiella, Escherichia coli, Neisseria gonorrhoeae, N. meningitidis, Haemophilus influenzae*

PHARMACOKINETICS

ROUTE	ONSET	PEAK	DURATION
PO	≤30 min	1-2.5 hr	Approx 6 hr; dose dependent

DISTRIBUTION
Widely distributed; CSF levels higher with inflammation

ELIMINATION
Primarily excreted in urine; half-life 1-1.5 hr, prolonged with renal impairment

INDICATIONS

Respiratory tract infections, sinusitis, otitis media • Urinary tract, skin, soft tissue infections • Not to replace penicillin for treatment of streptococcal or staphylococcal infections • Non-beta-lactamase–producing bacterial infections should be treated with amoxicillin without clavulanate.

PRECAUTIONS/ CONTRAINDICATIONS

Precautions: Bacterial or fungal overgrowth may occur.
Use caution with: Hypersensitivity to cephalosporins or other drugs; risk of allergic reaction • Renal insufficiency; lower dose/frequency
B Pregnancy category: Safety not clearly established
Contraindications: Hypersensitivity to any penicillin or clavulanate • Immediate hypersensitivity to cephalosporins or other beta-lactam antibiotics • Infectious mononucleosis

ADVERSE EFFECTS

CNS: Agitation, hyperactivity
GI: *Nausea, vomiting, diarrhea,* epigastric pain, gastritis, elevated AST (SGOT)/ALT (SGPT), pseudomembranous colitis

---

italic = common side effects   **bold** = life-threatening reactions

Hema: Eosinophilia, hemolytic anemia, other blood dyscrasias
Derm: *Rash,* urticaria, pruritus
Misc: *Hypersensitivity,* including **anaphylaxis,** serum sickness; superinfection, colonization

TOXICITY/OVERDOSE

Symptoms: Neuromuscular excitability • Acute allergic reaction, including anaphylaxis
Management: Discontinue drug. Initiate symptomatic and supportive measures. • After recent ingestion, implement guidelines for management of acute overdose (Appendix I). For acute allergic reaction, see Appendix H. • Hemodialysis is effective in drug removal; minimal removal with peritoneal dialysis.

INTERACTIONS

allopurinol ↑ Incidence of "ampicillin rash"
aminoglycosides (e.g., amikacin, gentamicin) Synergistic antibacterial activity
probenecid Higher/prolonged amoxicillin blood levels
tetracycline Inhibition of bactericidal activity

PATIENT CARE IMPLICATIONS

• Obtain specimens for culture and sensitivity before initiating antibiotic therapy. Therapy may be started before results received.
• Determine previous antibiotic use, including reactions to penicillins, cephalosporins. Cross-reactivity with cephalosporin allergies may occur.
• Have epinephrine, antihistamine, resuscitation equipment

available for use with severe allergic reaction.
• May be administered without regard to meals.
• Stagger doses if chloramphenicol or tetracycline also prescribed.

Vital signs/hemodynamics: Monitor VS at beginning and throughout therapy. • Monitor I&O for imbalance; older, debilitated, seriously ill, or renal-impaired patients at greater risk for nephrotoxicity.

Physical assessment: Assess for improvement in primary infection or symptoms of super/suprainfection: appearance of sputum, urine, stool, wound drainage; presence of fever, candidiasis, vaginitis; WBC. • Observe for symptoms of hypersensitivity: rash, pruritus, wheezing, laryngeal edema, hypotension. • Observe for "ampicillin rash," a nonallergic, maculopapular rash generally appearing 3-14 days after initiation of therapy.

Laboratory tests: Monitor: electrolytes, BUN, creatinine, CBC with differential with prolonged use; particularly important in patients with renal or cardiac impairment and elderly or debilitated patients • **May cause:** Falsely elevated serum albumin

PATIENT/FAMILY TEACHING

Purpose of drug is to limit growth of infection-causing bacteria. • Immediately report rash, swelling, intense itching, difficulty breathing, other signs of allergic reaction. • Report diarrhea, fever, vaginal itching or discharge, furry growth on tongue.

Outpatient: Take at evenly spaced intervals over each 24-hr period. • Take all of medication exactly as prescribed. Do not stop taking medicine even if you feel better. Failure to take all of antibiotic may result in recurrent or additional infection. Do not save or share unused medicine.

AVAILABLE FORMS

Film-coated scored tablets (for adults) • Chewable tablets • PO suspension

---

amphotericin B
(am-foe-ter′i-sin)
Fungizone

Classification: Antifungal antibiotic

USUAL DOSE

IV, intermit inf, adults: Initial test dose of 1 mg in 50-100 ml D_5W administered over 30 min or 2-4 hr. If well tolerated, start therapy of 0.1-0.3 mg/kg once daily. If significant reaction, initiate therapy with small initial dose of 5-10 mg. Gradually increase dose by 5-10 mg/day increments; may increase more rapidly for life-threatening infections. • Maintenance: 0.5-1.0 mg/kg/24 hr. Rarely, 1.5 mg/kg/24 hr; never exceed 1.5 mg/kg/24 hr • Therapy usually required for ≥30 days
Unlabeled/investigational:
Has been given intrathecally, intraarticularly, intrapleurally, and as an irrigant

ADMINISTRATION

IV, intermit inf: Test dose: Infuse over 30 min or 2-4 hr. Carefully monitor HR, RR, BP, temperature every 30 min during and for 4 hr after initial infusion. Too rapid infusion may cause dysrhythmias, ↓ BP, shock. • Subsequent doses: Infuse over 6 hr with close monitoring of VS. • **Administration precautions:** Flush NaCl solutions from IV line/catheter before initiating infusion. Do not filter or use filter ≥1.0 μm. Use infusion pump. Protect prolonged infusions (>8 hr) from light. Stop infusion for any adverse reaction. Reduce risk of thrombophlebitis by using large veins, small catheters/needles, and rotating infusion sites.

PREPARATION

IV: Reconstitute each 50-mg vial with 10 ml sterile water *without bacteriostatic agent.* Other diluents may cause precipitation. Concentration is 5 mg/ml • **Test dose:** withdraw 0.2 ml (1 mg) and further dilute in 50-100 ml D_5W for infusion. • **Maintenance dose:** Further dilute prescribed dose by adding D_5W for final concentration of 0.1 mg/ml or less.
Compatible fluids: D_5W, sterile water *without bacteriostic agent*
Stability: Stable at room temperature for at least 8 hr; when protected from light, stable for 24 hr

ACTIONS

Broad-spectrum antifungal agent; usually fungistatic but may be fungicidal in high concentrations against susceptible organisms; binds with sterol in fungal cell membranes, resulting in loss of cellular integrity. Human erythrocytes and certain

---

italic = common side effects   **bold** = life-threatening reactions

kidney cells contain sterols, accounting for drug toxicity. • Active against most fungi, including *Aspergillus fumigatus, Candida albicans, Cryptococcus neoformans, Coccidioides, Sporotrichum, Histoplasma capsulatum, Blastomyces dermatitidis* • Not active against bacteria, rickettsiae, viruses

PHARMACOKINETICS

ROUTE	ONSET	PEAK	DURATION
IV	Immed	End of infusion	Approx 24-48 hr

DISTRIBUTION

Multicompartmental; poor distribution to pleural, pericardial, peritoneal fluids; intrathecal use necessary for therapeutic CSF levels

ELIMINATION

Half-life ≥24 hr, up to 15 days with long-term therapy

INDICATIONS

Choice agent for treatment of serious or disseminated candidal infections, cryptococcal infections (meningitis requires addition of flucytosine), coccidioidomycosis, histoplasmosis, sporotrichosis • Because of frequent, serious adverse reactions, indicated only for treatment of progressive, potentially fatal fungal infections in hospitalized or closely supervised patients • Not indicated for treatment of oral-esophageal candidiasis or other conditions when less toxic agents (e.g., fluconazole, ketoconazole) could be used

PRECAUTIONS/ CONTRAINDICATIONS

Precautions: High incidence of serious adverse reactions, including nephrotoxicity, hypotension, dysrhythmias • Cardiac arrest is possible with rapid

infusion/overdosage • Optimize hydration, correct electrolyte imbalance before therapy
Use caution with: Reduced renal function • Concurrent use of other nephrotoxic agents, diuretics, corticosteroids
B Pregnancy category: Safe use not established; use only if safer alternative unavailable.
Contraindications: Hypersensitivity to amphotericin B

ADVERSE EFFECTS

CNS: *Headache, malaise,* peripheral neuropathy, **seizures**
CV: *Hypotension,* **CHF, ventricular fibrillation, cardiac arrest**
Resp: *Tachypnea,* dyspnea, **pulmonary edema**
GI: *Anorexia, nausea, vomiting, dyspepsia, cramping, epigastric pain,* elevated liver enzymes
GU: **Nephrotoxicity,** *hypokalemia,* proteinuria, hematuria, hypomagnesemia, hypocalcemia, decreased creatinine clearance, **acute renal failure**
Hema: Anemia, blood dyscrasias, coagulopathy
Local: *Injection site pain,* phlebitis, thrombophlebitis
Misc: *Chills; fever;* hypersensitivity, including **anaphylaxis**

TOXICITY/OVERDOSE

Symptoms: Nephrotoxicity, including severe hypokalemia, azotemia, renal failure, in up to 80% of patients • Acute febrile reactions • Severe hypotension, dysrhythmias, shock
Management: Initiate symptomatic/supportive measures, including airway management/ventilation. • Optimize hydration. Correct electrolyte imbalance • Urinary alkalinization,

---

mannitol, sodium loading to reduce nephrotoxicity • Corticosteroids before therapy may decrease severity of febrile reactions. • For acute allergic reaction, see Appendix N.

INTERACTIONS

aminoglycosides (e.g., amikacin, gentamicin) ↑ Risk of nephrotoxicity

cisplatin ↑ Risk of nephrotoxicity

corticosteroids Severe potassium depletion; CHF

cyclosporine ↑ Risk of nephrotoxicity

digoxin Amphotericin-related hypokalemia with ↑ risk of digitalis toxicity

pentamidine ↑ Risk of nephrotoxicity

polymyxin B ↑ Risk of nephrotoxicity

skeletal muscle relaxants (e.g., succinylcholine) ↑ Intensity/duration of muscle relaxation

vancomycin ↑ Risk of nephrotoxicity

Y-SITE COMPATIBILITIES

Diltiazem, heparin, zidovudine

Y-SITE INCOMPATIBILITIES

Sodium chloride solutions, and many agents. Consider incompatible with all agents, except those listed above. Avoid mixing or piggyback administration with other agents.

PATIENT CARE IMPLICATIONS

• Obtain specimens for culture and sensitivity; confirm diagnosis before initiating therapy. Start therapy before culture results in critically ill patients.
• Optimize hydration (at least 2,000-3,000 ml/day), correct electrolyte imbalance before initiating therapy.
• Very small initial test dose and many precautions necessary during administration (see Usual dose, Administration).
• Have epinephrine, antihistamine, corticosteroids, resuscitation equipment readily available for use with severe allergic reaction.
• Measures such as urinary alkalinization, mannitol administration, sodium loading may reduce nephrotoxic risk.
• Reduce vein irritation by using small catheters/needles in large veins and rotating infusion sites. Observe site frequently. Heparin added to solutions may reduce risk of thrombophlebitis.

Vital signs/hemodynamics: Monitor RR, HR, BP, temperature for febrile or other adverse reactions during and immediately after infusion. • Monitor VS for indicators of infection or complications. • Carefully monitor UO and evaluate I&O ratio. Decreasing urine volume or cloudy or pink urine may indicate nephrotoxicity. Keep patient well hydrated by oral or parenteral fluids of sufficient volume to produce adequate UO; older, debilitated, seriously ill, or renal-impaired patients at greater risk for toxicity. Decrease dose or discontinue therapy if BUN or creatinine is double baseline value.

Physical assessment: Assess for improvement in primary infection or resistance to therapy, as evidenced by recurrent infection or failure to respond. • Observe for symptoms of hypersensitivity: rash, pruritus, wheezing, hypotension. • Observe for onset of fever, chills,

---

italic = common side effects   **bold** = life-threatening reactions

nausea, vomiting, which typically occur 1-3 hr after infusion initiated. Usually reaction subsides within 4 hr, incidence decreases with subsequent infusions. Antiinflammatory agents or antihistamines before therapy may reduce severity of reaction. If corticosteroids used, closely monitor for hypokalemia, impaired renal function, CHF. **Laboratory tests: Monitor:** Potassium every 3-4 days • Electrolyte profile, including magnesium/CBC, every week • Urinalysis, BUN, creatinine, creatinine clearance before and weekly during therapy; follow more closely in critically ill patients, older adults, those with renal impairment or receiving high-dose/prolonged therapy • Liver enzymes, bilirubin • **May cause:** Severe hypokalemia immediately after administration • Decreased magnesium, Hgb, Hct • Elevated BUN/creatinine • Elevated liver enzymes/bilirubin

PATIENT/FAMILY TEACHING

Purpose of drug is to limit growth of infection-causing fungal organisms. • Immediately report palpitations, flushing, rash, lightheadedness, difficulty breathing, other signs of allergic reaction. • Drink plenty of fluids.

AVAILABLE FORMS

Parenteral for IV use • Lotion/ointment for topical use

---

ampicillin sodium
(am-pi-sill'in)
Omnipen, Polycillin, Principen, Totacillin, Ampicin ✽, Apo-Ampi ✽, Novo-Ampicillin ✽, Nu-Ampi ✽

Classifications: Penicillin antibiotic, aminopenicillin

USUAL DOSE

Ⓟ PO, adults/children >20 kg: 250-500 mg q6h
Ⓟ PO, children 1 mo-20 kg: 25-100 mg/kg/24 hr in equally divided doses q6h • **Renal impairment:** Reduce dose and/or frequency.
Ⓟ IV/IM, adults/children >40 kg: 250-500 mg q6h. For severe infections, 8-14 g/24 hr given in equally divided doses q4-6h
Ⓟ IV/IM, children 1 mo-40 kg: 100-200 mg/kg/24 hr in equally divided doses q6h • **Serious infections, including meningitis:** 200-400 mg/kg/24 hr in equally divided doses q4-6h • Maximum dose, 12 g/24 hr

ADMINISTRATION

IM injection: Inject deep into large muscle mass (e.g., gluteus maximus, lateral thigh).
Ⅴ Direct IV: ≤500 mg dose over 3-5 min. Do not exceed rate of 100 mg/min. Too rapid injection may cause seizures. Intermit. inf. recommended.
IV, intermit inf: Infuse prepared solution over 10-15 min; complete within 2 hr of reconstitution.

PREPARATION

IM injection: Reconstitute 125-500 mg vial with 5 ml sterile water for injection; use 7.4 ml for 1-g vial, 14.8 ml for 2-g vial. Shake to dissolve.

IV, intermit inf: Reconstitute as above and add to 50-100 ml compatible solution.

Compatible fluids: 0.9% NaCl, LR; mixing in dextrose causes some loss of antimicrobial activity and is not recommended.

Stability: Reconstituted solution stable for ≥2 hr at room temperature; dilute solutions more stable

Dilution for IM injection

VIAL SIZE	VOLUME OF DILUENT	CONCENTRATION
250 mg	1.0 ml	250 mg/ml
500 mg	1.8 ml	250 mg/ml
1 g	3.5 ml	250 mg/ml
2 g	6.8 ml	250 mg/ml

ACTIONS

Semisynthetic aminopenicillin with bactericidal action; interferes with bacterial cell wall synthesis/division • Greater activity against gram-negative bacteria than natural penicillins (e.g., penicillin G) and penicillinase-resistant penicillins (e.g., nafcillin, oxacillin) • Active against most gram-positive/gram-negative aerobic cocci (except penicillinase-producing strains), some gram-positive bacilli, some spirochetes • Notable activity against streptococci, pneumococci, enterococci, *Proteus mirabilis, Salmonella, Shigella, Escherichia coli,* non–penicillinase-producing *Neisseria gonorrhoeae, Haemophilus influenzae, Corynebacterium diphtheriae, Listeria mon-*

ocytogenes • Greater activity than other penicillins against *Enterococcus faecalis*

PHARMACOKINETICS

ROUTE	ONSET	PEAK	DURATION
PO	≤30 min	1-2 hr	Approx
IM	Rapid	<1 hr	4-6 hr;
IV	Immed	End infusion	dose dependent

DISTRIBUTION

Widely distributed; CSF levels higher with inflammation

ELIMINATION

Primarily excreted in urine; half-life 1-1.5 hr, prolonged with renal impairment

INDICATIONS

PO: Mild to moderate infections of respiratory or GU tract, infectious diarrhea, otitis media

Parenteral: Severe infections such as septicemia, meningitis, endocarditis, severe pneumonia, others; with aminoglycosides (e.g., gentamicin) for enterococcal endocarditis • Bacterial endocarditis prophylaxis before specific procedures • Not to replace penicillin for treatment of streptococcal or staphylococcal infections

PRECAUTIONS/ CONTRAINDICATIONS

Precautions: Bacterial or fungal overgrowth may occur.

Use caution with: Hypersensitivity to cephalosporins or other drugs; risk of allergic reaction • Renal insufficiency; lower dose/frequency

ᴮ Pregnancy category: Safety not clearly established

Contraindications: Hypersensitivity to any penicillin • Immediate hypersensitivity to cephalosporins or other beta-lactam antibiotic • Infectious mononucleosis

---

italic = common side effects   **bold** = life-threatening reactions

ADVERSE EFFECTS

CNS: Neurotoxicity, **seizures** (rare), especially with high dose/renal insufficiency; nerve irritation/paralysis with IM injection

GI: *Nausea, vomiting, diarrhea,* gastritis, elevated AST (SGOT)/ALT (SGPT); pseudomembranous colitis

Hema: Eosinophilia, hemolytic anemia, other blood dyscrasias

Derm: *Rash,* urticaria, pruritus

Local: *Pain* (IM injection)

Misc: *Hypersensitivity,* including **anaphylaxis,** serum sickness; superinfection, colonization

TOXICITY/OVERDOSE

Symptoms: Neurotoxicity, including seizures, particularly with high-dose therapy/renal insufficiency • Acute allergic reaction, including anaphylaxis **Management:** Discontinue drug. Initiate symptomatic/supportive measures • After recent ingestion, implement guidelines for management of acute overdose (Appendix I). • For acute allergic reactions, see Appendix N. • Hemodialysis may be effective.

INTERACTIONS

allopurinol ↑ Incidence of "ampicillin rash"

aminoglycosides (e.g., amikacin, gentamicin) Synergistic antibacterial activity

oral contraceptives ↓ contraceptive effectiveness

probenecid Higher/prolonged ampicillin blood levels

tetracycline Inhibition of bactericidal activity

Y-SITE COMPATIBILITIES

Acyclovir, enalaprilat, esmolol, famotidine, heparin, insulin, labetalol, magnesium sulfate, meperidine, morphine, potassium chloride, vitamin B complex with C

Y-SITE INCOMPATIBILITIES

Aminoglycosides (e.g., amikacin, gentamicin, tobramycin), epinephrine, fluconazole, hydralazine, metoclopramide, ondansetron, verapamil

PATIENT CARE IMPLICATIONS

• Obtain specimens for culture and sensitivity before initiating antibiotic therapy. Therapy may be started before results received.

• Determine previous antibiotic use, including reactions to penicillins, cephalosporins. Cross-reactivity with cephalosporin allergies may occur.

• Have epinephrine, antihistamine, resuscitation equipment readily available for use with severe allergic reaction.

• Do not discharge patient for at least 30 min after IV/IM antibiotic administration.

• To optimize absorption, administer PO dose at least 1 hr before or 2 hr after meals.

• To avoid drug incompatibility/interaction, administer at separate site and stagger schedules when aminoglycosides (e.g., gentamicin), tetracycline, or chloramphenicol also prescribed.

IV injection/infusion: Reduce risk of thrombophlebitis by using large veins, small catheters/needles, and rotating infusion sites. • IV route must be used

---

for severe infections or when shock present.

Vital signs/hemodynamics: Monitor VS at beginning and throughout therapy. • Monitor I&O for imbalance; older, debilitated, seriously ill, or renal impaired patients at greater risk for nephrotoxicity.

Physical assessment: Assess for improvement in primary infection or symptoms of super/suprainfection: appearance of sputum, urine, stool, wound drainage; presence of fever, candidiasis, vaginitis. • Observe for symptoms of hypersensitivity: rash, pruritus, wheezing, laryngeal edema, hypotension. • Observe for "ampicillin rash," nonallergic, maculopapular rash generally appearing 3-14 days after initiation of therapy.

Laboratory tests: Monitor: Electrolytes, BUN, creatinine, CBC with differential with IV or prolonged use; particularly important in patients with renal or cardiac impairment and elderly or debilitated patients • **May cause:** Falsely elevated serum albumin

PATIENT/FAMILY TEACHING

Purpose of drug is to limit growth of infection-causing bacteria. • Immediately report rash, swelling, intense itching, difficulty breathing, other signs of allergic reaction. • Report diarrhea, fever, vaginal itching or discharge, furry growth on tongue.

Outpatient: Take medication at least 1 hr before or 2 hr after meals. Take at evenly spaced intervals over each 24-hr period. • Take all of medication exactly as prescribed. Do not stop taking medicine even if you feel better. Failure to take all of antibiotic may result in recurrence or additional infection. Do not save or share unused medicine.

AVAILABLE FORMS

Parenteral for IV/IM use • Capsules • PO suspension

---

amrinone
(am′ri-none)
Inocor

Classification: Inotrope (increases myocardial contractility)

USUAL DOSE

Direct IV, adults: Initial loading dose of 0.75 mg/kg (approx 50 mg for 70-kg adult); repeat initial bolus in 30 min, if necessary.

IV, cont inf, adults: 5-10 μg/kg/min; up to 20 μg/kg/min as necessary • Titrate for desired CO. Usual daily dose not to exceed 10 mg/kg (700 mg for 70-kg adult) including boluses; higher doses (up to 18 mg/kg daily) used for short periods with CHF.

ADMINISTRATION

▼**Direct IV:** Slowly inject initial loading dose over 2-3 min

IV, cont inf: Adjust by 2-3 μg/kg/min q10min until desired CO, BP, PCWP, UO achieved. Must use infusion pump. See infusion rate table, Appendix Q.

PREPARATION

Compatible solution: 0.45% or 0.9% NaCl • Dilution with dextrose solutions causes loss of potency; acceptable to inject bolus dose through rapidly flowing IV dextrose.

---

italic = common side effects   **bold** = life-threatening reactions

DILUTION	CONCENTRATION
500 mg/500 ml	1,000 µg/ml
400 mg/250 ml	1,600 µg/ml
800 mg/250 ml	3,200 µg/ml

ACTIONS

Increases myocardial contractility and causes vasodilation; results in increased CO • HR usually remains unchanged except at doses >20 µg/kg/min, which produce tachycardia. • Less likely to exacerbate ischemia in patients with ischemic heart disease than other inotropic agents • **Hemodynamics:** CO increases up to 60% without increasing myocardial O_2 consumption or changes in arteriovenous O_2 difference; decreases LVEDP, PCWP, SVR, systemic arterial pressure; slight increases in conduction velocity through AV node with increased ventricular response rate possible in undigitalized patients.

PHARMACOKINETICS

ROUTE	ONSET	PEAK	DURATION
IV	2-5 min	10 min	Dose related; 30 min-2 hr

DISTRIBUTION

Protein bound; increased levels with impaired renal/hepatic perfusion

ELIMINATION

Metabolized in liver; half-life 4-6 hr; prolonged with CHF

INDICATIONS

Short-term relief of CHF, depressed myocardial contractility, when response to other measures such as digitalis, dobutamine, diuretics, and/or vasodilators unsatisfactory • Sometimes used concurrently with other inotropic agents (e.g., digitalis, dobutamine, diuretics) • Decreases need for diuretics in some patients

Unlabeled/investigational:
Alternative therapy during ACLS to improve CO

PRECAUTIONS/ CONTRAINDICATIONS

Precautions: Dose-related, reversible thrombocytopenia possible; discontinue for bleeding complications or dangerously low platelet counts (<50,000/ mm³). • Liver damage possible; discontinue for symptoms of hepatic impairment. • Commercial preparations may contain sulfites, which can cause serious allergic reactions.

Use caution with: Ventricular dysrhythmias • Acute MI; experience limited • Undigitalized atrial flutter/fibrillation; AV conduction increased • Children <18 yr: Safety/efficacy not clearly established

c Pregnancy category: Use only if safer alternative unavailable.

Contraindications: Hypersensitivity to amrinone; signs/ symptoms of hypersensitivity reaction variable, including pericarditis, pleuritis, ascites, myositis, vasculitis, jaundice • Severe pulmonic or aortic stenosis • Subaortic obstruction

ADVERSE EFFECTS

CV: **Dysrhythmias, hypotension**
GI: Nausea, vomiting, abdominal pain, anorexia, hepatic enzyme elevation
Hema: Dose-dependent thrombocytopenia
Misc: Fever, burning at infusion site

TOXICITY/OVERDOSE

Symptoms: Hypotension, dysrhythmias

Management: Hypotension: Reduce rate or discontinue.
• **Dysrhythmias:** Follow ACLS recommendations (Appendix P).
• Short duration of action; other treatment usually unnecessary

INTERACTIONS

digoxin Potentiation of inotropic effects
disopyramide Potentiation of inotropic effects

Y-SITE COMPATIBILITIES

Aminophylline, atropine, bretylium, calcium chloride, cimetidine, digoxin, dobutamine, dopamine, epinephrine, famotidine, hydrocortisone sodium succinate, isoproterenol, lidocaine, metaraminol, methylprednisolone sodium succinate, nitroglycerine, nitroprusside, norepinephrine, phenylephrine, potassium chloride, procainamide, propranolol, verapamil

Y-SITE INCOMPATIBILITIES

Furosemide, sodium bicarbonate

PATIENT CARE IMPLICATIONS

• Correct hypovolemia before initiating therapy and reevaluate throughout therapy.
• Optimize tissue oxygenation via supplemental oxygenation according to patient condition.
• Establish clear criteria for titration (e.g., desired CO, PCWP, UO). Use lowest effective dose.
• Evaluate fluid volume status; monitor UO, notify physician if ≥5 ml/kg/hr or ≤30 ml/hr. ↑ CO and subsequent diuresis may cause hypokalemia, especially if concurrent diuretic therapy. Administer supplemental potassium as necessary.

• Digitalize patients with atrial fibrillation/flutter before administering amrinone; ehanced AV conduction could cause dangerous dysrhythmias.
• **IABP:** ↑ Risk of drug-related thrombocytopenia
• **CHF,** ↓ **renal/hepatic perfusion:** Closely monitor hemodynamic response; use lowest effective dose, because plasma concentrations increase with these conditions.
Vital signs/hemodynamics: Initially monitor BP, HR q5-15 min; progressively advance according to titration schedule, hemodynamic stability. • Continuously monitor ECG for dysrhythmias, ischemic changes.
• Monitor central hemodynamics/CO frequently, as available; significant changes in CO may occur with minimal changes in HR or BP.
Physical assessment: Assess for resolution of signs/symptoms of CHF (peripheral edema, dyspnea, orthopnea, crackles, rales, weight gain). • Assess for evidence of thrombocytopenia: unusual bruising, bleeding from gums or venipuncture sites, dark or tarry stools, "coffee grounds" appearance of gastric drainage, pink-tinged urine. • Assess for jaundice, ascites, and other symptoms of hepatotoxicity.

LABORATORY TESTS

Monitor: CBC, esp. platelet count; consult physician for platelet count <150,000/mm³.
• Electrolytes, BUN, creatinine; potassium particularly important because hypokalemia may trigger cardiac dysrhythmias.
• Liver enzymes, bilirubin

---

italic = common side effects   **bold** = life-threatening reactions

PATIENT/FAMILY TEACHING

Purpose of drug is to improve heart's blood-pumping ability.
• Immediately report chest pain or discomfort, palpitations.
• Change positions slowly to minimize dizziness, prevent injury

AVAILABLE FORMS

Parenteral for IV injection/infusion

amyl nitrite
(am'il ni'trit)

Classifications: Antianginal, vasodilator, nitrite

USUAL DOSE

Nasal inhal, adults: Cyanide poisoning: 0.3-ml ampule inhaled each min until sodium nitrite IV solution available
• Angina pectoris, adults: 0.18–0.30-ml ampule inhaled prn

ADMINISTRATION

Nasal inhal: Crush covered ampule between fingers and hold to nostrils for inhal.

ACTIONS

Relaxes vascular smooth muscle, promotes vasodilation • Venous/arteriolar dilation reduces preload (CVP, PCWP), afterload (SVR), myocardial O_2 consumption. • In cyanide toxicity, nitrite ions combine with hemoglobin to form methemoglobin, which binds with cyanide and assists in cyanide elimination.

PHARMACOKINETICS

ROUTE	ONSET	PEAK	DURATION
Nasal inhal	Immed	<3 min	3-5 min

DISTRIBUTION
Widely distributed
ELIMINATION
Metabolized in liver; eliminated in urine

INDICATIONS

Relief of acute angina pectoris (infrequently used because of cost, adverse effects) • Initially in management of cyanide toxicity
Unlabeled/investigational:
To produce reflect tachycardia and aid in diagnosis of stenotic vs. regurgitant heart murmurs. Illicitly used to enhance sexual pleasure ("poppers")

PRECAUTIONS/
CONTRAINDICATIONS

Precautions: High incidence of adverse effects (orthostatic hypotension, headache, tachycardia), offensive odor, rapid tolerance, inhibit use for management of angina pectoris. • Alcohol ingestion intensifies hypotensive effects.
Use caution with: Hypovolemia
• Severe renal/hepatic impairment • Acute MI; safety/efficacy not well established; reductions in SBP/DBP may cause myocardial, cerebral hypoperfusion.
P • Children: Safety/efficacy not well established
✗ Pregnancy category: Marked reductions in maternal BP may harm fetus; do not use in pregnancy/lactation.
Contraindications: Hypersensitivity to amyl nitrate • Increased ICP, inadequate cerebral perfusion, CVA • Severe anemia • Hypotension

---

P pediatric   **G** geriatric   **V** Direct IV

ADVERSE EFFECTS

CNS: *Headache, dizziness, weakness,* nervousness, uncoordination, visual disturbances

Resp: Bronchitis, pneumonia, dyspnea

CV: **Hypotension, increased chest pain or pressure,** *tachycardia,* paradoxical bradycardia, palpitations, dysrhythmias, syncope

GI: *Nausea,* vomiting, diarrhea, abdominal pain

Derm: Sweating, flushing

Misc: Hemolytic anemia, **methemoglobinemia**

TOXICITY/OVERDOSE

Symptoms: Hypotension, tachycardia, circulatory collapse, increased ICP with confusion/fever, symptoms of methemoglobinemia (acidosis, cyanosis, coma, seizures), death

Management: Support breathing as needed with O_2 and/or mechanical ventilation. • **Hypotension:** Elevate legs, administer IV fluids; if unresponsive to fluid replacement, use vasopressors (i.e., norepinephrine). • Inotropic agents (e.g., dobutamine, dopamine) may be used to stimulate contractility. • Avoid epinephrine (ineffective in correcting hypotension).

INTERACTIONS

alcohol Severe hypotension; CV collapse

aspirin Nitrate accumulation, increased effects

calcium channel blockers Orthostatic/profound hypotension

epinephrine Blocked alpha-adrenergic effects with unopposed beta effects (tachycardia, hypotension)

hypotensive agents Profound hypotension

phenothiazines Profound hypotension

PATIENT CARE IMPLICATIONS

• Correct hypovolemia before administration.
• Patient should be supine before administration.
• Use in well-ventilated room.
• Use extreme caution when administering to patients with ethanol intoxication.
• Protect patients from injury associated with falls caused by orthostatic hypotension.
• If headache develops, administer acetaminophen or other analgesic. Consult physician for severe or persistent headache.

Vital signs/hemodynamics: Monitor BP, HR before and after administration. • Continuous ECG monitoring recommended; report new ST segment depression, elevated/inverted T wave, serious dysrhythmias.

Physical assessment: Assess for perfusion/oxygenation deficit: chest discomfort, decreased level of consciousness, activity intolerance, hypotension, dizziness.

PATIENT/FAMILY TEACHING

Purpose of drug is to relieve chest pain or help in management of cyanide toxicity. • May cause low BP, dizziness; use when lying down. Be careful when changing positions, walking. Symptoms more likely to occur with alcohol, hot weather, vigorous activity, standing.
• May cause headaches; take

---

italic = common side effects   **bold** = life-threatening reactions

acetaminophen or other prescribed analgesic as needed.

AVAILABLE FORMS

Crushable ampules for inhal

---

anistreplase
(an-ih-strep'layz)
**anisoylated
plasminogen
streptokinase
activator complex,
APSAC**
Eminase, Iminase ✤

Classification: Thrombolytic
agent

USUAL DOSE

Direct IV, adults: • Coronary
artery thrombolysis: 30 U
within 6 hr of onset of acute MI
symptoms

ADMINISTRATION

V Direct IV, adults: • Coronary
artery thrombolysis: Inject
each dose directly into vein or
freely flowing IV line over 2-5
min.

PREPARATION

Slowly add 5 ml sterile water
without preservative to each
vial; direct stream of diluent to
sides of vial. Gently invert or
swirl to mix; do not shake. • Do
not dilute or add to infusion fluids. Administer within 30 min
of preparation. • Prepared solution is colorless to pale yellow
and transparent.

ACTIONS

Inactive derivatives of thrombolytic enzyme synthesized
from streptokinase and lysplas-
minogen • Promotes thrombolysis (clot dissolution) after activation within body • Converts
plasminogen into proteolytic enzyme, plasmin. Plasmin degrades fibrin clots, fibrinogen,
other clotting factors, thus dissolving clots and improving
blood flow through previously
occluded arteries. • Duration of
action longer than with other
thrombolytics; maintains activity
for 4-6 hr • Prompt reperfusion
of myocardial tissue promotes
improved ventricular function.
• Reductions in circulating clotting factors may cause significant bleeding complications.
• Repeated administration triggers antibodies that reduce drug
effectiveness, cause serious allergic reactions.

PHARMACOKINETICS

ROUTE	ONSET	PEAK	DURATION
IV	Immed	Approx 45 min	4-6 hr

DISTRIBUTION
Rapid, wide
ELIMINATION
Slow rate of degradation; half-life 94 min

INDICATIONS

**Thrombolysis in evolving
acute MI:** restoration of coronary perfusion to limit infarct
size, improve ventricular function, reduce incidence of CHF/
other complications; indicated
only during initial phase of
acute MI, preferably within 6 hr
of symptom onset. Concomitant
anticoagulant therapy (e.g., heparin) and platelet-aggregation
inhibitors (e.g., aspirin, dipyridamole) reduces incidence of
reocclusion.

P pediatric   **G** geriatric   **V** Direct IV

PRECAUTIONS/ CONTRAINDICATIONS

Precautions: Bleeding, bruising, hematomas may occur, especially at vascular access sites, after invasive procedures, with IM injections. • Cerebral/other serious or fatal spontaneous bleeding may occur. • Atrial/ventricular dysrhythmias may occur during coronary reperfusion. • May trigger serious allergic reactions; patients with recent (5 days-6 mo) streptococcal infection or treatment with streptokinase or anistreplase have elevated levels of antibodies, may fail to respond to therapy, are at greater risk for hypersensitivity reactions.

G Use caution with: Older adults, history of cerebrovascular disease, increased risk of cerebral hemorrhage

C Pregnancy category: Safety not established; use only if safer alternative unavailable.

Minor relative contraindications: Recent (within 10 days) minor trauma, including CPR • History of cerebrovascular disease • Pregnancy • Likelihood of left-sided heart thrombus (e.g., atrial fibrillation, severe left ventricular dyskinesia) • Acute pericarditis • Subacute bacterial endocarditis • Hemostatic defects (including those associated with liver/renal dysfunction), anticoagulant therapy • Diabetic hemorrhagic retinopathy, other hemorrhagic ophthalmic conditions • **G** Age >75 yr • Septic thrombophlebitis or occluded AV cannula at seriously infected site • Any condition in which serious bleeding likely or would be difficult to control

Major relative contraindications: Recent (within 10 days) major surgery, serious trauma, obstetric delivery, organ biopsy, puncture of noncompressible vessels • GI/GU bleeding within 10 days • Hypertension (SBP >180 or DBP >110 mm Hg)

Absolute contraindications: Hypersensitivity to antistreplase or streptokinase • Active internal bleeding • Recent CVA • Recent (within 2 mo) intracranial neoplasm • Arteriovenous malformation/aneurysm • Recent (within 2 mo) intracranial/intraspinal surgery or trauma • Bleeding diathesis • Severe, **P** uncontrolled hypertension • Children: Safety not established

ADVERSE EFFECTS

CNS: **Cerebral hemorrhage**
EENT: Epistaxis, gingival bleeding, eye hemorrhage
Resp: Hemoptysis, noncardiogenic pulmonary edema
CV: *Reperfusion dysrhythmias* (e.g., accelerated idioventricular rhythm, PVCs, **ventricular tachycardia/fibrillation,** PACs, atrial fibrillation, junctional rhythm, sinus bradycardia), **hypotension**
GI: *Nausea/vomiting,* bleeding
GU: Hematuria
Hema: *Puncture site bleeding, soft tissue bleeding, bruising, ecchymosis/hematoma,* thrombocytopenia
Derm: Urticaria (allergic)
Misc: Mild to severe allergic reactions, including **anaphylaxis,** delayed hypersensitivity, serum sickness

TOXICITY/OVERDOSE

Symptoms: Bleeding, bruising, hematomas; spontaneous

---

italic = common side effects   **bold** = life-threatening reactions

bleeding from cerebral, retro-peritoneal, GU, GI, soft tissue sources • Dose-dependent depletion of clotting proteins, production of fibrin degradation products

Management: Stop infusion. • Initiate local measures such as manual compression followed by pressure dressings. • Administer plasma volume expanders (avoid dextran), packed RBCs, fresh-frozen plasma, cryoprecipitate, as indicated by blood loss, clotting studies. • Antifibrinolytics (e.g., aminocaproic acid) may be used for life-threatening bleeding (e.g., intracranial hemorrhage). • For management of acute allergic reaction, see Appendix N.

INTERACTIONS

aminocaproic acid ↓ Fibrinolysis
anticoagulants (e.g., heparin, warfarin) ↑ Bleeding risk
aspirin other NSAIDs ↑ Bleeding risk
cephalosporins may ↑ bleeding risk
dipyridamole ↑ Bleeding risk
streptokinase (within 5 days-6 mo) Failed thrombolytic therapy; ↑ risk of hypersensitivity reactions

INCOMPATIBILITIES

Do not admix, dilute, infuse with other agents.

PATIENT CARE IMPLICATIONS

Before starting therapy

• Obtain baseline 12-lead ECG.
• Review history for contraindications.
• Have emergency resuscitation equipment, including epinephrine, lidocaine, atropine, immediately available.

• Apply pressure dressings to unsuccessful venipuncture attempts.
• Start 2 or more 18-gauge or larger catheters for laboratory samples; medications, fluids, emergency use.

During/immediately after therapy

• Avoid unnecessary venipuncture, invasive procedures, IM injections.
• If venipuncture necessary, hold manual pressure over site for 20 min or until bleeding stops, then apply pressure dressing. Inspect frequently for bleeding.
• If arterial puncture necessary, avoid femoral site and hold manual pressure over puncture site for 30 min or until bleeding stops. Apply pressure dressing; inspect frequently for bleeding.
• Avoid arterial/venous invasive procedures in areas inaccessible to manual compression (e.g., internal jugular, subclavian).
• Transient dysrhythmias, reduced chest pain, reduction of ST segment elevation suggest successful thrombolysis, coronary reperfusion.
• Report significant dysrhythmias, unusual or excessive bleeding, change in neurologic status, unrelieved or recurrent chest pain, allergic reactions.

Vital signs/hemodynamics: Initially, monitor BP, HR at 5–15-min intervals; when stable, progress to 30–60-min intervals during and for several hr after infusion. Hypotension may result from reperfusion dysrhythmias, hemorrhage, or impaired myocardial contractility; carefully evaluate each case. • Immediately report severe or uncontrolled hypertension (SBP

P pediatric   **G** geriatric   **V** Direct IV

>180 or DBP >110 mm Hg).
Prepare to initiate hypotensive
therapy. • Continuously monitor
ECG for dysrhythmias, changes
in ST segment elevation. Anticipate reperfusion dysrhythmias;
if symptomatic, manage according to ACLS guidelines (Appendix P).
Physical assessment: Assess/
document chest pain intensity,
character, location, radiation,
duration. Note any associated
symptoms. • Monitor all vascular access sites; assess for
bleeding q15min immediately
after injection, then q4h for 24
hr. If bleeding occurs, apply
pressure, continue to monitor
closely. • Assess peripheral
pulses for diminished intensity,
especially those distal to arterial
puncture or other invasive procedures. • Assess neurologic
status before initiating therapy
and frequently immediately after
injection. Immediately report
changes. • Assess for retroperitoneal bleeding (e.g., low back
pain, flank ecchymosis). • Note
blood in urine, other body fluids. Check emesis/stools for occult blood.
Laboratory tests: Monitor:
CPK, CBC, PT, PTT, fibrinogen
before and after therapy • Cardiac enzymes for coronary
thrombolysis • **May cause:** Unreliable results with coagulation
studies; notify lab and consider
use of aprotinin.

PATIENT/FAMILY TEACHING

Purpose of drug is to dissolve
clots blocking blood flow to
heart muscle. • Frequent monitoring is necessary because of
many side effects. • Immediately report chest pain or discomfort, unusual bleeding (e.g.,

from venipunctures, nose,
mouth, urine), breathing difficulty, itching. • Remain on bed-
rest throughout therapy.
• Avoid potential trauma caused
by shaving, toothbrushing, excessive activity for 24 hr after
therapy.

AVAILABLE FORMS

Powder to be reconstituted for
IV injection

---

aspirin
(as′pir-in)

**acetylsalicylic acid,
ASA**
Aspergum, Bufferin,
Ecotrin, Empirin,
Maxiprin, Sloprin,
Entrophen ✹, Novasen ✹
aspirin with buffers
Ascriptin, Buffex
**aspirin with codeine
phosphate, (15, 30, 60
mg)**
Empirin No. 2-4
**aspirin with
oxycodone**
Codoxy, Percodan,
Roxiprin

Classifications: NSAID, nonnarcotic analgesic, antipyretic, antiplatelet

USUAL DOSE

PO/rectal, adults: Mild pain
or fever: 235-650 mg q4h as
needed; single doses up to 1g
may be used, but do not exceed
4 g/24 hr. • **Arthritic/inflam-
matory conditions:** 2.4-5.4 g/
day in divided doses. • **Thrombosis prevention:** 160-325 mg
once daily to prevent recurrence

---

or extension of MI; up to 1.3 g/ day in divided doses to reduce risk of recurring TIAs and CVA

P **PO/rectal, children** (as specifically directed by physician): **Mild pain or fever:** q4h; approximate doses as follows:

AGE (yr)	DOSE (mg)
2-3	160
4-5	240
6-8	325
9-10	400
11	480
>11	325-650

Juvenile rheumatoid arthritis: Initially 60-90 mg/kg/day in **P** divided doses for children <25 kg or 2.4-3.6 g/day in divided **P** doses for children >25 kg; usual maintenance dose, 80-100 mg/kg daily

ACTIONS

Inhibits cyclooxygenase, decreases production of prostaglandins, which are associated with pain/inflammatory response; results in suppression of pain, inflammation; analgesic effects primarily peripheral, but hypothalamic or other CNS mechanisms may be involved • Inhibits platelet aggregation, prolongs bleeding time by altering liver synthesis of vitamin K-dependent coagulation factors • Reduces fever by inhibiting prostaglandins that mediate effect of endogenous pyrogen in hypothalamus • Other effects, including decreased renal blood flow and gastric mucosal damage, attributed to prostaglandin inhibition

PHARMACOKINETICS

ROUTE	ONSET	PEAK	DURATION
PO	5-30 min; food delays absorption	15 min-2 hr	3-6 hr

DISTRIBUTION
Rapid and wide into most body tissues

ELIMINATION
Metabolized in GI mucosa, liver, excreted by kidneys; half-life 15-20 min

Therapeutic level (serum salicylate):
100-300 μg/ml

INDICATIONS

Relief of mild to moderate pain, especially that associated with inflammation (e.g., arthritis); used concomitantly with opiate-agonist analgesics (e.g., codeine, oxycodone) to produce greater analgesia than either agent alone • Fever reduction • Reduction of inflammation • Prophylactically to reduce risk of death or recurrent MI, immediately after acute MI and with unstable angina • Prevention of arterial/venous thrombosis

PRECAUTIONS/ CONTRAINDICATIONS

Precautions: Chronic use, especially with high doses or other NSAIDS, may result in GI ulcerations, bleeding, perforation. • Alcohol use increases risk of GI bleeding. • Allergic reactions more likely with history of asthma, chronic urticaria, chronic rhinitis

Use caution with: Ulcer disease, gastritis, other GI disorder • Impaired renal/hepatic function • Asthma, reactive airway disease • History of liver disease, anticoagulant therapy, thrombocytopenia, other bleed-**P** ing disorders • Dehydrated children

D Pregnancy category: Use only if safer alternative unavailable and risks explained to woman.

Contraindications: Hypersensitivity to aspirin, other NSAIDs, tartazine dye (FD&C yellow no. 5) • Active GI bleeding, ulcer disease • Children/adolescents with varicella or influenza, unless specifically directed by physician; risk of Reye's syndrome

ADVERSE EFFECTS

GI: Nausea, vomiting, heartburn, diarrhea, epigastric/abdominal pain, reversible hepatoxicity, **GI bleeding, gastritis, peptic ulceration/ perforation**

GU: Transient decrease in renal blood flow

Hema: Iron-deficiency anemia, thrombocytopenia, prolonged bleeding time

Misc: Tinnitus, hearing loss; sensitivity reactions: bronchospasm, urticaria, angioedema, severe rhinitis, **shock**

TOXICITY/OVERDOSE

Symptoms: Chronic: Tinnitus, hearing loss, dimness of vision, dizziness, mental confusion, sweating, thirst, hyperventilation, tachycardia, vomiting, GI irritation • Acute: Symptoms of chronic toxicity; acid-base/electrolyte disturbances, usually respiratory alkalosis followed by metabolic acidosis; dehydration; hyperthermia; hyper/hypoglycemia; CNS stimulation followed by depression/coma; respiratory insufficiency, pulmonary edema, possible CV collapse; acute renal failure; bleeding problems

Management: After recent ingestion, implement guidelines for management of acute overdose (Appendix I); activated charcoal extremely effective.
• Administer O_2 support ventilation as needed. • Monitor UO; correct fluid, electrolyte, acid-base disturbances; rehydrate with 5%-10% dextrose. • **Seizures:** Control with IV diazepam. • **Prolonged bleeding time:** Administer vitamin K.
• **Hyperthermia:** Use cooling blanket, tepid baths. • If intoxication severe, enhance elimination with forced alkaline diuresis and hemodialysis.

Toxic level: >300 µg/ml

INTERACTIONS

acetazolamide ↑ Acetazolamide levels; CNS toxicity

alcohol ↑ Risk of gastric mucosal damage; additive prolongation of bleeding time

antacids ↓ Serum salicylate levels with high-dose salicylate therapy

anticoagulants, oral ↑ **Risk of bleeding; avoid concurrent use**

antidiabetic agents (e.g., sulfonylureas, insulin) ↑ Hypoglycemic effects with high-dose aspirin therapy

heparin Excessive bleeding

methotrexate ↑ **Methotrexate levels, risk of toxicity**

NSAIDs ↑ Risk of adverse effects

phenytoin High-dose aspirin therapy alters phenytoin levels; monitor closely.

probenecid Inhibition of uricosuric effects

sulfinpyrazone Inhibition of uricosuric effects

thrombolytics ↑ Risk of bleeding

zidovudine ↑ Risk of zidovudine toxicity

---

italic = common side effects   **bold** = life-threatening reactions

PATIENT CARE IMPLICATIONS

• Effectiveness for secondary prevention of recurrent MI is improved if administered within 24 hr of onset of acute MI symptoms.
• Co-administer with centrally acting opiate agonists (e.g., codeine) for greater analgesia.
• Relief of arthritic pain may take 1-2 wk of continuous therapy.

P • Do not use in children/adolescents with varicella or influenza, unless specifically directed by physician; use increases risk of developing Reye's syndrome

Vital signs/hemodynamics: Antipyretic activity may mask fever associated with infection.
• Monitor temperature before and 1-2 hr after administration when used as antipyretic.
• Measure/record UO. Assess for evidence of renal insufficiency, especially in older adults
G with renal/hepatic disease.

Physical assessment: Observe for unusual bleeding, especially with coagulation disorders or use of thrombolytics or anticoagulants. • Test stools, emesis for occult blood. Report positive results. • Assess for levels of pain, range of motion (as indicated) before and 1-2 hr after administration.

Laboratory tests: Monitor: CBC, bleeding time/PT with concurrent thrombolytic, anticoagulant or high-dose therapy
• Therapeutic levels with long-term therapy • **May cause:** Prolonged bleeding time, prolonged PT for 4-7 days, particularly with high-dose therapy

PATIENT/FAMILY TEACHING

Purpose of drug is to relieve pain, reduce swelling, reduce fever, or prevent dangerous blood clots from forming. • Take with food, milk, or antacids to decrease stomach irritation. • For stomach upset, use enteric-coated or extended-release tablets. Use of alcohol increases stomach irritation. • Do not crush, break, or chew enteric-coated or extended-release tablets. • Inform dentist or physician of aspirin use before treatment or surgery. • Report tinnitus, bruising, unusual bleeding, bleeding of gums, black stools, vomiting of blood.
• Avoid repeated doses of bismuth subsalicylate–containing antidiarrheal preparations (e.g., Pepto-Bismol), which could lead to salicylate intoxication.
• Avoid buffered or effervescent preparations (e.g., Alka-Seltzer) if on sodium-restricted diet.
• Tablets: Store in cool, dry place; discard tablets with strong, vinegar-like odor.
• Gum: Chew thoroughly for 15 min, then remove from mouth.

AVAILABLE FORMS

Tablets, capsules alone and in multiple formulations: buffered, coated, extended release, in combination with acetaminophen, caffeine, codeine, meprobamate, oxycodone, pentazocine, propoxyphene, pseudoephedrine, other agents
• Gum • Suppositories

---

atenolol
(a-ten'oh-lole)
Tenormin, Apo-Atenolol ✣
Novo-Atenolol ✣

atenolol with chlorthalidone
Tenoretic

Classifications: Class II antidysrhythmic, cardioselective beta-adrenergic blocker, antihypertensive, antianginal

USUAL DOSE
PO, adults: 50-200 mg daily • **Acute MI:** 50 mg 10 min after completion of IV dose; repeat in 12 hr; thereafter, 50 mg bid or 100 mg once daily for 7 days • **Older adults, renal impairment:** 25-50 mg daily, monitor carefully.
Direct IV, adults: 5 mg; repeat dose in 10 min if tolerated; follow with PO therapy. • More effective if therapy initiated within 12 hr of first MI symptoms.

ADMINISTRATION
▼Direct IV: Inject slowly at rate not >1 mg/min; 5-mg dose given over 5 min. Dilution not necessary • Monitor ECG, BP throughout injection. Discontinue for symptomatic bradycardia, HR <45 bpm, 2nd or 3rd degree heart block, hypotension.
Compatible fluids: D_5W, 0.9% NaCl

ACTIONS
Blocks stimulation of beta-1-adrenergic receptors of myocardium; in usual doses has little effect on beta-2 receptors of vasculature and bronchial smooth muscle; higher doses less cardioselective • ↓ HR, BP, force of contraction, myocardial O_2 consumption • Reduced O_2 consumption, other effects diminish risk of myocardial reinfarction. • Depresses AV conduction/myocardial automaticity, particularly in SA node • Suppresses renin-angiotensin-aldosterone system

PHARMACOKINETICS

ROUTE	ONSET	PEAK	DURATION
PO	<30 min	2-4 hr	24 hr
IV	Immed	<5 min	<12 hr

DISTRIBUTION
Widely distributed into most tissue, except CSF, brain

ELIMINATION
Eliminated by liver, kidneys, half-life 6-7 hr. prolonged with renal impairment

INDICATIONS
Control of hypertension, chronic stable angina pectoris • Reduction of mortality, risk of reinfarction in acute MI patients *Unlabeled/investigational:* With benzodiazepines in managing acute alcohol withdrawal.

PRECAUTIONS/ CONTRAINDICATIONS
Precautions: May cause bradycardia, hypotension, CHF, particularly with preexisting heart disease • Abrupt cession of therapy may induce angina, ventricular dysrhythmias, and/or acute MI.
Use caution with: Heart failure, valvular heart disease; may precipitate/worsen heart failure • Peripheral or mesenteric vascular disease; may worsen arterial insufficiency • Asthma, COPD; ↓ dose; monitor for bronchospasm. • General anesthesia; additive impairment of cardiac contractility; consider

---

withdrawal before elective surgery. • Diabetes; beta-blocking effects mask hypoglycemic symptoms. • Hyperthyroidism; beta-blocking effects mask symptoms. • Renal/hepatic impairment; reduce dose. • Children: Safety/efficacy not established

D Pregnancy category: Use only if safer alternatives unavailable.

Contraindications: Hypersensitivity to atenolol. • Severe bradycardia • 2nd or 3rd degree heart block • CHF (unless resulting from tachycardia) • Cardiogenic shock

ADVERSE EFFECTS

CNS: *Fatigue, dizziness, depression,* drowsiness.
Resp: Dyspnea, wheezing
CV: ***Bradycardia, hypotension, heart failure, heart block, ventricular tachycardia, SVT***
GI: Elevated liver enzymes
Endo: Blocked symptoms of hypoglycemia/hyperthyroidism (e.g., absence of tachycardia, hypertension)
Hema: Thrombocytopenia
Derm: Rash, pruritus, alopecia
Misc: Lupus syndrome

TOXICITY/OVERDOSE

Symptoms: Profound bradycardia/hypotension, loss of consciousness, heart failure, advanced heart block, bronchospasm, hypoglycemia
Management: After recent ingestion, implement guidelines for management of acute overdose (Appendix I) • **Symptomatic bradycardia, heart block:** Atropine, isoproterenol according to ACLS guidelines (Appendix P) • **Bronchospasm:** Isoproterenol, amino-

phylline • **Heart failure:** Inotropic agents (e.g., dobutamine), diuretics, possibly digoxin • **Hypotension:** Elevate legs, administer IV fluids; use vasopressors (e.g., dopamine, norepinephrine) if severe and refractory to inotropic agents. • Hemodialysis may be helpful.

INTERACTIONS

amiodarone   Severe bradycardia; ventricular dysrhythmias
anesthetics, local   Hypertension, particularly if anesthetic contains epinephrine
antidiabetics (insulin, oral agents)   Prolonged recovery from hypoglycemic episodes; inhibition of hypoglycemia-associated tachycardia
calcium channel blockers   ↓ BP, slowed AV conduction, extreme bradycardia
disopyramide   Additive negative inotropy, ↓ CO
epinephrine   Beta effects of epinephrine blocked, resulting in unopposed alpha stimulation (severe hypertension, bradycardia, dysrhythmias); ↓ effectiveness in anaphylaxis
isoproterenol   ↓ Bronchodilatory effectiveness
lidocaine   ↑ Lidocaine levels; negative inotropy; ↓ CO
NSAIDS   ↓ Hypotensive effectiveness
phenothiazines   ↓ BP; enhanced effects of either agent
prazosin   ↓ BP, especially with initial dose
quinidine   Additive cardiac depression
rifampin   ↑ Beta-blocker metabolism
theophylline   ↑ Theophylline levels; possible ↓ bronchodilation

Y-SITE COMPATIBILITIES
Meperidine, morphine

PATIENT CARE IMPLICATIONS
• PO, IV doses not interchangeable; carefully check dose, route.
• Identify patients with COPD, asthma. Monitor closely; avoid high-dose therapy (>100 mg/day), which may precipitate bronchospasm.
• Gradually withdraw therapy to avoid rebound hypertension, angina, possible acute MI.
• Observe hyperthyroid patients for symptoms of thyrotoxicosis (e.g., tachycardia, hypertension) when withdrawing therapy.

IV use in acute MI:
• Begin therapy as soon as eligibility established and patient hemodynamically stable, usually within 12 hr of onset of MI symptoms.
• Closely monitor ECG, BP, during and immediately after injection.

Vital signs/hemodynamics:
As available, observe ECG for heart block, significant bradycardia, prolonged PR, widened QRS. If present, consult physician before administering next dose • Measure CVP, PAP, PCWP, CO, as available. Consult physician for ↓ CO or ↑ filling pressures associated with other symptoms of heart failure. • Monitor frequently if other antidysrhythmics or antihypertensive agents used.

Physical assessment:
Assess for perfusion/oxygenation deficit: ↓ level of consciousness, activity intolerance, hypotension, chest discomfort, dizziness.
• Auscultate lung fields for bi-basilar crackles. • When used for angina, assess/response, including frequency, duration of chest pain. • Assess for respiratory distress in patients with history of COPD or cardiac impairment. • Assess patients with diabetes for sweating, because tachycardia/tremors associated with hypoglycemia may be blocked by therapy.

Laboratory tests:
Monitor: Blood glucose, liver enzymes, creatinine, cholesterol, triglycerides, CBC • Blood glucose frequently in patients with diabetes.

PATIENT/FAMILY TEACHING
Purpose of medication is ↓ BP or reduce workload of heart muscle. • Frequent monitoring for adverse effects is required for IV use. • Change positions slowly to avoid dizziness and low BP, particularly when getting out of bed in morning.
• Report breathing difficulty, palpitations, dizziness, activity intolerance, chest pain, depression, rash, unusual bleeding, persistent fever, sore throat.
• Avoid excessive amounts of coffee, tea, caffeinated soft drinks, which may counteract drug's BP-lowering effects.

Outpatient:
Take medication exactly as prescribed. Do not stop taking medicine even if you feel better. If medication is abruptly discontinued, you may develop dangerously high BP, serious heartbeat irregularities, chest pain. • Check/resting pulse each day, BP each week. Contact health care provider if pulse <50 bpm or BP significantly different. • Medication is not cure for high BP, and other therapies, including life-style modi-

---

italic = common side effects   **bold** = life-threatening reactions

fications, must be continued.
• Medication may cause drowsiness; avoid driving and other activities requiring mental alertness until individual response to drug known. • Alcohol ingestion may cause extreme dizziness, drowsiness. • Consult health care provider before taking non-prescription preparations
• Carry medical ID card identifying drug, dosage, specific indication. • Notify physician/dentist of therapy before any treatment. • Medicine blocks ↑ HR and ↑ BP, so hyperthyroid and patients with diabetes must be aware of other symptoms of crisis.

AVAILABLE FORMS

Parenteral for IV injection
• Tablets

---

atracurium besylate
(a-tra-kyoo-ree′um)
Tracrium

Classification: Nondepolarizing neuromuscular blocking agent

USUAL DOSE

P **Direct IV, adults/children:** Initial bolus dose, 0.4-0.5 mg/kg; use lower initial dose of 0.3-0.4 mg/kg if history of CV disease, asthma, severe allergic reactions, or after succinylcholine **P** use. • **Children <2 yr:** 0.2-0.5 mg/kg • Maintenance, 0.08-0.1 mg/kg given 20-45 min after initial dose, and at 15–25-min intervals thereafter. • **Renal insufficiency:** Dosage adjustment not necessary
P **IV, cont inf, adults/children >2 yr:** Administer initial bolus dose. Maintenance, start at 9-10 µg/kg/min; adjust to individual requirements. Dose range is 2-15 µg/kg/min; 11-13 µg/kg/min typically required for adult intensive care unit (ICU) patients; **P** **children** may need higher rates

ADMINISTRATION

V **Direct IV:** Inject each dose over 60 sec; dilution not necessary. *Causes immediate respiratory paralysis; means for continuous artificial ventilation must be in place or provided immediately after injection.* Use nerve stimulator to monitor neuromuscular blockade. Avoid additional doses until there is a certain response to T_1 (first twitch).
IV, cont inf: Infusion pump necessary. Titrate for minimal dose required to maintain 90% (using nerve stimulator) or desired neuromuscular blockade. Avoid additional doses until there is a certain response to T_1 (first twitch). If no response, discontinue infusion until response returns. Using dilution of 500 µg/ml, infusion rate of 84 ml/hr will deliver 10 µg/kg/min to a 70-kg person. • See Infusion Rate Table, Appendix Q.

PREPARATION

DILUTION	CONCENTRATION
20 mg/100 ml	200 µg/ml (0.2 mg/ml)
50 mg/100 ml	500 µg/ml (0.5 mg/ml)

Compatible fluids: D_5W, 0.9% NaCl, prepared combinations of these solutions. Unstable in LR, alkaline solutions
Stability: Diluted solution stable for 24 hr at room temp.

ACTIONS

Causes skeletal muscle paralysis by interfering with transmission

---

of nerve impulses at neuromuscular junction. • Competes with/blocks activity of acetylcholine (neurotransmitter normally producing electrical depolarization) • Eye, face, neck muscles affected first; followed by limbs, abdomen, chest, diaphragm. Recovery occurs in reverse order • May trigger histamine release; likelihood increased if recommended dose exceeded • No analgesic/sedative effects • Shorter duration than pancuronium

PHARMACOKINETICS

ROUTE	ONSET	PEAK	DURATION
IV	2-2.5 min	3-5 min	Recovery: 25% in 30 min, 95% in 70 min

DISTRIBUTION
Throughout extracellular fluid

ELIMINATION
Inactivated in plasma; excreted in urine, bile

INDICATIONS

With general anesthesia to produce skeletal muscle relaxation during surgery • Facilitate ET intubation • In critical care to facilitate mechanical ventilation • No effects on consciousness/pain threshold • Used only after induction of general anesthesia or with analgesics/anxiolytic

PRECAUTIONS/CONTRAINDICATIONS

Precautions: *Causes respiratory paralysis; must use with artificial airway, ventilatory support* • Recommended for use with nerve stimulator • May trigger histamine release • Patients with major burns may develop resistance to neuromuscular blockade; increased doses usually needed • Neuromuscular

excitability, including seizures, have been reported after prolonged administration in ICU patients with head trauma, encephalopathy, cerebral edema.
Use caution with: Significant CV disease, asthma, previous severe allergic reaction, any other condition in which histamine release would be especially harmful • Myasthenia gravis, severe electrolyte disorders; drug effects potentiated by these conditions
C Pregnancy category: Use only if safer alternative not available.
Contraindications: Hypersensitivity to atracurium

ADVERSE EFFECTS

CNS: *muscle weakness, **paralysis,*** prolonged blockade
Resp: dyspnea, bronchospasm, excessive secretions
CV:vasodilation, hypotension, tachycardia, *bradycardia,* **asystole**
Derm: flushing, redness, itching, hives
Misc: anaphylaxis

TOXICITY/OVERDOSE

Symptoms: Bronchospasm, wheezing, flushing, hypotension, hives, itching, other manifestations of histamine releases • Prolonged neuromuscular blockade
Management: Provide continuous artificial ventilation. • Reverse effects with anticholinesterase agent such as neostigmine, edrophonium, pyridostigmine in conjunction with anticholinergic such as atropine, glycopyrrolate • **Hypotension:** Elevate legs, administer IV fluids; use dopamine, other pressors if necessary. • Benefits of

---

italic = common side effects **bold** = life-threatening reactions

hemodialysis not established
• For management of acute allergic reaction, see Appendix N

INTERACTIONS

Aminoglycosides (amikacin, gentamicin), amphotericin B, beta-blockers, calcium channel blockers, corticosteroids, diuretics, inhalation anesthetics, lidocaine, magnesium, procainamide, quinidine Potentiate/prolong neuromuscular blockade
digoxin ↑ Risk of dysrhythmias
opiate analgesics Respiratory depression
succinylcholine Quickens onset, ↑ depth of neuromuscular blockade; avoid atracurium until patient recovered from succinylcholine

Y-SITE COMPATIBILITIES

Bretylium, cefuroxime, cimetidine, dobutamine, dopamine, epinephrine, esmolol, fentanyl, hydrocortisone sodium succinate, isoproterenol, lidocaine, lorazepam, midazolam, morphine, nitroglycerin, potassium chloride, procainamide, trimethoprim-sulfamethoxazole, vancomycin

Y-SITE INCOMPATIBILITIES

Alkaline solutions, aminophylline, barbiturates, cefazolin, diazepam, gentamicin, heparin, quinidine, ranitidine, nitroprusside

PATIENT CARE IMPLICATIONS

• Has no effect on consciousness/pain threshold; patient is fully awake and feels all sensations. *Use only with general anesthesia or analgestics (e.g., morphine) and anxiolytics (e.g., midazolam).*
• Causes respiratory paralysis, apnea; *use only for patients under direct observation and continuous mechanical ventilation.*
• Prevent corneal drying by instillation of artificial tears, eye patching.
• Cholinesterase inhibitors such as neostigmine, edrophonium used to reverse effects; multiple doses may be necessary
• Long-term use may cause prolonged paralysis, skeletal muscle weakness (although less likely than with other NMBAs because of nonrenal/hepatic elimination); use lowest effective dose.
• Patients thought to have recovered from neuromuscular blockade may develop apnea when given certain drugs that potentiate NMBAs (see Interactions).
Vital signs/hemodynamics: Monitor ECG continuously. Observe for bradycardia (unlike some other NMBAs, will not counter bradycardia caused by anesthetics or vagal stimulation), tachycardia. • Monitor BP, observing for hypotension, q3-5 min during initiation of therapy and frequently thereafter. • Use continuous pulse oximetry to monitor oxygenation during recovery from neuromuscular blockade.
Physical assessment: Closely monitor respiratory status (rate, depth, pattern of ventilation) until fully recovered. Secretions may be increased; suction as necessary. • Paralysis of muscle groups usually occurs in the following order: eye, face, neck muscles affected first; followed by limbs, abdomen, chest, dia-

---

phragm. Recovery occurs in reverse order. Assess frequently for residual muscle weakness, respiratory distress until fully recovered from effects. • Use peripheral nerve stimulator to monitor effectiveness of NMBAs. *Avoid additional doses of NMBAs until there is a response to T_1 (first twitch). If no response, discontinue infusion until response returns.* When continuous infusion used in ICU, recovery to train-of-four ratio >75% (ratio of height of fourth to first twitch) occurs in approximately 60 min. • Monitor I&O; Foley catheter required.

Laboratory tests: Monitor: Potassium; drug action potentiated by hypokalemia. Magnesium; drug action potentiated by hypermagnesemia. Calcium; drug action potentiated by hypocalcemia. Acid-base status; imbalance alters drug action. ABGs; to evaluate adequacy of ventilation.

PATIENT/FAMILY TEACHING

Purpose of medication is to paralyze body muscles temporarily to facilitate procedures, surgery. • When recovering from effects, it may be difficult to swallow, talk; these effects temporary. • Drug does not affect consciousness: explain all procedures.

AVAILABLE FORMS

Parenteral for direct IV
Storage: Intact vials stable for 14 days at room temp.; refrigerate if stored for longer periods.

---

atropine sulfate
(a'troe-peen)
Atropen, Minims ✦,
Atropine ✦

Classifications: Anticholinergic, antimuscarinic, parasympatholytic, antidysrhythmic, ophthalmic-mydriatic

USUAL DOSE

IM/SC, adults: Preop: 0.4-0.6 mg

℗ IM/SC, children: Preop: According to body weight

WEIGHT	DOSE
3 kg	0.1 mg
7-9 kg	0.2 mg
12-16 kg	0.3 mg

Direct IV/ET, adults: Bradycardia: 0.5-1.0 mg; repeat q3-5min until desired response (usually HR >60 bpm) or up to total of 0.04 mg/kg. • Doses >2.0 mg usually not necessary • Avoid doses <0.5 mg; may cause paradoxical ↓ HR • **Asystole:** 1 mg repeat q3-5min up to total of 0.04 mg/kg • **Poisoning antidote (IV):** Initially 1-2 mg; additional 2-mg doses q5-60 min as needed; up to 50 mg may be necessary in first 24 hr.

Direct IV/ET/intraosseous, ℗ children: Bradycardia: 0.01-0.03 mg/kg; repeat at 5-min intervals up to total of 1.0 mg in young children, 2.0 mg in adolescents. • Avoid does <0.1 mg; may cause paradoxical ↓ HR. • **Poisoning antidote (IV):** 0.05 mg/kg; may repeat q10-30 min as needed

Inhal, adults: Bronchospasms: 0.025 mg/kg 3-4 times daily, up to 2.5 mg/day

---

italic = common side effects   **bold** = life-threatening reactions

P Inhal, children: Broncho-spasm: 0.05 mg/kg three to four times daily

P Ophth, adults/children: Cycloplegic refractions: 1-2 drops • Use 1% solution for adults, 0.5% solution for children.

ADMINISTRATION

V Direct IV: Inject rapidly over 1 min. Slow injection may cause paradoxical slowing of HR.

ET instillation, adults: Dilute 1-2 mg atropine in 10 ml normal saline. Hyperventilate, then expel directly into ETT. Follow with 5 additional full breaths to distribute medication.

P ET instillation, children: Dilute desired dose of atropine in volume of 1-2 ml normal saline. Hyperventilate, then expel atropine directly into ETT. Follow with 5 additional full breaths to distribute medication.

ACTIONS

Inhibits action of acetylcholine at parasympathetic neuroeffector junction sites within myocardium, smooth muscle, secretory glands, CNS; blocks vagal stimuli • Low doses reduce sweating, salivation, respiratory secretions. • Intermediate to large doses increase HR, decrease GI/GU motility, dilate pupils, promote cycloplegia (loss of visual accommodation). • **CV effects:** Blocks normal vagal inhibition of SA node, stimulates AV pacemaker, accelerates HR; facilitates AV/nodal conduction • At low doses, parasympathomimetic actions may induce paradoxical bradycardia.

PHARMACOKINETICS

ROUTE	ONSET	PEAK	DURATION
IM	<5 min	30 min	≥12.5 hr
IV	Immed	2-4 min	4-6 hr
Inhal	15-30 min	30-170 min	3-5 hr

DISTRIBUTION

Wide: readily crosses blood-brain barrier; crosses placenta

ELIMINATION

Metabolizes in liver, excreted in urine; half-life 2.5 hr

INDICATIONS

Bradycardia: Initial therapy for patients with symptomatic bradycardia (e.g., associated with hypotension, ventricular ectopy, other hemodynamic compromise); sometimes used for HRs within "physiologic" range when sinus tachycardia would be more appropriate (e.g., patient with acute MI, symptomatic hypotension, HR 70 bpm) • Minimal effect on sinus bradycardia caused by intrinsic SA nodal disease • Usually effective for type I 2nd degree AV block; type II may not respond.
• **Asystole:** Sometimes restores AV nodal conduction, may promote electrical activity • **Poisoning antidote:** Counters sinus bradycardia, other cholinergic effects induced by drugs or toxic substances (e.g., pilocarpine, organophosphate pesticides, *Amanita muscaria* mushrooms) • **Preop:** Inhibits salivation, excessive respiratory secretions; prevents cholinergic effects (e.g., bradycardia, hypotension) during surgery • **Bronchospasm:** With chronic bronchitis/emphysema, to reduce bronchial smooth muscle tone when beta-adrenergic therapy has been ineffective or longer duration of action desired; less

---

effective in treatment of bronchospasm associated with asthma • **Ophth:** To produce mydriasis, cycloplegic refraction; may be used for inflammatory conditions of iris, uvea.

PRECAUTIONS/ CONTRAINDICATIONS

Precautions: Excessive doses may cause delirium, tachycardia, ataxia, coma. • Older patients, infants/children more susceptible to adverse effects • Commercial preparations may contain sulfites, which can cause serious allergic reactions. **Use caution with:** CAD, CHF, tachydysrhythmias; ↑ HR may contribute to infarction or failure. • COPD; mucous plugs possible from reduced bronchial secretions • Gastric ulcer, esophageal reflux, intestinal infections, partial obstruction, other GI disorders in which intestinal motility may be harmful • Fever or exposure to high environmental temperature; risk of hyperthermia • Hyperthyroidism, hepatic/renal disease, hypertension

c Pregnancy category: Use only if safer alternative unavailable.

Contraindications: Hypersensitivity to atropine • Narrow-angle glaucoma • Acute hemorrhage • Tachycardia associated with cardiac insufficiency or thyrotoxicosis • Severe ulcerative colitis, toxic megacolon, paralytic ileus, GI obstruction • Myasthenia gravis (unless used to reduce adverse effects of anticholinesterase agent)

ADVERSE EFFECTS

CNS: *Drowsiness,*confusion, dizziness, headache, nervousness, insomnia

EENT: *Blurred vision, dilated pupils,* dry eyes, photophobia

CV: *Tachycardia,* dysrhythmias including **ventricular tachycardia/fibrillation,** palpitations

GI: *Dry mouth, slowing of GI motility,* constipation, nausea/ vomiting

GU: *Urinary hesitancy,* retention

Derm: *Hot flushed skin,* urticaria, rash

Misc: Diminished or absent sweating

TOXICITY/OVERDOSE

Symptoms: Tachycardia, ventricular dysrhythmias, extrasystoles, widened QRS complex, prolonged QT interval, depressed ST segment • Dilated unreactive pupils, hot dry skin, blurred vision, nausea/vomiting, hyptertension, increased RR, acute psychosis, hyperactivity, hyperreflexia • **Severe overdose:** CNS depression, coma, skeletal muscle paralysis, hyperpyrexia, hypotension, death from respiratory failure or cardiac depression

Management: Symptomatic/ supportive, including airway maintenance/assisted ventilations as indicated, continuous ECG monitoring, IV fluids, cooling blanket • **Delirium, excitement:** Administer diazepam; avoid phenothiazines, which contribute to anticholinergic effects. • **SVT:** Administer IV propranolol. • Because of severe adverse effects (e.g., seizures, bronchospasm, bradycardia, asystole), physostigmine reserved for serious manifestations such as severe sinus tachycardia, SVT, repetitive seizures, extreme hyperthermia, extreme agitation with potential for self-inflicted injury

INTERACTIONS

amantadine, antiparkinsonian agents, meperidine, phenothiazines, procainamide, quinidine, TCAs Additive anticholinergic effects

Y-SITE COMPATIBILITIES

Compatibilities: Amrinone, famotidine, heparin, nafcillin potassium chloride

In-syringe compatibilities: Butorphanol, chlorpromazine, diphenhydramine, droperidol, fentanyl, hydroxyzine, meperidine, metoclopramide, midazolam, morphine, nalbuphine, prochlorperazine, promethazine

INCOMPATIBILITIES

Aminophylline, metaraminol, norepinephrine, pentobarbital, sodium bicarbonate

PATIENT CARE IMPLICATIONS

IV/ET

• Paradoxical bradycardia (caused by slow injection or injection of smaller-then-recommended doses) usually resolves with 2 min.
• Consult physician for sustained tachydysrhythmias, angina, ectopy, signs of cardiac failure.

Opth

• Dim lights in room or provide dark glasses for patient because of pupil dilation.

Vital signs/hemodynamics: Monitor for excessive tachycardia, hyperthermia. • Carefully monitor I&O because of possible urinary retention. • IV/ET: Continuously monitor ECG; document response to therapy with rhythm strip. • Monitor VS immediately after injection and q5-15min until stable.

Physical assessment: Assess every 4-8 hr for bowel sounds, abdominal distention. Note bowel elimination patterns.
• Monitor character, amount of respiratory secretions. • Monitor breathing patterns, lung sounds for evidence of improved gas exchange (inhal therapy)

PATIENT/FAMILY TEACHING

Purpose of medication is to ↑ HR, ↓ salivation/respiratory secretions before surgery, improve breathing, aid in eye examination/healing. • Oral rinses, gum, or hard candy may help relieve dry mouth. • Intense but harmless flushing may occur 15-20 min after IV administration.
G • Inform older men and those with benign prostatic hypertrophy that atropine may cause urinary hesitancy, retention. Changes in urination patterns should be reported.

Outpatient: Avoid activities requiring mental alertness, visual acuity (e.g., operating car or other machinery). • Increase dietary fiber and fluid intake to help prevent/alleviate constipation (with prolonged therapy).
• Caution patient that atropine impairs heat regulation; encourage patient to avoid vigorous activity in hot environment.
• Wear dark glasses to protect eyes from bright or outdoor light. • Consult with health care provider before taking nonpre-

scription medications. • Ophthalmic preparations may temporarily blur vision and impair ability to judge distances. • For patients receiving inhal therapy, instruct in use of inhaler or other device.

AVAILABLE FORMS

Parenteral for IV/IM/SC use • Ophthalmic ointment, solution

azithromycin dihydrate
(ay-zi-thro-mye'sin)
Zithromax

Classification: Semisynthetic macrolide antibiotic

USUAL DOSE

PO, adults: 500 mg as single dose on day 1 of therapy; 250 mg once daily on days 2-5. Alternately, single 1-g dose may be used for *Chlamydia trachomatis* genital infections • **Renal insufficiency:** No adjustment necessary with creat. cl. ≥40 ml/min; studies not conducted on patients with more severe renal impairment

ADMINISTRATION

Give at least 1 hr before or 2 hr after a meal

ACTION

Usually bacteriostatic but may be bactericidal in high doses against particularly susceptible organisms • Penetrates bacterial cell wall, inhibits protein synthesis; effective against many gram-positive bacteria and some aerobic gram-negative organisms • Significant activity against staphylococci, streptococci, *Chlamydia trachomatis, Gardnerella vaginalis* • Excellent activity against *Haemophilus influenzae;* superior to erythromycin/clarithromycin • Not effective against methicillin-resistant *Staphylococcus aureus,* Enterobacteriaceae, *Pseudomonas* species

PHARMACOKINETICS

ROUTE	ONSET	PEAK	ONSET
PO	1-2 hr	3-4 hr	≥24 hr; dose-dependent

DISTRIBUTION
Wide; low CSF concentrations

ELIMINATION
Biliary excretion of unchanged drug. Half-life 11-14 hr after single dose, 2-4 days after several doses

INDICATIONS

Alternative treatment for patients with community-acquired upper or lower respiratory tract infections, otitis media, skin or soft tissue infections, particularly when allergies to penicillin, cephalosporins, cotriaximole are present, or when erythromycin is not tolerated • Choice agent for treatment of uncomplicated chlamydial urethritis, cervicitis, particularly if compliance with 7-day regimen cannot be assured • Not for use with severe or nosocomially acquired infections; elderly, immunocompromised, or debilitated patients

G

PRECAUTIONS/ CONTRAINDICATIONS

Precautions: Bacterial or fungal overgrowth may occur. • Not effective against gonorrhea/syphilis at recommended doses; use may mask symptoms of these infections • Allergic reactions may recur after treatment in patients without addi-

---

tional exposure to azithromycin; prolonged hypersensitivity response may be related to long half-life of azithromycin.
• Pseudomembranous colitis has occurred with other macrolide antibiotics. • Ventricular tachycardia/torsades de pointes have occurred in patients with prolonged QT interval treated with other macrolides, but has not been reported with azithromycin.

Use caution with: Hepatic or biliary disease; biliary excretion major route of elimination

B Pregnancy category: Use only if safer alternative not available

Contraindications: Hypersensitivity to azithromycin, erythromycins, or other macrolides

ADVERSE EFFECTS

CNS: Headache, dizziness
CV: Palpitations, chest pain
GI: Abdominal pain, nausea, vomiting, diarrhea, candidiasis
GU: Vaginitis, monilia
Misc: Allergic reactions, including rash, angioedema, **bronchospasm, anaphylaxis**

TOXICITY/OVERDOSE

Symptoms: Extension of side effects/adverse reactions
Management: Discontinue drug; initiate symptomatic/supportive measures. • After recent ingestion, implement guidelines for management of acute overdosage (Appendix I) • For acute allergic reaction, see Appendix N.

INTERACTIONS

antacids, aluminum/magnesium-containing ↓ Azithromycin concentration; avoid concurrent administration

digoxin ↑ Digoxin levels
ergotamine Ischemic reactions; peripheral vasospasm
theophylline Possible ↑ theophylline levels/toxicity

PATIENT CARE IMPLICATIONS

• Obtain culture and sensitivity (C&S) before initiating treatment; start treatment after specimens collected
• Obtain cultures for gonorrhea and serologic tests for syphilis before initiation of azithromycin therapy for *C. trachomatis.* Symptoms of gonorrhea/syphilis could be masked, resulting in delays in treatment if these infections are present.
• Food decreases absorption. Administer 1 hr before or 2 hr after meals.

Vital signs/hemodynamics: Monitor VS for indicators of infection, complications.

Physical assessment: Assess for improvement in primary infection or symptoms of super/suprainfection: appearance of sputum, urine, stool, wound drainage; presence of fever, candidiasis, vaginitis; WBC

Laboratory tests: Monitor: Liver enzymes, bilirubin • C&S results

PATIENT/FAMILY TEACHING

Purpose of medication is to limit growth of infection-causing bacteria. • Report diarrhea, fever, vaginal itching or discharge, furry growth on tongue. • Take medication at the same time each day. • Take at least 1 hr before or 2 hr after meals. • Do not take with aluminum/magnesium-containing antacids. • Do not crush, chew, or divide capsules. • Take all of

medication exactly as prescribed. Do not stop taking
medicine even if you feel better.
Failure to take all of antibiotic
may result in recurrence or additional infection. Do not save
or share unused medicine.

AVAILABLE FORMS
Capsules

bisoprolol fumarate
(bis-oh'proe-lole)
Zebeta
bisoprolol fumarate and hydrochlorothiazide
Ziac

Classification: Class II antidysrhythmic, cardioselective beta-
adrenergic blocker, antihypertensive

USUAL DOSE
PO, adults: Initially, 2.5-5 mg
once daily; may increase to 10-
20 mg once daily as necessary
• **Renal/hepatic impairment:**
Start at 2.5 mg once daily; increase cautiously as necessary.

ACTION
Blocks stimulation of beta-1-
adrenergic receptors of myocardium; in usual doses has little
effect on beta-2 receptors of
vasculature and bronchial
smooth muscle; doses >20 mg
are less cardioselective and may
increase airway resistance • Decreases HR, force of contraction, CO; reduces BP, myocardial O_2 consumption • Reduces
centrally mediated sympathetic
stimulation • Depresses IV con-
duction/myocardial automaticity,

particularly in SA node • Suppresses renin-angiotensin-
aldosterone system

PHARMACOKINETICS

ROUTE	ONSET	PEAK	DURATION
PO	<2 hr	2-4 hr	≥24 hr

DISTRIBUTION
30% protein bound

ELIMINATION
Kidneys and other pathways. Half-life
9-12 hr.

INDICATIONS
Hypertension; alone, and in
combination with diuretics,
other agents

PRECAUTIONS/ CONTRAINDICATIONS
Precautions: Symptomatic
bradycardia, hypotension, CHF
possible, particularly with preexisting heart disease • Abrupt
cessation of therapy may induce
angina, ventricular dysrhythmias, and/or acute MI.
Use caution with: Heart failure, valvular heart disease
• Asthma, COPD; use low dose;
monitor for bronchospasm • Peripheral or mesenteric vascular
disease; may worsen arterial insufficiency • General anesthesia;
additive impairment of cardiac
contractility; consider withdrawal before elective surgery
• Diabetes; beta-blocking effects
mask hypoglycemic symptoms
• Hyperthyroidism; beta-blocking effects mask symptoms
• Renal/hepatic impairment; reduce dose • Children: Safety/ef-
ficacy not established
c Pregnancy category: Use
only if safer alternative not
available
Contraindications: Hypersensitivity to bisoprolol • Severe
bradycardia; 2nd or 3rd degree

---

italic = common side effects   **bold** = life-threatening reactions

heart block • CHF (unless resulting from tachycardia) • Cardiogenic shock

ADVERSE EFFECTS

CNS: *Headache,* dizziness, depression, drowsiness
Resp: Dyspnea, wheezing
CV: ***Bradycardia,*** hypotension, chest pain, peripheral edema, **CHF**
GI: diarrhea, elevated liver enzymes
Endo: Blocked symptoms of hypoglycemia/hyperthyroidism
Hema: Thrombocytopenia
Misc: Lupus syndrome

TOXICITY/OVERDOSE

Symptoms: Symptomatic bradycardia, profound hypotension, heart failure, advanced heart block, bronchospasm, hypoglycemia
Management: After recent ingestion, implement guidelines for management of acute overdosage (Appendix I) • **Symptomatic bradycardia, heart block:** Atropine, isoproterenol according to ACLS guidelines (Appendix P) • **Bronchospasm:** Isoproterenol, aminophylline • **Heart failure:** Inotropic agents (e.g., dobutamine, dopamine), diuretics, possible digoxin • **Hypotension:** Elevate legs, administer IV fluids; use vasopressors (e.g., norepinephrine) if severe and refractory to inotropic agents

INTERACTIONS

antidiabetics Prolonged recovery from hypoglycemic episodes; inhibition of hypoglycemia-associated tachycardia
antihypertensives Profound hypotension

calcium channel blockers ↓ BP, slowed AV conduction, extreme bradycardia
disopyramide Additive negative inotropy, reduced CO
epinephrine Beta effects of epinephrine blocked, resulting in unopposed alpha stimulation (severe hypertension, dysrhythmias); reduced effectiveness in anaphylaxis
lidocaine ↑ Lidocaine levels; negative inotropy; decreased CO

PATIENT CARE IMPLICATIONS

• Identify patients with COPD, asthma. Monitor closely; avoid high-dose therapy (>20 mg/day), which may precipitate bronchospasm.
• Gradually withdraw therapy to avoid rebound hypertension, angina, possible acute MI.
• Observe patients with hyperthyroidism for symptoms of thyrotoxicosis (e.g., tachycardia, hypertension) when withdrawing therapy.
Vital signs/hemodynamics: As available, observe ECG for heart block, significant bradycardia, prolonged PR, widened QRS. If present, consult physician before administering next dose • Measure CVP, PAP, PCWP, CO as available. Report decreased CO or increased filling pressures associated with other symptoms of heart failure • Monitor frequently if antidysrhythmics or other antihypertensive agents used.
Physical assessment: •Assess for perfusion/oxygenation deficit: decreased level of consciousness, activity intolerance, hypotension, chest discomfort, dizziness. • Auscultate lung fields for basilar crackles, espe-

cially with CHF or cardiomyopathy. • Assess for respiratory distress in patients with history of COPD or cardiac impairment. • Assess patients with diabetes for sweating, because tachycardia/tremors associated with hypoglycemia may be blocked by therapy.

Laboratory tests: Monitor: Blood glucose, liver enzymes, creatinine, cholesterol, triglycerides, CBC • Blood glucose frequently in patients with diabetes

PATIENT/FAMILY TEACHING

Purpose of medication is to lower high BP • Change positions slowly to avoid dizziness and low BP, particularly when getting out of bed in morning. • Report breathing difficulty, palpitations, dizziness, activity intolerance, chest pain, depression, rash, unusual bleeding. • Avoid excessive amounts of coffee, tea, caffeinated soft drinks, which may counteract drug's BP-lowering effects.

Outpatient: Take exactly as prescribed. Do not stop taking medicine even if you feel better. If medication is abruptly discontinued, you may develop dangerously high BP, irregular heart beats, chest pain. • Check resting pulse each day, BP each week. Contact health care provider if pulse <50 or BP significantly different • Medication is not a cure for high BP; other therapies, including life-style modifications, must be continued. • May cause drowsiness; avoid driving and other activities requiring mental alertness until individual response to drug known • Alcohol ingestion may cause extreme dizziness/drowsiness. • Consult

health care provider before taking nonprescription preparations. • Carry medical ID card identifying drug, dosage, health information. • Notify physician/dentist of therapy before any treatment. • Medicine blocks elevated HR and BP, so hyperthyroid patients and patients with diabetes must be aware of other symptoms of crisis.

AVAILABLE FORMS

Tablets

---

bretylium tosylate
(bre-til'ee-um to-sol'ate)
Bretylate ✦, Bretylol

Classifications: Antidysrhythmic, membrane-stabilizer, Vaughan-Williams Class III

USUAL DOSE

IM, adults: 5-10 mg/kg, undiluted; repeat q1-2h to suppress dysrhythmias; maintenance, 5-10 mg/kg q6h • Do not use IM route during cardiac arrest.

Direct IV, adults: Life-threatening dysrhythmias: Initial bolus of 5 mg/kg (350-500 mg): If not converted, increase next dose to 10 mg/kg (700-1,000 mg); repeat as necessary, usually q15-30min up to maximum of 30 mg/kg/24 hr (2.1-3.0 g) • Use lowest possible dose for dysrhythmia control.

Direct IV, children (unlabeled/investigational): Life-threatening dysrhythmias: Initial bolus of 2.5-5 mg/kg; if not converted may increase to 10 mg/kg; repeat as needed at 1-2 hr intervals up to maximum of 40 mg/kg/24 hr.

---

italic = common side effects   **bold** = life-threatening reactions

IV, intermit inf, adults: Non–life-threatening dysrhythmias: 5-10 mg/kg q1-2h to suppress dysrhythmias; maintenance, 5-10 mg/kg q6h or continuous infusion
IV, cont inf: 1-2 mg/min; titrate to control ventricular dysrhythmias. • Indicated only after successful suppression of ventricular dysrhythmias with IV bolus or loading dose

ADMINISTRATION

IM: Administer no more than 5 ml at one injection site. Rotate subsequent injection sites.
• Avoid injection near a major nerve.
V Direct IV: Life-threatening dysrhythmias: Administer as bolus over 1 min. • Non–life-threatening dysrhythmias: Administer dilute solution over at least 8 min. • Rapid administration may cause nausea/vomiting.
IV, cont inf: Start at 1 mg/min, increase to 2 mg/min as needed for dysrhythmia control.

PREPARATION

IV, cont inf: Dilute 500 mg in 50 ml D_5W or 0.9% NaCl.
• Use infusion pump.

DILUTION	CONCENTRATION
500 mg/500 ml	1 mg/ml
500 mg/250 ml	2 mg/ml

More concentrated solutions may be used if necessary to limit fluid intake.
Compatible fluids: D_5W, 0.9% NaCl, LR, prepared combinations of these solutions.
Stability: Solution stable for 48 hr at room temperature

ACTIONS

Delays repolarization; prolongs action potential duration, effective refractory period; conduction velocity not affected • Decreases disparity in action potential duration between ischemic/infarcted tissue and normal myocardium; assists in control of reentrant tachycardias • Initially causes release of stored endogenous norepinephrine from postganglionic nerve terminals, resulting in transient tachycardia, BP elevation, possible dysrhythmias; in approximately 20 min, sympathetic blockade ensues, blocking further norepinephrine release.

PHARMACOKINETICS

ROUTE	ONSET	PEAK	DURATION
IM	20-120 min	Within 6 hr	Up to 24 hr
IV	Minutes	Within 1 hr	6-24 hr

DISTRIBUTION
Wide; selectively accumulates in sympathetic ganglia
ELIMINATION
Excreted unchanged by kidneys; half-life 5-10 hr

Therapeutic level: 0.5-1.5 µg/ml

INDICATIONS

Suppression/prevention of ventricular fibrillation, pulseless ventricular tachycardia, other serious ventricular dysrhythmias when first-line antidysrhythmics (e.g., lidocaine) ineffective

PRECAUTIONS/ CONTRAINDICATIONS

Precautions: Norepinephrine-related dysrhythmias and ↑ BP may occur during first 20 min after administration. • ↓ BP often occurs when sympathetic blockade ensues (after first 20

B

min). • Consider dosage reduction in patients with renal failure to avoid toxicity.

Use caution with: Fixed CO (e.g., severe pulmonary hypertension, aortic stenosis), because of ↓ ability to compensate for drug-related ↓ BP • Digitalized patients; use only if dysrhythmia life-threatening and not related to cardiac glycoside toxicity. • Children: Safety/efficacy not established

ⓒ Pregnancy category: Use only if safer alternatives not available.

Contraindications: Hypersensitivity to bretylium • Commercially prepared solution contraindicated with hypersensitivity to corn

ADVERSE EFFECTS

CNS: Dizziness, vertigo, syncope

CV: **Initial exacerbation of dysrhythmias** (e.g., bradycardia, tachycardia, PVCs); *hypertension; hypotension,* angina, chest pressure

GI: *Nausea/vomiting* (rapid Direct IV), diarrhea, hiccups

Derm: *Soreness at IM injection site,* rash, flushing

TOXICITY/OVERDOSE

Symptoms: ↑ BP, ↓ BP, dysrhythmias, nausea/vomiting

Management: Hypertension: Use short-acting hypotensive agent such as nitroprusside; monitor closely because hypotension follows initial hypertension. • **Symptomatic hypotension:** Elevate legs, administer IV fluids; use vasopressors (e.g., dopamine, norepinephrine) if unresponsive to initial measures. Use cautiously because pressor effects are enhanced by bretylium.

INTERACTIONS

antidysrhythmics (e.g., lidocaine, procainamide, propranolol, quinidine) Additive or antagonistic effects; ↑ risk of toxicity

antihypertensives Excessive hypotension

Y-SITE COMPATIBILITIES

Amiodarone, amrinone, diltiazem, dobutamine, famotidine, isoproterenol, potassium chloride, ranitidine

Y-SITE INCOMPATIBILITIES

Phenytoin

PATIENT CARE IMPLICATIONS

• Correct hypoxia, electrolyte/acid-base imbalance before and throughout therapy; O_2 therapy usually indicated

• Anticipate/prepare for possible nausea/vomiting in conscious patients.

• Keep bed in low position with side rails up for at least 12 hr after infusion discontinued. Use caution with initial ambulation.

• For continuous infusion, use infusion pump.

Vital signs/hemodynamics: Continuously monitor ECG for resolution of ventricular dysrhythmias, onset of new dysrhythmias. • Evaluate bedside and 12-lead ECG (as available) for ST segment depression/elevation. • Monitor BP, HR q5min throughout bolus injection or IV loading and frequently (according to stability, titration schedule) during IV infusion. • Monitor O_2 saturation via pulse oximeter, as available.

---

italic = common side effects   **bold** = life-threatening reactions

Physical assessment: Assess for perfusion/oxygenation deficit: ↓ level of consciousness, chest pain, breathing difficulty, hypotension, dizziness.
Laboratory tests: Monitor: ABGs, electrolytes • Plasma levels; therapeutic level, 0.5-1.5 µg/ml

PATIENT/FAMILY TEACHING

Purpose of medication is to regulate heartbeats; frequent monitoring necessary because of serious side effects. • Call for assistance with position changes. Do not get out of bed until instructed by nurse. • Report chest pain, breathing difficulty, palpitations, dizziness.

AVAILABLE FORMS

Concentrate for IV/IM use • Prepared solution for IV infusion

bumetanide
(byoo-met'a-nide)
Bumex

Classification: Sulfonamide-type loop diuretic

USUAL DOSE

PO, adults: 0.5-2.0 mg once daily in AM; may repeat in 4-5 hr if initial diuretic effect insufficient • **Long-term therapy:** Administer qod or once daily for 3-4 days, then 1-2 days without therapy. • Maximum daily dose, 10 mg
Direct IV/IM, adults: 0.5-1.0 mg; repeat q2-3h as needed up to maximum daily dose of 10 mg. • Initiate PO therapy as soon as possible.

IV, cont inf, adults: 2-3 mg/hr (33-50 µg/min) • Maximum daily dose, 10 mg • Initiate PO therapy as soon as possible.

ADMINISTRATION

▼**Direct IV, adults:** Inject each dose slowly over 1-2 min. Dilution not necessary
IV, cont inf, adults: Titrate infusion of 2-3 mg/hr (33-50 µg/min) to desired diuresis and preload reduction. For example, infuse 25 mg/250 ml solution at 20 ml/hr to yield dose of 2 mg/hr (33 µg/min). Use rate-controlling device.

PREPARATION

IV, cont inf: Generally, concentrated solutions such as 25 mg/250 ml (0.1 mg/ml) used to limit total fluid intake; other concentrations may be used.
Compatible fluids: D_5W, 0.9% NaCl, LR, prepared combinations of these solutions; use within 24 hr of mixing.

ACTIONS

Produces rapid diuresis • Inhibits reabsorption of electrolytes in ascending limb of loop of Henle; decreases sodium, chloride reabsorption; increases excretion of sodium, chloride, potassium, calcium, magnesium, hydrogen, ammonium, bicarbonate, phosphate • Excessive losses of potassium, hydrogen, chloride may induce metabolic alkalosis. • Beneficial effects for patients with CHF include reduced plasma volume, decreased BP, increased Hct. • Potency 40 times that of furosemide

---

P pediatric   **G** geriatric   ▼ Direct IV

PHARMACOKINETICS

ROUTE	ONSET	PEAK	DURATION
PO	30-60 min	1-2 hr	4-6 hr
IV	5-10 min	15-45 min	4-6 hr

DISTRIBUTION

90% protein bound; crosses placenta

ELIMINATION

Metabolized in liver, eliminated in urine; half-life 60-90 min, ↑ with renal failure

INDICATIONS

To decrease edema associated with CHF, other conditions • As adjunct in treatment of acute pulmonary edema • Cautiously used when pulmonary edema is complication of cardiogenic shock, because overaggressive diuresis may result in reduced CO • Used as adjunct to dialysis, other therapy to reduce edema in patients with acute/chronic renal failure • Used cautiously to reduce edema associated with nephrotic syndrome, hepatic cirrhosis

PRECAUTIONS/CONTRAINDICATIONS

Precautions: Excessive diuresis may cause hypovolemia, hypokalemia, hypomagnesemia; severe hypotension, malignant dysrhythmias, sudden death may ensue • BUN, creatinine may be elevated, particularly in renal impairment, dehydration.
• Hearing impairment may occur, especially with high doses, rapid IV administration, concommitant use of other ototoxic agents (e.g., aminoglycosides). **Use caution with:** Renal impairment; reduced plasma volume may decrease GFR. • Cirrhotic, nephrotic, digitalized patients; profound hypokalemia possible. • Cirrhosis, hepatic failure; rapid fluctuations in fluids/electrolytes may prompt hepatic coma. • Sulfonamide sensitivity; may cause allergic reaction • Children: Safety/effectiveness not well established

c Pregnancy category: Use only if safer alternative unavailable.

Contraindications: Hypersensitivity to bumetanide • Anuria, increasing azotemia, oliguria • Untreated severe hepatic coma • Severe uncorrected electrolyte depletion

ADVERSE EFFECTS

CNS: Dizziness, headache
EENT: Tinnitus, hearing impairment
Resp: Alkalosis, compensatory respiratory depression
CV: *Orthostatic hypotension,* **hypotension,** ECG changes, dysrhythmias (PACs, PVCs, VT/VF), hypovolemia, hemoconcentration, **thromboembolism**
GI: Nausea, ↑ liver enzymes/bilirubin, precipitation of **hepatic coma** (preexisting liver disease)
GU: ↑ BUN/creatinine, **renal failure** (rare)
Endo: Hyperglycemia, glycosuria
Derm: Photosensitivity, rash, itching
F&E: *Hypokalemia, hypochloremia, hyponatremia,* metabolic alkalosis, hypophosphatemia, hypocalcemia
Hema: Anemia, leukopenia, thrombocytopenia
Misc: *Asymptomatic hyperuricemia, muscle cramps*

TOXICITY/OVERDOSE

Symptoms: Hypotension, dehydration, circulatory collapse • Electrolyte loss with weak-

---

italic = common side effects   **bold** = life-threatening reactions

ness, dizziness, mental confusion, dysrhythmias, cramps
Management: After recent ingestion, implement guidelines for management of acute overdose (Appendix I). • Replace electrolytes; closely monitor sodium, potassium balance.
• Support respiration as needed with O_2 and/or mechanical ventilation. • **Hypotension:** Elevate legs, administer IV fluids; if unresponsive to fluid replacement, use vasopressors (i.e., dopamine, norepinephrine). • Hemodialysis may be moderately effective.

INTERACTIONS
aminoglycosides ↑ Risk of ototoxicity
amphotericin B Severe potassium depletion
beta-blockers ↑ Risk of hypotension
calcium channel blockers ↑ Risk of hypotension
corticosteroids Severe potassium depletion
digitalis preparations Hypokalemia, hypomagnesemia, predisposition to digoxin toxicity, fatal cardiac dysrhythmias
diuretics Profound diuresis, severe hypokalemia
diuretics, potassium sparing Enhanced diuretic effects with less potassium loss
hypotensive agents ↑ Risk of hypotension
indomethacin, possibly other NSAIDs ↓ Diuretic effectiveness
nondepolarizing NMBAs (e.g., pancuronium) Prolonged neuromuscular blockade
phenytoin ↓ Diuretic response
probenecid ↓ Diuretic response

Y-SITE COMPATIBILITIES
Diltiazem, meperidine, morphine, piperacillin-tazobactam

Y-SITE INCOMPATIBILITIES
Dobutamine, milrinone

PATIENT CARE IMPLICATIONS
• Correct electrolyte/acid-base imbalance before initiating therapy.
• Potassium supplements are often necessary, especially in digitalized patients.
• Consider use of potassium-sparing diuretic (e.g., spironolactone, amiloride) if other diuretics will be used concomitantly.
• Insert Foley catheter before or immediately after initiation of IV therapy.
• Weigh patient daily.
• Adjust dose according to response to therapy; consider diuresis, edema, fluid balance, weight, electrolytes.
• If patients with pre–renal failure become progressively more oliguric or azotemic, discontinue use.
Vital signs/hemodynamics: Monitor BP frequently, especially with high-dose or parenteral therapy. • With parenteral therapy: Monitor VS, UO hourly with parenteral therapy; As available, continuously monitor ECG. Note presence of PVCs, dysrhythmias, hypokalemic ECG changes (e.g., flattened ST segment, T wave inversion, U wave). If present, check potassium level, correct as necessary. Digitalized patients should be carefully monitored for these and other dysrhythmias associated with

---

toxicity. • Hemodynamic monitoring strongly recommended for patients with severe CHF, cardiac failure associated with acute MI, cardiogenic shock, hemodynamic instability; monitor closely for overaggressive diuresis/excessive lowering of preload, which could produce ↓ CO.

Physical assessment: Assess for improvement in pulmonary edema: clear breath sounds, reduced neck vein distention. • Assess extremities, face, sacrum for improvement in edema. • Assess for signs/symptoms of electrolyte imbalance; dysrhythmias, confusion, dizziness, weakness, muscle cramps, fatigue, faintness, headache, paresthesias, thirst, vomiting. • Assess for perfusion/oxygenation deficit caused by hypovolemia: chest discomfort, ↓ level of consciousness, breathing difficulty, hypotension, dizziness. • Assess hearing, particularly in older adults, with parenteral or high-dose therapy, with concurrent use of other ototoxic agents (e.g., aminoglycosides).

Laboratory tests: Monitor: Electrolytes frequently, especially during parenteral or high-dose therapy. Promptly correct imbalances. • BUN, creatinine, bilirubin, liver enzymes, CBC **May cause:** Severe hypokalemia with dysrhythmias: ↑ / ↓ effects of other drugs, including cardiac glycosides, antidiabetic agents

PATIENT/FAMILY TEACHING

Purpose of drug is to encourage elimination of excess body fluid. • May cause dizziness, especially during initiation of therapy; use caution when changing positions, walking. • Immediately report signs/symptoms of heart failure: breathing difficulty, palpitations, dizziness, activity intolerance, chest pain; electrolyte imbalance: confusion, weakness, dizziness, fatigue, faintness, headache, tingling/numbness, muscle cramps, persistent thirst, nausea, vomiting.

Outpatient: Take medication in morning. Never double doses. • Continue taking medication as prescribed even if you feel better. Drug controls but does not cure hypertension/CHF. • If GI upset occurs, take with food or milk. • Alcohol, hot weather, vigorous activity, prolonged standing make dizziness more likely. • Take potassium supplements as prescribed, particularly if also taking digoxin. • Use sunscreen, wear protective clothing to prevent photosensitivity reactions. • Weigh twice/wk, report weight gain or edema.

AVAILABLE FORMS

Parenteral for IV admixture/IM use • Tablets

calcium chloride

Classification: Electrolyte replacement agent

USUAL DOSE

IV, adult: 500 mg-1 g or 7-14 mEq (5-10 ml) of 10% solution, up to 2 g with acute calcium channel blocker toxicity. 10 ml 10% solution (1 g) contains 272 mg or 1.36 mEq of calcium. In cardiac resuscitation may repeat q10min; otherwise base dose on

---

calcium deficit • **Hyperkalemic ECG changes:** 100 mg-1 g (1-10 ml); titrate to ECG changes.

🅟 IV, children: 15-50 mg/kg/dose. In cardiac resuscitation may repeat q10min; otherwise base dose on calcium deficit.

ADMINISTRATION

Verify catheter placement before injection/infusion; inadvertent perivascular injection may cause severe tissue necrosis.

▼ Direct IV: Injection recommended only in emergency situations when rapid calcium replacement is necessary • Inject dilute (5%) or undiluted (10%) solution SLOWLY at rate not to exceed 50-100mg/min (0.5-1.0 ml/min). • Dilution recommended to reduce vein irritation • Stop or slow injection for burning or discomfort.
• Use large vein, small needle/catheter. • Do not administer **🅟** via scalp veins in children
• *Rapid injection may cause hypotension, bradycardia, cardiac arrest.*
IV, intermit inf: Preferred route • Administer dilute solution over 30-60 min. • Use large vein, small needle/catheter.

PREPARATION

Direct IV: May dilute each ml with equal amount of sterile water for injection to yield 5% solution (recommended)
IV, intermit inf: Dilute in 50-100 ml compatible IV solution.
Compatible fluids: D_5W, 0.9% NaCl, LR, most common IV solutions

ACTIONS

Basic element essential for growth/maintenance of nerve, muscle, bone tissue • Necessary for transmission of nerve impulses; contraction of cardiac, smooth, skeletal muscles; renal function; respiration; blood clotting • Important in regulation of neurotransmitters, hormones, amino acid metabolism • IV administration improves vascular tone/myocardial contractility in hypocalcemic states; CO, BP usually increase. • 10 ml calcium chloride contains 13.6 mEq calcium, 3 times amount contained in same volume of calcium gluconate.

PHARMACOKINETICS

ROUTE	ONSET	PEAK	DURATION
IV	Immed	Rapid	Up to 2 hr

DISTRIBUTION
Wide; 45% bound to plasma proteins
ELIMINATION
Excreted in feces and urine

INDICATIONS

IV: Rapid electrolyte replacement in severe hypocalcemia or emergency situations; calcium gluconate preferred in nonemergency situations • Hypocalcemic tetany, such as that associated with parathyroid deficiency
• Hypocalcemia associated with transfusion of citrated blood
• Hypotension associated with overdose of calcium channel blockers • Antidote for magnesium sulfate • Hyperkalemic ECG changes • Immediately after cardiac surgery to improve vascular tone, myocardial contractility • In seriously hypotensive patients who respond poorly to fluids/vasopressors when hypocalcemia possible
• During cardiac resuscitation, only for hypocalcemia, hyperkalemia, calcium channel blocker

toxicity • To relieve muscle spasms associated with insect bites/stings (e.g., black widow spider) • To decrease capillary permeability in sensitivity reactions
Unlabeled/investigational:
To antagonize neuromuscular blockade associated with use of aminoglycoside antibiotics

PRECAUTIONS/CONTRAINDICATIONS
Precautions: Carefully adjust dose to serum calcium levels. • For IV use only; may cause tissue necrosis with IM, SC, perivascular injection • Rapid injection may cause hypotension, dysrhythmias, bradycardia, cardiac arrest. • 3 times potency of calcium gluconate
Use caution with: Renal impairment; avoid overtreatment of hypocalcemia; contributes to acidosis. • Sarcoidosis • Cardiac disease • Concurrent use of cardiac glycosides • COPD, cor pulmonale, respiratory acidosis, respiratory failure; because of acidifying effects
c **Pregnancy category:** Use only if safer alternative unavailable.
Contraindications: Ventricular fibrillation • Hypercalcemia

ADVERSE EFFECTS
CV: Hypotension, hot or flushing sensation, bradycardia, shortened ST segment/QT interval, prolonged PR interval, **ventricular dysrhythmias, cardiac arrest**
GI: Chalky taste, nausea, vomiting
Local: *Pain, burning at injection site;* necrosis with extravasation

TOXICITY/OVERDOSE
Symptoms: Hypotension, dysrhythmias, cardiac arrest with IV use • Hypercalcemia: anorexia, nausea, vomiting • Lethargy, weakness, confusion, paresthesias, coma
Management: After recent ingestion, implement guidelines for management of acute overdose (Appendix I). • **Critical overdose:** Consider use of disodium edetate as chelating agent.

INTERACTIONS
digoxin Dysrhythmias, ↑ risk of digoxin toxicity
tetracyclines Tetracycline inactivation when administered together

Y-SITE COMPATIBILITIES
Amrinone, dobutamine, epinephrine, esmolol, morphine

Y-SITE INCOMPATIBILITIES
Potassium phosphate (concentration dependent), sodium bicarbonate, tetracycline, tobramycin

PATIENT CARE IMPLICATIONS
• Vitamin D deficiency contributes to hypocalcemia in critically ill patients who are likely to be chronically ill, are malnourished, and have limited exposure to sunlight.
IV
• Many precautions necessary with IV use; see Administration.
• Hypotensive patients who respond poorly to fluids/vasopressors may be hypocalcemic. Restoration of serum calcium may improve vascular tone, myocardial contractility.

---

italic = common side effects   **bold** = life-threatening reactions

• Avoid use of IV calcium in patients receiving digoxin, other cardiac glycosides. If use necessary, administer slowly in small increments with continuous ECG monitoring. Monitor for digoxin toxicity.

Vital signs/hemodynamics: IV: Continuously monitor ECG for bradycardia, ECG changes associated with hypercalcemia: shortened ST segment/QT interval, prolonged PR interval, ventricular dysrhythmias. If present, slow or stop injection, consult physician. • Assess BP frequently with large doses or rapid administrations. of large doses or written short periods (e.g., <1 hr). • As available, measure CO/CI, SV for improved contractility.

Physical assessment: Assess for hypocalcemia: numbness/tingling of fingers and around mouth, Chvostek's or Trousseau's sign, muscle twitching, tetany, seizures • Assess for hypercalcemia: anorexia, nausea, vomiting, lethargy, confusion, weakness. • Assess for improved myocardial contractilitiy: mentation, peripheral perfusion, UO ≥5 ml/kg/hr.

Laboratory tests: Monitor: Serum calcium levels • Albumin in critically ill patients • Digoxin levels with concurrent cardiac glycoside therapy • Only ionized serum calcium is physiologically active; approx 45% bound to plasma proteins. Change in albumin of 1 g/dl results in serum calcium change of 0.8 mg/dl. • Calcium administration results in higher-than-normal levels in patients who have received transfusions of citrated blood; however, most calcium bound to citrate and inactive.

PATIENT/FAMILY TEACHING

Purpose of medication is to replace calcium. • Remain recumbent for 30-60 min after IV dose.

AVAILABLE FORMS

Parenteral for IV use

---

calcium gluconate
Kalcinate

Classification: Electrolyte replacement

USUAL DOSE

PO, adults: 1-2 g once daily
P PO, children: 45-65 mg/kg once daily
IV, adult: 500 mg-2 g or 2.3-9.3 mEq (5-20 ml of 10% solution); up to 6 g (60 ml) may be given in IV infusion. 10 ml of 10% solution is equivalent to 1 g, or 4.5 mEq of calcium.
• **Magnesium intoxication:** 4.5-9 mEq or 1-2 g (10-20 ml)
• **Calcium replacement with massive transfusion:** 500 mg (5 ml) for each 500 ml citrated blood; usually after ≥2 U transfused
P IV, children: 100-200 mg/kg/dose. In cardiac resuscitation may repeat q10min; otherwise base dose on calcium deficit.

ADMINISTRATION

PO: Administer 1-1.5 hr after meals or with milk to improve absorption.
V Direct IV: Injection recommended only in emergency situations when rapid calcium replacement necessary • SLOW-

LY inject each dose of 50 mg or less (0.5 ml) over 1 min • Dilution recommended to reduce vein irritation • Stop or slow injection for burning or discomfort. • Use large vein, small needle/catheter. • Do not administer via scalp veins in children. • *Rapid injection may cause hypotension, bradycardia, cardiac arrest.*

IV, cont inf: Preferred route • Administer dilute solution over 30-60 min or 12-24 hr if diluted in large volume of fluid. • Use large vein, small needle/catheter.

PREPARATION

Direct IV: May dilute each ml with equal amount of sterile water for injection (recommended)
IV, intermit inf: Dilute in 50-100 ml compatible IV solution.
Compatible fluids: D_5W, 0.9% NaCl, LR, most common IV solutions

ACTIONS

Basic element essential for growth/maintenance of nerve, muscle, bone tissue • Necessary for transmission of nerve impulses; contraction of cardiac, smooth, skeletal muscles; renal function; respiration; blood clotting • Important in regulation of neurotransmitters, hormones, amino acid metabolism • IV administration improves vascular tone/myocardial contractility in hypocalcemic states; CO, BP usually increase. • Recent data show BP-lowering effects with PO use in young adults, pregnant women, some hypertensive patients. • 10 ml calcium gluconate contains 4.6 mEq calcium, 1/3 amount contained in same volume of calcium chloride.

PHARMACOKINETICS

ROUTE	ONSET	PEAK	DURATION
PO	Var	Var	6-8 hr
IV	Immed	Rapid	Up to 2 hr

DISTRIBUTION
Wide; 45% bound to plasma proteins
ELIMINATION
Most excreted in feces

INDICATIONS

PO: Treatment/prevention of calcium deficiency, such as occurs with hypoparathyroidism, vitamin D deficiency, achlorhydria, chronic diarrhea, steatorrhea, sprue, pregnancy/lactation, menopause, pancreatitis, renal failure, alkalosis, hyperphosphatemia, diuretic/anticonvulsant therapy
IV: Electrolyte replacement with hypocalcemia • Hypocalcemic tetany, such as that associated with parathyroid deficiency • Hypocalcemia associated with transfusion of citrated blood • Antidote for magnesium sulfate • To relieve muscle spasms associated with insect bites/stings (e.g., black widow spider) • To decrease capillary permeability in sensitivity reactions
Unlabeled/investigational: To antagonize neuromuscular blockade associated with use of aminoglycoside antibiotics

PRECAUTIONS/ CONTRAINDICATIONS

Precautions: READ LABEL CAREFULLY; DO NOT CONFUSE WITH CALCIUM CHLORIDE. • Carefully adjust dose to serum calcium levels. • Rapid injection may cause hypotension, dysrhythmias, brady-

---

cardia, cardiac arrest. • Absorp-
G tion of PO doses ↓ in older
adults

Use caution with: Renal impairment; avoid overtreatment of hypocalcemia; contributes to acidosis. • Sarcoidosis • Cardiac disease • Concurrent use of cardiac glycosides • COPD, cor pulmonate, respiratory acidosis, respiratory failure; contributes to acidosis

c **Pregnancy category:** Use only if safer alternative unavailable.

Contraindications: Ventricular fibrillation • Hypercalcemia

ADVERSE EFFECTS

CV: Hypotension, hot or flushing sensations, bradycardia, shortened ST segment/QT interval, prolonged PR interval, **ventricular dysrhythmias, cardiac arrest**
GI: Chalky taste, *constipation,* nausea, vomiting, gastric irritation
Local: *Burning, pain at injection site;* phlebitis

TOXICITY/OVERDOSE

Symptoms: Hypotension, dysrhythmias, cardiac arrest with IV use • Hypercalcemia: anorexia, nausea, vomiting • Lethargy, weakness, confusion, paresthesias, coma
Management: After recent ingestion, implement guidelines for management of acute overdose (Appendix I). • **Critical overdose:** Consider use of disodium edetate as chelating agent.

INTERACTIONS

digoxin Dysrhythmias, ↑ risk of digoxin toxicity

tetracyclines Tetracycline inactivation when administered together

Y-SITE COMPATIBILITIES

Cefazolin, ciprofloxacin, dobutamine, enalaprilat, epinephrine, famotidine, heparin, labetalol, netilmicin, piperacillin-tazobactam, potassium chloride, sodium bicarbonate

Y-SITE INCOMPATIBILITIES

Ampicillin, cephalothin, cefazolin, fluconazole, potassium phosphate (concentration dependent), tobramycin

PATIENT CARE IMPLICATIONS

• Vitamin D deficiency contributes to hypocalcemia in critically ill patients who are likely to be chronically ill, are malnourished, and have limited exposure to sunlight.
PO
• Administer 1-1.5 hours after meals or with milk to improve absorption.
• Absorption of PO calcium increases during pregnancy, with acidic intestinal pH; decreases with alkaline pH, steatorrhea,
G advanced age.
IV
• Hypotensive patients who respond poorly to fluids/vasopressors may be hypocalcemic. Restoration of serum calcium may improve vascular tone, myocardial contractility.
• Avoid use of IV calcium in patients receiving digoxin, other cardiac glycosides. If use necessary, administer slowly in small increments with continuous ECG monitoring. Monitor for digoxin toxicity

Vital signs/hemodynamics:
IV: Continuously monitor ECG for bradycardia, ECG changes associated with hypercalcemia: shortened ST segment/QT interval, prolonged PR interval, ventricular dysrhythmias. If present, slow or stop injection, consult physician. • Assess BP frequently with IV administration of large doses or within short periods (e.g., <1 hr). • As indicated, measure CO/CI, SV for improved contractility.

Physical assessment: Assess for hypocalcemia: numbness/tingling of fingers and around mouth, Chvostek's or Trousseau's sign, muscle twitching, tetany, seizures. • Assess for hypercalcemia: anorexia, nausea, vomiting, lethargy, confusion, weakness. • Assess for improved myocardial contractility: LOC, peripheral perfusion, UO ≥5 ml/kg/hr.

Laboratory tests: Monitor: Serum calcium levels • Albumin in critically ill patients • Digoxin levels with concurrent cardiac glycoside therapy • Only ionized serum calcium is physiologically active; approx 45% bound to plasma proteins. Change in albumin of 1 g/dl results in serum calcium change of 0.8 mg/dl. • Calcium administration results in higher-than-normal levels in patients who have received transfusion of citrated blood; however, most calcium bound to citrate and inactive.

PATIENT/FAMILY TEACHING

Purpose of medication is to replace calcium. • Remain recumbent for 30-60 min after IV dose. • Take PO formulations 1-1.5 hrs after meals. • Vitamin D aids absorption.

AVAILABLE FORMS

Parenteral for IV injection • Tablets

captopril
(kap'toe-pril)
Capoten, Apo-Capto ✦
captopril with hydrochlorothiazide
Capozide

Classifications: Angiotensin-converting enzyme (ACE) inhibitor, antihypertensive

USUAL DOSE

PO, adults: 25-150 mg bid-tid; start with 25-mg and increase as needed to control BP, improve heart failure. • Up to 450 mg/day has been used in hypertensive crisis (with constant monitoring). Use lower dose with concurrent diuretic therapy

PO, older adults/renal impairment: 6.25-12.5 mg bid-tid • Gradually increase dose to control BP, improve heart failure. Usual dose, 25 mg tid

ACTIONS

Inhibits ACE, which prevents conversion of angiotensin I to angiotensin II, a potent vasoconstrictor • BP reduced directly by decreased vascular tone, indirectly by reduction in aldosterone secretion and therefore decreased sodium/water retention; bradykinin accumulation/prostaglandin release may contribute to hypotensive effects; generally reduces SBP, DBP by 15%-20% • Little or no effect on HR or contractility (in ab-

---

italic = common side effects   **bold** = life-threatening reactions

sence of heart failure) • In CHF patients, SVR, PVR, MAP, PCWP, right atrial pressure are decreased, creating reductions in both preload, afterload. • Renal blood flow may increase slightly, but GFR usually unchanged. • Unlike some other ACE inhibitors, captopril does not require conversion in liver to be activated.

PHARMACOKINETICS

ROUTE	ONSET	PEAK	DURATION
PO, std	15 min	1-2 hr	2-6 hr; up to 12 hr with high doses

DISTRIBUTION

Widely distributed except into CNS tissue; 25%-30% protein bound

ELIMINATION

Eliminated in urine; half-life <2 hr, but increases to 6½ days in severe renal failure

INDICATIONS

BP reduction in mild to severe hypertension; may be used in conjunction with other hypotensive agents, diuretics; effective in patients with renovascular/malignant hypertension • Along with cardiac glycosides, diuretics to improve cardiac function, relieve symptoms, improve exercise tolerance in CHF patients

PRECAUTIONS/ CONTRAINDICATIONS

Precautions: Initial dose may cause profound hypotension or severe allergic reaction, probably related to bradykinin accumulation. • May cause hyperkalemia, esp. with renal insufficiency, diabetes mellitus, use of potassium-sparing diuretics/potassium supplements

Use caution with: Renal impairment; reduce dose. • Colla-

gen vascular disease, immunosuppression, renal impairment; risk of bone marrow depression • Diuretic use, hypovolemia, hyponatremia, surgery, anesthesia; may cause severe hypotension • Coronary artery/cerebrovascular disease, CHF, aortic stenosis; hypotensive episodes may worsen condition. • Patients with diabetes may precipitate **(P)** hypoglycemia • Children: Safety/efficacy of use not established

C Pregnancy category: C: First trimester–Use only if safer alternative unavailable. D: Second/Third trimester–can cause fetal death

Contraindications: Hypersensitivity to this or other ACE inhibitors • Bilateral renal artery stenosis

ADVERSE EFFECTS

CNS: *Headache, dizziness, fatigue,* confusion, depression
CV: *Transient or orthostatic hypotension,* **severe hypotension,** tachycardia, palpitations, chest pain, **MI** (rare)
Resp: *Cough,* nasal congestion, bronchospasm, dyspnea, **angioedema/stridor** (allergic reaction)
GI: *Loss of taste,* anorexia, **hepatitis** (rare)
GU: Proteinuria, **decreased renal function, nephrotic syndrome**
Derm: *Rash,* pruritus, urticaria
Hema: Neutropenia, agranulocytosis, eosinophilia
Misc: Muscle cramps, hyponatremia, hyperkalemia, photosensitivity

TOXICITY/OVERDOSE

Symptoms: Hypotension, ↓ LOC, severe hypotension may cause MI or CVA

Management: After recent ingestion, implement guidelines for management of acute overdose (Appendix I). • Support respiration as needed with O_2 and/or mechanical ventilation. • **Hypotension:** Elevate legs, administer IV fluids; usually responsive to intravascular volume expansion using 0.9% NaCl or LR. • Hemodialysis facilitates drug removal.

INTERACTIONS

alcohol ↑ Risk of hypotension
antacids ↓ Captopril absorption
calcium channel blockers Profound hypotension
digoxin ↑ Serum digoxin levels
diuretics Additive hypotension
diuretics, potassium-sparing Hyperkalemia
indomethacin, other NSAIDS ↓ Captopril effectiveness
lithium ↑ lithium levels/ ↑ risk of toxicity
phenothiazines Hypotension
potassium supplements Hyperkalemia
probenecid Potentiation of captopril effects
sympathetic blockers Profound hypotension

PATIENT CARE IMPLICATIONS

• Correct hypovolemia before administration
• Evaluate renal function before initiating therapy.
• Protect patient from injury associated with orthostatic hypotension, especially when initiating therapy.

• Vomiting, diarrhea, excessive perspiration, dehydration may cause excessive ↓ in BP.
• Monitor fluid balance; weigh daily.
• Food reduces absorption. Administer 1 hr before or 2 hr after meals.

Vital signs/hemodynamics: Monitor BP, HR at 1–2 hr intervals when initiating therapy and with hypertensive crisis, with acute CHF, when hypotensive agents/diuretics also used, until patient stable. • Administer IV 0.9% NaCl as needed for transient hypotensive episodes during initial therapy. • As available, continuously monitor ECG for PVCs, ST segment elevation/depression, especially when initiating therapy in patients with CHF or CAD.

Physical assessment: Assess for perfusion/oxygenation deficit: chest discomfort, ↓ level of consciousness, breathing difficulty, activity intolerance, hypotension, dizziness. • Frequently assess neurologic status until BP controlled. • Assess for fluid volume overload (bibasilar crackles, dyspnea, peripheral edema, neck vein distention, weight gain). • Assess for progressive edema, proteinuria, other evidence of nephrotic syndrome.

Laboratory tests: Monitor: BUN, creatinine, bilirubin, liver enzymes, CBC with differential • Electrolytes for hyperkalemia, hyponatremia: • ↑ risk of hyperkalemia with renal impairment, CHF, diabetes mellitus, or use of potassium-sparing diuretics, potassium supplements, salt substitutes • Blood glucose levels in patients with diabetes

---

italic = common side effects   **bold** = life-threatening reactions

• Digoxin, lithium levels as appropriate

PATIENT/FAMILY TEACHING

Purpose of drug is to lower BP and/or relieve symptoms of heart failure. • May cause orthostatic hypotension/dizziness, especially during initiation of therapy; use caution when changing positions, walking. Alcohol, hot weather, vigorous activity, vomiting, diarrhea, dehydration, prolonged standing make these symptoms more likely. • Lie down immediately if lightheaded or dizzy. • Medication is not a cure for high BP, and other therapies, including lifestyle modifications, must be continued. • Promptly report rash; swelling of extremities; fever, sore throat, infection; chest pain; swelling of face, lips, tongue, throat; difficulty breathing. • May interfere with taste perception or cause persistent coughing; report these effects if bothersome.

Outpatient: Take medication exactly as prescribed. Do not stop taking medicine even if you feel better. If medication abruptly discontinued, you may develop dangerously high BP. • Avoid driving and other activities requiring mental alertness until individual response to drug known. • Avoid salt substitutes or other foods high in potassium unless otherwise directed. • Weigh twice/wk; report weight gain or edema. • Consult physician or pharmacist before taking cough, cold, or allergy preparations.

AVAILABLE FORMS

Tablets

---

cefaclor
(sef'a-klor)
Ceclor

Classification: Cephalosporin antibiotic, 2nd generation

USUAL DOSE

Administer with food or milk.
PO, adults; 250 mg q8h • **Severe infection:** 500 mg q8h
• **Severe renal impairment:** Use reduced dose and monitor closely.
 PO, children >1 mo: 20 mg/kg/24 hr in divided doses q8h
• **Severe infection:** 40 mg/kg/24 hr in divided doses: do not exceed 1 g/24 hr. Shake suspensions thoroughly before administration.

ACTIONS

2nd generation cephalosporin antibiotic; interference with bacterial cell wall synthesis/division results in bactericidal effects.
• Excellent activity against many gram-positive cocci, including penicillinase-producing and non–penicillinase-producing staphylococci/streptococci, but not methicillin-resistant staphylococci/enterococci • Active against *Haemophilus influenzae,* including ampicillin-resistant strains • Minimal activity against gram-negative organisms

---

PHARMACOKINETICS

ROUTE	ONSET	PEAK	DURATION
PO	30 min	30-60 min; slower when taken with food	Dose dependent

DISTRIBUTION

Widely distributed; CSF concentrations low

ELIMINATION

Excreted unchanged in urine; half-life 30-60 min

INDICATIONS

Otitis media, uncomplicated respiratory tract infections, especially when caused by *H. influenzae* or when penicillins, sulfonamides contraindicated • Mild to moderate infections of skin, soft tissue, urinary tract caused by susceptible organisms; often as follow-up therapy after parenteral cephalosporins • Penicillin preferred for treatment of streptococcal respiratory tract infections because of superior efficacy in preventing rheumatic fever

PRECAUTIONS/CONTRAINDICATIONS

Precautions: Bacterial or fungal overgrowth may occur.
Use caution with: Hypersensitivity to penicillin, other drugs; risk of allergic reaction • GI disease, especially colitis; risk of pseudomembranous colitis • Renal impairment
B Pregnancy category: Safety not clearly established
Contraindications: Hypersensitivity to cefaclor, any cephalosporin • Avoid use with history of immediate penicillin reaction.

ADVERSE EFFECTS

CNS: Hyperactivity, nervousness, confusion

GI: *Diarrhea,* nausea, vomiting, oral thrush, transient increases in AST/ALT/alkaline phosphatase, **pseudomembranous colitis**
GU: Vaginitis, transient increase in BUN or creatinine
Hema: Eosinophilia, thrombocytopenia, other blood dyscrasias
Derm: Rash, urticaria, pruritus
Misc: Superinfection, colonization; anaphylaxis, serum sickness, other allergic reactions

TOXICITY/OVERDOSE

Symptoms: Nausea, vomiting, epigastric distress, diarrhea, hematuria • Acute allergic reaction, including anaphylaxis • Pseudomembranous colitis with abdominal pain/diarrhea
Management: Discontinue drug. Initiate symptomatic/supportive measures. • After recent ingestion, implement guidelines for management of acute overdose (Appendix I). • For management of acute allergic reaction, see Appendix N. • Treat severe pseudomembranous colitis with oral vancomycin or metronidazole. • Hemodialysis probably is unnecessary.

INTERACTIONS

aminoglycosides (e.g., amikacin, gentamicin) Synergistic antibacterial activity; risk of nephrotoxicity
probenecid ↑ Cephalosporin blood levels

PATIENT CARE IMPLICATIONS

• Obtain specimens for culture and sensitivity before initiating antibiotic therapy. First dose may be given before results received.

---

italic = common side effects   **bold** = life-threatening reactions

• Determine previous antibiotic use, including reactions to penicillins, cephalosporins, Cross-reactivity with penicillin allergies may occur.
• Administer with food or milk to minimize gastric irritation. Food may slow onset of action but does not affect efficacy.

Vital signs: Monitor temperature for elevation at beginning and throughout therapy.

Physical assessment: Assess for improvement in primary infection or symptoms of super/suprainfection: appearance of sputum, urine, stool, wound drainage; presence of fever, candidiasis, vaginitis; WBC. • Observe for symptoms of hypersensitivity: rash, pruritus, wheezing, laryngeal edema, hypotension.
• Assess for pseudomembranous colitis: blood/mucus in stool, diarrhea, fever, abdominal pain. Symptoms may not appear for several weeks after cessation of therapy.

Laboratory tests: Monitor: Liver enzymes (e.g., ALT, AST, alkaline phosphatase) • Electrolytes, BUN, creatinine, especially in seriously ill/renal impaired patients, older adults
G • CBC with differential • **May cause:** False-positive urinary glucose using copper sulfate method (Clinitest, others); use enzyme-based test (Clinistix, Tes-Tape). • Positive direct antiglobulin (Coombs') test

PATIENT/FAMILY TEACHING

Purpose of drug is to limit growth of infection-causing bacteria. • Immediately report rash, swelling, intense itching, difficulty breathing, other signs of allergic reaction. • Report diarrhea, blood/mucus in stool, fever, abdominal pain, vaginal itching or discharge, furry growth on tongue. Do not take medicine for diarrhea without consulting health care provider.

Outpatient: Take with food or milk to minimize gastric irritation. • Take all of medication exactly as prescribed. Do not stop taking medicine even if you feel better. Failure to take all of antibiotic may result in recurrence or additional infection. Do not save or share unused medicine. • Keep oral suspensions refrigerated and shake well before use.

AVAILABLE FORMS

Capsules • PO suspension

cefazolin sodium
(sef'a-zoe-lin)
Ancef, Kefzol, Zolicef

Classification: Cephalosporin antibiotic, 1st generation

USUAL DOSE

IV/IM, adults: 250 mg-1.5 g q6-8h • **Severe infection:** Up to 12 g/24 hr in divided doses • **Renal impairment:** Initially 500 mg; maintenance dose according to creat. cl.

P **IV/IM, children >1 mo:** 25-50 mg/kg/24 hr in divided doses q6-8h • **Severe infection:** Up to 100 mg/kg/24 hr in divided doses

ADMINISTRATION

IM: Inject deep into large muscle mass (e.g., gluteus maximum, lateral thigh).
V **Direct IV:** Slowly inject each dose over 3-5 min

IV intermit: Infuse prepared solution over 15-30 min; 0.22-μm filter recommended.

PREPARATION

IM: Dilute with 2.0-2.5 ml of sterile water for injection or bacteriostatic water for injection; shake to dissolve. Do not use 0.9% NaCl for dilution of 1 g dose because hyperosmolar solution results (see table).

A	B	C	D
250 mg	2 ml	2 ml	125 mg/ml
500 mg	2 ml	2.2 ml	225 mg/ml
1 g	2.5 ml	3 ml	330 mg/ml

A, Vial size; B, volume of diluent; C, withdrawn volume; D, concentration of solution.

Direct IV: Reconstitute as described under IM injection. Further dilute with at least 10 ml sterile water for injection.

IV intermit: Reconstitute as described under IM injection. Further dilute by adding to 50- or 100-ml piggyback bags of D_5W or 0.9% NaCl.

Compatible fluids: D_5W, 0.9% NaCl, LR, prepared combinations of these solutions

Appearance: Light yellow to yellow

Stability: Reconstituted solution stable for 24 hr at room temperature

ACTIONS

First-generation cephalosporin antibiotic; interferes with bacterial cell wall synthesis/division • Excellent activity against gram-positive cocci, including penicillinase-producing and non–penicillinase-producing staphylococci/streptococci, but not methicillin-resistant staphylococci/enterococci • Limited activity against gram-negative bacteria; however, some strains of *Escherichia coli, Klebsiella pneumoniae, Proteus mirabilis* possibly susceptible • Not active against *Pseudomonas aeruginosa, Bacteroides fragilis,* many other gram-negative organisms • Poor CNS penetration

PHARMACOKINETICS

ROUTE	ONSET	PEAK	DURATION
IM	≤60 min	1-2 hr	Dose dependent
IV	Immed	5 min	Dose dependent

DISTRIBUTION

Widely distributed; CSF concentrations low

ELIMINATION

Excreted unchanged in urine; half-life 1.2-2.2 hr

INDICATIONS

Prevention of infection in clean, contaiminated surgery (e.g., cholecystectomy) or when infection could result in serious consequences (e.g., CV surgery, joint replacements) • Serious infections of lower respiratory tract, skin/soft tissue, abdomen/peritoneum, biliary tract, bones/joints, GU tract; septicemia caused by susceptible organisms • Preferred over 2nd/3rd generation cephalosporins for treatment of susceptible gram-positive infections • Limited use in gram-negative bacterial infections • Not indicated for meningitis because CNS penetration poor

PRECAUTIONS/ CONTRAINDICATIONS

Precautions: Bacterial or fungal overgrowth may occur.

Use caution with: Hypersensitivity to penicillin or other drugs; risk of allergic reaction • GI disease, especially colitis;

---

risk of pseudomembranous colitis • Renal impairment

B Pregnancy category: Safety not clearly established

Contraindications: Hypersensitivity to cefazolin, any cephalosporin • Avoid use with history of immediate penicillin reaction.

ADVERSE EFFECTS

CNS: Headache, dizziness, fatigue, **seizures** (high dose/renal insufficiency)

GI: *Diarrhea;* nausea, vomiting, abdominal pain, oral thrush, transient increases in AST/ALT/alkaline phosphatase, **pseudomembranous colitis**

GU: Transient increase in BUN or creatinine, **nephrotoxicity** (rare), vaginitis

Hema: Neutropenia, thrombocytopenia, other blood dyscrasias

Derm: Rash, hives, itching

Local: Pain at IM site, phlebitis at IV site

Misc: Superinfection, colonization; anaphylaxis, serum sickness, other allergic reactions

TOXICITY/OVERDOSE

Symptoms: Neuromuscular excitability/seizures, particularly in renal impairment • Acute allergic reaction, including anaphylaxis • Pseudomembranous colitis with abdominal pain/diarrhea

Management: Discontinue drug. Initiate symptomatic/supportive measures, including airway protection/anticonvulsant therapy. • For management of acute allergic reaction, see Appendix N. • Treat severe pseudomembranous colitis with PO vancomycin or metronidazole. • Hemodialysis or peritoneal dialysis may be effective in drug removal.

INTERACTIONS

aminoglycosides (e.g., amikacin, gentamicin) Synergistic antibacterial activity; risk of nephrotoxicity

chloramphenicol ↓ Bactericidal activity

probenecid ↑ Cephalosporin blood levels

Y-SITE COMPATIBILITIES

Acyclovir, atracurium, calcium gluconate diltiazem, enalaprilat, esmolol, famotidine, fluconazole, hydromorphone, insulin, labetalol, lidocaine, magnesium sulfate, meperidine, metronidazole, morphine, multivitamins, ondansetron, pancuronium bromide, vecuronium

Y-SITE INCOMPATIBILITIES

Amiodarone, aminoglycosides (e.g., amikacin, gentamicin, tobramycin), hetastarch, hydromorphone

PATIENT CARE IMPLICATIONS

• Obtain specimens for culture and sensitivity before initiating antibiotic therapy. First dose may be given before results received.

• Determine previous antibiotic use, including reactions to penicillins, cephalosporins. Cross-reactivity with penicillin allergies may occur.

• Have epinephrine, antihistamine, resuscitation equipment readily available for use with severe allergic reaction.

• Do not discharge patient for at least 30 min after antibiotic administration.

• High sodium content may contribute to edema, electrolyte

abnormalities, dysrhythmias, heart failure.

• Administer at separate site from aminoglycosides (e.g., amikacin, gentamicin, tobramycin); stagger schedules if both antibiotics prescribed.

Direct IV

• Reduce risk of thrombophlebitis by using large veins and small catheters/needles, rotating infusion sites, using 0.22-μm filter.

• IV route is preferred over IM route, and must be used for severe infections or when shock present.

Vital signs/hemodynamics: Monitor VS for indicators of infection, complications. • Monitor I&O for imbalance; Older, debilitated, seriously ill, or renal-impaired patients at greater risk for nephrotoxicity.

Physical assessment: Assess for improvement in primary infection or symptoms of super/suprainfection: appearance of sputum, urine, stool, wound drainage; presence of fever, candidiasis, vaginitis. • Observe for symptoms of hypersensitivity: rash, pruritus, wheezing, laryngeal edema, hypotension. • Assess for pseudomembranous colitis: blood/mucus in stool, diarrhea, fever, abdominal pain. Symptoms may not appear for several weeks after cessation of therapy.

Laboratory tests: Monitor: Liver enzymes (e.g., ALT, AST, alkaline phosphatase) • Electrolytes, BUN, creatinine, creat. cl., especially in seriously ill/renal-impaired patients, older adults • CBC with differential **May cause:** Falsely elevated serum albumin. • Positive direct antiglobulin (Coombs') test

PATIENT/FAMILY TEACHING

Purpose of drug is to limit growth of infection-causing bacteria. • Immediately report rash, swelling, intense itching, difficulty breathing, other signs of allergic reaction. Report diarrhea, blood/mucus in stool, fever, abdominal pain, vaginal itching or discharge, furry growth on tongue.

AVAILABLE FORMS

Parenteral for IV/IM use • Premixed solution of IV infusion

cefoperazone sodium
(sef-oh-per′a-zone)
Cefobid

Classification: Cephalosporin antibiotic, 3rd generation

USUAL DOSE

IV intermit inf/IM, adults: 1-2 g q12h **Severe infection:** 6-12 g/24 hr in divided doses, q6-12h • **Hepatic, biliary disease/renal impairment:** Use lower dose range; monitor serum levels if higher doses used. • **Dialysis:** Schedule dose at end of dialysis.

ADMINISTRATION

IM: Inject deep into large muscle mass (e.g., gluteus maximus, lateral thigh). Give in two different large muscles if 2-g dose used; IV route preferred for 2-g dose.

IV, intermit inf: Infuse prepared solution over 15-30 min. Discontinue primary IV line during infusion; 0.2-μm filter recommended.

IV, cont inf: Use concentration of 2-25 mg/ml.

---

italic = common side effects   **bold** = life-threatening reactions

PREPARATION

IM: Step 1: Dilute with sterile water for injection, shake vigorously to dissolve. Step 2: Add 2% lidocaine HC1 (see table).

A	B	C	D	E
1g	2.0 ml	0.6 ml	3 ml	333 mg/ml
	2.8 ml	1.0 ml	4ml	250 mg/ml
2g	3.8 ml	1.2 ml	6 ml	333 mg/ml

A, Vial size; B, volume of sterile water; C, volume of 2% lidocaine; D, withdrawn volume; E, concentration of solution.

IV: Dilute each 1 g with 5 ml sterile water for injection, D₅W, or 0.9% NaCl. Difficult to dissolve; prolonged, vigorous shaking is required. Wait for solution to clear, then further dilute by adding to 50- or 100-ml piggyback bags of D₅W or 0.9% NaCl or by adding 20-40ml compatible solution to 1-g piggyback vial or 40-80 ml to 2-g vial.

Compatible fluids: D₅W, 0.9% NaCl, LR, prepared combinations of these solutions
Stability: Reconstituted solution stable for 24 hr at room temperature

ACTIONS

Broad-spectrum, 3rd generation cephalosporin antibiotic; interferes with bacterial cell wall synthesis/division • Good activity against gram-positive aerobes, including *Staphylococcus aureus, S. epidermidis, Streptococcus pneumoniae,* but not methicillin-resistant staphylococci/most enterococci • Good activity against *Pseudomonas aeruginosa,* but less than with aminoglycosides, ceftazidime • Moderate activity against many gram-negative aerobes, including *Escherichia coli, Shi-gella, Salmonella, Serratia, Citrobacter, Klebsiella pneumoniae, Neisseria* • Some activity against anaerobes, including *Bacteroides fragilis* • Does not penetrate CNS well

PHARMACOKINETICS

ROUTE	ONSET	PEAK	DURATION
IM	≤60 min	1-2 hr	Approx 12 hr
IV	Immed	30 min	Approx 12 hr

DISTRIBUTION

Widely distributed; CSF concentrations low unless inflammation present

ELIMINATION

Primarily excreted in bile; half-life 2.0 hr, prolonged with hepatic impairment

INDICATIONS

Serious infections of lower respiratory tract, skin soft tissue, abdomen/peritoneum, GU tract; septicemia caused by susceptible organisms • Not indicated for gram-positive bacterial infections when penicillin or 1st generation cephalosporin (e.g., cefazolin) could be used

PRECAUTIONS/ CONTRAINDICATIONS

Precautions: Bacterial or fungal overgrowth may occur.
• Possible prolonged PT, especially with chronic liver disease, malnutrition • Disulfiram (Antabuse)-like reaction to alcohol (severe headache, dyspnea, vomiting) may occur.
Use caution with: Hypersensitivity to penicillin, other drugs; risk of allergic reaction • GI disease, especially colitis; risk of pseudomembranous colitis • Hepatic disease, biliary obstruction • Children: Safety not clearly established
B Pregnancy category: Safety not clearly established

Contraindications: Hypersensitivity to cefoperazone or any cephalosporin • Avoid use with history of immediate penicillin reaction.

ADVERSE EFFECTS

CNS: Headache, **seizures** (large doses)

GI: *Diarrhea,* nausea, vomiting, oral thrush, ↑ liver enzymes, bilirubin, **pseudomembranous colitis**

GU: ↑ BUN or creatinine, vaginitis

Hema: ↓ Hgb/Hct, neutropenia, other blood dyscrasias, prolonged PT

Derm: Rash, urticaria, pruritus

Local: Pain at IM site, phlebitis at IV site

Misc: Superinfection, colonization; hypersensitivity, including **anaphylaxis, TEN,** serum sickness

TOXICITY/OVERDOSE

Symptoms: Neuromuscular excitability/seizures • Acute allergic reaction, including anaphylaxis • Pseudomembranous colitis with abdominal pain/diarrhea

Management: Discontinue drug. Initiate symptomatic/supportive measures, including airway protection/anticonvulsant therapy. • For management of acute allergic reaction, see Appendix N. • Treat severe pseudomembranous colitis with PO vancomycin or metronidazole. • Hemodialysis is effective in drug removal.

INTERACTIONS

alcohol Disulfiram-like reaction

aminoglycosides (e.g., amikacin, gentamicin) Synergistic antibacterial activity; risk of nephrotoxicity

anticoagulants (e.g., heparin, warfarin) Bleeding abnormalities

aspirin Bleeding abnormalities

chloramphenicol ↓ Bactericidal activity

probenecid ↑ Cephalosporin blood levels

Y-SITE COMPATIBILITIES

Acyclovir, enalaprilat, esmolol, famotidine, heparin, hydromorphone, magnesium sulfate, morphine

Y-SITE INCOMPATIBILITIES

Aminoglycosides (e.g., amikacin, gentamicin, tobramycin), diltiazem, hetastarch, labetalol, meperidine, ondansetron, perphenazine, promethazine

PATIENT CARE IMPLICATIONS

• Obtain specimens for culture and sensitivity before initiating antibiotic therapy. First dose may be given before results received.

• Determine previous antibiotic use, including reactions to penicillins, cephalosporins. Cross-reactivity with penicillin allergies may occur.

• Have epinephrine, antihistamine, resuscitation equipment readily available for use with severe allergic reaction.

• Do not discharge patient for at least 30 min after antibiotic administration.

• High sodium content may cause edema, electrolyte abnormalities, dysrhythmias, and contribute to heart failure.

• Administer at separate site from aminoglycosides (e.g., amikacin, gentamicin, tobramycin); stagger schedules if both antibiotics prescribed.

• Hypoprothrombinemia/bleeding may be reversed by phytonadione (vitamin K₁). Prophylactic phytonadione may be given to critically ill, debilitated, hepatic-impaired patients.

IV K₁

• Reduce risk of thrombophlebitis by using large veins and small catheters/needles, rotating infusion sites, using 0.22-μm filter.

• IV route preferred over IM route and must be used for severe infections or when shock present.

Vital signs/hemodynamics: Monitor temperature for elevation at beginning and throughout therapy. • Monitor I&O for [G] imbalance; older, debilitated, seriously ill, hepatic or renal impaired patients at greater risk for nephrotoxicity.

Physical assessment: Assess for improvement in primary infection or symptoms of super/suprainfection: appearance of sputum, urine, stool, wound drainage; presence of fever, candidiasis, vaginitis. • Observe for symptoms of hypersensitivity: rash, pruritus, wheezing, laryngeal edema, hypotension. • Assess for pseudomembranous colitis: blood/mucus in stool, diarrhea, fever, abdominal pain. Symptoms may not appear for several weeks after cessation of therapy. • Assess for bleeding abnormalities: bruising, oozing from venipuncture sites, blood in urine/stool.

Laboratory tests: Monitor: Liver enzymes (e.g., ALT, AST, alkaline phosphatase), total bilirubin • Electrolytes, BUN, creatinine, creat. cl., especially in

seriously ill/renal-impaired pa-[G] tients, older adults • CBC with differential • Serum levels if high-dose therapy used with severe hepatic/renal disease • PT [G] in older adults, debilitated patients, those with chronic liver disease or malnutrition • **May cause:** False-positive urinary glucose. • Positive antiglobulin (Coombs') test, and may interfere with cross-matching.

PATIENT/FAMILY TEACHING

Purpose of drug is to limit growth of infection-causing bacteria. • Immediately report rash, swelling, intense itching, difficulty breathing, other signs of allergic reaction. • Report diarrhea, blood or mucus in stool, fever, abdominal pain, vaginal itching or discharge, furry growth on tongue. • Do not drink alcohol for at least 2-3 days after last antibiotic dose.

AVAILABLE FORMS

Parenteral for IV/IM use • Premixed solution for IV infusion

---

cefotaxime sodium
(sef-oh-taks'eem)
Claforan

Classification: Cephalosporin antibiotic, 3rd generation

USUAL DOSE

IV/IM, adults: 1-2 g q6-12h
Life-threatening infection: 2 g q4h; Maximum dose, 12 g/24 hr • **Renal impairment:** Usual dose if creat. cl. ≥20 ml/min; reduce by half for creat cl. <20 ml/min. • **Hemodialysis:** 0.5-2 g in single daily dose; adminis-

ter supplemental doses after each dialysis.

℗ IV, children 1 mo-12 yr: 50-200 mg/kg/24 hr in 3-6 divided doses; use usual adult dose for children >50 kg, but do not exceed 12 g/24 hr.

ADMINISTRATION

IM injection: Inject deep into large muscle mass (e.g., gluteus maximus, lateral thigh). Give in two different large muscles if 2-g dose used; IV route recommended for 2-g dose.

▼ Direct IV: Slowly inject each dose over 3-5 min.

IV, intermit inf: Infuse prepared solution over 20-30 min; 0.22-μm filter recommended.

Intraperitoneal: Add reconstituted solution to peritoneal dialysis solution for concentration of 250 mg/2 L.

PREPARATION

IM injection: Dilute with sterile water for injection (see table). Shake well; wait for solution to clear.

A	B	C	D
500 mg	2 ml	2.2 ml	230 mg/ml
1g	3 ml	3.4 ml	300 mg/ml
2g	5 ml	6.0 ml	330 mg/ml

A, vial size; B, volume of diluent; C, withdrawn volume; D, concentration of solution.

IV: Dilute with 10 ml sterile water for injection. Shake well; wait for solution to clear. Further dilute by adding to 50 or 100 ml piggyback bags of D_5W Or 0.9% NaCl. Alternately, if using piggyback vials, first dilute with 10 ml/g to dissolve drug, then further dilute to 50 or 100 ml with compatible fluid for IV infusion.

Compatible fluids: IV solutions: D_5W, $D_{10}W$, 0.9% NaCl, LR, prepared combinations of these solutions • Peritoneal dialysis solutions: 2.5% dextrose and electrolytes, Dianeal 137, PD2 (heparin, 500 U/L also added) • Do not dilute in solutions with pH >7.5

Appearance: Light yellow to amber

Stability: Reconstituted solution stable for 24 hr at room temperature

ACTIONS

Broad-spectrum, 3rd generation cephalosporin antibiotic; inhibits bacterial cell wall synthesis/division • Bactericidal activity greater against gram-negative organisms than with 1st or 2nd generation cephalosporins • Generally, less active against staphylococci than 1st generation cephalosporins • Similar in spectrum of activity to ceftizoxime, ceftriaxone. • Excellent activity against gram-negative aerobes, including *Escherichia coli, Serratia marcescens, Klebsiella pneumoniae,* other Enterobacteriaceae; penicillinase-producing *Neisseria gonorrhoeae* (PPNG); *Haemophilus influenzae* • Moderate activity against *Streptococcus pneumoniae,* other gram-positive organisms, except enterococci • Active against some anaerobes, including *Bacteroides fragilis* • Not active against most strains of *Pseudomonas aeruginosa*

---

italic = common side effects   **bold** = life-threatening reactions

PHARMACOKINETICS

ROUTE	ONSET	PEAK	DURATION
IM	≤30 min	0.5 hr	Dose dependent
IV	Immed	≤30 min	

DISTRIBUTION

Widely distributed throughout body tissue; crosses blood-brain barrier

ELIMINATION

Partially metabolized in liver, excreted in urine via tubular secretion; half-life 0.9-1.7 hr

INDICATIONS

Serious infections of abdomen/peritoneum, pelvis, endometrium, lower respiratory tract, skin/soft tissue, bone/joints, urinary tract, especially when hospital acquired, caused by Enterobacteriaceae resistant to other antibiotics, or use of aminoglycosides undesired • Prevention of infection in clean, contaminated surgery (e.g., cholecystectomy) or when infection could result in serious consequences (e.g., CV procedures, joint replacements) • CNS infections, including meningitis; septicemia with susceptible organisms • Choice agent for uncomplicated gonorrheal infections of urethra, cervix, rectum, especially if suspected to be penicillinase-producing strain • Should not be used as sole therapy for *Pseudomonas aeruginosa* • Not indicated for gram-positive bacterial infections when penicillin or 1st generation cephalosporin (e.g., cefazolin) could be used

PRECAUTIONS/ CONTRAINDICATIONS

Precautions: Bacterial or fungal overgrowth may occur.

• Prolonged PT may occur, particularly with chronic liver disease, malnutrition.
Use caution with: Hypersensitivity to penicillin, other drugs; risk of allergic reaction • GI disease, especially colitis; risk of pseudomembranous colitis • Renal impairment; reduce dose.
B Pregnancy category: Safety not clearly established
Contraindications: Hypersensitivity to cefotaxime, any cephalosporin • Avoid use with history of immediate penicillin reaction

ADVERSE EFFECTS

CNS: Headache, agitation, confusion, **seizures** (high dose/renal insufficiency)
GI: *Diarrhea,* nausea, vomiting, oral thrush, ↑ liver enzymes/bilirubin, **pseudomembranous colitis**
GU: ↑ BUN/creatinine, vaginitis
Hema: Neutropenia, granulocytosis, leukopenia, eosinophilia, thrombocytopenia, other blood dyscrasias, prolonged PT (rare)
Derm: Rash, urticaria, pruritus
Local: Pain/induration at IM site; phlebitis at IV site
Misc: Superinfection, colonization; hypersensitivity, including **anaphylaxis, TEN,** serum sickness

TOXICITY/OVERDOSE

Symptoms: Neuromuscular excitability/seizures, particularly in renal impairment • Pseudomembranous colitis with abdominal pain/diarrhea • Acute allergic reaction, including anaphylaxis
Management: Discontinue drug. Initiate symptomatic/supportive measures, including air-

---

P pediatric   **G** geriatric   **V** Direct IV

way protection/anticonvulsant therapy. • Treat severe pseudo-membranous colitis with PO vancomycin or metronidazole. • For management of acute allergic reaction, see Appendix N. • Hemodialysis is effective in drug removal.

INTERACTIONS

aminoglycosides (e.g., amikacin, gentamicin) Synergistic antibacterial activity; risk of nephrotoxicity
chloramphenicol ↓ Bactericidal activity
furosemide, other potent diuretics Risk of nephrotoxicity
probenecid ↑ Cephalosporin blood levels

Y-SITE COMPATIBILITIES

Acyclovir, diltiazem, famotidine, hydromorphone, magnesium sulfate, meperidine, morphine, ondansetron

Y-SITE INCOMPATIBILITIES

Alkaline solutions, aminoglycosides (e.g., amikacin, gentamicin, tobramycin), aminophylline, hetastarch, sodium bicarbonate

PATIENT CARE IMPLICATIONS

• Obtain specimens for culture and sensitivity before initiating antibiotic therapy. First dose may be given before results received.
• Determine previous antibiotic use, including reactions to penicillins, cephalosporins. Cross-reactivity with penicillin allergies may occur.
• Have epinephrine, antihistamine, resuscitation equipment readily available for use with severe allergic reaction.

• Do not discharge patient for at least 30 min after antibiotic administration.
• High sodium content may cause edema, electrolyte abnormalities, dysrhythmias, and contribute to heart failure.
• Administer at separate site from aminoglycosides (e.g., amikacin, gentamicin, tobramycin); stagger schedules if both antibiotics are prescribed.
• Hypoprothrombenemia/bleeding may be reversed by phytonadione (vitamin K_1).
• Pelvic inflammatory disease (PID): One-time IM dose followed by doxycycline or tetracycline.

Direct IV:
• Reduce risk of thrombophlebitis by using large veins and small catheters/needles, rotating infusion sites, using 0.22-µm filter.
• IV route preferred over IM route and must be used for severe infections or when shock present.

Vital signs/hemodynamics: Monitor temperature for elevation at beginning and throughout therapy. • Monitor I&O for imbalance; older, debilitated, seriously ill, renal impaired patients and those receiving nephrotoxic agents at greatest risk for renal toxicity.

Physical assessment: Assess for improvement in primary infection or symptoms of super/suprainfection: appearance of sputum, urine, stool, wound drainage; presence of fever, candidiasis, vaginitis. • Observe for symptoms of hypersensitivity: rash, pruritus, wheezing, laryngeal edema, hypotension. • Assess for psuedomembranous colitis: blood/mucus in stool,

---

diarrhea, fever, abdominal pain. Symptoms may not appear for several weeks after cessation of therapy. • Assess for bleeding abnormalities: bruising, oozing from venipuncture sites, blood in urine/stool.

Laboratory tests: Monitor: Liver enzymes (e.g., ALT, AST, alkaline phosphatase), total bilirubin • Electrolytes, BUN, creatinine, creat. cl., especially in seriously ill/renal-impaired patients, older adults • CBC with differential • PT in older adults, debilitated patients, those with chronic liver disease or malnutrition • May cause: Positive antiglobulin (Coombs') test and interference with cross-matching

PATIENT/FAMILY TEACHING

Purpose of drug is to limit growth of infection-causing bacteria. • Immediately report rash, swelling, intense itching, difficulty breathing, other signs of allergic reaction. • Report diarrhea, blood/mucus in stool, fever, abdominal pain, vaginal itching or discharge, furry growth on tongue.

AVAILABLE FORMS

Parenteral for IV/IM use • Frozen premixed solution for IV infusion

---

cefotetan disodium
(sef'oh-tee-tan)
Cefotan

Classification: Cephalosporin antibiotic, 2nd generation

USUAL DOSE

IM injection: Inject deep into large muscle mass (e.g., gluteus maximus, lateral thigh).
IV/IM, adults: 1-2 g q12h
• **Severe infection:** 2-3 g q12h; maximum dose, 6 g/24 hr
• **Renal impairment:** Reduce dose or frequency according to creat. cl.

ADMINISTRATION

▼Direct IV: Slowly inject each dose over 3-5 min
IV, intermit inf: Infuse prepared solution over 15-30 min; 0.22-μm filter recommended. Discontinue other solutions during infusion.

PREPARATION

IM: Dilute with sterile water for injection. Alternatively, 0.9% NaCl or lidocaine HCl 0.5%-1% may be used (see Table). Shake well; wait for solution to clear before injecting.
IV: Dilute 1 or 2 g vial with 10 ml sterile water for injection. Add diluent to vial, shake well, wait for solution to clear. Further dilute by adding to 50- or 100-ml piggyback bags of D_5W or 0.9% NaCl. For infusion bottles, add 50-100 ml D_5W or 0.9% NaCl; shake to dissolve, infuse when clear.

A	B	C	D
1 g	2 ml	2.5 ml	400 mg/ml
2 g	3 ml	4 ml	500 mg/ml

A, vial size; B, volume of diluent; C, withdrawn volume; D, concentration of solution.

Compatible fluids: D_5W, 0.9% NaCl
Appearance: Clear and colorless to yellow

Stability: Reconstituted solution stable for at least 24 hr at room temperature

ACTIONS

Broad-spectrum, 2nd generation cephalosporin antibiotic; inhibits bacterial cell wall synthesis/division; activity similar to cefoxitin, but with advantage of q12h dosing • Expanded activity against gram-negative bacteria, including *Escherichia coli, Proteus mirabilis, Klebsiella pneumoniae* • Active against many anaerobes, including most strains of *Bacteroides fragilis* • Less effective than cefotaxime, ceftriaxone against gram-positive cocci, *Haemophilus, Neisseria,* Enterobacteriaceae • Less active against staphylococci than 1st generation cephalosporins • Inactive against *Pseudomonas aeruginosa*

PHARMACOKINETICS

ROUTE	ONSET	PEAK	DURATION
IM	10 min	1.5-3 hr	Approx 10-12 hr; dose dependent
IV	Immed	5 min	

DISTRIBUTION
Widely distributed; poor CSF penetration
ELIMINATION
Most excreted unchanged via urine; half-life 3-4.6 hr

INDICATIONS

Gynecologic/intraabdominal infections; with doxycycline in management of pelvic inflammatory disease (PID) • Serious infections of lower respiratory tract, skin/soft tissue, bone/joints, GU tract • Perioperative infection prophylaxis • Not indicated for gram-positive bacterial infections when penicillin or 1st generation cephalosporin (e.g., cefazolin) could be used

PRECAUTIONS/CONTRAINDICATIONS

Precautions: Bacterial or fungal overgrowth may occur. • Prolonged PT may occur, particularly with chronic liver disease, malnutrition. • Disulfiram (Antabuse)-like reaction to alcohol (severe headache, dyspnea, vomiting) may occur.
Use caution with: Hypersensitivity to penicillin, other drugs; risk of allergic reactions • GI disease, especially colitis; risk of pseudomembranous colitis • Renal insufficiency • Children: Safety not clearly established
B Pregnancy category: Safety not clearly established
Contraindications: Hypersensitivity to cefotetan, any cephalosporin • Avoid use with history of immediate penicillin reaction.

ADVERSE EFFECTS

GI: *Diarrhea,* nausea, oral thrush, ↑ liver enzymes/bilirubin, **pseudomembranous colitis**
GU: ↑ BUN or creatinine, vaginitis
Hema: Eosinophilia, thrombocytosis, anemia, other blood dyscrasias, prolonged PT
Derm: Rash, wheals, itching
Local: Painful injection, phlebitis at IV site
Misc: Superinfection, colonization; hypersensitivity, including **anaphylaxis, TEN,** serum sickness

TOXICITY/OVERDOSE

Symptoms: Nausea, vomiting, diarrhea, hematuria • Acute al-

---

italic = common side effects   **bold** = life-threatening reactions

lergic reaction, including anaphylaxis • Pseudomembranous colitis with abdominal pain/diarrhea

Management: Discontinue drug. Initiate symptomatic/supportive measures. • Treat severe pseudomembranous colitis with PO vancomycin or metronidazole. • For management of acute allergic reaction, see Appendix O. • Hemodialysis is effective in drug removal.

INTERACTIONS

alcohol Disulfiram-like reaction
aminoglycosides (e.g., amikacin, gentamicin) Synergistic antibacterial activity; risk of nephrotoxicity
anticoagulants (e.g., heparin, warfarin) Bleeding abnormalities
aspirin Bleeding abnormalities
chloramphenicol ↓ Bactericidal activity

Y-SITE COMPATIBILITIES

Aminophylline, ampicillin, atropine, digoxin, diltiazem, dopamine, epinephrine, famotidine, fluconazole, furosemide, insulin, meperidine, morphine, multivitamins, oxytocin, penicillin G potassium, piperacillin, ticarcillin, vitamin B complex with C

Y-SITE INCOMPATIBILITIES

Aminoglycosides (e.g., amikacin, gentamicin, tobramycin), heparin, netilmicin, tetracycline

PATIENT CARE IMPLICATIONS

• Obtain specimens for culture and sensitivity before initiating antibiotic therapy. First dose may be given before results received.

• Determine previous antibiotic use, including reactions to penicillins, cephalosporins. Cross-reactivity with penicillin allergies may occur.
• Have epinephrine, antihistamine, resuscitation equipment readily available for use with severe allergic reaction.
• Do not discharge patient for at least 30 min after antibiotic administration.
• High sodium content may cause edema, electrolyte abnormalities, dysrhythmias, and contribute to heart failure.
• Administer at separate site from aminoglycosides (e.g., amikacin, gentamicin, tobramycin); stagger schedules if both antibiotics prescribed.
• Hypoprothrombinemia/bleeding may be reversed by phytonadione (vitamin K₁). Prophylactic phytonadione may be given to critically ill, debilitated patients or those with liver impairment.
• PID: One time IM dose followed by doxycycline or tetracycline.
IV
• Reduce risk of thrombophlebitis by using large veins and small catheters/needles, rotating infusion sites, using 0.22-μm filter.
• IV route preferred over IM route, and must be used for severe infections or when shock present.
Vital signs/hemodynamics: Monitor temperature for elevation at beginning and throughout therapy. • Monitor I&O for imbalance; older, debilitated, seriously ill, or renal impaired patients at greater risk for nephrotoxicity.

Physical assessment: Assess for improvement in primary infection or symptoms of super/suprainfection: appearance of sputum, urine, stool, wound drainage; presence of fever, candidiasis, vaginitis. • Observe for symptoms of hypersensitivity: rash, pruritus, wheezing, laryngeal edema, hypotension. • Assess for pseudomembranous colitis: blood/mucus in stool, diarrhea, fever, abdominal pain. Symptoms may not appear for several weeks after cessation of therapy. • Assess for bleeding abnormalities: bruising, oozing from venipuncture sites, blood in urine/stool.

Laboratory tests: Monitor: Liver enzymes (e.g., ALT, AST, alkaline phosphatase), total bilirubin • Electrolytes, BUN, creatinine, creat. cl., especially in seriously ill/renal-impaired patients, older adults • CBC with differential • PT in older adults, debilitated patients, those with chronic liver disease or malnutrition • May cause: False increases in serum or urinary creatinine using Jaffé's test • Positive direct antiglobulin (Coombs') test and interference with cross-matching

PATIENT/FAMILY TEACHING

Purpose of drug is to limit growth of infection-causing bacteria. • Immediately report rash, swelling, intense itching, difficulty breathing, other signs of allergic reaction. • Report diarrhea, blood/mucus in stool, fever, abdominal pain, vaginal itching or discharge, furry growth on tongue. • Do not drink alcohol for at least 3 days after last antibiotic dose.

AVAILABLE FORMS

Parenteral for IV/IM use

C

cefoxitin sodium
(se-fox'i-tin)
Mefoxin

Classification: Cephalosporin antibiotic, 2nd generation

USUAL DOSE

IV/IM, adults: 1-2 g q6-8h **Severe infection:** 2-3 g q4-6th; maximum dose 12 g/24 hr **Renal impairment:** Loading dose of 1-2 g followed by reduced dose according to creat. cl.

IV, children 3 mo-12 yr: 80-160 mg/kg/24 hr; give q4-6h in divided doses. • Maximum dose, 12 g/24 hr

ADMINISTRATION

IM injection: Inject deep into large muscle mass (e.g., gluteus maximus, lateral thigh).

Direct IV: Slowly inject each dose over 3-5 min

IV, intermit inf: Infuse prepared solution over 15-30 min; 0-22-μm filter recommended. Discontinue other solutions during infusion.

PREPARATION

IM: Dilute with sterile water for injection. Alternatively, lidocaine HCl 0.5%-1% may be used as IM diluent. (see table) Shake well; wait for solution to clear before injecting.

A	B	C	D
1 g	2 ml	2.5 ml	400 mg/ml
2 g	4 ml	5 ml	400 mg/ml

A, vial size; B, volume of diluent; C, withdrawn volume; D, concentration of solution.

---

italic = common side effects   **bold** = life-threatening reactions

IV inf: Dilute each 1 g with 10 ml sterile water for injection or other compatible solution. Shake well, wait for solution to clear. May further dilute by adding to 50-or 100-ml piggyback bags of D_5W or 0.9% NaCl.

Compatible fluids: D_5W, 0.9% NaCl, LR, prepared combinations of these solutions; peritoneal dialysis solution with 2.5% dextrose and electrolytes

Appearance: Clear and colorless to light amber

Stability: Reconstituted solutions stable for at least 24 hr at room temperature

ACTIONS

Broad-spectrum, 2nd generation cephalosporin antibiotic; inhibits bacterial cell wall synthesis/division • Active against many gram-negative bacteria, including *Escherichia coli, Proteus mirabilis, Klebsiella pneumoniae* • Active against most strains of *Bacteroides fragilis,* penicillinase-producing *Neisseria gonorrheae* • Less effective than cefamandole, cefuroxime against *Haemophilus influenzae* • Active against many gram-positive cocci, including penicillinase-producing and non–penicillinase-producing staphylococci/streptococci, but not methicillin-resistant staphylococci • Inactive against *Pseudomonas aeruginosa,* enterococci

PHARMACOKINETICS

ROUTE	ONSET	PEAK	DURATION
IM	≤30 min	20-30 min	Dose dependent
IV	Immed	5 min	

DISTRIBUTION
Widely distributed throughout body tissue

ELIMINATION
Most excreted unchanged via urine; half-life 40-60 min

INDICATIONS

Serious infections of lower respiratory tract, skin/soft tissue, bone/joints, GU tract; septicemia • Gynecologic/intraabdominal infections; with doxycycline in management of pelvic inflammatory disease (PID) • Uncomplicated gonorrheal infections, although ceftriaxone usually considered cephalosporin of choice • Perioperative infection prophylaxis • Not indicated for gram-positive bacterial infections when penicillin or 1st generation cephalosporin (e.g., cefazoline) could be used

PRECAUTIONS/ CONTRAINDICATIONS

Precautions: • Bacterial or fungal overgrowth may occur.

Use caution with: Hypersensitivity to penicillin, other drugs; risk of allergic reaction • GI disease, especially colitis; risk of pseudomembranous colitis • Renal insufficiency

B **Pregnancy category:** Safety not clearly established

Contraindications: Hypersensitivity to cefoxitin, any cephalosporin • Avoid use with history of immediate penicillin reaction.

ADVERSE EFFECTS

GI: *Diarrhea,* nausea, vomiting, oral thrush, ↑ liver enzymes/

bilirubin, **pseudomembranous colitis**

GU: ↑ BUN or creatinine, vaginitis

Hema: Eosinophilia, leukopenia, neutropenia, anemia, other blood dyscrasias

Derm: Rash, wheals, itching

Local: Pain/induration at IM site, thrombophlebitis at IV site

Misc: Superinfection, colonization; hypersensitivity, including **anaphylaxis, TEN;** serum sickness

TOXICITY/OVERDOSE

Symptoms: Nausea, vomiting, diarrhea, hematuria • Acute allergic reaction, including anaphylaxis • Pseudomembranous colitis with abdominal pain/diarrhea

Management: Discontinue drug. Initiate symptomatic/supportive measures. • Treat severe pseudomembranous colitis with PO vancomycin or metronidazole. • For management of acute allergic reaction, see Appendix N.

INTERACTIONS

aminoglycosides (e.g., amikacin, gentamicin) Synergistic antibacterial activity; risk of nephrotoxicity

chloramphenicol ↓ Bactericidal activity

probenecid ↑ Cefoxitin levels

Y-SITE COMPATIBILITIES

Acyclovir, diltiazem, famotidine, fluconazole, hydromorphone, magnesium sulfate, meperidine, morphine, ondansetron, sodium bicarbonate, verapamil

Y-SITE COMPABILITIES

Aminoglycosides (e.g., amikacin, gentamicin, tobramycin), hetastarch

PATIENT CARE IMPLICATIONS

• Obtain specimens for culture and sensitivity before initiating antibiotic therapy. First dose may be given before results received.

• Determine previous antibiotic use, including reactions to penicillins, cephalosporins. Cross-reactivity with penicillin allergies may occur.

• Have epinephrine, antihistamine, resuscitation equipment readily available for use with severe allergic reaction.

• Do not discharge patient for at least 30 min after antibiotic administration.

• High sodium content may cause edema, electrolyte abnormalities, dysrhythmias and contribute to heart failure.

• Administer at separate site from aminoglycosides (e.g., amikacin, gentamicin, tobramycin); stagger schedules if both antibiotics prescribed.

• Hypoprothrombinemia/bleeding may be reversed by phytonadione (vitamin K_1).

• PID: One-time IM dose should be followed by doxycycline or tetracycline.

Direct IV/infusion

• Reduce risk of thrombophlebitis by using larger veins and small catheters/needles, rotating infusion sites, using 0.22-μm filter.

• IV route preferred over IM route and must be used for severe infections or when shock present.

---

italic = common side effects   **bold** = life-threatening reactions

Vital signs/hemodynamics:
Monitor temperature for elevation at beginning and throughout therapy. • Monitor I&O for **G** imbalance; older, debilitated, seriously ill, or renal-impaired patients at greater risk for nephrotoxicity.

Physical assessment: Assess for improvement in primary infection or symptoms of super/suprainfection: appearance of sputum, urine, stool, wound drainage; presence of fever, candidiasis, vaginitis. • Observe for symptoms of hypersensitivity: rash, pruritus, wheezing, laryngeal edema, hypotension. • Assess for pseudomembranous colitis; blood/mucus in stool, diarrhea, fever, abdominal pain. Symptoms may not appear for several weeks after cessation of therapy.

Laboratory tests: Monitor: Liver enzymes (e.g., ALT, AST, alkaline phosphatase), total bilirubin • Electrolytes, BUN, creatinine, creat. cl. especially in seriously ill/renal-impaired patients, and older adults • CBC **G** with differential. May cause: False increases in serum or urinary creatinine • Positive antiglobulin (Coombs') test and interference with cross-matching

PATIENT/FAMILY TEACHING

Purpose of drug is to limit growth of infection-causing bacteria. • Immediately report rash, swelling, intense itching, difficulty breathing, other signs of allergic reaction. • Report diarrhea, blood/mucus in stool, fever, abdominal pain, vaginal itching or discharge, furry growth on tongue.

AVAILABLE FORMS

Parenteral for IV/IM use • Frozen premixed solution for IV infusion

ceftazidime
(sef'tay-zi-deem)
Ceptaz, Fortaz, Pentacef, Tazicef, Tazidime

Classification: Cephalosporin antibiotic, 3rd generation

USUAL DOSE

IV/IM, adults: 250 mg-1 g q8-12h; **Severe infections:** 2 g q8-12h, do not exceed 6 g/day or 1 g in single IM dose. • **Renal impairment:** Reduce dose or frequency, according to creatinine clearance. • Dialysis: Administer loading dose, schedule additional doses after dialysis. **P IV, children 1 mo-12 yr:** 30-50 mg/kg q8h, using sodium carbonate formulation • Maximum daily dose, 6 g

ADMINISTRATION

IM injection: Inject deep into large muscle mass (e.g., gluteus maximus, lateral thigh).
V Direct IV: Slowly inject each dose over 3-5 min.
IV, intermit inf: Infuse prepared solution over 15-30 min. Discontinue primary IV line during infusion; 0.22 μm filter recommended.
Intraperitoneal: Add reconstituted solution to peritoneal dialysis solution for concentration of 250 mg/2 L.

PREPARATION

IM injection: Add 1.5 ml sterile water for injection to 500-mg vial or 3 ml for 1-g vial.

Alternately, bacteriostatic water for injection or lidocaine HCl 0.5% or 1% may be used. Shake well; wait for solution to clear. Invert vial, completely depress plunger of syringe, insert needle, withdraw. CO_2 gas forms during dilution; keep needle in solution to avoid aspiration of gas into syringe. Expel any bubbles in syringe before injection.

Direct IV: Add 5.0 ml sterile water for injection to 500-mg vial. Use 10 ml for 1- or 2-g vial. Shake well; wait for solution to clear. Invert vial, completely depress plunger of syringe, insert needle, withdraw. CO_2 gas forms during dilution; keep needle in solution to avoid aspiration of gas into syringe. Expel any bubbles in syringe before injection.

IV, intermit inf: Constitute as directed above. Further dilute by adding to 50- or 100-ml piggyback bags of D_5W or 0.9% NaCl. Alternately, if using piggyback vials, first dilute with 10 ml to dissolve drug, then shake well, allow solution to clear. Next, vent to remove accumulated gas, add 90 ml compatible solution for IV infusion.

Compatible fluids: D_5W, 0.9% NaCl, prepared combinations of these solutions • **Peritoneal dialysis solution:** Dianeal with dextrose 1.5%

Appearance: Slightly yellow to amber

Stability: Reconstituted solutions stable for 18 hr at room temperature

ACTIONS

Broad-spectrum, bactericidal, 3rd generation cephalosporin antibiotic; interferes with bacterial cell wall synthesis/division • Effective against many gram-negative, gram-positive, anaerobic organisms, including *Pseudomonas aeruginosa, Serratia marcescens, Acinetobacter* • Effective against many otherwise resistant organisms • Most potent cephalosporin available against *Pseudomonas, Serratia* • No activity against *Enterococcus faecalis*

PHARMACOKINETICS

ROUTE	ONSET	PEAK	DURATION
IM	≤30 min	0.5-1.5 hr	8-12 hr
IV	Immed	15 min	8-12 hr*

DISTRIBUTION
Widely distributed throughout body tissue
ELIMINATION
Excreted in urine; half-life 1.4-2 hr, prolonged with renal impairment

*Longer with renal impairment.

INDICATIONS

Serious infections of lower respiratory tract, skin/soft tissue, bones/joints, urinary tract • Intraabdominal, gonorrheal infections; septicemia/meningitis caused by susceptible organisms • To prevent resistance, generally reserved for treatment of multiantibiotic-resistant or hospital-acquired infections as alternative to aminoglycosides in patients with impaired renal function or older adults • Not indicated for gram-positive bacterial infections when penicillin or 1st generation cephalosporin (e.g., cefazolin) could be used

PRECAUTIONS/ CONTRAINDICATIONS

Precautions: Elevated plasma levels may cause serious neurotoxicity in renal impairment; use reduced dose and/or frequency.

• Bacterial or fungal overgrowth may occur.
Use caution with: Hypersensitivity to penicillin, other drugs; risk of allergic reaction • GI disease, especially colitis; risk of pseudomembranous colitis • Older adults, renal impairment, concurrent therapy with nephrotoxic drugs; risk of renal toxicity • Children <12 yr: Safety of arginine formulation (Ceptaz, Pentacef) not established

B Pregnancy category: Safety not clearly established
Contraindications: Hypersensitivity to ceftazidime, any cephalosporin • Avoid use with history of immediate penicillin reaction.

ADVERSE EFFECTS

CNS: Headache, dizziness, neurotoxicity including asterixis, encephalopathy, **seizures** (high dose/renal insufficiency)
GI: *Diarrhea, nausea, vomiting,* metallic taste, oral thrush, ↑ liver enzymes/bilirubin, **pseudomembranous colitis**
GU: ↑ BUN or creatinine, vaginitis
Hema: Hemolytic anemia, eosinophilia, thrombocytosis, other blood dyscrasias
Derm: Rash, urticaria, pruritus
Local: *Pain/induration at IM site;* pain phlebitis, thrombophlebitis at IV site
Misc: ↑ / ↓ Serum glucose; serum albumin and/or total protein; superinfection, colonization; hypersensitivity, including serum sickness, **anaphylaxis, TEN**

TOXICITY/OVERDOSE

Symptoms: Neuromuscular excitability/seizures, particularly in renal impairment • Pseudomembranous colitis with abdominal pain/diarrhea • Acute allergic reaction, including anaphylaxis
Management: Discontinue drug. Initiate symptomatic/supportive measures, including airway protection/anticonvulsant therapy. • Treat severe pseudomembranous colitis with PO vancomycin or metronidazole. • For management of acute allergic reaction, see Appendix N. • Hemodialysis may be effective in drug removal.

INTERACTIONS

aminoglycosides (e.g., amikacin, gentamicin) Synergistic antibacterial activity; risk of nephrotoxicity
chloramphenicol ↓ Bactericidal activity
furosemside, other potent diuretics Risk of nephrotoxicity
probenecid ↑ Cephalosporin blood levels

Y-SITE COMPATIBILITIES

Acyclovir, ciprofloxacin, diltiazem, enalaprilat, esmolol, famotidine, hydromorphone, labetalol, meperidine, metronidazole, ↑ morphine, ondansetron, ranitidine, zidovudine

Y-SITE INCOMPATIBILITIES

Aminoglycosides, fluconazole, sodium bicarbonate, vancomycin

PATIENT CARE IMPLICATIONS

• Obtain specimens for culture and sensitivity before initiating antibiotic therapy. First dose may be given before results received.
• Determine previous antibiotic use, including reactions to peni-

---

cillins, cephalosporins. Cross-reactivity with penicillin allergies may occur.
• Have epinephrine, antihistamine, resuscitation equipment readily available for use with severe allergic reaction.
• Do not discharge patient for at least 30 min after antibiotic administration.
• High sodium content may cause edema, electrolyte abnormalities, dysrhythmias, and contribute to heart failure.
• Ceftazidime is used concomitantly with aminoglycosides, vancomycin, or clindamycin for life-threatening infections or in immunocompromised patients.
• Administer at separate site from aminoglycosides (e.g., amikacin, gentamicin, tobramycin); stagger schedules if both antibiotics prescribed.
• Hypoprothrombinemia/bleeding may be reversed by phytonadione (vitamin K₁).

Direct IV/inf
• Reduce risk of thrombophlebitis by using large veins and small catheters, rotating infusion sites, using 0.22-μm filter.
• IV route preferred over IM route and must be used for severe infections or when shock present.

Vital signs/hemodynamics: Monitor temperature for elevation at beginning and throughout therapy. • Monitor I&O for imbalance; older, debilitated, seriously ill, or renal-impaired patients and those receiving nephrotoxic agents at greatest risk for renal toxicity.

Physical assessment: Assess for improvement in primary infection or symptoms of super/suprainfection: appearance of sputum, urine, stool, wound

drainage; presence of fever, candidiasis, vaginitis. • Observe for symptoms of hypersensitivity: rash, pruritus, wheezing, laryngeal edema, hypotension. • Assess for pseudomembranous colitis: blood/mucus in stool, diarrhea, fever, abdominal pain. Symptoms may not appear for several weeks after cessation of therapy. • Assess for bleeding abnormalities: bruising, oozing from venipuncture sites, blood in urine/stool.

Laboratory tests: Monitor: Liver enzymes (e.g., ALT, AST, alkaline phosphatase), total bilirubin • Electrolytes, BUN, creatinine, creat. cl., especially in seriously ill/renal-impaired patients, older adults • CBC with differential • PT in older adults, debilitated patients, those with chronic liver disease or malnutrition

May cause: Positive antiglobulin (Coombs') test and interference with cross-mating

PATIENT/FAMILY TEACHING

Purpose of drug is to limit growth of infection-causing bacteria. • Immediately report rash, swelling, intense itching, difficulty breathing, other signs of allergic reactions. • Report diarrhea, blood in stool, fever, abdominal pain, vaginal itching or discharge, furry growth on tongue.

AVAILABLE FORMS

Parenteral for IV/IM use • Premixed solutions for IV infusion

ceftizoxime sodium
(sef-ti-zox'eem)
Cefizox

Classification: Cephalosporin
antibiotic, 3rd generation

USUAL DOSE
IV/IM, adults: 1-2 g q8-12h
• Life-threatening infection:
3-4 g q8h; up to 2 g q4h has
been used • Renal impair-
ment: Initially 500 mg-1 g;
maintenance dose according to
creat. cl.
P **IV, children >6 mo:** 33-50
mg/kg q6-8h • Severe infections: 200 mg/kg/24 hr in
equally divided doses; do not
exceed 12 g/24 hr.

ADMINISTRATION
IM injection: Inject deep into
large muscle mass (e.g., gluteus
maximus, lateral thigh). Give in
two different large muscles if 2
g dose used; IV route recommended for 2-g dose.
V **Direct IV:** Slowly inject each
dose over 3-5 min
IV, intermit inf: Infuse prepared solution over 15-30 min.

PREPARATION
IM: Dilute each 500 mg with
1.5 ml sterile water for injection
(see table). Shake well; wait for
solution to clear.
IV, intermit inf: Dilute each
500 mg with 5 ml sterile water
for injection (see table). Add
diluent to vial, shake well, wait
for solution to clear. Further dilute by adding to 50 or 100 ml
piggyback bags of D_5W or
0.9% NaCl. Alternately, if using
piggyback vials, first dilute with
10 ml/g to dissolve drug, then
further dilute to 50 or 100 ml

with compatible fluid for IV infusion.

VIAL SIZE	VOL DILUENT (IV)	VOL DILUENT (IM)
500 mg	5 ml	1.5 ml
1g	10 ml	3 ml
2g	20 ml	6 ml

Compatible fluids: D_5W;
0.9% NaCl; LR or prepared
combinations of the above solutions.
Appearance: Colorless to pale
yellow
Stability: Reconstituted solution stable for 24 hr at room
temperature

ACTIONS
Broad-spectrum, 3rd generation
cephalosporin antibiotic; inhibits
bacterial cell wall synthesis/divi-
sion • Bactericidal activity
greater against gram-negative organisms than 1st/2nd generation
cephalosporins; generally, less
active against staphylococci than
2nd generation cephalosporins;
similar in spectrum of activity
to cefotaxime, ceftriaxone
• Excellent activity against gram-
negative aerobes, including *Escherichia coli, Enterobacter
aerogenes, Klebsiella pneumoniae,* other Enterobacteriaceae;
penicillinase-producing *Neisseria
gonorrhoeae* (PPNG); *Haemophilus influenzae* • Moderate activity against *Streptococcus
pneumoniae,* other gram-positive
organisms, except enterococci
• Active against many anaerobes,
including *Bacteroides fragilis*
• Not active against most strains
of *Pseudomonas aeruginosa*

PHARMACOKINETICS

ROUTE	ONSET	PEAK	DURATION*
IM	≤ 30 min	0.5-1.5 hr	8-12 hr
IV	Immed	30 min	8-12 hr

DISTRIBUTION

Widely distributed throughout body tissue; crosses blood-brain barrier

ELIMINATION

Excreted in urine via glomerular filtration, tubular secretion; half-life 1.4-1.9 hr

*Dose dependent.

INDICATIONS

Serious infections of lower respiratory tract, skin/soft tissue, bones/joints, abdomen/peritoneum, urinary tract, especially when hospital acquired, caused by Enterobacteriaceae resistant to other antibiotics, or when use of aminoglycosides undesired • CNS infections (including meningitis), septicemia with susceptible organisms • Uncomplicated gonorrheal infections of urethra, cervix, rectum, especially if suspected to be penicillinase-producing strain • Should not be used as sole therapy for *Pseudomonas aeruginosa* • Not indicated for gram-positive bacterial infections when penicillin or 1st generation cephalosporin (e.g., cefazolin) could be used.

PRECAUTIONS/ CONTRAINDICATIONS

Precautions: Bacterial or fungal overgrowth may occur. • Prolonged PT may occur, particularly with chronic liver disease, malnutrition. • Possible nephrotoxicity with high-dose therapy
Use caution with: Hypersensitivity to penicillin, other drugs; risk of allergic reaction • GI disease, especially colitis; risk of pseudomembranous coli-

tis • Renal impairment; reduce dose.
B Pregnancy category: Safety not clearly established
Contraindications: Hypersensitivity to ceftizoxime, any cephalosporin • Avoid use with history of immediate penicillin reaction

ADVERSE EFFECTS

CNS: Headache, dizziness, tinnitus, **seizures** (high dose/renal insufficiency)
GI: *Diarrhea,* nausea, vomiting, metallic taste, abdominal pain, oral thrush, **pseudomembranous colitis,** ↑ liver enzymes/bilirubin
GU: ↑ BUN or creatinine, vaginitis
Hema: Eosinophilia, thrombocytosis, leukopenia, anemia, other blood dyscrasias; prolonged PT
Derm: Rash, hives, itching
Local: Pain/induration at IM site; phlebitis at IV site
Misc: Superinfection, colonization; hypersensitivity, including serum sickness, **anaphylaxis, TEN**

TOXICITY/OVERDOSE

Symptoms: Neuromuscular excitability/seizures • Pseudomembranous colitis with abdominal pain/diarrhea • Acute allergic reaction, including anaphylaxis
Management: Discontinue drug. Initiate symptomatic/supportive measures, including airway protection/anticonvulsant therapy. • Treat severe pseudomembranous colitis with PO vancomycin or metronidazole. • For management of acute allergic reaction, see Appendix N. • Limited removal by hemodialysis

---

italic = common side effects   **bold** = life-threatening reactions

INTERACTIONS

aminoglycosides (e.g., amikacin, gentamicin) Synergistic antibacterial activity; risk of nephrotoxicity

chloramphenicol ↓ Bactericidal activity

furosemide, other potent diuretics Risk of nephrotoxicity

probenecid ↑ Cephalosporin blood levels

Y-SITE COMPATIBILITIES

Acyclovir, enalaprilat, esmolol, famotidine, hydromorphone, labetalol, meperidine, morphine, odansetron

Y-SITE INCOMPATIBILITIES

Aminoglycosides (e.g., amikacin, gentamicin, tobramycin)

PATIENT CARE IMPLICATIONS

• Obtain specimens for culture and sensitivity before initiating antibiotic therapy. First dose may be given before results received.

• Determine previous antibiotic use, including reactions to penicillins, cephalosporins. Cross-reactivity with penicillin allergies may occur.

• Have epinephrine, antihistamine, resuscitation equipment readily available for use with severe allergic reaction.

• Do not discharge patient for at least 30 min after antibiotic administration.

• High sodium content may cause edema, electrolyte abnormalities, dysrhythmias, and contribute to heart failure.

• Administer at separate site from aminoglycosides (e.g., amikacin, gentamicin, tobramy-

cin); stagger schedules if both antibiotics prescribed.

• Hypoprothrombinemia/bleeding may be reversed by phytonadione (vitamin K_1).

• Pelvic inflammatory disease (PID): One-time IM dose is followed by doxycycline or tetracycline.

IV

• Reduce risk of thrombophlebitis by using large veins and small catheters/needles, rotating infusion sites, using 0.22-μm filter.

• IV route preferred over IM and must be used for severe infections or when shock present.

Vital signs/hemodynamics: Monitor temperature for elevation at beginning and throughout therapy. • Monitor I&O for **G** imbalance; older, debilitated, seriously ill, or renal-impaired patients at greater risk for nephrotoxicity.

Physical assessment: Assess for improvement in primary infection or symptoms of super/suprainfection: appearance of sputum, urine, stool, wound drainage; presence of fever, candidiasis, vaginitis. • Observe for symptoms of hypersensitivity: rash, pruritus, wheezing, laryngeal edema, hypotension. • Assess for pseudomembranous colitis: blood/mucus in stool, diarrhea, fever, abdominal pain. Symptoms may not appear for several weeks after cessation of therapy. • Assess for bleeding abnormalities: bruising, oozing from venipuncture sites, blood in urine/stool.

Laboratory tests: Monitor: Liver enzymes (e.g., ALT, AST, alkaline phosphatase), total bilirubin • Electrolytes, BUN, creatinine, creat. cl, especially in

---

P pediatric   **G** geriatric   **V** Direct IV

seriously ill, renal-impaired, and older adults • CBC with differential • PT in older adults, debilitation, chronic liver disease, malnutrition • May cause: Positive antiglobulin (Coombs') test and interference with cross-matching

PATIENT/FAMILY TEACHING

Purpose of drug is to limit growth of infection-causing bacteria. • Immediately report rash, swelling, intense itching, difficulty breathing, or other signs of allergic reaction. • Report diarrhea, blood or mucus in stool, fever, abdominal pain, vaginal itching or discharge, furry growth on tongue.

AVAILABLE FORMS

Parenteral for IV/IM use • Frozen premixed solution for IV infusion

ceftriaxone sodium
(sef-try′ax-on)
Rocephin

Classification: Cephalosporin antibiotic, 3rd generation

USUAL DOSE

IV/IM, adults: 500 mg-1 g q12-24h • **Severe infections:** 1-2 g q12h; maximum dose, 4 g/24 hr • **Renal/hepatic impairment:** Maximum dose, 2 g/24 hr; larger doses used with close monitoring

IV, children 1 mo-12 yr: 50-75 mg/kg/24 hr; q12-24 hr; maximum dose, 2 g/24 hr • **Severe infections:** 80-100 mg/kg/24 hr; q12-24h.

ADMINISTRATION

IM injection: Inject deep into large muscle mass (e.g., gluteus maximus, lateral thigh).
IV, intermit inf: Infuse prepared solution over 30 min.

PREPARATION

IV: Dilute each 250 mg with 2.4 ml sterile water for injection, or bacteriostatic water for injection (see table). Shake well, wait for solution to clear before withdrawing. Further dilute by adding to 50- or 100-ml piggyback bags of D_5W or 0.9% NaCl. Alternately, if using piggyback vials, first dilute with 10 ml/g to dissolve drug, then further dilute to 50 or 100 ml with compatible solution for IV infusion.

A	B	C	D	E
		CONC.		CONC.
VIAL SIZE	VOLUME DILUENT, IV	FOR IV USE*	VOLUME DILUENT, IM	FOR IM USE*
250 mg	2.4 ml	100 mg/ml	0.9 ml	250 mg/ml
500 mg	4.8 ml	100 mg/ml	1.8 ml	250 mg/ml
1 g	9.6 ml	100 mg/ml	3.6 ml	250 mg/ml
2 g	19.2 ml	100 mg/ml	7.2 ml	250 mg/ml

*Concentration.

IM: Dilute each 250 mg with 0.9 ml sterile water for injection or lidocaine HC1 1% (see table). Shake well; wait for solution to clear before withdrawing.
Compatible fluids: D_5W, 0.9% NaCl, LR, prepared combinations of these solutions
Appearance: Light yellow to amber
Stability: Most reconstituted solutions stable for at least 24 hr at room temperature

---

italic = common side effects   **bold** = life-threatening reactions

ACTIONS

Broad-spectrum, 3rd generation cephalosporin antibiotic; inhibits bacterial cell wall synthesis/division • Bactericidal activity greater against gram-negative organisms than with 1st/2nd generation cephalosporins • Similar in spectrum of activity to cefotaxime, ceftizoxime but has longer duration of activity and requires less frequent dosing • Excellent activity against *Escherichia coli, Klebsiella pneumoniae,* other Enterobacteriaceae; penicillinase-producing *Neisseria gonorrhoeae* (PPNG) • Moderate activity against *Staphylococcus aureus, S. epidermidis, Streptococcus pneumoniae,* other gram-positive organisms, except enterococci • Minimal activity against *Bacteroides fragilis* • Not active against many strains of *Pseudomonas aeruginosa*

PHARMACOKINETICS

ROUTE	ONSET	PEAK
IM	≤30 min	1.5-4.0 hr
IV	Immed	30-60 min

DURATION

Dose dependent; similar steady state obtained with q24h or q12h dosing

DISTRIBUTION

Widely distributed throughout body tissue; crosses blood-brain barrier

ELIMINATION

Excreted via urine, bile; half-life 5.4-10.9 hr

INDICATIONS

Serious infections of lower respiratory tract, skin/soft tissue, bone/joints, abdomen/peritoneum, urinary tract; septicemia; especially when hospital acquired, caused by Enterobacteriaceae resistant to other antibiotics, or use of aminoglycosides undesired • Prevention of infection in clean, contaminated surgery (e.g., cholecystectomy) or when infection could result in serious consequences (e.g., CV surgery, joint replacements) • CNS infections, including meningitis with susceptible organisms • Choice agent for uncomplicated gonorrheal infections, especially if suspected to be penicillinase-producing strain • Choice agent for chancroid genital ulcers • Not used as sole therapy for *Pseudomonas aeruginosa* • Not indicated for gram-positive bacterial infections when penicillin or 1st generation cephalosporin (e.g., cefazolin) could be used.

PRECAUTIONS/ CONTRAINDICATIONS

Precautions: Bacterial or fungal overgrowth may occur. • Prolonged PT may occur, especially with chronic liver disease, malnutrition. **Use caution with:** Hypersensitivity to penicillin, other drugs; risk of allergic reaction • GI disease, especially colitis; risk of pseudomembranous colitis • Liver, gallbladder, pancreatic disease; risk of gallbladder precipitates • Severe renal/hepatic disease

B **Pregnancy category:** Safety not clearly established **Contraindications:** Hypersensitivity to ceftriaxone, any cephalosporin • Avoid use with history of immediate penicillin reaction.

ADVERSE EFFECTS

CNS: Headache, dizziness, **seizures** (high dose/renal insufficiency)
GI: *Diarrhea,* nausea, vomiting, metallic taste, oral thrush,

pseudomembranous colitis, ↑ liver enzymes/bilirubin, gallbladder precipitates

GU: ↑ BUN or creatinine, vaginitis

Hema: Eosinophilia, thrombocytosis, leukopenia, other blood dyscrasias, prolonged PT (rare)

Derm: Rash, wheals, itching

Local: Pain/induration at IM site; phlebitis at IV site

Misc: Superinfection, colonization; hypersensitivity, including serum sickness, **anaphylaxis, TEN**

TOXICITY/OVERDOSE

Symptoms: Neuromuscular excitability/seizures, particularly in renal impairment • Pseudomembranous colitis with abdominal pain/diarrhea • Acute allergic reaction, including anaphylaxis

Management: Discontinue drug. Initiate symptomatic/supportive measures, including airway protection/anticonvulsant therapy. • Treat severe pseudomembranous colitis with PO vancc. cin or metronidazole. • For management of acute allergic reaction, see Appendix O. • Hemodialysis is not effective in drug removal.

INTERACTIONS

aminoglycosides (e.g., amikacin, gentamicin) Synergistic antibacterial activity; risk of nephrotoxicity

anticoagulants (e.g., heparin, warfarin) ↑ Risk of bleeding abnormalities

aspirin ↑ Risk of bleeding abnormalities

chloramphenicol ↓ Bactericidal activity

furosemide, other potent diuretics Risk of nephrotoxicity

probenecid (high dose) ↑ Serum concentrations of ceftriaxone

Y-SITE COMPATIBILITIES

Acyclovir, diltiazem, meperidine, morphine, zidovudine

Y-SITE INCOMPATIBILITIES

Aminoglycosides (e.g., amikacin, gentamicin, tobramycin), fluconazole, vancomycin

PATIENT CARE IMPLICATIONS

• Obtain specimens for culture and sensitivity before initiating antibiotic therapy. First dose may be given before results received.

• Determine previous antibiotic use, including reactions to penicillins, cephalosporins. Cross-reactivity with penicillin allergies may occur.

• Have epinephrine, antihistamine, resuscitation equipment readily available for use with severe allergic reaction.

• Do not discharge patient for at least 30 min after antibiotic administration.

• High sodium content may cause edema, electrolyte abnormalities, dysrhythmias and contribute to heart failure.

• Administer at separate site from aminoglycosides (e.g., amikacin, gentamicin, tobramycin); stagger schedules if both antibiotics prescribed.

• Pelvic inflammatory disease (PID): One-time IM dose is followed by doxycycline or tetracycline.

• History of liver, biliary, pancreatic disorders: Serial abdomi-

---

italic = common side effects   **bold** = life-threatening reactions

nal ultrasounds used to detect gallbladder precipitates

IV
• Hypoprothrombinemia/bleeding may be reversed by phytonadione (vitamin K₁).
• Reduce risk of thrombophlebitis by using large veins and small catheters, rotating infusion sites, using 0.22-μm filter.
• IV route preferred over IM route and must be used for severe infections or when shock present.

Vital signs/hemodynamics: Monitor temperature for elevation at beginning and throughout therapy. • Monitor I&O for **G** imbalance; older, debilitated, seriously ill, or renal-impaired patients at greater risk for nephrotoxicity.

Physical assessment: Assess for improvement in primary infection or symptoms of super/suprainfection: appearance of sputum, urine, stool, wound drainage; presence of fever, candidiasis, vaginitis. • Observe for symptoms of hypersensitivity: rash, pruritus, wheezing, laryngeal edema, hypotension. • Assess for pseudomembranous colitis: blood/mucus in stool, diarrhea, fever, abdominal pain. Symptoms may not appear for several weeks after cessation of therapy. • Assess for biliary symptoms: colic, nausea, vomiting, anorexia. Consult physician if present. • Assess for bleeding abnormalities: bruising, oozing from venipuncture sites, blood in urine/stool.

Laboratory tests: Monitor: Liver enzymes (e.g., ALT, AST, alkaline phosphatase), total bilirubin • Electrolytes, BUN, creatinine, creatinine clearance, es-

pecially in seriously ill/
G renal-impaired patients, older adults • CBC with differential
• Serum levels if high-dose therapy used with severe hepatic
G disease • PT in older adults, debilitated patients, those with chronic liver disease or malnutrition. • **May cause:** Positive antiglobulin (Coombs') test and interference with cross-matching.

PATIENT/FAMILY TEACHING

Purpose of drug is to limit growth of infection-causing bacteria. • Immediately report rash, swelling, intense itching, difficulty breathing, other signs of allergic reaction. • Report diarrhea, blood/mucus in stool, fever, abdominal pain, vaginal itching or discharge, furry growth on tongue.

AVAILABLE FORMS

Parenteral for IV/IM use • Frozen premixed solution for IV infusion

cefuroxime sodium, IV/IM
(se-fyoor-ox′eem)
Kefurox, Zinacef
cefuroxime axetil, PO
Ceftin

Classification: Cephalosporin antibiotic, 2nd generation

USUAL DOSE
PO, adults: 250-500 mg q12h
• **Gonorrhea:** 1 g single dose
P PO, children: 20-30 mg/kg/24 hr given in divided doses q12h
IV/IM, adults: 750 mg-1.5 g q6-8h; do not exceed 3 g q8h.
• **Renal impairment:** Reduce

dose and/or frequency according to creat. cl.

P IV, children >3 mo: 50-150 mg/kg/24 hr in divided doses q6-8h. • **Bacterial meningitis:** 200-240 mg/kg/24 hr in divided doses q6-8h; do not exceed 3 g q8h.

ADMINISTRATION

IM: Inject deep into large muscle mass (e.g., gluteus maximus, lateral thigh).

▼ Direct IV: Slowly inject each dose over 3-5 min.

IV, intermit inf: Infuse over 15-30 min.

PREPARATION

IM: Dilute 750 mg vial with 3.6 ml sterile water for injection: shake well and withdraw entire contents. Resulting suspension contains 200 mg/ml. Shake gently immediately before injection.

IV: Dilute 750-mg vial with 8 ml sterile water for injection; use 16 ml for 1.5-g vial. Shake well, wait for solution to clear. Solution contains 90 mg/ml. For infusion, further dilute by adding to 100 ml piggyback bags of D_5W or 0.9% NaCl.

Compatible fluids: D_5W, 0.9% NaCl, LR

Appearance: Light yellow to amber

Stability: Reconstituted suspensions/solutions stable for at least 24 hr at room temperature

ACTIONS

Broad-spectrum, 2nd generation cephalosporin antibiotic; inhibits bacterial cell wall synthesis/division • Expanded activity against gram-negative bacteria, including some resistant to cefamandole • Susceptible organisms: *Escherichia coli, Kleb-*

siella, Enterobacter, Neisseria, Haemophilus influenzae, many Enterobacteriaceae • Spectrum of activity narrower than with most 3rd generation cephalosporins • Broad spectrum of activity against many gram-positive aerobes, including most staphylococci/streptococci, but not methicillin-resistant staphylococci/enterococci • Inactive against *Pseudomonas aeruginosa, Bacteroides fragilis* • Penetrates CSF, although most 3rd generation cephalosporins provide broader coverage

PHARMACOKINETICS

ROUTE	ONSET	PEAK
PO		2 hr
IM	<15 min	15-60 min
IV	Immed	15 min

DURATION
Dose dependent; IV/IM: 5-8 hr

DISTRIBUTION
Widely distributed

ELIMINATION
Most excreted unchanged via urine; half-life 1-2 hr

INDICATIONS

PO route for infections of lower respiratory tract, GU tract, skin/soft tissue, otitis media, pharyngitis, tonsillitis; also after initial parenteral therapy • Parenteral route for serious infections of lower respiratory tract, skin/soft tissue, GU tract; also for bone/joint infections, septicemia, meningitis, especially ampicillin-resistant *Haemophilus in-*
P *fluenzae* in children • Perioperative infection prophylaxis • Not indicated for gram-positive bacterial infections when penicillin or 1st generation cephalosporin (e.g., cefazolin) could be used • Lack of liquid formulation **P** limits PO use in children.

---

italic = common side effects   **bold** = life-threatening reactions

PRECAUTIONS/CONTRAINDICATIONS

Precautions: Bacterial or fungal overgrowth may occur.
• Prolonged PT may occur, particularly with chronic liver disease, malnutrition.
Use caution with: Hypersensitivity to penicillin, other drugs; risk of allergic reaction
• GI disease, especially colitis; risk of pseudomembranous colitis • Renal insufficiency
B Pregnancy category: Safety not clearly established
Contraindications: Hypersensitivity to cefuroxime, any cephalosporin • Avoid use with history of immediate penicillin reaction.

ADVERSE EFFECTS

CNS: Headache, dizziness, **seizures** (high dose/renal insufficiency)
GI: *Diarrhea,* nausea, vomiting, oral thrush, **pseudomembranous colitis,** ↑ liver enzymes; PO: epigastric burning, GI bleeding
GU: ↑ BUN or creatinine, vaginitis
Hema: Decreased Hgb/Hct, eosinophilia, other blood dyscrasias, prolonged PT
Derm: Rash, urticaria, pruritus
Local: *Painful IM injection;* pain/thrombophlebitis at IV site
Misc: Superinfection, colonization; hypersensitivity, including serum sickness, **anaphylaxis, TEN**

TOXICITY/OVERDOSE

Symptoms: Neuromuscular excitability/seizures, particularly in renal impairment • Pseudomembranous colitis with abdominal pain/diarrhea • Acute allergic reaction, including anaphylaxis
Management: Discontinue drug. Initiate symptomatic/supportive measures, including airway protection/anticonvulsant therapy. • After recent ingestion, implement guidelines for management of acute overdose (Appendix I). • Treat severe pseudomembranous colitis with PO vancomycin or metronidazole.
• For management of acute allergic reaction, see Appendix N.
• Hemodialysis is effective in drug removal.

INTERACTIONS

aminoglycosides (e.g., amikacin, gentamicin) Synergistic antibacterial activity; risk of nephrotoxicity
anticoagulants (e.g., heparin, warfarin) Bleeding abnormalities
aspirin Bleeding abnormalities
chloramphenicol ↓ Bactericidal activity
probenecid ↑ Cefuroxime levels

Y-SITE COMPATIBILITIES

Acyclovir, atracurium, diltiazem, famotidine, heparin, hydromorphone, meperidine, morphine, ondansetron, pancuronium, potassium chloride, vecuronium

Y-SITE INCOMPATIBILITIES

Aminoglycosides (e.g., amikacin, gentamicin, tobramycin), doxapram, fluconazole, sodium bicarbonate

PATIENT CARE IMPLICATIONS

• Obtain specimens for culture and sensitivity before initiating antibiotic therapy. First dose may be given before results received.

P pediatric   **G** geriatric   **V** Direct IV

C

• Determine previous antibiotic use, including reactions to penicillins, cephalosporins. Cross-reactivity with penicillin allergies may occur.

PO

• Administration with food or milk increases absorption, reduces adverse gastric effects.

Parenteral

• Have epinephrine, antihistamine, resuscitation equipment readily available for use with severe allergic reaction.

• Do not discharge patient for at least 30 min after parenteral antibiotic administration.

• High sodium content of parenteral form may contribute to edema, electrolyte abnormalities, dysrhythmias, heart failure.

• Administer parenteral form at separate site from aminoglycosides (e.g., amikacin, gentamicin, tobramycin); stagger schedules if both antibiotics prescribed.

IM

• Administration in buttock less painful than in thigh

IV

• Hypoprothrombinemia may be reversed by phytonadione (vitamin K_1).

• Reduce risk of thrombophlebitis by using large veins and small catheters/needles, rotating infusion sites, using 0.22-µm filter.

• IV route preferred over IM route and must be used for severe infections or when shock present.

Vital signs/hemodynamics: Monitor temperature for elevation at beginning and throughout therapy. • Monitor I&O for **G** imbalance; older, debilitated, seriously ill, or renal-impaired pa-

tients at greater risk for nephrotoxicity.

Physical assessment: Assess for improvement in primary infection or symptoms of super/suprainfection: appearance of sputum, urine, stool, wound drainage; presence of fever, candidiasis, vaginitis. • Observe for symptoms of hypersensitivity: rash, pruritus, wheezing, laryngeal edema, hypotension. • Assess for pseudomembranous colitis: blood/mucus in stool, diarrhea, fever, abdominal pain. Symptoms may not appear for several weeks after cessation of therapy. • Assess for bleeding abnormalities: bruising, oozing from venipuncture sites, blood in urine/stool.

Laboratory tests: Monitor: Liver enzymes (e.g., ALT, AST, alkaline phosphatase), total bilirubin • Electrolytes, BUN, creatinine, creatine clearance, especially in seriously ill/renal-impaired patients, older adults **G** • CBC with differential • PT in **G** older adults, debilitated patients, those with chronic liver disease or malnutrition

May cause: Positive antiglobulin (Coombs') test and interference with cross-matching

PATIENT/FAMILY TEACHING

Purpose of drug is to limit growth of infection-causing bacteria. • Immediately report rash, swelling, intense itching, difficulty breathing, other signs of allergic reaction. • Report diarrhea, blood/mucus in stool, fever, abdominal pain, vaginal itching or discharge, furry growth on tongue.

Outpatient: Take with food or milk to minimize gastric irritation. • Take all of medication

---

italic = common side effects   **bold** = life-threatening reactions

exactly as prescribed. Do not stop taking medicine even if you feel better. Failure to take all of antibiotic may result in recurrence or additional infection. Do not save or share unused medicine.

AVAILABLE FORMS

Cefuroxime sodium: Parenteral for IV/IM use • Cefuroxime axetil: Tablets, oral suspension

---

cephalexin
(sef-a-lex'in)
Cefanex, Keflex, Keflet, Novo-Lexin ✤
Nu-Cephale ✤
cephalexin HCl
Keftab

Classification: Cephalosporin antibiotic, 1st generation

USUAL DOSE

PO, adults: 250 mg q6h or 500 mg q12h; up to 4 g/24 hr may be given in divided doses. • **Renal impairment:** Initially 250 mg; maintenance dose lowered according to creat. cl.
Ⓟ **PO, children:** 25-50 mg/24 hr in divided doses q6h; up to 50-100 mg/kg/24 hr may be given in divided doses.

ADMINISTRATION

PO: Give with food or milk to minimize gastric irritation. Food may slow onset of action but will not affect efficacy.
Enteral formula compatibilities: Ensure, Ensure HN, Ensure Plus, Isocal, Osmolite, Osmolite HN, Sustacal, Sustacal HC, Vital

ACTIONS

First-generation cephalosporin antibiotic; interferes with bacterial cell wall synthesis/division • Excellent activity against gram-positive cocci, including penicillinase-producing and non-penicillinase-producing staphylococci/streptococci, but not methicillin-resistant staphylococci/enterococci • Very limited activity against gram-negative organisms • Usually not active against *Haemophilus influenzae* • Poor CNS penetration

PHARMACOKINETICS

ROUTE	ONSET	PEAK	DURATION
PO	≤60 min	1 hr	Dose dependent

DISTRIBUTION
Widely distributed; CSF concentrations low
ELIMINATION
Excreted unchanged in urine; half-life 0.5-1.2 hr, prolonged in children <1 yr

INDICATIONS

Mild to moderate infections of skin/soft tissue, bones/joints, urinary tract caused by susceptible organisms; often as follow-up therapy after parenteral cephalosporins • Otitis media, uncomplicated respiratory tract infections (e.g., pharyngitis, tonsillitis), especially when penicillins/sulfonamides contraindicated • Pencillin preferred for treatment of streptococcal respiratory tract infections because of superior efficacy in preventing rheumatic fever

PRECAUTIONS/
CONTRAINDICATIONS

Precautions: Bacterial or fungal overgrowth may occur.
Use caution with: Hypersensitivity to penicillin, other

---

drugs; risk of allergic reaction • GI disease, especially colitis; risk of pseudomembranous colitis • Renal impairment

B Pregnancy category: Safety not clearly established

Contraindications: Hypersensitivity to cephalexin, any cephalosporin • Avoid use with history of immediate penicillin reaction.

ADVERSE EFFECTS

CNS: Headache, dizziness, **seizures** (high dose/renal insufficiency)

GI: *Diarrhea,* nausea, vomiting, oral thrush, **pseudomembranous colitis,** increased liver enzymes

GU: Vaginitis, transient increase in BUN or creatinine, **nephrotoxicity** (rare)

Hema: Leukopenia thrombocytopenia, other blood dyscrasias, anemia (rare)

Derm: Rash, urticaria, pruritus

Misc: Superinfection, colonization, other allergic reactions including **anaphylaxis, TEN,** serum sickness

TOXICITY/OVERDOSE

Symptoms: Nausea, vomiting, diarrhea, hematuria • Acute allergic reaction, including anaphylaxis • Pseudomembranous colitis with abdominal pain/diarrhea

Management: Discontinue drug. Initiate symptomatic/supportive measures. • After recent ingestion, implement guidelines for management of acute overdose (Appendix I). • For management of acute allergic reaction, see Appendix N. • Treat severe pseudomembranous colitis with PO vancomycin or met-

ronidazole. • Hemodialysis probably is not needed.

INTERACTIONS

aminoglycosides (e.g., amikacin, gentamicin) Synergistic antibacterial activity; risk of nephrotoxicity

probenecid ↑ Cephalosporin levels

PATIENT CARE IMPLICATIONS

• Obtain specimens for culture and sensitivity before initiating antibiotic therapy. First dose may be given before results received.

• Determine previous antibiotic use, including reactions to penicillins, cephalosporins. Cross-reactivity with penicillin allergies may occur.

Vital signs/hemodynamics: Monitor temperature for elevation at beginning and throughout therapy. • Monitor I&O for imbalance: older, debilitated, seriously ill, or renal-impaired patients at greater risk for nephrotoxicity.

Physical assessment: Assess for improvement in primary infection or symptoms of super/suprainfection: appearance of sputum, urine, stool, wound drainage; presence of fever, candidiasis, vaginitis. • Observe for symptoms of hypersensitivity: rash, pruritus, wheezing, laryngeal edema, hypotension. • Assess for pseudomembranous colitis: blood/mucus in stool, diarrhea, fever, abdominal pain. Symptoms may not appear for several weeks after cessation of therapy.

Laboratory tests: Monitor: Liver enzymes (e.g., ALT, AST, alkaline phosphatase) • Electrolytes, BUN, creatinine, creat. cl. in seriously ill/renal-impaired **G** patients, older adults • CBC with differential • **May cause:** Positive antiglobulin (Coombs') test and interference with cross-matching

PATIENT/FAMILY TEACHING

Purpose of drug is to limit growth of infection-causing bacteria. • Immediately report rash, swelling, intense itching, difficulty breathing, other signs of allergic reaction. • Report diarrhea, blood/mucus in stool, fever, abdominal pain, vaginal itching or discharge, furry growth on tongue. Do not take medicine for diarrhea without consulting health care provider. **Outpatient:** Take with food or milk to minimize gastric irritation. • Take all of medication exactly as prescribed. Do not stop taking medicine even if you feel better. Failure to take all of antibiotic may result in recurrence or additional infection. Do not save or share unused medicine. • Keep oral suspensions refrigerated; shake well before use.

AVAILABLE FORMS

Capsules, tablets • PO suspension • Pediatric drops

---

charcoal, activated
Acta-Char, Actidose, Charcoaid, Insta-Char, Liqui-Char

Classification: Adsorbent

USUAL DOSE

P **PO/NG, adults/children:** 30-100 g (20-30 g = ½ cup lightly packed powder) • Dose is 5-10 times estimated weight of ingested poison; larger dose used for patients who have recently eaten. • Multiple doses often used

ADMINISTRATION

Do not administer with milk, ice cream, sherbet. • If ipecac also prescribed, administer ipecac before charcoal. • For greatest effectiveness, administer as soon as possible.

PREPARATION

Slurry: Mix each 20-30 g of powder with ≥240 ml tap water; avoid more concentrated slurries. Thickening agent or small amount of flavoring (e.g., fruit juice concentrate, chocolate powder) may be added. Charcoal may also be mixed with sorbitol, saline cathartics. • Do not mix with milk, ice cream, or sherbet, which can ↓ effectiveness of charcoal.

ACTIONS

Inhibits GI absorption of toxins by directly adsorbing wide variety of drugs, chemicals • Also adsorbs enzymes, vitamins, minerals, nutrients from GI tract • Does not adsorb cyanide; limited absorption of ethanol, methanol, ferrous sulfate, caustic alkalis, mineral acids

PHARMACOKINETICS

ROUTE	ONSET	PEAK/DURATION
PO	Immed	Dependent on type used, amount of toxin; food in stomach

DISTRIBUTION
Not absorbed
ELIMINATION
Excreted unchanged in feces

INDICATIONS

Antidote for most oral poisonings, except cyanide, corrosive agents, iron, mineral acids, organic solvents • Most effective when administered shortly after poison ingestion; however, late administration sometimes useful for agents not highly protein bound and with relatively low volumes of distribution (e.g., phenobarbital, theophylline) • Effectiveness enhanced by emptying stomach (e.g., induced emesis with ipecac syrup or gastric lavage) before administration • Hemoperfusion through columns of activated charcoal used to remove endogenous toxins (e.g., in uremia, hepatic failure) and exogenous toxins • Used in drainage devices as deodorant for foul-smelling wounds or drainage

PRECAUTIONS/ CONTRAINDICATIONS

Precautions: Not effective for all drugs, toxins; avoid use with corrosives, petroleum distillates. • Use before endoscopy may obscure findings.
c Pregnancy category: Use only if safer alternatives unavailable.
Contraindications: Hypersensitivity to charcoal • CNS depression with unprotected airway

ADVERSE EFFECTS

GI: *Black stools, vomiting,* constipation, diarrhea

TOXICITY/OVERDOSE

Minimal risk of toxicity

INTERACTIONS

ipecac ↓ Absorption/effectiveness of ipecac
laxatives ↓ Absorption/effectiveness of laxative
medications ↓ Absorption/effectiveness of most medications

PATIENT CARE IMPLICATIONS

• Assess neurologic status; avoid administration to patients with CNS depression unless airway protected.
• To increase effectiveness, empty stomach by induced emesis with ipecac or gastric lavage before administration.
• Have airway management, resuscitation equipment immediately available.
• Administer with laxative or sorbitol to prevent constipation. Delayed intestinal transit could result in systemic absorption of some drugs from intestinal charcoal.
• Food in stomach reduces effectiveness; do not administer with food products.
• Store all preparations in tightly closed container.
• Tablets/granules are less effective than powder, should not be used in acute poisoning.
Vital signs: Monitor VS frequently, ECG continuously according to substance ingested, patient stability.
Physical assessment: Assess for CNS depression. Be prepared to protect airway if patient becomes lethargic, unresponsive, or lacks gag reflex.
• After administration, monitor amount, consistency, frequency of bowel elimination.

---

italic = common side effects   **bold** = life-threatening reactions

PATIENT/FAMILY TEACHING

Purpose of medication is to absorb toxins or medications in stomach, upper intestine.
• Stools are black until all charcoal eliminated. • Gritty residue in mouth may be removed by rinsing with water.

AVAILABLE FORMS

Powder for oral suspension
• Commercially prepared PO suspensions in sorbitol, water
• Tablets for nonemergency use
• Tablets with simethicone for non-emergency use

---

chlordiazepoxide, chlordiazepoxide HCl
(klor-dye-az-e-pox'ide)
CDP, H-tran, Librium, Libritabs, Mitran, Spaz-10

Classifications: Benzodiazepine, sedative/hypnotic, antianxiety (anxiolytic) agent
Schedule IV controlled substance

USUAL DOSE

PO, adults: 5-25 mg 3-4 times daily according to degree of anxiety; start with small initial dose, increase gradually as needed. • Acute alcohol withdrawal: 50-100 mg; may repeat up to maximum dose of 300 mg/24 hr.
G PO, older adults/debilitated patients: 5 mg bid-qid; increase cautiously as needed.
P PO, children >6 yr: 5 mg 2-4 times daily; increase cautiously; maximum dose 10 mg bid-tid.
IV/IM, adults: Acute or severe anxiety: Initially 50-100 mg, IV or IM (preferred); then 25-50 mg q6-8h as necessary; convert to PO therapy as soon as possible. • Maximum dose 300 mg/24 hr
G IV/IM, older adults/debilitated patients: 25-50 mg, IV or IM (preferred); convert to PO therapy as soon as possible.
P IV/IM, children >12 yr: 25-50 mg or 0.5 mg/kg/24 hr in equally divided doses, q6-8h, IV or IM (preferred); convert to PO therapy as soon as possible.

ADMINISTRATION

V Direct IV: Inject each dose of 100 mg or less slowly over 1-3 min. *Too rapid administration may cause hypotension, respiratory depression, apnea, CV collapse*
IM: Inject deeply into large muscle mass (upper outer quadrant of gluteus preferred); administer slowly.

PREPARATION

IM: Use 2 ml special IM diluent provided by manufacturer to reconstitute immediately before use. DO NOT USE OTHER DILUENTS, WHICH MAY CAUSE PAIN ON INJECTION. Add diluent slowly to prevent bubble formation; shake gently until dissolved. Concentration is 50 mg/ml. Discard unused portion.
Direct IV: Reconstitute immediately before use with 5 ml 0.9% NaCl or sterile water for injection. DO NOT USE IM DILUENT PROVIDED BY MANUFACTURER. Shake gently until dissolved. Concentration is 20 mg/ml. Discard unused portion.

ACTIONS

Acts in CNS to facilitate action of gamma-aminobutyric acid (GABA, major inhibitory neuro-

---

P pediatric   **G** geriatric   **V** Direct IV

transmitter; produces antianxiety, sedative-hypnotic, tranquilizing effects • May have weak analgesic effects • When given PO or IM in usual doses, has few effects on respiratory, CV, autonomic nervous systems.

PHARMACOKINETICS

ROUTE	ONSET	PEAK	DURATION
PO	30-60 min	30 min-4 hr	12-24 hr
IM	15-30 min	Approx 60 min	4-6 hr
IV	1-5 min	<15 min	15-60 min

DISTRIBUTION

Widely distributed; crosses blood-brain barrier

ELIMINATION

Metabolized in liver, eliminated by kidneys; half-life 5-30 hr, prolonged in older adults, liver disease

INDICATIONS

Anxiety disorders; short-term relief of anxiety symptoms • Relief of apprehension, anxiety before surgery, procedures • To reduce agitation, tremors, hallucinations, other symptoms associated with acute alcohol withdrawal

PRECAUTIONS/ CONTRAINDICATIONS

Precautions: Adverse effects more likely in first few days of therapy • Paradoxical excitement with acute rage may occur, especially in psychiatric patients, hyperactive children. • Seizures may result with sudden cessation of prolonged or high-dose parenteral therapy. • *IV administration may cause hypotension/respiratory depression,* especially in older adults/debilitated patients and when administered too rapidly.

Use caution with: Hepatic/renal disease, older adults, children, debilitation, low serum albumin; reduced dose indicated

Pregnancy category: Risk of congenital malformation, prolonged CNS depression, withdrawal symptoms in newborn; avoid use in pregnancy/lactation.

Contraindications: Hypersensitivity to chlordiazepoxide • Acute alcohol intoxication with VS depression • Acute angle-closure glaucoma • Depressive neuroses, psychotic reactions when anxiety not prominent • Avoid IV administration in shock, coma, respiratory depression, or with recent administration of other respiratory depressants.

ADVERSE EFFECTS

CNS: *Drowsiness, ataxia, dizziness, fatigue,* syncope, blurred vision, confusion, paradoxical excitation, especially in children, psychiatric patients

Resp: Respiratory depression with IV use

CV: Tachycardia, hypotension, edema, **CV collapse** (IV)

GI: Nausea, constipation, hepatic dysfunction, jaundice

Hema: Blood dyscrasias

Derm: Skin eruptions

Local: Injection site pain

Misc: Tolerance, psychologic/ physical dependence

TOXICITY/OVERDOSE

Symptoms (acute toxicity): Somnolence, impaired coordination, slurred speech, confusion, coma, diminished reflexes • Hypotension, seizures, respiratory depression, apnea, especially with IV administration • Toxic-

---

italic = common side effects   **bold** = life-threatening reactions

ity more likely with concurrent ingestion of alcohol, other CNS depressants

Management: After recent ingestion, implement guidelines for management of acute overdose (Appendix I). • Flumazenil reverses sedation, partially reverses respiratory depression. • Maintain airway/support ventilation as necessary. • *Hypotension:* Elevate legs, administer IV fluids; use vasopressors (e.g., norepinephrine, metaraminol) as necessary. • Do not use barbiturates for paradoxical excitation. • Hemodialysis is not generally useful.

INTERACTIONS

alcohol, ethyl, antihistamines, barbiturates, beta-blockers, cimetidine, disulfiram, isoniazid, ketoconazole, opiate analgesics, probenecid propoxyphene Excessive sedation
antacids Altered absorption
digoxin ↑ Digoxin levels, toxicity possible
flumazenil ↓ Sedation
levodopa ↓ Antiparkinsonian effectiveness
rifampin ↓ Sedation
theophylline ↓ Sedation

Y-SITE COMPATIBILITIES

Heparin, hydrocortisone sodium, potassium chloride, vitamin B complex with C

Y-SITE INCOMPATIBILITIES

Cefepime

PATIENT CARE IMPLICATIONS

• Individualize dosage, increase slowly. Always use smallest effective dose.
• Adverse effects more likely in first few days of therapy

• Administer with food to reduce gastric irritation.
• Avoid sudden cessation of therapy, especially in patients who have received therapy for several months or longer (may cause withdrawal symptoms, including seizures).
• Limit quantities prescribed for patients with severe depression, suicidal tendencies, history suggesting likelihood of substance abuse.
• Reserve IM use to urgent/emergency situations or when PO therapy contraindicated, such as perioperatively. IV use indicated only in emergency situations and with continuous monitoring; convert to PO therapy as soon as possible.

G Older adults
• Use lower dose, increase cautiously, closely monitor for adverse effects such as impaired psychomotor/mental performance.
• Periodically assess need for continued therapy.

IV
• Hypotension/respiratory depression are possible, especially with rapid IV administration and in older adults/debilitated patients; have resuscitation equipment immediately available.
• Monitor frequently for 3-4 hr after IV administration. Patient should remain in bed for at least 3 hr and requires assistance with initial ambulation.

Vital signs/hemodynamics: Monitor VS at frequent intervals in heavily sedated patients (e.g., those also receiving opiates) or during immediate postop period. • Continuous pulse oximetry recommended for heavily sedated patients. • Mon-

itor HR, RR, BP during and frequently for 3-4 hr after parenteral administration.
Physical assessment: Assess neurologic status for excessive sedation, impaired physical co-ordination. Reduce dose as necessary. • Assess for effectiveness: relief of anxiety, control of agitation/tremors in acute alcohol withdrawal.
Laboratory tests: Monitor: Liver enzymes, bilirubin • CBC

PATIENT/FAMILY TEACHING

Purpose of medication is to reduce anxiety/agitation. • Medication may cause drowsiness. Call for assistance when getting out of bed, walking. • Report possibility of pregnancy.
Outpatient: Avoid driving and other activities requiring mental alertness or physical coordination until response to medication established. • This medication may cause psychologic/physical dependence. Withdrawal symptoms, including seizures, may develop if you abruptly stop taking this medication. Consult health care provider before increasing dose or abruptly discontinuing. • Avoid concurrent use of alcohol or other drugs that cause sedation while taking this medication. • Take with food if desired to minimize gastric irritation.

AVAILABLE FORMS

Powder for reconstitution and IM/IV use • Tablets, capsules

chlorothiazide
(klor-oh-thye'a-zide)
Diachlor, Diurigen, Diuril

Classifications: Thiazide diuretic, antihypertensive

C

USUAL DOSE

℗ PO, adults/children >12 yr: 0.5-2.0 g once daily in AM or bid; may give 3-5 times/wk • Maximum dose, 2 g/24 hr
℗ PO, children 6 mo-12 yr: 10-20 mg/kg/day once daily in AM or bid.
IV, adults: 0.5-1.0 g once daily or q12h; initiate PO therapy as soon as possible.

ADMINISTRATION

▼ Direct IV, adults: Inject prepared solution at rate of 100 mg/min or more slowly. 500-mg dose is given over at least 5 min. • IV infusion recommended
IV, intermit inf, adults: Infuse prepared solution over 15-30 min. • Do not exceed 100 mg/min.

PREPARATION

IV: Reconstitute powder with 18 ml sterile water; concentration is 25 mg/ml. Do not use less than 18 ml. May add to desired volume (usually 30-50 ml) of D_5W or 0.9% NaCl.
Compatible solutions: D_5W, or 0.9% NaCl, LR, prepared combinations of these solutions
Stability: Stable at room temperature for 24 hr after reconstitution

ACTIONS

Interferes with sodium transport, resulting in increased excretion of sodium, chloride, water • Increases excretion of potassium, bicarbonate, magnesium, phosphate • Reduces calcium, ammonia, uric acid excretion • Increases plasma renin activity, causing slight elevation in aldosterone secretion • Reduces BP in hypertensive patients; augments action of other antihypertensives • In diabetes insipidus, paradoxically reduces UO • Affects glucose metabolism; may cause elevated blood glucose

PHARMACOKINETICS

ROUTE	ONSET	PEAK	DURATION
PO	1-2 hr	4 hr	6-12 hr
IV	<15 min	30 min	2 hr

DISTRIBUTION
Widely distributed; crosses placenta

ELIMINATION
Excreted unchanged in urine; delayed excretion with CHF impairment; renal half-life 45-120 min

INDICATIONS

To reduce BP in hypertensive patients; used alone or to enhance effects of other agents • To reduce edema associated with right-sided/mild left-sided heart failure, liver cirrhosis, nephrotic syndrome • May not be effective in long-term management of edema in patients with significant renal impairment
Unlabeled/investigational:
To reduce excessive UO associated with diabetes insipidus; treatment of electrolyte disturbances associated with renal tubular acidosis

PRECAUTIONS/ CONTRAINDICATIONS

Precautions: Hypokalemia, hypochloremic alkalosis may occur. • Digitalis toxicity more likely in hypokalemic patients;

potassium supplements indicated • Dilutional hyponatremia may slowly develop in patients receiving chronic therapy.
• Uric acid elevation, gout may occur.
Use caution with: Renal impairment; reduced plasma volume may decrease GFR, precipitate azotemia. • Cirrhosis, hepatic failure; rapid fluctuations in fluids/electrolytes may prompt hepatic coma. • Patients with diabetes, prediabetes; may produce hyperglycemia • SLE; may exacerbate condition
B Pregnancy category: Safety of IV route not clearly established
Contraindications: Hypersensitivity to chlorothiazide, other thiazides, sulfonamides • Anuria • Untreated severe hepatic coma • Severe uncorrected **P** electrolyte depletion • Children: Safety of IV route not clearly established

ADVERSE EFFECTS

CNS: Dizziness, headache, yellow vision, paresthesias
Resp: Cough, sore throat, rhinorrhea, alkalosis, compensatory respiratory depression
CV: Orthostatic hypotension, **hypotension, dysrhythmias, pulmonary edema**
GI: Nausea, vomiting, anorexia, diarrhea, constipation, abdominal pain/cramping, precipitation of **hepatic coma, cholestatic jaundice, pancreatitis** (rare)
GU: ↑ BUN/creatinine, progressive azotemia
Endo: Hyperglycemia, glycosuria
F&E: *Hypokalemia, hypochloremia,* hyponatremia, metabolic

alkalosis, hypercalcemia, ↑ ammonia

Derm: Photosensitivity, rash, wheals, itching, purpura

Misc: Weakness, ↑ cholesterol; hyperuricemia, gout

TOXICITY/OVERDOSE

Symptoms: Hypotension, dehydration, circulatory collapse • Electrolyte loss with weakness, dizziness, mental confusion, vomiting, muscle cramps **Management:** After recent oral ingestion, implement guidelines for management of acute overdose (Appendix I). • Support respiration as needed. • Administer IV fluids, replace electrolytes; closely monitor sodium, potassium balance. • **Hypotension:** Elevate legs, administer IV fluids; if unresponsive to fluid replacement, use vasopressors (i.e., dopamine, norepinephrine) • Avoid administration of cathartics, which could contribute to fluid/electrolyte imbalance.

INTERACTIONS

alcohol Hypotension

amphetamines ↓ Renal clearance; risk of toxicity

amphotericin B Severe potassium depletion

antidiabetic agents Interference with glucose-lowering effects

barbiturates Hypotension

beta-blockers Hypotension

calcium channel blockers Hypotension

corticosteroids Severe potassium depletion

digoxin Hypokalemia, hypomagnesemia, predisposition to digoxin toxicity

diuretics Risk of severe hyokalemia

diuretics, potassium sparing Enhanced diuretic effects with less potassium loss

hypotensive agents Hypotension

insulin Interference with glucose-lowering effects

NSAIDs (i.e., ibuprofen, indomethacin) Fluid retention; NSAID-induced renal failure

nondepolarizing IMBAs (e.g., pancuronium) Prolonged neuromuscular blockade

opiates Hypotension

probenecid Blockage of thiazide-related uric acid retention

quinidine ↓ Quinidine excretion; risk of toxicity

Y-SITE INCOMPATIBILITIES

multivitamins

PATIENT CARE IMPLICATIONS

• Evaluate response to therapy, considering diuretic response, fluid balance, weight, electrolytes. Adjust dose accordingly.
• Potassium supplements are frequently necessary, especially in digitalized patients.
• Consider use of potassium-sparing diuretic, i.e., spironolactone, amiloride, if other diuretics will be used concomitantly.
• Avoid combination formulas with potential for profound hypotension when initiating therapy.

Vital signs/hemodynamics: Monitor BP, HR, UO frequently with parenteral therapy. Consult physician for hypotension, oliguria. • As available, continuously monitor ECG with parenteral therapy. Note presence of PVCs, dysrhythmias, hypokalemic ECG changes: flattened ST segment, T wave inversion, U wave. If present, check potassium level, correct as necessary. Digitalized patients should be carefully monitored for these and other dysrhythmias associated with digitalis toxicity. • Hemodynamic monitoring strongly recommended for patients with severe CHF, cardiac failure associated with acute MI, cardiogenic shock, hemodynamic instability; monitor closely for overaggressive diuresis with excessive lowering of preload and ↓ CO.

Physical assessment: Assess extremities, face, sacrum for improvement in edema. • Assess for signs/symptoms of electrolyte imbalance: dysrhythmias, confusion, dizziness, weakness, muscle cramps, faintness, headache, paresthesias, thirst, anorexia, vomiting. • Assess for perfusion/oxygenation deficit caused by hypovolemia: chest discomfort, ↓ level of consciousness, activity intolerance, hypotension, dizziness. • Assess hyperuricemic patients for toe or foot pain, suggesting gout. • Weigh patient daily. • **CHF:** Assess for improvement: clear breath sounds, reduced neck vein distention, resolution of edema.

Laboratory tests: Monitor: Electrolytes, particularly sodium, potassium, chloride, calcium, magnesium • BUN, creatinine • Bilirubin, liver enzymes • CBC • Blood glucose levels, especially in diabetic patients • Promptly correct imbalances. • Adverse effects of hypokalemia include severe dysrhythmias, increased/decreased effects of other drugs, including cardiac glycosides, antidiabetic agents.

PATIENT/FAMILY TEACHING

Purpose of drug is to encourage elimination of excess body fluid and lower BP. • May cause dizziness, especially when starting therapy; use caution when changing positions, walking. • Report breathing difficulty, palpitations, dizziness, activity intolerance, chest pain, confusion, weakness, faintness, muscle cramps, persistent thirst, vomiting.

Outpatient: Alcohol, hot weather, vigorous activity, prolonged standing may cause dizziness, faintness. • Take potassium supplements as prescribed • Take medication in AM. Never double doses. • Continue taking medication as prescribed even if you feel better. Drug controls but does not cure hypertension. • Take with food or milk for gastric irritation. • Do not take ibuprofen or other nonprescription drugs without consulting health care provider. • Use sunscreen, wear protective clothing to prevent photosensitivity reactions. • Routine follow-up exams are important to detect/prevent serious side effects. • **Patients with diabetes:** Blood glucose levels may increase; insulin dose may need adjustment.

AVAILABLE FORMS

Powder for IV use • Tablets

chlorpromazine
(klor-proe′ma-zeen)
Largactil ✤, Ormazine,
Thorazine

Classifications: Antipsychotic,
antiemetic, tranquilizer, phenothiazine

USUAL DOSE

PO, adults: Initially 10-25 mg
bid, tid, or qid; increase dose
gradually as necessary. Psychiatric patients may require 400
mg/day. • **Sustained release:**
Administer bid; dose based on
total daily dosage of standard
formulation
Ⓟ PO, children >6 mo: 0.55
mg/kg q4-6h
Rectal, adults: 100 mg q6-8h
Ⓟ Rectal, children >6 mo: 1.1
mg/kg q6-8h
IM, adults: 12.5-50 mg q3-4h
• **Severe psychiatric disturbances:** 25 mg; may repeat
dose in 1 hr; up to 400 mg q4-
6h has been used. • Convert to
PO therapy as soon as possible.
Ⓟ IM, children >6 mo: 0.55
mg/kg q6-8h • Convert to PO
therapy as soon as possible.
IV, intermit inf, adults: 25-50
mg • **Perioperative:** 2 mg at
2-min intervals; do not exceed
total dose of 25 mg • IV
ROUTE ONLY FOR TETA-
NUS, SEVERE HICCUPS,
PERIOPERATIVE USE
**Ⓖ Older adults, debilitated pa-
tients:** Start with ¼-⅓ usual
dose; increase gradually as
needed. • Monitor closely; reduce dose for hypotension, extrapyramidal reactions.

ADMINISTRATION

IM: Inject slowly, deep into upper outer quadrant of buttock.

IV inf: Administer dilute solution very slowly at rate of 0.5-1
mg/min. Give 25 mg dose over
25-50 min. Infusion pump or
rate-controlling device necessary. • Patient should be supine.
• Stop infusion for hypotension,
dysrhythmias, ECG changes.
Enteral formula compatibilities
(concentrated solution): vital

PREPARATION

Avoid contact with solution;
may cause contact dermatitis.
PO concentrate: Add to at
least 60 ml of juice, or other
beverage, coffee, tea, semisolid
food. Administer immediately.
IM: May be diluted with 0.9%
NaCl or 2% procaine HCl to reduce irritation
IV: Dilute each mg with at least
1 ml 0.9% NaCl (e.g., 25 mg/25
ml). May be further diluted in
50-1000 ml of 0.9% NaCl. Appearance: clear to slightly yellow. Discard dark or markedly
discolored solutions.

ACTIONS

Dopamine receptor antagonist;
depresses part of CNS affecting
wakefulness, basal metabolism,
temperature regulation, vasomotor tone, emesis, hormonal balance • Results in decreased anx-
iety/tension, muscle relaxation,
sedation • Relative to other phenothiazines, has strong antiemetic, strong anticholinergic
(e.g., dry mouth, blurred vision), strong sedative, moderate
extrapyramidal (e.g., dystonia,
motor restlessness, parkinsonism) effects • Strong peripheral
alpha-adrenergic blocking activity, may cause hypotension
• Potentiates CNS, respiratory
depressant, analgesic effects of

C

opioid analgesics, sedatives, hypnotics, anesthetics

PHARMACOKINETICS

ROUTE	ONSET	PEAK	DURATION*
PO	30-60 min	2-4 hr	4-6 hr
PO, sus rel	30-60 min	2-4 hr	10-12 hr
IM	10-20 min	20 min	3-6 hr
IV	Immed	10 min	2-4 hr

DISTRIBUTION

Widely distributed; readily crosses blood-brain barrier, 92%-97% protein bound

ELIMINATION

Metabolized by liver, excreted in urine and feces; half-life 10-30 hr

---

*Duration of effectiveness in most patients; levels detectable for up to 6 mo after therapy.

INDICATIONS

Preop to decrease tension/anxiety, enhance anesthetic induction, potentiate anesthetic agents, reduce postop vomiting • Prevention/control of nausea/vomiting; relief of intractable hiccups • As adjunct in treatment of acute tetanus • To reduce hallucinations, autonomic hyperactivity, other symptoms in schizophrenia, psychotic disorders • Symptomatic control during manic phase of bipolar disorder • Severe behavioral P problems in children manifested by extreme hyperexcitability or hyperactivity • Acute intermittent porphyria

PRECAUTIONS/ CONTRAINDICATIONS

Precautions: Serious adverse CNS effects possible: irreversible tardive dyskinesia, potentially fatal neuroleptic malignant syndrome (see Adverse Effects) • Initiate long-term therapy only if need clearly established; use smallest effective dose, shortest possible duration • Lowers seizure threshold, may precipitate seizures • Antiemetic effects may delay diagnosis of disorders when vomiting is prominent feature (e.g., intestinal obstruction, Reye's syndrome).

Use caution with: CNS depressants, severe CV disease, hepatic/renal disease, seizure G disorder, older adults, debilitation, glaucoma, prostatic hypertrophy, exposure to organophosphate insecticides, thermoregulatory failure, hypocalcemia; lower dose indicated • COPD, asthma, acute respiratory infections, limited ventilatory reserve; causes CNS depression • Obtunded patients or when vomiting/aspiration likely; suppresses cough reflex

c **Pregnancy category:** Use only if safer alternative unavailable.

Contraindications: Hypersensitivity to chlorpromazine, other phenothiazines • Severe CNS depression, coma, bone marrow depression, severe hypertension, hypotension, Reye's syndrome P • Children <6 mo, pediatric surgery • First trimester of pregnancy • Commercial parenteral preparations may contain sulfites, which can cause serious allergic reactions.

ADVERSE EFFECTS

CNS: *Drowsiness,* depression, weakness, insomnia, restlessness, paradoxical excitation, headache, cerebral edema, **seizures,** *extrapyramidal reactions* including (1) dystonia (e.g., neck/back muscle rigidity, carpedal spasm, difficulty swallowing/talking), (2) motor restlessness, (3) parkin-

---

P pediatric   G geriatric   V Direct IV

sonian signs/symptoms (e.g., tremors, shuffling gait), (4) tardive dyskinesia (e.g., rhythmic involuntary movements of tongue, face, mouth, jaw, extremities), (5) **neuroleptic malignant syndrome:** hyperthermia, severe hypertonicity, ↓ level of consciousness, autonomic instability (e.g., tachycardia, dysrhythmias, BP instability)

Resp: Nasal congestion, bronchospasm, dyspnea

CV: *Hypotension, orthostatic hypotension,* tachycardia, syncope, Q and T wave ECG changes, **circulatory collapse, sudden death**

GI: *Constipation, dry mouth,* **adynamic ileus, hepatitis**

GU: Urinary retention, pink or brownish discoloration of urine

Hema: Blood dyscrasias, including agranulocytosis/leukopenia

Derm: *Photosensitivity,* rashes, changes in pigmentation, contact dermatitis

Syst: Thermoregulatory failure with hypo/hyperthermia

Misc: Allergic/hypersensitivity reactions, ocular changes

TOXICITY/OVERDOSE
Symptoms (acute toxicity):
Somnolence, CNS depression, coma • Hypotension, dysrhythmias, especially with IV administration • Extrapyramidal symptoms, seizures, hypo/hyperthermia, paradoxical excitation, autonomic reactions • Toxicity more likely with concurrent ingestion of alcohol, other CNS depressants

Management: After recent ingestion of large amounts, consider gastric lavage with airway protection; lavage may be useful even several hours after ingestion because phenothiazines slow gastric motility; *induction of vomiting not recommended, since dystonic reaction of head or neck could result in aspiration of vomitus.* • Saline cathartics may be used to evacuate sustained-release capsules. • Maintain airway/support ventilation; administer IV fluids. • Observe closely for dystonia, extrapyramidal reactions, which could lead to airway difficulties. • **Hypotension:** Elevate legs, administer IV fluids; use vasopressors (e.g., norepinephrine, phenylephrine) as necessary if unresponsive to volume replacement. Avoid epinephrine, similar vasopressors because phenothiazines may reverse vasopressor effects, causing profound hypotension.
• Manage acute dystonic reactions with parenteral diphenhydramine or parenteral benztropine (Cogentin). • For extrapyramidal symptoms, use diphenhydramine, barbiturates, anticholinergic antiparkinsonians agents. • Control seizures with diazepam or pentobarbital.
• Phenytoin may be used for ventricular dysrhythmias. • Dialysis is not likely to be helpful.

INTERACTIONS
alcohol, ethyl ↑ Sedation
amphetamines Mutual inhibition of therapeutic effects
antacids Altered absorption
anticholinergics Inhibition of antipsychotic effect; additive anticholinergic effects
antihistamines ↑ Sedation
barbiturates ↓ Levels of chlorpromazine

---

italic = common side effects   **bold** = life-threatening reactions

beta-blockers ↑ Levels/enhanced effects of both agents, hypotension possible

epinephrine Blocked alpha effects with unopposed beta effects; profound hypotension

levodopa ↓ Antiparkinsonian effectiveness

meperidine Profound hypotension; excessive sedation

opiate analgesics ↑ Sedation

propoxyphene ↑ Sedation

TCAs ↑ Levels of both agents; additive anticholinergic effects; toxicity

Y-SITE COMPATIBILITIES

Fluconazole, heparin, hydrocortisone, odansetron, potassium chloride

SYRINGE COMPATIBILITIES

Atropine, butorphanol, diphenhydramine, droperidol, fentanyl, glycopyrrolate, hydroxyzine, meperidine, metoclopramide, midazolam, morphine, pentazocine, prochlorperazine, promethazine

Y-SITE INCOMPATIBILITIES

Alkaline solutions, cefepime, piperacillin-tazobactam

PATIENT CARE IMPLICATIONS

P G • Children/older adults more likely to develop extrapyramidal reactions, paradoxical excitation, other adverse reactions. Use lowest effective dose; monitor closely.

• Avoid skin contact with syrup/solution for injection, which may cause contact dermatitis.

• Drowsiness, orthostatic hypotension possible, especially during 1st week of therapy; use safety precautions. When feasible, administer at bedtime.

• Large quantities should not be prescribed for patients with severe depression, suicidal tendencies, history of substance abuse.

• Administer antacids 1 hr before or 2 hr after chlorpromazine administration.

• Do not break/crush sustained-release capsules.

• Reserve parenteral therapy for urgent/emergency situations or when PO route unacceptable

IV inf

• Adverse CV effects (e.g., hypotension, tachycardia, dizziness, syncope) more likely

• Monitor frequently for 1-2 hr after IV administration. Patient should remain in bed for at least 1 hr and requires assistance with initial ambulation.

• Have resuscitation equipment immediately available.

G Older adults

• Individualize dose; closely monitor for adverse effects.

• Periodically assess need for continued therapy.

Vital signs/hemodynamics: Monitor VS frequently in heavily sedated patients (e.g., those also receiving opiates) or during immediate postop period. • Continuous pulse oximetry recommended for heavily sedated patients • IV inf: Monitor HR, BP during and frequently after administration. • As available, monitor ECG for increased QT interval, ST segment depression, AV conduction disturbances, dysrhythmias during and immediately after infusion.

Physical assessment: Assess neurologic status for excessive sedation, dizziness, impaired physical coordination. Dose reduction may be necessary. • As-

sess for respiratory distress in patients with history of COPD or cardiac impairment.
Laboratory tests: Monitor: Liver enzymes • BUN, creatinine • CBC regularly throughout therapy • **May cause:** False-positive pregnancy test

PATIENT/FAMILY TEACHING

Purpose of medication is to reduce anxiety, promote relaxation, prevent nausea/vomiting. • Medication may cause dizziness, drowsiness. Call for assistance when getting out of bed, walking. Change positions slowly. These reactions are less likely to occur after 1st week of therapy. • Urine may turn pink or reddish brown. • Inform health care provider if you may be pregnant or are considering pregnancy.
Outpatient: Avoid driving and other activities requiring mental alertness, physical coordination. • May contribute to development of heatstroke; avoid hot weather, seek air conditioning. • Avoid alcohol or other drugs that cause sedation while taking this medication. • Take antacids 1 hr before or 2 hr after taking this drug. • Do not break or chew sustained-release capsules. • If syrup used, avoid skin contact.
Long-term therapy: Report sore throat, mouth, or gums or other signs of infection; yellowing of skin or whites of eyes; tremors or muscle twitching; problems with eyesight. • Avoid prolonged exposure to sunlight; use sunscreen wear protective clothing. • This medication may cause withdrawal symptoms in patients receiving long-term therapy. Consult health care provider before changing dose or abruptly discontinuing.

AVAILABLE FORMS

Parenteral for IM/IV use • Tablets, capsules, syrup, concentrated solution • Rectal suppositories

cimetidine
cimetidine HCl
(sye-met′i-deen)
Tagamet, Nu-Cimet ✦, Peptol ✦, Tagan ✦

Classifications: Antisecretory agent, histamine H$_2$ receptor antagonist

USUAL DOSE

PO, adults: Initially 800 mg daily, usually hs; 1.6 g dosage used for heavy smokers/large ulcers. Maintenance dose is 400 mg daily. Other dosing schedules used. • **Pathologic hypersecretory conditions:** 300 mg four times daily with meals and hs; larger doses used; total dose not to exceed 2.4 g/day • **Renal impairment:** 300 mg q12h; schedule dose immediately after dialysis.
IV/IM, adults: 300 mg q6-8h; adjust dose to maintain gastric pH ≥5; do not exceed 2.4 g daily. • **Renal impairment:** 300 mg q12h; schedule dose immediately after dialysis.
IV, cont inf, adults: Initially 150 mg loading dose (optional); follow with continuous infusion at 50 mg/hr. Titrate to desired gastric pH; as much as 600 mg/hr used in pathologic hypersecretory conditions.

italic = common side effects   **bold** = life-threatening reactions

ADMINISTRATION

▼Direct IV: Dilute in 20 ml sterile water or 0.9% NaCl; inject slowly over at least 5 min. Too rapid injection may cause bradycardia, dysrhythmias, hypotension.

IV, intermit inf: Infuse premixed or prepared solution over 15-20 min.

IV, cont inf: Use infusion pump or rate-controlling device; start at 35-50 mg/hr and titrate to desired gastric pH, usually ≥5.

PREPARATION

IV, intermit inf: Mix 300 mg in 50-100 ml compatible solution.

IV, cont inf: Dilute as follows:

COMMON DILUTIONS	CONCENTRATION
900 mg/500 ml	1.8 mg/ml
900 mg/250 ml	3.6 mg/ml
900 mg/100 ml	9 mg/ml

Compatible fluids: D_5W, 0.9% NaCl
Stability: Stable at room temperature for 48 hr

ACTIONS

Inhibits action of histamine on H_2 receptors of parietal cells, thus reducing gastric acid secretion • Decreases volume of gastric juice, resulting in reduced pepsin secretion • Weak antiandrogenic effects (gynecomastia, impotence) • No anticholinergic properties • Reduces hepatic metabolism of some drugs; many medication interactions (see Interactions)

PHARMACOKINETICS

ROUTE	ONSET	PEAK	DURATION
PO	<1 hr	1 hr	4-8 hr*
IM	Rapid	Rapid	4-6 hr
IV	Immed	Immed	4 hr

DISTRIBUTION
Wide distribution; 15%-20% protein bound

ELIMINATION
Excreted in urine, feces; half-life 2 hr

*Dose related.

INDICATIONS

Short-term treatment of active benign gastric, duodenal ulcers to reduce pain/other symptoms, promote healing • In reduced doses to reduce ulcer recurrence • To reduce acid secretion, promote ulcer healing in hypersecretory conditions (Zollinger-Ellison syndrome, postop hypersecretion, short-gut syndrome) • Symptomatic relief of gastroesophageal reflux that fails to respond to conventional therapy alone • Prevention of upper GI bleeding in critically ill patients
Unlabeled/investigational:
Preoperatively to reduce risk of aspiration pneumonia • Concomitantly with antihistamines (H_1 receptor antagonists) to relieve allergic symptoms, urticaria in patients who are unresponsive to H_1 receptor antagonists alone • With other therapy in management of acetaminophen overdose to reduce hepatotoxicity

PRECAUTIONS/ CONTRAINDICATIONS

Precautions: Rapid IV injection may cause bradycardia, other dysrhythmias, hypotension. • Reversible mental confu-

---

C

sion possible, especially with advanced age, renal/hepatic disease, critical illness
Use caution with: Renal dysfunction • Hepatic dysfunction • Increases AST, ALT, other liver enzymes
Pregnancy category: Safety not clearly established
Contraindications: Hypersensitivity to cimetidine, other histamine H_2 blockers • Children: Safety not established

ADVERSE EFFECTS

CNS: *Headache, malaise,* dizziness, sleepiness, reversible mental confusion, particularly in critical illness
CV: With IV use: bradycardia; AV block, tachycardia, PVCs, **ventricular tachycardia/fibrillation, cardiac arrest,** hypotension
GI: Diarrhea; ↑ liver enzymes; hepatitis/pancreatitis (rare)
GU: ↑ *Creatinine*
Derm: Urticarial, macropapular, or acneiform rash; rarely, severe dermatologic reactions
Misc: Sexual impotence/gynecomastia in males, fever, transient pain at IM injection site, **anaphylaxis**

TOXICITY/OVERDOSE

Symptoms: Similar to adverse effects; death reported after ingestion of >40 g
Management: After recent ingestion, implement guidelines for management of acute overdose (Appendix I). • Initiate supportive/antidysrhythmic therapy according to ACLS guidelines (Appendix P).

INTERACTIONS

alcohol ↑ Alcohol intoxication
antacids ↓ Cimetidine absorption
anticoagulants, oral **Excessively prolonged PT; risk of bleeding**
benzodiazepines ↑ Benzodiazepine levels
beta-blockers: alprenolol, oxprenolol, propranolol ↑ Levels/effects of some beta-blockers
calcium channel blockers ↑ Levels of calcium channel blocker
ketoconazole ↓ Ketoconazole levels
lidocaine ↑ Lidocaine levels; toxicity
meperidine, other opiate analgesics ↑ Opiate analgesic effects; monitor closely; morphine less likely to interact
phenytoin ↑ Phenytoin levels; risk of toxicity
procainamide ↑ Procainamide levels; toxicity
quinidine ↑ Quinidine levels; toxicity
theophylline ↑ **Theophylline levels; risk of fatal toxicity**
TCAs ↑ Tricyclic levels; toxicity

Y-SITE COMPATIBILITIES

Acyclovir, aminophylline, amrinone, atracurium, diltiazem, enalaprilat, esmolol, fluconazole, haloperidol, heparin, hetastarch, labetalol, ondansetron, pancuronium, piperacillin-tazobactam, vecuronium, zidovudine

Y-SITE INCOMPATIBILITIES

Amphotericin B, cefepime, theophylline

PATIENT CARE IMPLICATIONS

• Do not administer within 1 hr of antacids.
• Administer IV doses as intermittent infusion when possible.
Vital signs/hemodynamics: Monitor BP, HR for orthostatic

---

italic = common side effects   **bold** = life-threatening reactions

changes in acutely ill patients.
• **Direct IV:** Observe for brady-cardia, dysrhythmias, hypoten-sion during administration.

Physical assessment: Assess for epigastric or abdominal pain; consult physician for per-sistent or severe pain. • Monitor for GI bleeding: occult blood in emesis or stool, orthostatic

G changes. • Assess older adults/severely ill patients for mental confusion.

Laboratory tests: Monitor: Liver enzymes (e.g., ALT, AST, alkaline phosphatase) • Creati-nine • CBC with differential

PATIENT/FAMILY TEACHING

Purpose of medication is to re-duce stomach acid. • May cause drowsiness, dizziness, mental

G confusion especially in elders; use caution and avoid activities requiring mental alertness until response to drug known. • Re-port black tarry stools, blood in stools, or emesis, dizziness, confusion. • Smoking decreases effectiveness of cimetidine, in-creases gastric acidity; smoking cessation programs/therapy rec-ommended.

Outpatient: Take all doses as prescribed, even if you feel bet-ter. • Do not take antacids with-in 1 hr of cimetidine. • Avoid coffee, caffeine, alcohol, aspirin, ibuprofen, other food or drugs that may cause gastric irritation. • Inform all health care provid-ers of cimetidine therapy to avoid possible drug interactions.

AVAILABLE FORMS

Parenteral for IM/IV use • Pre-mixed parenteral solution for IV infusion • Tablets • PO solution

---

ciprofloxacin
(sip-ro-floks´a-sin)
Cipro

Classification: Fluoroquinolone antibiotic

USUAL DOSE

PO, adults: 250-500 mg q12h
• **Renal insufficiency:** Reduce dose and/or frequency according to creat. cl.
IV, adults: 200-400 mg q12h
• **Renal insufficiency:** Reduce dose and/or frequency according to creat. cl.
Not for IM use

ADMINISTRATION

PO: Do not administer with dairy products, mineral supple-ments, sucralfate, antacids.
IV inf: Infuse prepared solution over 60 min; pain, local reac-tions likely with too-rapid infu-sion. Use dilute solution, large vein, small catheter/needle to reduce risk of vein irritation. Discontinue primary solution during administration.

PREPARATION

IV inf: Dilute 400-mg dose in ≥200 ml of compatible IV solu-tion; use 100 ml for 200-mg dose. Other volumes may be used, but final concentration should be ≤2 mg/ml.
Compatible fluids: D_5W, 0.9% NaCl • Peritoneal dialysis solution: Dianeal 137
Stability: Reconstituted solu-tion stable for at least 24 hr at room temperature

ACTIONS

Bactericidal; interferes with bac-terial enzyme necessary for DNA replication • Broad spec-

---

trum of activity against wide variety of gram-negative, gram-positive bacteria • Gram-negative activity includes *Pseudomonas aeruginosa,* most Enterobacteriaceae • Gram-positive activity includes penicillinase-producing and non–penicillinase-producing staphylococci, some methicillin-resistant staphylococci; most streptococci only moderately sensitive • Little or no activity against *Mycobacterium tuberculosis, Chlamydia trachomatis,* anerobic bacteria

PHARMACOKINETICS

ROUTE	ONSET	PEAK	DURATION
PO	Rapid	30-120 min	Approx 12 hr
IV	Immed	End infusion	

DISTRIBUTION
Widely distributed; low CSF levels

ELIMINATION
Metabolized in liver, eliminated in urine/feces; half-life 3-5 hr

INDICATIONS

Treatment of serious aerobic bacterial infections, particularly those caused by gram-negative organisms; often used for skin/bone infections, nosocomial pneumonia, complicated urinary tract infections • Choice drug for infectious diarrhea *(Escherichia coli, Campylobacter, Shigella)*
Unlabeled/investigational: Alternative therapy for gonorrhea

PRECAUTIONS/ CONTRAINDICATIONS

Precautions: Bacterial or fungal overgrowth possible • May cause urinary crystal formation, particularly with high-dose therapy/alkaline urine • Not indicated for community-acquired infections (e.g., otitis media, sinusitis, pneumonia) when a penicillin or cephalosporin could be used • Not used alone for infections involving anaerobic organisms

Use caution with: Epilepsy, cerebral arteriosclerosis, other CNS disorders; may precipitate seizures • Concurrent theophylline therapy; may cause dysrhythmias, seizures, respiratory failure, cardiac arrest • Hepatic/renal impairment; reduce dose/frequency.

C Pregnancy category: Use only if safer alternative unavailable.

Contraindications: Hypersensitivity to ciprofloxacin or other quinolones • Children <18 yr: Safety not established

ADVERSE EFFECTS

CNS: Headache, restlessness, dizziness, insomnia, drowsiness, tremor, paresthesias, **seizures** (rare), ↑ **ICP** (rare)
CV: Palpitations, dysrhythmias, hypertension, **MI** (rare)
Resp: Dyspnea, bronchospasm
GI: *Nausea, vomiting, diarrhea, abdominal pain,* anorexia, GI erosion, increased liver enzymes, oral candidiasis
GU: ↑ Creatinine/BUN, **nephritis,** crystalluria
Derm: Rash, wheals, itching, photosensitivity
Local: Irritation, pain
Misc: Hypersensitivity, including **anaphylaxis;** superinfection, colonization; joint inflammation, arthralgia

TOXICITY/OVERDOSE

Symptoms: Allergic reactions, including pharyngeal/pulmonary edema, CV instability/collapse, loss of consciousness • Toxic reactions: Vomiting, psychosis, CNS stimulation, seizures

Management: Initiate symptomatic/supportive measures, including airway management/ventilation. • After recent ingestion, implement guidelines for management of acute overdose (Appendix I). • For acute allergic reaction, see Appendix N. • Maintain hydration to reduce risk of crystalluria. • Hemodialysis may remove small amounts of drug.

INTERACTIONS

aminoglycosides ↑ Antibacterial activity in some patients

aminophylline, other xanthines ↑ Theophylline levels; ↑ adverse reactions, including dysrhythmias, seizures

antacids ↓ Ciprofloxacin absorption (PO)

anticoagulants, oral Prolonged PT

caffeine Exaggerated caffeine effects (e.g., tachycardia, anxiety)

Iron, mineral supplements ↓ PO absorption; ↓ antibiotic levels

penicillins, extended spectrum (e.g., piperacillin) ↑ Antibacterial activity against some gram-negative bacteria

probenecid ↓ Renal clearance/prolonged half-life of ciprofloxacin

sucralfate ↓ PO absorption; ↓ antibiotic levels

Y-SITE COMPATIBILITIES

Calcium gluconate, ceftazidime, digoxin, diltiazem, dobutamine, dopamine, gentamicin, hydroxyzine, lidocaine, metaclopromide, metronidazole, piperacillin, potassium chloride, promethazine, ranitidine, tobramycin, verapamil

Y-SITE INCOMPATIBILITIES

Aminophylline, floxacillin, furosemide, heparin, magnesium sulfate, mezlocillin, phenytoin, sodium bicarbonate

PATIENT CARE IMPLICATIONS

• Obtain specimens for culture and sensitivity before initiating antibiotic therapy. Therapy may be initiated before results received.

• With concurrent theophylline therapy, observe for evidence of theophylline toxicity, monitor theophylline levels, adjust dose as necessary. Excessive theophylline levels especially likely in **G** older adults. See theophylline for symptoms of toxicity and therapeutic levels.

• Do not discharge patient for at least 30 min after antibiotic administration.

• With concurrent sucralfate, antacid, or mineral supplement therapy, stagger schedules to avoid administration of these drugs within 2 hr of PO ciprofloxacin.

IV inf

• IV route must be used for severe infections or when shock present.

• Reduce risk of thrombophlebitis by using large veins and small catheters/needles, rotating infusion sites.

• Have epinephrine, antihistamine, resuscitation equipment readily available for use with severe allergic reaction.

Vital signs/hemodynamics: Monitor VS for indicators of infection, complications. • Carefully monitor UO, evaluate I&O

P pediatric   **G** geriatric   **V** Direct IV

ratio. Keep patient well hydrated by PO or parenteral fluids.

Physical assessment: Assess for improvement in primary infection or symptoms of super/suprainfection: appearance of sputum, urine, stool, wound drainage; presence of fever, candidiasis, vaginitis. • Observe for symptoms of hypersensitivity: rash, pruritus, wheezing, laryngeal edema, hypotension.

Laboratory tests: Monitor: Electrolytes, liver enzymes, PT, CBC with differential • Urinalysis, BUN, creatinine

PATIENT/FAMILY TEACHING

Purpose of drug is to limit growth of infection-causing bacteria. • Immediately report rash, swelling, intense itching, difficulty breathing, other signs of allergic reaction. • Report diarrhea, fever, vaginal itching or discharge, furry growth on tongue. • Drink plenty of fluid to avoid formation of crystals in urine.

Outpatient: Avoid concurrent use of alcohol, other CNS depressants. • Avoid excessive amounts of coffee, tea, soft drinks, other caffeinated beverages, chocolate; particularly important with CNS, cardiac disease. • Do not take with milk, yogurt, other dairy products. • Do not take antacids within 2 hr of taking this medication. • Avoid direct sunlight; severe sunburn possible. • Take at evenly spaced intervals over each 24-hr period. • Take all of medication exactly as prescribed. Do not stop taking medicine even if you feel better. Failure to take all of antibiotic may result in recurrence or ad-

ditional infection. Do not save or share unused medicine.

AVAILABLE FORMS
Parenteral for IV use • Tablets

clindamycin HCl
(klin-da-mye'sin)
Cleocin, Dalacin ✤
clindamycin palmitate HCl
Cleocin Pediatric
clindamycin phosphate
Cleocin

Classification: Miscellaneous antibiotic

USUAL DOSE
PO, adults: 150-450 mg q6h
PO, children >1 mo: 8-20 mg/kg/24 hr given q6-8h in evenly divided doses
IV/IM, adults: 600-2,700 mg/24 hr given q6, 8, or 12h in evenly divided doses • **Severe infections:** Up to 4.8 g/24 hr • Do not exceed single IM dose of 600 mg or IV dose of 1.2 g/hr. • **Severe renal/hepatic insufficiency:** Reduce dose and/or frequency.
IV/IM, children >1 mo: 15-40 mg/kg/24 hr given q6-8h in evenly divided doses

ADMINISTRATION
PO: Administer capsules with full glass of water to avoid esophageal irritation.
IM: Inject deep into large muscle mass (e.g., gluteus maximus, lateral thigh).
IV inf: Infuse each 300 mg of prepared solution over at least 10 min; maximum infusion rate,

30 mg/min. • Do not administer more than 1.2 g in 1 hr; too rapid administration may cause profound hypotension. • *Never administer as undiluted bolus injection.*
IV, cont inf: Initially, infuse at rate of 10-20 mg/min for 30 min. Follow by continuous infusion at 0.75-1.25 mg/min

PREPARATION

IV inf: Dilute 300-600 mg dose in 50 ml compatible solution, 900-1,200 mg dose in 100 ml. More concentrated solutions may be used; do not exceed concentration of 18 mg/ml.
Compatible fluids: D_5W, $D_{10}W$, 0.9% NaCl, LR, prepared combinations of these solutions; also, peritoneal dialysis solutions with or without heparin at 10 mg/L concentration.
Stability: Reconstituted solution stable for 24 hr at room temperature

ACTIONS

Bactericidal or bacteriostatic depending on drug concentration, susceptibility of bacterial strain; effects caused by inhibition of bacterial protein formation • Active against most aerobic gram-positive cocci, except *Enterococcus faecalis* • Active against many anaerobic bacteria, including *Actinomyces, Bacteroides, Peptococcus* • Gram-negative aerobic organisms, including *Pseudomonas aeruginosa,* are resistant.

PHARMACOKINETICS

ROUTE	ONSET	PEAK	DURATION
PO	Rapid	45-60 min	6 hr
IM	Rapid	<3 hr	6-8 hr
IV	Immed	End infusion	6-8 hr

DISTRIBUTION
Widely distributed; low CSF levels
ELIMINATION
Partially metabolized, remainder excreted unchanged; half-life 2-3 hr

INDICATIONS

Treatment of serious infections caused or believed to be caused by anaerobic or susceptible gram-positive organisms; particularly useful for intraabdominal, soft tissue, respiratory, pelvic, genital tract infections likely to be caused by susceptible organisms • Use generally reserved for patients with hypersensitivity reactions to penicillins • Considered by some the choice agent for *Bacteroides fragilis* infections • May be used with aminoglycoside to provide optimal coverage for mixed aerobic-anaerobic bacterial infections • Alternate agent for treatment of bacterial vaginosis • Not indicated for gram-positive bacterial infections if other less toxic antibiotics could be used

PRECAUTIONS/ CONTRAINDICATIONS

Precautions: Bacterial or fungal overgrowth possible, particularly with prolonged use • May cause serious or fatal colitis during or after treatment, particularly in older adults; preexisting GI disorders
Use caution with: Severe renal/hepatic impairment, advanced age • GI disease, especially colitis, ↑ risk of pseudo-

membranous colitis • Neonates/ infants; contains benzyl alcohol • Recent or concurrent use of NMBAs

c Pregnancy category: Use only if safer alternative unavailable.

Contraindications: Hypersensitivity to clindamycin, lincomycin or tartrazine dye (FD&C yellow no. 5) in 75-, 150-mg capsules • Treatment of meningitis; poor CNS penetration

ADVERSE EFFECTS

CV: **Hypotension, cardiac arrest** after rapid IV administration

GI: *Nausea, vomiting, diarrhea, abdominal pain,* anorexia, esophagitis, **pseudomembranous colitis,** ↑ bilirubin/liver enzymes

Derm: Rash, urticaria, pruritus

Hema: Leukopenia, neutropenia, eosinophilia, thrombocytopenia, agranulocytosis

Misc: Superinfection, colonization, hypersensitivity, including fever, hypotension, **anaphylaxis**

TOXICITY/OVERDOSE

Symptoms: Extensions of adverse effects • Pseudomembranous colitis with abdominal pain/ diarrhea • Acute allergic reaction, hypotension, anaphylaxis

Management: Discontinue drug. Initiate symptomatic/supportive measures, including airway management/ventilation.

• **Acute allergic reaction:** see Appendix N. • **Severe pseudomembranous colitis:** Administer PO vancomycin or metronidazole; corticosteroids systemically or by retention enema. Do not use opiates, diphenoxylate/ atropine (Lomotil) or other antiperistaltic/antidiarrheal agents.

• Hemodialysis is not likely to be helpful.

INTERACTIONS

aminoglycosides ↑ Risk of renal toxicity

erythromycin ↓ Antibiotic effectiveness

NMBAs Prolonged neuromuscular blockade

Y-SITE COMPATIBILITIES

Amiodarone, diltiazem, enalaprilat, esmolol, hydromorphone, labetalol, meperidine, morphine, multivitamins, ondansetron, perphenazine, piperacillin-tazobactam, potassium chloride, verapamil, vitamin B complex with C, zidovudine

Y-SITE INCOMPATIBILITIES

Aminophylline, ampicillin, barbiturates, calcium gluconate, fluconazole, magnesium sulfate, phenytoin

PATIENT CARE IMPLICATIONS

• Obtain specimens for culture and sensitivity before initiating antibiotic therapy. Therapy may be initiated before results received.

• IV route must be used for severe infections or when shock present.

• Administer capsules with full glass of water.

• Shake PO suspension well before using; refrigeration not required.

Vital signs: Monitor VS for indications of infection, complications.

Physical assessment: Assess for improvement in primary infection or symptoms of super/ suprainfection: appearance of

---

italic = common side effects   **bold** = life-threatening reactions

sputum, urine, stool, wound drainage; presence of fever, candidiasis, vaginitis. • Assess for colitis: severe diarrhea, blood/mucus in stools, abdominal cramping, fever. If present, consult physician before administering next dose. Continue therapy only if necessary and with close observation of patient. • *With recent use of NMBAs, use caution and assess for prolonged neuromuscular blockade.*
Laboratory tests: Monitor: Electrolytes, liver enzymes, PT, PTT, CBC with differential • Urinalysis, BUN, creatinine

PATIENT/FAMILY TEACHING

Purpose of drug is to limit growth of infection-causing bacteria. • Report rash, itching, diarrhea, abdominal cramping, fever, vaginal itching or discharge. • Expect a bitter or unpleasant taste with capsules, solution. Take with full glass of water and with meals or snack.

AVAILABLE FORMS

• Parenteral for IV/IM use • PO capsules • Granules for reconstitution and PO use (pediatrics)

---

clonidine HCl
(kloe'ni-deen)
Catapres, Dixarit ✦

clonidine HCl with clorthalidone
Combipres

Classifications: Antihypertensive, central alpha$_2$-adrenoreceptor agonist

USUAL DOSE

PO, adults: Initially 0.1 mg bid; gradually increase dose by 0.1-0.2 mg/day until BP controlled. • Given 2, 3, or 4 times daily • Maximum dose, 2.4 mg/day

G PO, older adults: Initially 0.5 mg bid; gradually increase dose by 0.1 mg/day until BP controlled. • Given 2, 3, or 4 times daily

Transdermal, adults: Initially, one 0.1 mg/24-hr system q7d; gradually increase dose every 1-2 wk until BP controlled. • Maximum dose, two 0.3-mg/24-hr systems q7d • **Renal impairment:** Reduce dose and/or frequency. Additional dose not required after hemodialysis

ADMINISTRATION

Transdermal: Use gentle pressure, especially around edges, to firmly apply to skin not covered by hair. Avoid distal extremities, open or irritated skin, calluses. Rotate sites to avoid skin irritation. Do not bend, cut, otherwise manipulate unit.

ACTIONS

Stimulates medullary alpha$_2$-adrenergic receptors, causing inhibition of sympathetic vasomotor centers; results in ↓ peripheral vascular resistance, ↓ SBP/DBP, HR slowing • May reduce plasma renin, decrease excretion of aldosterone, catecholamines • Postural reflexes maintained, orthostatic hypotension minimal • Causes sedation, reduces GI motility

---

PHARMACOKINETICS

ROUTE	ONSET	PEAK	DURATION
PO	30-60 min	3-5 hr	8 hr
Trans-dermal	2 days	2-3 days	7 days

DISTRIBUTION

Widely distributed

ELIMINATION

Metabolized by liver, eliminated in urine; half-life 16-20 hr

INDICATIONS

PO: Reduction of mild, moderate and severe hypertension • Considered step 2 drug • Used alone or in combination with other agents • Less likely to cause postural hypotension than many other agents
Unlabeled/investigational:
Rapid PO loading regimen used for nonemergency, severe hypertension; diagnosis of pheochromocytoma; migraine prophylaxis; management of opiate withdrawal

PRECAUTIONS/ CONTRAINDICATIONS

Precautions: Rebound hypertension, elevated catecholamines, agitation may occur with abrupt cessation of therapy.
Use caution with: Recent MI, severe CAD • Cerebrovascular disease • Renal failure; lower dose • Raynaud's disease • History of mental depression; may trigger further episodes
Contraindications: Hypersensitivity to clonidine • Children: Safety/efficacy not established
c Pregnancy category: Use only if safer alternative unavailable.

ADVERSE EFFECTS

CNS: *Drowsiness, sedation, dizziness,* weakness, headache, agitation, depression, sleep disturbances, ↓ visual acuity
CV: Orthostatic hypotension, palpitations, tachycardia, bradycardia, **CHF,** Raynaud's phenomenon, ECG conduction disturbances
GI: *Constipation, dry mouth,* nausea, vomiting, ↑ liver enzymes
Derm: Rash, wheals, itching, localized skin reactions with transdermal system
Misc: Muscle/joint pain, ↑ sensitivity to alcohol

TOXICITY/OVERDOSE

Symptoms: Hypotension, transient hypertension, bradycardia, dysrhythmias • Deep sedation or coma, seizures, respiratory depression
Management: After recent ingestion, implement guidelines for management of acute overdose (Appendix I). Gastric lavage with airway protection preferred over emesis because sedation likely • Establish/maintain airway; support breathing as needed with O_2 and/or mechanical ventilation • **Hypotension:** Elevate legs, administer IV fluids; if not responsive to volume expansion, use vasopressors (e.g., dopamine) • **Hypertension:** Use IV furosemide or diazoxide or alpha-adrenergic blockers (e.g., phentolamine). IV tolazoline (Priscoline) sometimes given to reverse clonidine effects • **Seizures:** Use IV diazepam or lorazepam. • **Dysrhythmias:** Manage according to ACLS guidelines (Appendix P). • Hemodialysis is generally ineffective.

---

italic = common side effects   **bold** = life-threatening reactions

INTERACTIONS

alcohol ↑ Sedation
antihypertensives Potentiation of hypotensive effects
barbiturates ↑ Sedation
beta-blockers Profound bradycardia
digoxin Profound bradycardia
diuretics Potentiation of hypotensive effects
guanethidine Profound bradycardia
opioid analgesics ↑ Sedation
TCAs ↓ Clonidine effectiveness

PATIENT CARE IMPLICATIONS

• Use precautions to protect sedated patients, especially when initiating therapy or increasing dose. Increase dose in evening to avoid daytime sedation.
• Use with diuretics increases effectiveness.
• Do not interrupt therapy for surgery; may use transdermal systems if PO therapy not possible.
• Abrupt cessation of therapy may result in rebound hypertension, elevated catecholamines, agitation, headache, tachycardia, GI dysfunction; tapered withdrawal necessary.

Transdermal:
• Dose of PO clonidine does not predict dose of transdermal system. Always initiate transdermal therapy with 0.1 mg/24 hr patch.
• Remove transdermal unit before defibrillation/cardioversion to avoid injury to patient or damage to equipment.

Vital signs/hemodynamics: Closely monitor BP, HR, especially with initial therapy and if used with other antihypertensives or diuretics.

Physical assessment: Assess for excessive sedation, lethargy, depression. Dose adjustment may improve these symptoms.
• Monitor fluid balance; weigh daily.

Laboratory tests: Monitor: BUN, creatinine • Liver enzymes, bilirubin • CBC with differential

PATIENT/FAMILY TEACHING

Purpose of drug is to lower BP. • May cause sedation and hypotension; change positions slowly. • Dry mouth relieved by frequent oral hygiene, sugarless gum or candy. • Medicine is not a cure for high BP; other therapies, including lifestyle modifications, must be continued.

Outpatient: Take medication exactly as prescribed. Do not stop taking medicine even if you feel better. If medication is abruptly discontinued, you may develop dangerously high BP and serious withdrawal symptoms. • Avoid alcohol, sedatives, antihistamines, other medications that cause drowsiness.
• Use caution in performing hazardous tasks requiring mental alertness or physical coordination. • Weigh twice/wk; notify health care provider of weight gain or edema. • Consult health care provider before taking cold, cough, or allergy preparations.

Transdermal: See Administration. Bathing and swimming do not affect unit. Physical activity, warm body temperature may cause more rapid release of medicine.

AVAILABLE FORMS

Tablets • Transdermal systems

codeine phosphate
codeine sulfate
(koe'deen)

codeine phosphate with acetaminophen
Phenaphen No. 2, 3, 4;
Tylenol No. 2, 3, 4
codeine phosphate with aspirin
Empirin No. 2 (15 mg), 3 (30 mg), 4 (60 mg)

Classifications: Opiate agonist, narcotic analgesic, antitussive
Schedule II controlled substance

USUAL DOSE
PO/IM/SC, adults: 30 mg q4h; range, 15-60 mg according to patient response • Use reduced **G** dose for older adults.
P PO/IM/SC, children ≥1 yr: 0.5 mg/kg q4-6h
PO/antitussive, adult: 10-20 mg q4-6h; do not exceed 120 mg/day.
P PO, antitussive, children: 2-6 yr: 2.5-5 mg q4-6h; do not exceed 12-18 mg/day. • 6-12 yr: 5-10 mg q4-6h; do not exceed 60 mg/day.

ACTIONS
Opium derivative that acts in CNS to inhibit pain perception; action similar to but milder than morphine • Reduces apprehension associated with pain • Suppresses coughing at lower doses than required for analgesia • Less likely than morphine or meperidine to cause respiratory depression, increased biliary pressures, spasm • Parenteral administration may cause orthostatic hypotension.

PHARMACOKINETICS

ROUTE	ONSET	PEAK	DURATION
PO	15-30 min	60 min	4-6 hr
SC	15-30 min	60 min	4-6 hr
IM	10-30 min	30-60 min	4-6 hr

DISTRIBUTION
Wide; readily crosses placenta
ELIMINATION
Metabolized in liver, CNS, other tissue; excreted in urine; half-life 3 hr

INDICATIONS
Relief of moderate pain not relieved by nonopiate analgesic • In low doses, suppression of nonproductive coughing caused by mechanical/chemical irritation

PRECAUTIONS/ CONTRAINDICATIONS
Precautions: May cause respiratory depression, especially with pulmonary disease • May cause hypotension, especially in hypovolemia, or when administered with phenothiazines, general anesthetics • Commercial preparations may contain sulfites, which can cause serious allergic reactions.
Use caution with: Pulmonary disease • Hepatic/renal dysfunction • Hypovolemia, shock • Addison's disease • Untreated myxedema • CNS depression, head injury, seizure disorder • Concurrent use of other CNS depressants • Acute alcoholism **G** • Prostatic hypertrophy • Older **P** adults, young children, debilitated patients; reduced dosage indicated
c Pregnancy category: Use only if safer alternative unavailable.
Contraindications: Hypersensitivity to codeine • Respiratory depression • Undiagnosed acute

---

abdominal conditions • Acute
ulcerative colitis • Diarrhea
caused by poisoning

ADVERSE EFFECTS

CNS: *Sedation, confusion,* dizziness, hallucinations, depression, euphoria, dysphoria, agitation, restlessness, coma,
seizures (rare)
EENT: Pupillary constriction,
visual disturbances
Resp: **Respiratory depression**
CV: *Orthostatic hypotension,* reflex tachycardia, sweating,
flushing
GI: *Constipation,* nausea, vomiting, delayed absorption of PO
agents
GU: Urinary retention
Derm: Pruritus, itching, wheals,
injection site pain
Misc: Hypothermia, tolerance,
physical/psychologic dependence

TOXICITY/OVERDOSE

Symptoms, acute: Profound
CNS depression • Respiratory
depression, apnea • Bradycardia,
hypotension, circulatory collapse, cardiopulmonary arrest
• Hypothermia with cool,
clammy skin
Management: After recent ingestion, implement guidelines
for management of acute overdose (Appendix I). • Gastric
lavage may be effective even
hours after ingestion, because
pylorospasm may cause much
of drug to remain in stomach.
• Establish/maintain airway; administer O$_2$. • **Hypotension:**
Elevate legs, administer IV fluids; if unresponsive to fluids,
use vasopressors (e.g., dopamine, norepinephrine). • Use
naloxone (opiate antagonist) to

reverse respiratory depression,
other symptoms.

INTERACTIONS

alcohol, ethyl; antihistamines;
anesthetics, general CNS depression
MAO inhibitors CNS depression
opiate agonist-antagonists (e.g.,
buprenorphine, butorphanol,
nalbuphine, pentazocine)
Acute withdrawal in opiate-dependent patients
opiate analgesics CNS depression
phenothiazines ↑ Analgesic effectiveness; CNS depression
sedatives CNS depression
tranquilizers CNS depression
quinidine ↓ Analgesic effectiveness
TCAs ↑ CNS depression

IN-SYRINGE
COMPATIBILITIES

Glycopyrrolate, hydroxyzine

PATIENT CARE
IMPLICATIONS

• Assess type, location, intensity of pain before and after administration.
• Use in smallest effective dose
to minimize development of tolerance, limit CNS depressant effects. PO doses are ⅔ as effective as IM/SC doses.
• Administer prn doses before
pain becomes severe; regularly
scheduled dosing more effective
than prn scheduling.
• Administer concurrently with
peripherally acting nonnarcotic
analgesics (e.g., acetaminophen,
ibuprofen) for additive analgesic
effects.
• Hospitalized patients receiving
codeine for acute pain control
do not usually develop dependence. As tolerance develops,

---

progressively higher doses may be necessary to relieve pain during long-term therapy.
• With long-term therapy, withdrawal symptoms may develop if drug abruptly discontinued.
Vital signs/hemodynamics: Assess BP, RR, pulse before and 30-60 min after IM/SC administration.
Physical assessment: Assess adequacy of ventilation by noting rate/depth of respirations, auscultating breath sounds, particularly in older adults/young children, with parenteral therapy. • Assess bowel function by auscultating for bowel sounds, and noting abdominal distention/elimination patterns. • Assess for urinary retention. Consult physician of diminished UO or bladder distention.

PATIENT/FAMILY TEACHING

Purpose of medication is to relieve moderate pain. • Request medication before pain becomes severe.
IM/SC: Change position slowly to minimize orthostatic hypotension. Call for assistance when ambulating.
Outpatient: Do not perform hazardous tasks requiring mental alertness or physical coordination. • Minimize constipation by increasing intake of fluids and dietary bulk and using stool softeners. Use laxatives only if necessary. • Avoid concurrent use of alcohol or other drugs that cause drowsiness while taking this medication.

AVAILABLE FORMS

Parenteral for IM/SC injection
• Tablets • PO solution

dalteparin
(dal-te′-par-in)
Fragmin

Classification: Anticoagulant, low-molecular-weight heparin

USUAL DOSE

SC, adult: 2,500 IU daily • Initiate therapy 1-2 hrs before surgery; continue for 5-10 days until deep vein thrombosis no longer a risk. • Dose adjustments for renal impairment, advanced age have not been established.

ADMINISTRATION

SC: Administer deep into subcutaneous tissue by grasping abdominal skin between thumb and forefinger and inserting entire length of needle into subcutaneous pocket of skin fold
• Patient should be lying down
• Use 25–27-gauge ⅝-inch needle; do not aspirate or massage when giving injection • Rotate injection sites from left to right anteriolateral, then left to right posterolateral abdominal wall.
• *Do not administer IM.*

ACTION

Augments the inhibitory effects of antithrombin III, thereby preventing the conversion of fibrinogen to fibrin and prothrombin to thrombin • Less effect on thrombin than unfractionated heparin • At usual doses does not significantly affect platelet aggregation, PT, APTT, fibrinogen level • Derived from porcine tissue

---

PHARMACOKINETICS

ROUTE	ONSET	PEAK	DURATION
SC	Rapid	4 hr	12-24 hr

DISTRIBUTION
Throughout plasma
ELIMINATION
Renal; half-life 3-5 hr

INDICATIONS

Prevention of deep vein thrombosis (which could lead to pulmonary embolism) after abdominal surgery

PRECAUTIONS/ CONTRAINDICATIONS

Precautions: Not for IM use • Cannot be used interchangeably with heparin, other low-molecular-weight heparins • May cause moderate thrombocytopenia; monitor closely
Use caution with: History of heparin-induced thrombocytopenia • Any condition associated with increased risk of hemorrhage: congenital or acquired bleeding disorder, severe hepatic or renal dysfunction, recent GI ulceration or bleeding, hemorrhagic CVA, severe hypertension, subacute bacterial endocarditis; recent brain, spinal, or ophthalmologic surgery
B **Pregnancy category:** Use only if safer alternative not available
Contraindications: Hypersensitivity to dalteparin, heparin, or pork products • Active major bleeding • Thrombocytopenia with positive antiplatelet antibody test • Safe and effective
P use in children has not been established.

ADVERSE EFFECTS

CNS: Confusion
CV: Edema
GI: Nausea
Hema: Thrombocytopenia, bleeding, bruising
Local: Injection site irritation, redness, pain, hematoma
Misc: Full range of hypersensitivity reactions, incl. anaphylaxis

TOXICITY/OVERDOSE

Symptoms: Hemorrhage, related complications
Management: Antidote is protamine sulfate, 1 mg for each mg dalteparin. Protamine can cause severe hypotension and anaphylaxis; use only if necessary; emergency medications and equipment must be readily available • For acute allergic reaction, see Appendix N.

INTERACTIONS

anticoagulants, incl. other heparins, thrombolytics, warfarin ↑ Risk of bleeding
antiplatelet agents, incl. NSAIDs, dipyridamole, ticlopidine ↑ Risk of bleeding

PATIENT CARE IMPLICATIONS

• Review history for contraindications. Do not administer if bleeding disorder is present.
• Inform all personnel caring for patient of anticoagulant therapy. Place highly visible written notice in patient's room.
• If unexplained decrease in Hct/Hgb, hypotension, or other evidence of hemorrhage, look for a bleeding site.
• Avoid unnecessary arterial and venous punctures, IM injections. If possible use saline or heparin lock for blood drawing. If venipuncture necessary, hold manual pressure over site until bleeding stops.

• Avoid arterial/venous invasive procedures in areas where direct pressure is difficult to apply: subclavian, jugular veins.
Vital signs/hemodynamics: Immediately consult physician for severe or uncontrolled hypertension: SBP >180 or DBP >110 mm Hg. Prepare to initiate hypotension therapy.
Physical assessment: Assess for unusual bleeding: petechiae, ecchymosis, bleeding from gums/mucous membranes, excessive bleeding from superficial injury. • Assess for occult bleeding: headache, altered mentation, paralysis, joint pain, shortness of breath, unexplained swelling, hypotension, shock. • Note blood in urine, other body fluids.
Laboratory tests: Monitor: Platelet count; Hgb/Hct; stools, gastric drainage/emesis for occult blood • May cause: Moderate thrombocytopenia, reversible elevations in AST/ALT

PATIENT/FAMILY TEACHING

Purpose of medication is to prevent clots from forming in leg veins. • Report unusual bruising or bleeding from IV sites, nose, mouth, or in urine/stools. • Remain on bed rest throughout therapy. • Avoid possible tissue damage from shaving, toothbrushing; avoid activities that may cause injury. • Inform laboratory personnel, other health care workers of anticoagulant therapy.

AVAILABLE FORMS

Parenteral for SC injection

dexamethasone
(dex-a-meth'a-sone)
Decadron, Dexone, Hexadrol

dexamethasone acetate
Dalalone LA, Decadron-LA, Dekasol LA, Dexasone-LA, Dexone LA, Solurex LA

dexamethasone sodium phosphate
Dalalone, Decadrol, Decadron, Dekasol, Dexasone, Hexadrol, Solurex

Classifications: Adrenal corticosteroid, glucocorticoid, antiinflammatory agent

USUAL DOSE

Dexamethasone: PO, adult: 0.75-9 mg daily in 2-4 equally divided doses • **PO, children:** 0.24-0.34 mg/kg daily in 4 equally divided doses
Dexamethasone sodium phosphate: IV/IM, adult: Severe shock: 1-6 mg/kg IV as single dose or 40 mg q2-6h until condition stabilizes • **Cerebral edema:** Initially 10 mg IV, followed by 4 mg IV/IM q6h; alternately, 20 mg IV loading dose, followed by IV infusion of 3 mg/kg/24 hr, which is 0.125 mg/kg/hr. • **Allergic reactions:** 4-8 mg IM, followed by 0.75-3 mg/24 hr in tapered PO doses • **IV, children:** Bacterial meningitis: 0.15 mg/kg q6h for first 4 days of antibiotic therapy • **Cerebral edema:** 0.5-1.5 mg/kg loading dose, followed by 0.2-0.5 mg/kg/24 hr in divided doses q4-6h for 5

days and then tapered doses for next 5 days

Dexamethasone acetate (parenteral suspension): IM, adult: 8-16 mg q1-3wk

ADMINISTRATION

Verify concentration of oral solution. Two strengths available: 0.5 mg/5 ml and 1 mg/ml (Intensol concentrate)

PO: When possible, administer with meals to minimize gastric irritation.

PO concentrate: May dilute in juice or semisolid food immediately before administration

▼ **Direct IV:** Administer each dose over 1-3 min. • Dilution not necessary. May be added to compatible solution for infusion • Check label carefully; use dexamethasone sodium phosphate; dexamethasone acetate not for IV administration.

Compatible fluids: D_5W, 0.9% NaCl, prepared combinations of these solutions

ACTIONS

Antiinflammatory glucocorticoid with complex action affecting almost all body systems • Stabilizes lysosomal membranes in leukocytes; prevents release of acid hydrolases; inhibits macrophage accumulation in inflamed tissues; reduces leukocyte adhesion to capillary walls; decreases capillary permeability/edema • Antagonizes histamine, kinin release • Suppresses immune response by producing lymphocytopenia, decreasing Ig/complement, reducing volume/activity of lymphatic system • Minimal mineralocorticoid activity; does not cause sodium retention • 7 times potency of prednisolone

PHARMACOKINETICS

ROUTE	ONSET	PEAK	DURATION
PO	<60 min	1-2 hr	Dose
IV	Rapid	Rapid	dependent

DISTRIBUTION
Widely distributed throughout body tissue

ELIMINATION
Metabolized in liver, eliminated by kidneys; half-life 36-54 hr

INDICATIONS

Severe allergic conditions • Reduction of cerebral edema • Profound shock unresponsive to conventional therapy • Acute life-threatening infections, along with massive antibiotics • Acute viral hepatitis • High-altitude sickness • Inflammatory respiratory, GI, neuromuscular disorders refractory to other therapies • Acute idiopathic thrombocytopenic purpura (ITP), hemolytic anemia • Autoimmune conditions such as SLE, polymyositis • Palliative management of leukemias, lymphomas • To prevent rejection of transplanted organs • Not used alone in treatment of adrenocortical insufficiency because of lack of mineralcorticoid properties

PRECAUTIONS/CONTRAINDICATIONS

Precautions: Prolonged therapy suppresses adrenocortical function, resulting in withdrawal symptoms with abrupt discontinuation. • May mask signs of infection, decrease resistance to infection • May cause edema, particularly in renal impairment • May worsen systemic fungal infections; use indicated only if reaction to amphotericin B • Peptic ulceration possible in high-risk patients (e.g., history of peptic ulcer, liver/intestinal dis-

ease, nephrotic syndrome, critical illness) • Commercial preparations may contain sulfites, which could cause severe allergic reactions in susceptible individuals.
Use caution with: Diabetes; insulin requirements may increase. • Renal disorders, CHF; fluid retention may be harmful • Osteoporosis • Seizure disorder • Concurrent anticholinesterase therapy • Acute MI • Recent CVA • Phlebitis • Active tuberculosis; use only in severe cases and as adjunct to chemotherapy • Cirrhosis, hypothyroidism; corticosteroid effects are enhanced • Chronic active hepatitis; may promote liver failure • Commercial preparations may contain sulfites and cause hypersensitivity reactions in susceptible individuals

c **Pregnancy category:** Use only if safer alternative unavailable.
Contraindications: Hypersensitivity to dexamethasone, any corticosteroid • Systemic fungal infections • Recent administration of live viral vaccine (e.g., smallpox) • IM route with ITP

ADVERSE EFFECTS

CNS: *Euphoria, insomnia, mood swings, depression,* aggravation of psychiatric disorder, psychosis, headache, paresthesias, **seizures, increased ICP** (children)

P

CV: *Hypertension,* thrombophlebitis, **thromboembolism, myocardial rupture** (recent MI)
GI: *Nausea,* vomiting, *anorexia,* weight gain, **peptic ulceration, GI bleeding**
Endo: *Adrenal suppression, menstrual irregularities,* hyperglycemia, suppression of

growth in children, "steroid-induced" diabetes mellitus
F&E: Hypokalemia, hypokalemic alkalosis, fluid retention
MS: *Muscle wasting, osteoporosis,* aseptic joint necrosis
Derm: *Diminished wound healing, petechiae, ecchymosis, hirsutism, acne, thinning of skin,* hypo/hyperpigmentation
Misc: *Cushingoid appearance, ↑ susceptibility to infection, ↓ symptoms of infection*

TOXICITY/OVERDOSE

Symptoms: Cushingoid: Moon face, central obesity, hirsutism, acne, hypertension, osteoporosis, diabetes mellitus, hyperlipidemia, peptic ulcers, myopathy, immunosuppression, fluid/electrolyte imbalance.
• Acute adrenal insufficiency: Fever, anorexia, malaise, nausea, dizziness, fainting, dyspnea, hypoglycemia, myalgia, arthralgia; follows rapid withdrawal of therapy
Management: After recent ingestion, implement guidelines for management of acute overdose (Appendix I). • Hypotension: Elevate legs, administer IV fluids; use vasopressor (e.g., dopamine, norepinephrine) or inotrope (e.g., dopamine, dobutamine) as appropriate. • Severe fluid overload: Administer diuretics; replace potassium as necessary. • Adrenal insufficiency: Supplement with additional corticosteroid; taper dose gradually before withdrawal.

INTERACTIONS

antidiabetics, oral; insulin ↑ Antidiabetic drug requirements
carbamazepine, phenytoin, rifampin ↓ Corticoid effects

---

italic = common side effects   **bold** = life-threatening reactions

Y-SITE COMPATIBILITIES

Acyclovir, famotidine, fluconazole, heparin, meperidine, morphine, ondansetron, piperacillin-tazobactam, potassium chloride, zidovudine

Y-SITE INCOMPATIBILITIES

Ciprofloxacin, vancomycin

PATIENT CARE IMPLICATIONS

• Precise dosage depends on condition, patient response.
• Administer daily dose in AM to coincide with physiologic peak in cortisol levels.
• Administer PO dose with meals to avoid gastric irritation.
• Dosage increases are necessary when patients subjected to severe emotional/physical stress.
• High dose/prolonged therapy suppresses hypothalamic-pituitary-adrenal axis, may lead to suppression of adrenal synthesis of glucocorticoids/mineralocorticoids. Abrupt discontinuation may cause adrenal insufficiency. Dosage must be gradually tapered.
• Drug-related immunosuppression may mask signs of infection. Monitor closely; initiate antibiotic therapy as soon as infection suspected.
• Use in management of shock is controversial; if used, therapy should be initiated in early rather than late phase.
Vital signs: Frequency of VS monitoring depends on patient condition rather than drug effects. Hypovolemic shock possible with adrenal crisis; VS should be monitored q15min or more often until condition stabilizes.

Physical assessment: Assess for adrenal insufficiency: hypotension, fever, anorexia, malaise, nausea, dizziness, fainting, dyspnea, hypoglycemia, myalgia, arthralgia. Presence of these symptoms indicates insufficient dosage or too rapid withdrawal of therapy. • Assess for cushingoid symptoms: moon face, central obesity, hirsutism, acne, hypertension, osteoporosis, diabetes mellitus, hyperlipidemia, peptic ulcers, myopathy, immunosuppression, fluid/electrolyte imbalance. Presence of these symptoms indicates excessive dosage. • Assess for weight gain, peripheral edema, dyspnea crackles (rales). Consult physician if present. • Check stools, emesis for occult blood. • Monitor I&O; weigh daily. • **Cerebral edema:** Assess neurologic status before and throughout therapy. Maintain cerebral perfusion pressure of 60-80 mm Hg or other specified range.
Laboratory tests: Monitor: Electrolytes, especially sodium, potassium, calcium • Blood glucose • CBC with differential

PATIENT/FAMILY TEACHING

Purpose of medication is to reduce inflammation of affected area or body system. • Take exactly as prescribed. Do not double up if dose missed. Sudden cessation of therapy may cause adrenal insufficiency: weakness, fatigue, nausea, low BP, low blood sugar. • Take with meals to minimize stomach upset.
• Drug causes suppression of immune system, may mask signs of infection. Avoid individuals with contagious illnesses. Report fever, prolonged malaise, any symptom of infec-

tion immediately. • Report rapid weight gain, unusual swelling, very dark or bloody stools, vomiting of blood, sores slow to heal, significant behavior changes. • Inform physicians, dentists, and other health care providers of medication regimen before treatment. • Carry medical ID describing medication regimen.

AVAILABLE FORMS

Parenteral solution for IV/IM injection • Parenteral suspension for IM injection • Tablets • PO solution • Concentrated PO solution

dextran, low molecular weight dextran 40
(dek'stran)
Gentran 40, Rheomacrodex, LMD

Classifications: Plasma volume expander, anticoagulant

USUAL DOSE

IV inf, adults: Shock: Initially 500 ml rapidly infused over 15-30 min with ongoing monitoring of CVP, PAPs; infuse more slowly when unable to monitor central pressures; administer additional doses as needed; total dose not to exceed 20 ml/kg during first 24 hr; thereafter, not to exceed 10 ml/kg/24 hr; do not continue therapy for more than 5 days. • Venous thrombosis/pulmonary embolism prophylaxis: Day of surgery, 500-1,000 ml or 10 ml/kg, usually given during surgery; followed by 500 ml/day for 2-3 days; thereafter, 500 ml every 2nd or 3rd day for approx 2 wk

IV inf, children: Shock: 5-10 ml/kg; total dose not to exceed 20 ml/kg/24 hr

ADMINISTRATION

IV inf: Rate varies according to clinical condition. • For profound shock, infuse up to 500 ml over 15-30 min; continuous hemodynamic monitoring recommended. • For other uses, infuse daily dose over 8-24 hr depending on indication. • Reduce infusion rate for ↑ CVP/PCWP

PREPARATION

Temperature fluctuations cause formation of flakes, which may be dissolved by heating in warm water or autoclaving at 110° C (230° F) for 15 min. Do not use solutions that are turbid or contain a deposit. Infuse within 4 hr of opening. Store at constant temperature, preferably 25° C (77° F).

ACTIONS

Maintains and restores plasma volume by drawing fluid from interstitial to intravascular space by colloidal osmotic effects; plasma volume expansion short-lived and slightly greater than volume infused • ↑ filling pressures, CO, BP, UO; ↓ HR, SVR, mean transit time • Improves microcirculation by ↓ blood viscosity, coating endothelial surfaces and blood cells. These effects reduce sludging and cellular aggregation seen in shock states • Not interchangeable with HMW dextran

PHARMACOKINETICS

ROUTE	ONSET	PEAK
IV	Rapid	Within minutes

DURATION

Dependent on plasma volume status, rate of renal clearance

DISTRIBUTION

Throughout plasma

ELIMINATION

Approx 70% excreted in urine within 24 hr; remainder degraded to glucose

INDICATIONS

Plasma volume expansion, maintenance of CO in hypovolemic shock or serious hypovolemia resulting from burns, hemorrhage, trauma, surgery, other conditions causing fluid volume deficit • Adjunct to blood/electrolyte therapy when blood not immediately available • To minimize microcirculatory sludging of blood • Priming fluid in pump oxygenators • Prophylaxis for venous thrombosis, pulmonary embolism

Unlabeled/investigational:
Microcirculatory improvement in acute MI, sickle cell crisis

PRECAUTIONS/ CONTRAINDICATIONS

Precautions: May cause anaphylaxis • Increases viscosity, specific gravity of urine; may result in tubular stasis/blockage, especially in dehydrated patients • Rapid or excessive infusion may cause circulatory overload. • Restoration of volume, improved microcirculatory flow in surgical, trauma, or bleeding patients may result in increased bleeding. • Large volumes may decrease Hct, plasma protein concentrations. • Large volumes of dextran 40 in 0.9% NaCl may cause hypernatremia, hyperchlo-

remic metabolic acidosis. • Interference with platelet function may prolong bleeding time.

Use caution with: Cardiac decompensation, concurrent corticosteroid therapy, other conditions associated with sodium retention/edema formation **G** • Older adults • Thrombocytopenia • Impaired renal function • Diabetes mellitus; may elevate blood sugar

c Pregnancy category: Use only if safer alternative unavailable.

Contraindications: Hypersensitivity to dextrans • Nonhypovolemic shock • Pulmonary edema • Increased intravascular volume • Renal disease with severe oliguria or anuria • Extreme dehydration • Marked thrombocytopenia, other serious bleeding disorders

ADVERSE EFFECTS

CV: **Circulatory overload;** ↑ CVP, PCWP

Resp: Dyspnea, **pulmonary edema**

GI: ↑ AST/ALT

GU: ↑ Viscosity, specific gravity of urine; nephrotoxicity

Hema: Hemodilution, prolonged bleeding time, hematoma, wound bleeding, hematuria, melena

Misc: Hypersensitivity; itching/ wheals, hypotension, vomiting, headache, fever, dyspnea, bronchospasm, **anaphylaxis**

TOXICITY/OVERDOSE

Symptoms: Circulatory overload, ↑ CVP/PCWP, pulmonary edema • Nephrotoxicity • Prolonged bleeding time, bleeding complications • Acute allergic reaction

Management: Stop infusion; consult physician. • **Oliguria, anuria:** Administer mannitol or other osmotic diuretic. • **Bleeding complications:** Treat symptomatically. • For management of acute allergic reaction, see Appendix N.

INTERACTIONS

corticosteroids Fluid retention
heparin, warfarin Prolonged bleeding

Y-SITE COMPATIBILITIES

Enalaprilat, famotidine

PATIENT CARE IMPLICATIONS

• Dose, rate of infusion vary according to clinical condition, fluid loss, VS, central hemodynamics, presence of venous or pulmonary congestion, plasma oncotic pressure, Hct.
• If rapid infusion indicated, use 20-gauge or larger needle-catheter.
• Not a replacement for transfusion therapy; for actively bleeding or anemic patients, use as adjunct to whole blood or packed cells.
• May cause severe anaphylaxis; observe closely during first few minutes of infusion. Have epinephrine, antihistamine, resuscitation equipment immediately available.

Vital signs/hemodynamics: Monitor BP, HR q5min for first 15 min of initial infusion. Thereafter, monitor at q1-2h depending on indication, rate of administration. Monitor more frequently with acute hypovolemia or rapid administration.
• Monitoring of CVP, PAPs, CO is recommended, particularly when used to restore fluid volume deficit. Administer at rate, dosage to restore intravascular fluid volume, avoid overload. Stop or slow infusion; consult physician of CVP >6 or PCWP >12 mm Hg or other preestablished range. • Monitor UO, note patient response before and after therapy. Anticipate ↑ UO; if no increase noted after 500 ml, stop infusion, consult physician. If oliguria or anuria develops, stop infusion, consider osmotic diuretic (e.g., mannitol).
• Measure urine specific gravity during therapy. Low values suggest poor clearance. Stop infusion, consult physician.

Physical assessment: Assess for circulatory overload, especially with rapid infusion. Auscultate for crackles (rales), S_3 gallop, neck vein distention, dyspnea. • When restoring volume to surgical, trauma, or bleeding patients, assess for ↑ bleeding due to ↑ intravascular pressure. • Assess for bleeding complications, such as melena, blood in urine, hematoma formation, bleeding from puncture sites, especially if patient receiving concurrent anticoagulants or has undergone surgery.

Laboratory tests: Monitor: Hgb, Hct • Electrolytes • AST, ALT • Blood glucose • Urine specific gravity • **May cause:** Elevation of blood glucose • Interference with laboratory tests for bilirubin, total protein, type/cross-match; when possible, collect blood for these tests before initiating therapy.

PATIENT/FAMILY TEACHING

Purpose of medication is to provide additional fluid within bloodstream or prevent clots from forming. • Report immedi-

---

italic = common side effects   **bold** = life-threatening reactions

ately breathing difficulty, itching, unusual bruising, blood in urine, bleeding.

AVAILABLE FORMS

10% dextran 40 in D_5W • 10% dextran 40 in 0.9% NaCl

---

dextran, high molecular weight
dextran 70; dextran 75
(dek'stran)
Gentran 70, Gentran 75, Macrodex

Classifications: Plasma volume expander, anticoagulant

USUAL DOSE

IV inf, adults: Shock: Initially 500 ml rapidly infused over 15-30 min with ongoing monitoring of CVP, PAPs; infuse more slowly when unable to monitor central pressures; administer additional doses as needed; total dose not to exceed 20 ml/kg during first 24 hr; thereafter, not to exceed 10 ml/kg/24 hr.

P IV inf, children: Shock: 5-10 ml/kg; total dose not to exceed 20 ml/kg/24 hr

ADMINISTRATION

IV inf: Dose, rate of infusion vary according to clinical condition. • **Profound shock:** Up to 500 ml infused over 15-30 min; continuous hemodynamic monitoring recommended • Slower rates (e.g., 250 ml/hr) used with normovolemia

PREPARATION

Temperature fluctuations may cause formation of flakes, which are dissolved by heating in warm water or autoclaving at 110° C (230° F) for 15 min.
• Do not use solutions that are turbid or contain a deposit. • Infuse within 4 hr of opening.
• Store at constant temperature, preferably 25° C (77° F).

ACTIONS

Maintains/restores plasma volume by drawing fluid from interstitial to intravascular space by colloidal osmotic effects; plasma volume expansion slightly greater than volume infused and sustained for up to 24 hr • Approx. same molecular weight and similar effects as human albumin. • Increases filling pressures, CO, BP, UO; Decreases HR, SVR, mean transit time • Improves microcirculation by ↓ blood viscosity, coating endothelial surfaces and blood cells. These effects reduce sludging and cellular aggregation seen in shock states. Not interchangeable with LMW dextran.

PHARMACOKINETICS

ROUTE	ONSET	PEAK
IV	Rapid	Approx. 1 hr after infusion completion

DURATION

Dependent on plasma volume status, rate of renal clearance

DISTRIBUTION

Throughout plasma

ELIMINATION

Approx 50% excreted in urine within 24 hr; remainder degraded to glucose

INDICATIONS

Plasma volume expansion/maintenance of CO in hypovolemic shock or serious hypovolemia resulting from burns, hemorrhage, trauma, surgery, or other conditions causing fluid volume deficit • Adjunct to blood and electrolyte therapy when blood not immediately available

PRECAUTIONS/CONTRAINDICATIONS

Precautions: May cause anaphylaxis • Rapid or excessive infusion may cause circulatory overload. • Restoration of volume, improved microcirculatory flow in surgical, trauma, or bleeding patients may result in increased bleeding. • Large volumes may decrease Hct, plasma protein concentrations. • Large volumes of dextran 70/75 in 0.9% NaCl may cause hypernatremia, hyperchloremic metabolic acidosis. • Doses >1000 ml may result in prolonged bleeding time.

Use caution with: Cardiac decompensation, concurrent corticosteroid therapy, other conditions associated with sodium retention/edema formation **G**• Older adults • Thrombocytopenia • Impaired renal function • Diabetes mellitus; may elevate blood sugar.

c Pregnancy category: Use only if safer alternative unavailable.

Contraindications: Hypersensitivity to dextrans • Nonhypovolemic shock • Pulmonary edema • Increased intravascular volume • Severe CHF • Severe renal disease • Marked thrombocytopenia, other serious bleeding disorders

ADVERSE EFFECTS

Resp: Dyspnea, **pulmonary edema**
CV: **Circulatory overload,** ↑ CVP, PCWP
GI: Nausea, vomiting, involuntary defecation

Hema: Prolonged bleeding time, hemodilution
Misc: Fever; arthralgia; hypersensitivity: itching/wheals, hypotension, bronchospasm, dyspnea, **anaphylaxis**

TOXICITY/OVERDOSE

Symptoms: Circulatory overload, elevated CVP/PCWP, pulmonary edema • Prolonged bleeding time, bleeding complications • Acute allergic reaction
Management: Stop infusion, consult physician. • Treat bleeding complications symptomatically. • For management of acute allergic reaction, see Appendix N.

INTERACTIONS

corticosteroids Fluid retention
heparin, warfarin Prolonged bleeding

Y-SITE COMPATIBILITIES

Enalaprilat, famotidine

PATIENT CARE IMPLICATIONS

• Dose, rate of infusion vary according to clinical condition, fluid loss, VS, central hemodynamics, presence of venous or pulmonary congestion, plasma oncotic pressure, Hct.
• If rapid infusion indicated, use 20-gauge or larger catheter.
• Not a replacement for transfusion therapy; for actively bleeding or anemic patients, use as adjunct to whole blood or packed cells.
• May cause severe anaphylaxis; observe patient closely during first few minutes of infusion. Have epinephrine, antihistamine, resuscitation equipment immediately available.

italic = common side effects   **bold** = life-threatening reactions

Vital signs/hemodynamics:
Monitor BP, HR q5min for first
15 min of initial infusion.
Thereafter, monitor q1-2h depending on indication, rate of
administration. Monitor more
frequently with acute hypovolemia or rapid administration.
• Monitoring of CVP, PAPs, CO
is recommended, particularly
when used to restore fluid volume deficit. Administer at rate,
dosage to restore intravascular
fluid volume, avoid overload.
Stop or slow infusion; consult
physician of CVP >6 or PCWP
>12 mm Hg or other preestab-
lished range. • Monitor UO,
note patient response before and
after therapy. Anticipate ↑ UO;
if no increase noted after 500
ml, stop infusion, consult physician.
Physical assessment: Assess
for circulatory overload, especially with rapid infusion. Auscultate for crackles (rales), S₃
gallop, neck vein distention,
dyspnea. • When restoring volume to surgical, trauma, or
bleeding patients, assess for ↑
bleeding due to ↑ intravascular
pressure. • Assess for bleeding
complications, such as melena,
blood in urine, hematoma formation, bleeding from puncture
sites, especially if patient receiving concurrent anticoagulants or has undergone surgery.
Laboratory tests: Monitor:
Hgb, Hct • Electrolytes • AST,
ALT • Blood glucose • Urine
specific gravity • **May cause:**
Elevation of blood glucose • Interference with laboratory tests
for bilirubin, total protein, type/
cross-match; when possible, collect blood for these tests before
initiating therapy.

PATIENT/FAMILY TEACHING

Purpose of medication is to provide additional fluid within
bloodstream or prevent clots
from forming. • Immediately report unusual bruising or bleeding, blood in urine, itching,
breathing difficulty.

AVAILABLE FORMS

6% dextran 70 in D₅W • 6%
dextran 70 in 0.9% NaCl • 6%
dextran 75 in D₅W • 6% dextran 75 in 0.9% NaCl

dextrose
(dek'stros)
glucose
Glutose, Insta-Glucose

Classifications: Caloric agent,
carbohydrate

USUAL DOSE

PO, adult: 10-20 g as gel or
chewable tablets • Each 25 g of
gel provides 10 g dextrose.
Direct IV, adult: 50% solution,
12.5-25 g (25-50 ml)
🅟 **Direct IV, children:** 25% solution, 200-500 mg/kg; maximum
dose is 1 g/kg.
IV, cont inf: 0.25%-10% solutions used; rate varies according
to condition, indication

ADMINISTRATION

🆅 **Direct IV, adults:** Inject slowly
at rate of 3 ml/min. • May be
injected more rapidly at rate of
10 ml/min if extreme emergency • 50% solution is hypertonic; use central vein if possible; may use large peripheral
vein if emergency.
IV, cont inf: Rate depends on
total volume to be infused, concentration. • 10%, 1,000 ml so-

lution must be given over at least 3 hr. • Infusion via central vein necessary for hypertonic solutions (≥10%); large peripheral veins may be used for 10% solutions if necessary.

Compatible fluids: D_5W, RL, 0.9% NaCl, prepared combinations of these solutions

ACTIONS

Readily metabolized monosaccharide that increases blood glucose concentrations, provides calories. D_5W contains 170 cal/liter; $D_{10}W$ contains 340 cal/liter. • Reduces rate of excess ketone production, slows or prevents protein/nitrogen loss, prevents electrolyte loss • Commercial products usually derived from corn

PHARMACOKINETICS

ROUTE	ONSET	PEAK	DURATION
PO	10 min	40 min	6-8 hr
IV	Immed	Rapid	1-6 hr

DISTRIBUTION

Throughout body tissue

ELIMINATION

Metabolized to CO_2, water

INDICATIONS

Peripheral infusions of 2.5%-10% used to provide calories, fluid • Central infusions of 10%-20% in parenteral nutrition provide calories in minimal volumes. • 50% injection used for emergency treatment of hypoglycemia; cerebral/meningeal edema related to eclampsia; acute glomerulonephritis • 20% solution/insulin used in hyperkalemia to shift potassium into cells • Gel, chewable tablets used for hypoglycemia in conscious patients with diabetes

PRECAUTIONS/CONTRAINDICATIONS

Precautions: Excessive IV administration may cause fluid volume or solute overload, electrolyte dilution, water intoxication, CHF, pulmonary edema • Hypertonic solutions may cause hyperglycemia, dehydration, hyperosmolar coma; insulin administration reduces hyperglycemia.

Use caution with: Diabetes • Carbohydrate intolerance • Renal insufficiency • Chronic alcoholics; administer thiamine first.

c Pregnancy category: Use only if safer alternative unavailable.

Contraindications (hyperosmolar solution): Hypersensitivity to corn, corn products • Diabetic coma • Anuria • Intracranial hemorrhage • Delirium tremens if dehydration also present

ADVERSE EFFECTS

CV: Hypertension, **CHF, pulmonary edema**

GU: Glycosuria, osmotic diuresis

F&E: Hypokalemia, hypophosphatemia, hypomagnesemia, fluid overload

Local: Pain, irritation (hypertonic solutions)

Misc: Hyperglycemia

TOXICITY/OVERDOSE

Symptoms: Hyperglycemia, dehydration, hyperosmolar coma

Management: Slow or discontinue infusion. • Administer insulin, fluids

---

italic = common side effects   **bold** = life-threatening reactions

PATIENT CARE IMPLICATIONS

• Evaluate changes in fluid balance, electrolytes, acid-base status during prolonged therapy and in patients with diabetes, renal insufficiency, heart failure, other disturbances in fluid volume balance.

• To prevent rebound hypoglycemia, substitute 10% dextrose solution when discontinuing concentrated dextrose solutions (e.g., TPN, 50% dextrose).

• Avoid simultaneous administration through same line as blood; clumping of blood cells will occur.

Physical assessment: Assess patients with chronic uremia or diabetes for hyperglycemia and/or hyperosmolar syndrome: mental confusion, dehydration, loss of consciousness. • Monitor I&O; weigh daily.

Laboratory tests: Monitor: Electrolytes • Blood glucose • BUN, creatinine • Prolonged IV administration may cause hypokalemia, hypophosphatemia, hypomagnesemia.

PATIENT/FAMILY TEACHING

Purpose of medication is to restore blood sugar to normal levels or provide additional calories. • Report breathing difficulty, mental confusion.

AVAILABLE FORMS

Parenteral for IV injection • Tablets • Gel

diazepam

(dye-az′e-pam)
Diazac (emulsified injection), Diazemuls ✹, Diazepam Intensol (conc. sol.), D-Tran ✹, E-Pam ✹, Meval ✹, Novodipam ✹, Stress-Pam ✹, Valium, Valrelease (ext. rel.), Vazepam, Vivol ✹, Zetran

Classifications: Benzodiazepine, sedative/hypnotic, antianxiety (anxiolytic) agent, anticonvulsant, skeletal muscle relaxant
Schedule IV controlled substance

USUAL DOSE

Individualize dosage; increase cautiously. When used with opiate analgesics, reduce dose by ⅓.

PO, adults: 2-10 mg 2-4 times daily • **Older adults, debilitation:** 2-2.5 mg 1-2 times daily; increase dose cautiously as needed.

PO, children >6 mo: 1-2.5 mg 3-4 times daily; increase gradually as needed.

PO, ext. rel., adults: 15 mg once daily; use only for patients tolerating ≥15 mg/day standard formulation.

IV/IM, adults: 2-20 mg, depending on indication, patient response; may repeat in 3-4 hr or after 1 hr in acute conditions; do not exceed 30 mg within 8-hr period. • **Older adults, debilitation, with other sedatives:** 2-5 mg; monitor frequently, increase dose gradually.

• **Status epilepticus:** Initially 5-10 mg; repeat as necessary at 10–15-min intervals up to max-

imum dose of 30 mg; use IV route whenever possible; may repeat therapy in 2-4 hr as necessary. • **Preprocedural:** 5-10 mg 30 min before scheduled procedure; use lower dose if narcotics also used.
IV, adults: Conscious sedation: 5-10 mg; administer in small increments, titrate to desired effect (e.g., slurred speech); up to 20 mg sometimes used. Reduce dose if narcotics also used.
IV/IM, infants >30 days/ children ≤5 yr: Status epilepticus: 0.2-0.5 mg q2-5min up to maximum dose of 5 mg • **Tetanus:** 1-2 mg q3-4h • Use IM route only if IV route impossible
IV/IM, children >5 yr: Status epilepticus: 1 mg q2-5min up to maximum dose of 10 mg • **Tetanus:** 5-10 mg q3-4h • Use IM route only if IV route impossible

ADMINISTRATION

PO: Administer with food to ↓ gastric irritation.
PO, conc: Measure dose using the calibrated dropper supplied with Diazepam Intensol. Mix with semisolid food or liquid; administer immediately. Discard unused portion.
Enteral Formula Compatibilities: Isocal, Sustacal, Sustacal HC
Direct IV, adults: Inject undiluted solution slowly at rate of 2-5 mg/min. • **Infants/children:** Inject each dose over 3-5 min. • *Too rapid administration may result in profound hypotension, respiratory depression, bradycardia, PVCs, cardiac arrest.* • Administer as close as possible to vein insertion prefer-

ably through a freely flowing IV. Use antecubital or other large vein; take care to avoid intraarterial administration or extravasation. Avoid small veins (e.g., hand, wrist). Emulsified injection (Diazac) causes less injection site pain/irritation than aqueous diazepam. Do not mix with other medications or fluids; may precipitate if added to IV solutions. Adsorption of diazepam may occur with polyvinyl chloride bags, IV tubing, cellulose IV filters.

ACTIONS

Acts in CNS to facilitate action of gamma-aminobutyric acid (GABA, major inhibitory neurotransmitter); reduces anxiety, causes sedation, promotes sleep, relaxes skeletal muscles, has anticonvulsant effects • Results in varying degrees of CNS depression, from mild sedation to hypnosis, coma • In usual doses, has few effects on respiratory, CV, autonomic nervous systems • No analgesic effects

PHARMACOKINETICS

ROUTE	ONSET	PEAK	DURATION
PO	30-60 min	1-2 hr	12-24 hr
PO, ext rel	ND	5 hr	≥24 hr
IM	Slow, erratic	30-90 min	2-6 hr
IV	1-5 min	5-15 min	15-60 min

DISTRIBUTION

Widely distributed; 70%-99% protein bound, readily crosses blood-brain barrier

ELIMINATION

Metabolized by liver, eliminated by kidneys; half-life 20-50 hr, longer in older adults, hepatic dysfunction

---

INDICATIONS

Anxiety disorders; short-term relief of anxiety symptoms • To relieve anxiety; provide sedation, light anesthesia; diminish patient recall after surgery, procedures • As IV anticonvulsant, considered choice agent for management of status epilepticus • To relieve skeletal muscle spasms caused by local inflammation or trauma; to reduce spasticity caused by upper motor neuron disorders, tetanus, other diseases • Adjunct for relief of acute musculoskeletal pain • To reduce agitation, tremors, hallucinations, other symptoms associated with acute alcohol withdrawal

Unlabeled/investigational:
To reduce requirements for opiate analgesics; neonatal opiate withdrawal

PRECAUTIONS/ CONTRAINDICATIONS

Precautions: Adverse effects more likely in first few days of therapy • Sudden cessation of therapy in patients with epilepsy may increase frequency/severity of seizures. • *Profound hypotension, respiratory depression possible with IV administration, especially in* older adults, debilitation, limited pulmonary reserve, rapid administration • Safe use of PO diazepam in infants <6 mo and parenteral diazepam in infants <30 days not established

Use caution with: COPD, limited pulmonary reserve • Hepatic/renal dysfunction, older adults, children, debilitation, low serum albumin; use reduced dose.

Pregnancy category: Risk of congenital malformations, prolonged CNS depression, withdrawal symptoms in newborn; use only if safer alternative unavailable and risk explained to woman.

Contraindications: Hypersensitivity to diazepam • Hypersensitivity to soy protein (emulsified injection) • Acute alcohol intoxication with depression of VS • Acute angle-closure glaucoma • Pregnancy/lactation • Depressive neuroses or psychotic reactions when anxiety not prominent

ADVERSE EFFECTS

CNS: *Drowsiness, ataxia, fatigue,* confusion, syncope, anterograde amnesia, headache, mental depression, bizarre/abnormal behavior, paradoxical excitation (especially children, psychiatric patients)

Resp: IV—respiratory depression, decreased gag reflex, dyspnea, hyperventilation, laryngospasm, **apnea**

CV: Edema; hypotension; IV—PVCs, other dysrhythmias, **hypotension, bradycardia, cardiac arrest**

GI: Nausea, constipation; rarely, hepatitis/jaundice

GU: Retention, incontinence, difficulty with micturition

Derm: Rash, itching, wheals, nonthrombocytopenic purpura

Local: IV—pain, swelling, thrombophlebitis

Misc: Tolerance, psychologic/ physical dependence

TOXICITY/OVERDOSE

Symptoms (acute toxicity):
Somnolence, confusion, coma, diminished reflexes, hypotension, seizures, respiratory de-

pression, apnea, especially with IV administration • Respiratory depression more likely with concurrent ingestion of alcohol, other CNS depressants **Management:** After recent ingestion, implement guidelines for management of acute overdose (Appendix I). • Maintain airway/support ventilation as necessary • Antidote: Administer flumazenil to reverse diazepam effects. • **Hypotension:** Elevate legs, administer IV fluids; use vasopressors (e.g., norepinephrine, dopamine) if not responsive to fluids. • Do not use barbiturates for paradoxical excitation. • Forced diuresis may be helpful. • Hemodialysis generally is not useful.

INTERACTIONS

alcohol, ethyl ↑ Sedation
antacids Altered absorption
antihistamines ↑ Sedation
barbiturates ↑ Sedation
beta-blockers ↑ Sedation
cimetidine ↑ Sedation
digoxin ↑ Digoxin levels; toxicity possible
erythromycin ↑ Diazepam levels, ↑ sedation
isoniazid ↑ Sedation
ketoconazole ↑ Sedation
opiate analgesics ↑ Sedation
probenecid ↑ Sedation
propoxyphene ↑ Sedation
rifampin ↓ Sedation
theophylline ↓ Sedation

INCOMPATIBILITIES

Numerous; do not mix in syringe or solution or administer at Y site with other agents.

PATIENT CARE IMPLICATIONS

• Adverse effects more likely in 1st few days of therapy

• Always use smallest effective dose. Reduce dose by ⅓, administer in small increments when used with opiate analgesics.
• Reserve parenteral therapy for urgent/emergency situations. Convert to PO therapy as soon as possible.
• Avoid sudden cessation of therapy, especially in patients who have received therapy for several months or longer (may cause withdrawal symptoms, including seizures).
• Large quantities should not be prescribed for patients with severe depression, suicidal tendencies, history of substance abuse.
• Use only for short-term seizure control. Seizure activity may recur; be prepared to readminister diazepam.

G Older adults
• Use lower, individualized dose; closely monitor for adverse effects.
• Periodically assess need for continued therapy.

IV
• May result in hypotension, respiratory depression, excessive sedation, especially in older adults, debilitated patients, those with limited pulmonary reserve; monitor VS, level of consciousness frequently.
• Rapid administration may result in hypotension, dysrhythmias, apnea, cardiac arrest; have resuscitation equipment, flumazenil immediately available.
• May cause burning and irritation at injection site; emulsified injection (Dizac) less likely to cause vein irritation
• Patient should remain in bed for at least 3 hr after administration and requires assistance with initial ambulation.

---

italic = common side effects   **bold** = life-threatening reactions

• Avoid IV administration in shock, coma, respiratory depression or with recent administration of other respiratory depressants. • Many precautions necessary; see Administration.

Vital signs/hemodynamics: Monitor VS frequently in heavily sedated patients (e.g., those also receiving opiates) or during immediate postop period. • As available, use continuous pulse oximetry for heavily sedated patients. • IV injection: Monitor HR, RR, BP q2-5min during and immediately after administration. • Continuously monitor ECG for bradycardia, PVCs.

Physical assessment: Assess neurologic status for excessive sedation, impaired physical coordination. Reduce dose as necessary. • Assess for respiratory distress in patients with history of COPD, cardiac impairment. **Laboratory tests:** Monitor: Liver enzymes, BUN, creatinine, CBC

PATIENT/FAMILY TEACHING

Purpose of medication is to reduce anxiety and relax muscles. • May cause drowsiness, dizziness, especially during first few days of therapy; use caution with activity until individual effects recognized. • Cigarette smoking interferes with drug effectiveness. • Inform health care provider if you may be pregnant or are considering pregnancy.

Outpatient: Avoid concurrent use of alcohol or other drugs that cause sedation while taking this medication. • Avoid driving and other activities requiring mental alterness or physical coordination. • This medication may cause psychologic/physical dependence. Seizures may develop if you abruptly stop taking prescribed medications. Consult health care provider before increasing or abruptly discontinuing dose. • Do not break or chew extended-release capsules. • Take with food if desired to minimize gastric irritation. • If used for seizure control, wear Medic-Alert ID.

AVAILABLE FORMS

PO solution (1 mg/ml) • Concentrated PO solution (5 mg/ml) • Aqueous solution for IM/IV use • Emulsified injection for IV use • Tablets • Capsules, extended release

---

diazoxide
(dye-az-ox′ide)
Hyperstat (parenteral),
Proglycem (PO)

Classifications:
Antihypertensive/vasodilator,
hyperglycemic

USUAL DOSE

P PO, adults/children: Initially 3 mg/kg daily in 3 equally divided doses (e.g., 70 mg q8h, for 70-kg patient • Maintenance: 3-5 mg/kg/24 hr in 2 or 3 equally divided doses; individualize to control blood glucose.
Direct IV, adults: Initially 1-3 mg/kg, or approx 50-150 mg; repeat q5-15min as needed to control severe hypertension; second injection likely to have greater effect. • May follow with short-term maintenance doses of 50-150 mg q4-24h • Do not use >10 days.

P pediatric   **G** geriatric   **V** Direct IV

ADMINISTRATION

▼Direct IV: Inject each dose of up to 150 mg rapidly over 10-30 sec. Slow administration reduces hypotensive effectiveness. Avoid extravasation, which causes burning/cellulitis. Patient must be recumbent.

ACTIONS

PO: Inhibition of pancreatic insulin/increases blood glucose.
• BP generally unaffected; may be slightly decreased
IV: Promotes direct relaxation of arteriolar smooth muscle, vasodilation, reduced BP • Hypotensive effectiveness greatest with malignant hypertension
• HR, CO, left ventricular ejection increase in response to reduced peripheral vascular resistance • Coronary, cerebral blood flow usually unchanged; renal blood flow transiently decreased, then increased • Unlike thiazide diuretics, causes sodium/water retention, diminished UO, fluid volume expansion and may precipitate edema/CHF; concurrent diuretic therapy reverses these effects.
• Inhibits pancreatic insulin; may increase blood glucose, particularly in patients with diabetes

PHARMACOKINETICS

ROUTE	ONSET	PEAK*	DURATION
PO, caps	<1 hr	8 hr	8 hr
PO, susp	<1 hr	4 hr	8 hr
IV	<1 min	2-5 min	3-12 hr

DISTRIBUTION
Widely distributed; >90% protein bound
ELIMINATION
Metabolized by liver, eliminated in urine; half-life 20-36 hr

*Refers to hypotensive effects for IV route, hyperglycemic effects with PO route.

INDICATIONS

PO: Elevation of blood glucose in hypoglycemic patients with hyperinsulinism caused by pancreatic/islet cell adenoma or carcinoma, extrapancreatic malignancy, other conditions
IV: Rapid reduction of BP in hypertensive crises, severe hypertension • Especially effective for resistant renal-impaired patients with resistance to other hypotensive agents • Used only as short-term measure

PRECAUTIONS/CONTRAINDICATIONS

Precautions: Sudden, severe drop in BP possible • Parenteral solution highly alkaline; IM/SC injection may cause tissue damage. • Sodium/water retention may cause refractoriness to hypotensive effects.
Use caution with: Cardiac impairment; fluid retention may trigger CHF. • Cerebral, coronary, renal vascular disease; severe hypotension may cause ischemia. • Acute myocardial ischemia; tachycardia may be detrimental. • Renal/hepatic impairment, diabetes, hypokalemia, concurrent use of other blood glucose–elevating medications; severe hyperglycemia possible
• Severe renal failure; greater sensitivity to drug effects
• *Concurrent administration of other antihypertensive agents; sudden profound hypotension possible*
C Pregnancy category: Use only if safer alternative unavailable.
Contraindications: Hypersensitivity to thiazide diuretics, sulfonamides, diazoxide • Compensatory hypertension (e.g.,

italic = common side effects   **bold** = life-threatening reactions

arteriovenous shunt, coarctation of aorta) • Pheochromocytoma (ineffective) • Hypoglycemia not caused by hyperinsulinism

ADVERSE EFFECTS

CNS: *Dizziness, weakness,* headache, **cerebral ischemia, seizures,** transient tinnitus

CV: ***Hypotension,** edema, weight gain,* **CHF,** IV: **dysrhythmias, myocardial ischemia**

GI: *Nausea, vomiting,* abdominal pain, pancreatitis

GU: Nocturia, worsening of renal insufficiency, azotemia

Derm: Flushing, rash, dermatitis

Local: Burning, irritation at injection site

Misc: *Hyperglycemia,* ketoacidosis, hyperosmolar nonketotic coma, ↑ uric acid, fever, muscle cramping

TOXICITY/OVERDOSE

Symptoms: Hypotension, hyperglycemia

Management: After recent ingestion, implement guidelines for management of acute overdose (Appendix J). • **Hypotension:** Elevate legs, administer 0.9% NaCl as necessary for volume expansion; if unresponsive to IV fluids, use dopamine or norepinephrine. • **CHF, fluid volume excess:** Limit fluid intake; consider diuretics. • **Hyperglycemia:** Administer insulin • Long half-life; monitor closely at least 24 hr. • Hemodialysis is unlikely to be effective.

INTERACTIONS

antihypertensives* Potentiation of hypotensive effects

corticosteroids Hyperglycemia

diuretics Potentiation of hypotensive, hyperglycemia, hyperuricemic effects

phenothiazines Hyperglycemia

phenytoin ↑ or ↓ phenytoin levels, phenytoin toxicity; hyperglycemia

thiazide diuretics Hyperuricemia

warfarin, other highly proteinbound agents Displacement from protein-bound sites with ↑ or ↓ drug effects, possible toxicity

---

*Manufacturer recommends IV diazoxide not be given within 6 hr of administration of beta-adrenergic blockers, hydralazine, methyldopa, minoxidil, nitrites, prazosin, reserpine, papaverine-like agents, because excessive hypotension may result.

Y-SITE INCOMPATIBILITIES

Hydralazine, propranolol

PATIENT CARE IMPLICATIONS

• *Parenteral/PO preparations not interchangeable*

• Loop diuretics often administered with diazoxide to counter sodium/water retention

Parenteral

• Patient must remain in bed with appropriate safety precautions during and at least 1 hr after parenteral administration. If furosemide also given, patient must remain supine for 8-10 hr. Use caution with initial ambulation.

• Do not discontinue until BP controlled by other (preferably PO) agent.

• Extravasation may cause cellulitis and/or phlebitis. Use warm, moist compresses to relieve pain.

Vital signs/hemodynamics: Parenteral: Monitor BP, HR q1-5min initially, then q15-30min until controlled. • As available, monitor ECG, noting tachycardia, bradycardia, ischemic ECG changes.

Physical assessment: Assess for perfusion/oxygenation deficit: chest discomfort, shortness of breath, ↓ level of consciousness, confusion, dizziness. • Assess for CHF: dyspnea, bibasilar crackles, peripheral edema, weight gain, S_3 gallop, neck vein distention. • Assess for hyperglycemia: drowsiness, confusion, increased urination, thirst, ketone breath. • Monitor fluid balance; weigh daily.

Laboratory tests: Monitor: Renal, hepatic, hematologic status before initiating therapy and at intervals thereafter; in hypertensive crisis, do not delay therapy for test results. Blood sugar esp. in patients with diabetes and when frequent IV doses are required • Uric acid

PATIENT/FAMILY TEACHING

Purpose of drug is to lower BP or reduce elevated blood sugar. • Report immediately dizziness, chest discomfort, breathing difficulty. • Report joint soreness or sensitivity in feet, which may indicate gout.

IV: May cause dizziness, very low BP; do not attempt to get out of bed without assistance.

Outpatient: Monitor blood glucose, daily or more often as directed. • Report immediately signs/symptoms of hypo/hyperglycemia.

PREPARATIONS

Parenteral for IV injection
• Capsules, PO suspension

---

digoxin
(di-jox'in)
Lanoxin, Lanoxicaps

Classifications: Cardiac glycoside, antidysrhythmic

D

USUAL DOSE

Narrow range between therapeutic and toxic levels requires individual dosage adjustment. Management of atrial dysrhythmias generally necessitates larger doses than heart failure. Soft capsules are more completely absorbed; use 80% of tablet dose.

Loading dose IV/PO, adults: 0.5-1.0 mg total in divided doses as follows: initially ½ total loading dose; then 0.25 mg q4-8h until total dose administered.

Maintenance dose IV/PO, adults: 10-15 µg/kg, or approx 0.25 mg daily

G Older adults: Reduce dose, usually 0.125-0.25 mg once daily, once every other day, or less frequently.

P Loading dose IV/PO, children: 10-50 µg/kg total in divided doses as follows: initially ½ loading dose; then ¼ loading dose 8-12 hr later; give remaining ¼ 8-12 hr after second dose (see table).

Maintenance dose IV/PO, P children: 5-10 µg/kg, or 25%-35% of total loading dose; administer in two divided daily doses, or once daily when compliance is problem (see table).

---

italic = common side effects   **bold** = life-threatening reactions

P Usual loading/maintenance doses of digoxin in children/infants with normal renal function

AGE	IV LOADING DOSE* µg/kg	MAINTENANCE DOSE* µg/kg/day divided q 12h
Term neonate	10-30	8-10
1 mo <2 yrs	30-40	10-12
2-10 yrs	20-30	8-10
≥10 yrs	8-12	3-10

*Dose based on lean (ideal) body weight.

ADMINISTRATION

IV/PO: Assess/document clinical response (e.g., apical pulse, dysrhythmias) before administering. Hold dose, consult physician if apical pulse significantly different from patient's usual pulse, if symptomatic bradycardia present or if bradycardiac with atrial fibrillation/flutter.
Enteral formula compatibility: Ensure, Ensure HN, Ensure Plus, Ensure Plus HN, Osmolite
▼ Direct IV: Administer each dose over at least 5 min. Continuous ECG monitoring is recommended. Rapid injection causes systemic/coronary arteriolar vasoconstriction.

PREPARATION

IV: May be given undiluted, or dilute in ≥4 ml D_5W or 0.9% NaCl. Dilution recommended to improve accuracy of measurement when giving small doses. Use diluted solution immediately. Dilution in <4 ml may result in precipitation.

ACTIONS

Increases cardiac contractility by depressing myocardial sodium-potassium pump, thereby increasing availability of calcium ions, which improve contractility • Vagal-like reduction in HR caused by SA nodal depression, prolonged conduction through AV node, increased AV nodal refractory period • Contractility and CO improved • With heart failure, systolic emptying more complete, elevated LVEDP reduced, elevated PAPs reduced • Peripheral vascular resistance reflexively decreases as CO improves. • Higher doses cause sympathetic stimulation; atrial/ventricular rates may increase. • Plasma steady state necessary for full effects

PHARMACOKINETICS

ROUTE	ONSET	PEAK	DURATION
PO	30-120 min	2-6 hr	after attainment of steady state
IV	5-30 min	1-5 hr	6-8 days

DISTRIBUTION
Widely distributed; 20%-25% protein bound

ELIMINATION
Small amounts metabolized in liver and by intestinal bacteria, remainder excreted in urine; half-life 34-44 hr

Therapeutic level: 0.5-2.5 ng/ml

INDICATIONS

CHF, cardiogenic shock, other low CO states when improved myocardial contractility desired • HR reduction in patients with rapid atrial rhythms (e.g., atrial fibrillation/flutter, paroxysmal atrial tachycardia), especially when ventricular response also elevated

PRECAUTIONS/CONTRAINDICATIONS

Precautions: Dysrhythmias associated with toxicity may be similar to those that warranted therapy. • Electrolyte imbalances (e.g., hypokalemia, hypomagnesemia, hypercalcemia) promote serious dysrhythmias in digitalized patients.

Use caution with: Heart block; may advance block • WPW syndrome, atrial fibrillation; enhanced conduction along accessory pathways may result in tachycardia. • Hepatic/renal impairment, hypothyroidism; reduce dose

c Pregnancy category: Use only if safer alternative unavailable.

Contraindications: Hypersensitivity to digoxin • Ventricular tachycardia/fibrillation • Beriberi heart disease • Hypersensitive carotid sinus syndrome

ADVERSE EFFECTS

CNS: *Headache,* weakness, drowsiness, apathy, confusion, psychosis

EENT: *Yellow-green or blurred vision,* photophobia, diplopia

CV: PVCs, **ventricular, tachycardia, AV block/dissociation,** accelerated junctional rhythm, atrial tachycardia; ECG changes: PR prolongation, ST depression

GI: *Anorexia, nausea, vomiting,* diarrhea, abdominal pain

Syst: Hyperkalemia, hypokalemia, muscle weakness

TOXICITY/OVERDOSE

Symptoms: CNS dysfunction • Yellow-green or blurred vision • Severe ventricular dysrhythmias, bradycardia, heart block • Anorexia, GI upset, particularly in older adults • Hyperkalemia (acute overdose), hypokalemia (chronic toxicity) • Pediatric toxicity usually manifested by heart block, supraventricular/

ventricular dysrhythmias; CNS, GI symptoms

Management: Reduce or discontinue digoxin until symptoms resolve. • Obtain potassium level; administer supplements according to levels and for suppression of dysrhythmias. • Do not exceed 20 mEq/hr in adults, 0.5 mEq/kg hr in children; use lower dose in renal impairment. Do not administer to hyperkalemic or heart block patients (unless hypokalemic) • After recent ingestion, implement guidelines for management of acute overdose (Appendix I). Avoid gastric emptying in patients with heart block or sinus bradycardia; may increase vagal tone, worsen dysrhythmia. • Activated charcoal helpful, even if administered late • Dysrhythmias (bradycardias, PVCs, SVT) may not respond to conventional ACLS therapy. • Avoid elective cardioversion; may cause resistant ventricular tachycardia, fibrillation. If necessary, start with low energy levels; gradually increase until successful. • **Resistant ventricular/supraventricular dysrhythmias:** Administer phenytoin, 0.5 mg/kg IV, at 50 mg/min q1-2h as needed up to 10 mg/kg/24 hr. • **Severe sinus bradycardia, AV block:** May respond to atropine • Use IV sympathomimetics with extreme caution; may contribute to dysrhythmias. • **Potentially life-threatening toxicity:** Administer digoxin immune Fab • Dialysis is ineffective in removing cardiac glycosides.

Toxic serum level: >2.5 ng/ml associated with symptoms of toxicity

---

INTERACTIONS

amiodarone ↑ Digoxin levels; bradycardia

amphotericin B ↑ Risk of digoxin toxicity from hypokalemia

antacids ↓ Digoxin absorption

calcium, IV Risk of acute digoxin toxicity/fatal dysrhythmias

calcium channel blockers ↑ Digoxin levels; risk of toxicity

corticosteroids Potassium deficiency with ↑ risk of dysrhythmias/toxicity

diuretics, thiazide/potassium losing Potassium deficiency with ↑ risk of dysrhythmias/toxicity

magnesium sulfate Altered cardiac conduction

neomycin, PO ↓ Digoxin absorption

phenytoin ↓ Digoxin levels

propafenone ↑ Digoxin levels; risk of toxicity

quinidine ↑ Digoxin levels; risk of toxicity

rifampin ↓ Digoxin levels

spironolactone ↑ Digoxin levels

sucralfate ↓ Digoxin adsorption

verapamil ↑ Digoxin levels; slowed AV conduction

COMPATIBILITIES

Amrinone, ciprofloxacin, diltiazem, famotidine, floxacillin, heparin, lidocaine, meperidine, milrinone, morphine, potassium chloride

INCOMPATIBILITIES

Fluconazole, insulin

PATIENT CARE IMPLICATIONS

• Do not administer at same time as antacids (aluminum hydroxide, magnesium hydroxide) or other agents that may inhibit absorption (see Interactions).

• Radiation, chemotherapy may reduce absorption; use of elixir/capsules recommended in these patients.

• If digoxin toxicity suspected, avoid elective cardioversion, which may result in ventricular tachycardia/fibrillation resistant to cardioversion. If necessary, start with low energy levels, gradually increase until successful.

• Avoid IV administration of calcium. If necessary, administer slowly, in small doses.

Vital signs/hemodynamics: Assess/document apical pulse before administering. Hold dose, consult physician for apical pulse significantly different from patient's usual pulse or of bradycardia that is symptomatic or associated with atrial fibrillation/flutter. • As available during initial therapy, monitor ECG for resolution of atrial dysrhythmias, development of other dysrhythmias. • If tachydysrhythmia develops, hold digoxin, delay elective cardioversion until drug level obtained. • During parenteral loading, continuously monitor ECG, carefully observe for dysrhythmias so that lowest effective dose used. • Monitor ECG continuously in patients with suspected toxicity. • Hemodynamic monitoring recommended for patients with heart failure, multiple therapies (e.g., dobutamine, dopamine, diuretics)

Physical assessment: Observe for early toxic effects: anorexia, nausea, vomiting, headache, drowsiness, disorientation, yellow-green or blurred vision, sinus bradycardia, AV conduction disturbances; drowsiness often **P** first symptom in children; anorexia or disorientation often first **G** symptom in older adults. Withhold further doses; consult physician. Narrow margin between effective and toxic doses results in high incidence of sometimes fatal toxicity. • Assess for perfusion/oxygenation deficit: decreased level of consciousness, activity intolerance, hypotension, chest discomfort, dizziness. • Auscultate lung fields for evidence of pulmonary edema (bibasilar crackles), especially in patients with history of CHF, cardiomyopathy.

Laboratory tests: Monitor: Electrolytes, particularly potassium, magnesium, calcium; correct before initiating therapy. • Serum digoxin levels • Consult physician of electrolyte abnormalities or digoxin levels >2.5 ng/ml.

PATIENT/FAMILY TEACHING

Purpose of medication is to regulate and improve heart functioning. • Immediately report breathing difficulty, palpitations, dizziness, activity intolerance, chest pain. • Immediately report symptoms of toxicity: poor appetite, nausea, vomiting, persistent headache, drowsiness, disorientation, yellow-green or blurred vision, palpitations.

Outpatient: Check/record resting pulse for 1 min before taking next dose. Report changes >15 bpm from usual pulse, especially if associated with symptoms of toxicity. • Take medication at same time each day. Take missed doses within 12 hr. Never double doses. Contact physician if dose missed for ≥2 days. • Failure to take potassium supplements as prescribed could result in serious toxicity. • Consult physician or pharmacist before using any over-the-counter treatments, including cold or allergy remedies, antacids. • Do not take antacids or kaolin-pectin (Kapectolin) antidiarrheals within 2 hr of digoxin administration. • Inform all health care providers of digoxin therapy. • Carry MedicAlert ID briefly describing dosage, indication for digoxin.

AVAILABLE FORMS

Tablets, capsules • PO elixir
• Parenteral for IV injection, adult formulation (0.25 mg/ml)
• Parenteral for IV injection, pediatric formulation (0.10 mg/ml)

digoxin immune Fab
(di-jox'in)
antidigoxin Fab fragments, digoxin-specific Fab antibody fragments
Digibind

Classifications: Serum, monovalent antibodies; antidote

USUAL DOSE

P **IV, intermit inf, adults/children:** Dosage based on body weight, serum digoxin level or estimate of ingested dose of digoxin (see tables)

Approx digoxin immune Fab dosage (mg) based on serum digoxin levels

WEIGHT (kg)	SERUM DIGOXIN LEVEL (ng/ml)					
	2	4	8	12	16	20
3	2	5	9	13	18	22
5	4	8	15	22	30	40
10	8	15	30	40	60	80
20	15	30	60	80	120	160
40	40	80	200	200	240	320
60	40	80	200	280	360	440
80	80	120	240	360	480	600
100	80	160	320	440	600	760

Approx digoxin immune Fab dosage (40-mg vials) based on acute ingestion of 0.25-mg tablets or 0.2-mg capsules

NO. INGESTED	NO. VIALS
10	4
25	9
50	17
100	34
150	50

ADMINISTRATION

Obtain blood for serum digoxin levels before administration.

▼ **Direct IV, imminent cardiac arrest only:** Rapidly inject undiluted dose. USE 0.22-μm IN-LINE FILTER TO REMOVE PROTEIN AGGREGATES. Rapid IV injection associated with higher rate of allergic reaction than infusion.
IV, intermit inf, recommended: Add reconstituted solution to ≥50 ml 0.9% NaCl; infuse entire dose over 15-30 min. USE 0.22-μm IN-LINE FILTER TO REMOVE PROTEIN AGGREGATES.

PREPARATION

Reconstitute by adding 4 ml sterile water to vial; mix gently. Solution contains 10 mg/ml. Reconstituted solution should be clear, colorless. Keep reconstituted solution refrigerated; use within 4 hr.

ACTIONS

Solution of digoxin-specific antigen-binding fragments (Fab) prepared from sheep serum • Fragments bind to free (unbound) digoxin to block or reverse all drug effects/symptoms of toxicity. • Digoxin effects on electrical conduction pathways, myocardial contractility reversed; electrical dysfunction resolves before mechanical dysfunction. Promotes immediate potassium shift into cells; hypokalemia is possible.

PHARMACOKINETICS

ROUTE	ONSET	PEAK	DURATION
IV	≤30 min	ND	16-50 hr

DISTRIBUTION
Widely distributed into plasma, interstitial fluids

ELIMINATION
Bound complex eliminated by kidneys; half-life 14-20 hr

INDICATIONS

Reversal of life-threatening cardiotoxic effects of cardiac glycoside intoxication, including severe bradycardias, advanced heart block, ventricular tachycardia/fibrillation, severe hyperkalemia

PRECAUTIONS/ CONTRAINDICATIONS

Precautions: Increased risk of hypersensitivity in following: previous exposure to ovine (sheep) proteins, known allergies to papaya extracts or any antibiotic • Rapid shifts in potassium from extracellular to intracellular compartment may occur as toxicity resolved; hypokalemia, dysrhythmias may ensue. • Response in renal-impaired patients similar to that in nonimpaired patients.

c Pregnancy category: Use only if safer alternative unavailable.

Contraindications: Hypersensitivity to digoxin immune Fab • Non–life-threatening digoxin toxicity

ADVERSE EFFECTS

CV: Rapid ventricular response in atrial fibrillation, **worsening of CHF**

Misc: *Hypokalemia,* hypersensitivity reactions

TOXICITY/OVERDOSE

Symptoms: Sensitivity, allergic, febrile, and delayed serum sickness reactions increase with use of higher-than-necessary dose. Redigitalization may be impaired with excessive administration.

Management: For management of acute allergic reactions, see Appendix N.

INTERACTIONS

cardiac glycosides ↓ Effectiveness of cardiac glycoside

INCOMPATIBILITIES

Do not mix, administer with other agents.

PATIENT CARE IMPLICATIONS

• Obtain history of allergies, previous exposure to ovine (sheep) proteins, especially digoxin immune Fab. Intradermal or scratch sensitivity test may be prescribed before use; risk of hypersensitivity increased in patients with previous exposure to drug.

• Have epinephrine, antihistamine, resuscitation equipment immediately available at time of injection.

• Use sympathomimetics (e.g., dobutamine, dopamine, epinephrine) cautiously, because they may contribute to dysrhythmias in patients with digitalis toxicity.

• Postpone redigitalization, if possible, for 3-7 days after administration.

Vital signs/hemodynamics: Monitor VS before and regularly after infusion complete.

• Monitor BP, HR at 10-min intervals during and after infusion, until stable. • Continuously monitor ECG for resolution of dysrhythmias, ECG evidence of hypokalemia (ST depression, flat T waves, presence of U wave, ventricular dysrhythmias) or hyperkalemia (peaked T waves, prolonged PR interval, ST depression, widened QRS, loss of P wave).

• Anticipate possible CO decrease when therapy initiated. Hemodynamic monitoring recommended for hypotensive or unstable patients; to improve CO, use dobutamine, dopamine, or vasodilators. Be aware that catecholamine use may ↑ dysrhythmias. Avoid using other cardiac glycosides.

Physical assessment: Assess for perfusion/oxygenation deficit: ↓ level of consciousness, activity intolerance, hypotension, chest discomfort, dizziness.

• Auscultate lung fields for evidence of pulmonary edema (bibasilar crackles), especially in patients with history of CHF, cardiomyopathy. • Assess for allergic reactions: chills, fever,

---

sweating, itching, rash, laryngeal edema, wheezing.
Laboratory tests: *Obtain blood for serum digoxin level before administration.* Digoxin immune Fab interferes with digoxin immunoassay measurements; results inaccurate until Fab fragments cleared, usually within 3 days, but up to 7 days with renal impairment.
• Monitor potassium frequently until toxicity resolved. Digoxin-related hyperkalemia usually present because of potassium shifts from within to outside cell. After digoxin immune Fab, potassium returns to cell, resulting in hypokalemia/possible dysrhythmias. Manage hyperkalemia with extreme caution.

PATIENT/FAMILY TEACHING

Purpose of medication is to bind excess digoxin and reduce dangerously high blood levels.
• Immediately report chills, fever, sweating, itching, breathing difficulty. • If digoxin immune Fab required in future, inform physician of prior dose. • Be certain that patient/family knowledgeable regarding use, administration of digoxin. See digoxin monograph for additional information.

AVAILABLE FORMS

Parenteral for IV use

---

diltiazem HCl
(dil-tye´a-zem)
Cardizem, Cardizem CD,
Cardizem SR, Dilacor XR

Classifications: Calcium channel blocker, antidysrhythmic, antianginal, antihypertensive

---

USUAL DOSE

PO standard, adult: 30-90 mg q6-8h
PO sust rel (Cardizem SR), adult: 60-120 mg q12h; may increase up to 180 mg q12h
PO controlled dose (Cardizem CD, Dilacor XR), adult: 180-480 mg once daily
Direct IV, adult: Initially 0.25 mg/kg (approx 20 mg for average adult) • If inadequate HR reduction, may administer second dose of 0.35 mg/kg (approx 25 mg) after 15 min • Additional boluses at individually adjusted doses may be administered until rapid HR controlled.
IV, cont inf, adult: 5-15 mg/hr for up to 24 hr

ADMINISTRATION

▼ Direct IV: Inject each dose slowly over at least 2 min.
IV inf: Start infusion at 5-10 mg/hr (see table); increase in 5-mg increments as necessary to control rapid HR.

PREPARATION

Recommended dilutions/ infusion rates for diltiazem

DILUTION	CONCENTRATION (mg/ml)	DOSE (mg/hr)	INFUSION (ml/hr)
125 mg/	1	10	10
125 ml*		15	15
250 mg/	0.83	10	12
300 ml†		15	18
250 mg/	0.45	10	22
550 ml‡		15	33

*Add 25 ml to 100-ml bag.
†Add 50 ml to 250-ml bag.
‡Add 50 ml to 500-ml bag.

Compatible fluids: D₅W, 0.9% NaCl, prepared combinations of these solutions.

Stability: Refrigerate parenteral solution before and after dilution. Dilute solution stable at room temperature for 24 hr. Unopened vials may be stored at room temperature for up to 1 mo.

ACTIONS

Inhibits movement of calcium ions across myocardium, vascular smooth muscle • Dilates coronary/systemic arteries; SA node automaticity ↓ • HR, myocardial contractility ↓ ; Reduces BP by ↓ peripheral vascular resistance • AV conduction time prolonged; ↑ refractoriness of AV node and selectively reduces HR during tachycardias involving AV node • Afterload reduction decreases myocardial O_2 demand. • Serum calcium levels unchanged • Negative inotropic properties not usually seen clinically unless prior ventricular dysfunction

PHARMACOKINETICS

ROUTE	ONSET	PEAK	DURATION
PO	30-60 min	2-3 hr	3-4 hr
PO, sus rel	30-60 min	6-11 hr	8-12 hr
PO*	2 hr	10-14 hr	24 hr
IV	Immed	≤15 min	

DISTRIBUTION

Wide; 70%-80% bound to plasma protein

ELIMINATION

Metabolized in liver, eliminated by kidneys; half-life 3.5-7 hr

*Controlled dose.

Therapeutic level: 50-200 ng/ml

INDICATIONS

Management of vasospastic/chronic stable angina in non-emergency situations • Sustained release used exclusively for management of essential hypertension • IV route used for temporary control of rapid ventricular response in patients with atrial fibrillation/flutter, paroxysmal SVT.

PRECAUTIONS/ CONTRAINDICATIONS

Precautions: May cause transient hypotension when therapy initiated • Negative inotropic effects may exacerbate heart failure • PVCs may occur after conversion to sinus rhythm.

Use caution with: Cardiac pacemakers, underlying conduction disorders; severe bradycardia or worsening of heart block possible • Recent (within 2 hr) administration of IV beta-blocker • Older adults, liver/renal impairment; dosage reduction may be necessary

C Pregnancy category: Use only if safer alternative unavailable.

Contraindications: Hypersensitivity to diltiazem • Acute MI • Pulmonary congestion • Severe hypotension • Cardiogenic shock • Sick sinus syndrome, 2nd/3rd degree heart block unless functional ventricular cardiac pacemaker in place or readily available • Ventricular tachycardia (QRS ≥0.12 sec); may cause ventricular fibrillation

ADVERSE EFFECTS

CNS: *Dizziness, headache, muscle weakness,* paresthesias
Resp: Dyspnea
CV: *Peripheral edema, AV heart block, bradycardia,* **hypotension,** angina, abnormal ECG, syncope, ventricular

---

italic = common side effects   **bold** = life-threatening reactions

dysrhythmias, sinus node dysfunction, CHF
GI: Nausea, elevated liver enzymes
Hema: Rarely—thrombocytopenia, anemia, leukopenia
Derm: Rash, pruritus, flushing,
sweating, gingival hyperplasia

TOXICITY/OVERDOSE

Symptoms: Profound hypotension • Dysrhythmias: bradycardia, 2nd/3rd degree heart block
• CHF • Dizziness, drowsiness,
confusion
Management: After recent ingestion, implement guidelines
for management of acute overdose (Appendix I). • **Hypotension:** Elevate legs, administer
IV fluids. Except with hypertrophic cardiomyopathy, use beta-
adrenergic agonists, IV calcium
chloride; vasopressors (e.g., norepinephrine, dopamine) used if
unresponsive to other measures.
With hypertrophic cardiomyopathy or IHSS, alpha-adrenergic
agents (e.g., methoxamine,
phenylephrine) may be used for
hypotension. • **Symptomatic
bradycardia, heart block:**
Use IV atropine, calcium, epinephrine, or possibly isoproterenol; consider temporary pacemaker. • **Other dysrhythmias:**
Rapid ventricular response from
antegrade conduction (e.g.,
WPW, LGL) managed with
direct-current cardioversion or
IV lidocaine or procainamide;
other dysrhythmias managed according to ACLS guidelines
(Appendix P). • Calcium may
be helpful in reversing adverse
hemodynamic effects but may
not always reverse electrophysiologic toxicity. • Dialysis is
not likely to be helpful.

INTERACTIONS

amiodarone ↑ Negative inotropy; bradycardia
antihypertensives/vasodilators
Profound hypotension
barbiturates ↓ Diltiazem levels
(PO)
beta-blockers Profound hypotension; exacerbation of heart block
calcium ↓ Diltiazem effectiveness
cimetidine ↑ Diltiazem levels/
toxicity
digoxin Exacerbation of heart
block; ↑ digoxin levels
fentanyl Profound hypotension
NMBAs (e.g., pancuronium)
Prolonged neuromuscular blockade
procainamide ↑ Negative inotropy
quinidine Quinidine toxicity
theophylline ↑ Theophylline
levels/toxicity

Y-SITE COMPATIBILITIES

Albumin, amikacin, amphotericin B, bretylium, bumetanide,
cefazolin, cefotaxime, cefotetan,
cefoxitin, ceftazidime, ceftriaxone, cefuroxime, cimetidine,
ciprofloxacin, digoxin, dobutamine, dopamine, epinephrine,
esmolol, fluconazole, gentamicin, hetastarch, imipenem-
cilastatin, lidocaine, lorazepam,
meperidine, metoclopramide,
morphine, nitroglycerin, nitroprusside, norepinephrine, oxacillin, penicillin G potassium, piperacillin, potassium chloride,
ranitidine, theophylline, ticarcillin, tobramycin, vancomycin

Y-SITE INCOMPATIBILITIES

Acyclovir, aminophylline, ampicillin, cefoperazone, diazepam,
furosemide, heparin, insulin,

nafcillin, phenytoin, sodium bi-carbonate

PATIENT CARE IMPLICATIONS

G • Older adults may experience profound hypotension. Use lowest effective dose; monitor closely.
• Use cautiously in patients with atrial fibrillation/flutter associated with WPW, LGL, other preexcitation syndromes.
• Never crush or break sustained-release or controlled-dose tablets for NG administration or other purpose; dangerous overdose could result.
Vital signs/hemodynamics: Monitor BP, HR. Hold next dose, consult with physician for hypotension, symptomatic bradycardia. • When initiating therapy in acutely ill patients, check VS frequently, continuously monitor ECG for signs of ischemia (e.g., T wave inversion, ST segment elevation), heart block. **Direct IV inf:** Monitor ECG for resolution of tachycardia, development of heart block. • Monitor BP at 2–5-min intervals until stable and frequently thereafter, according to titration schedule, patient condition.
Physical assessment: Assess for evidence of pulmonary edema: bibasilar crackles (rales), neck vein distention, S_3 gallop, breathing difficulty, especially in patients with CHF, cardiomyopathy. • Assess for perfusion/oxygenation deficit: ↓ level of consciousness, ↓ BP, activity intolerance, chest discomfort.
Laboratory tests: Monitor: CBC with differential • Liver enzymes

PATIENT/FAMILY TEACHING

Purpose of medication is to control high BP, relieve angina pain, or slow rapid heartbeat. **Initiation of therapy:** May cause dizziness; use caution, change positions slowly.
• Sustained-release or controlled-dose tablets should never be broken, chewed, or crushed. **IV:** Remain in bed during and for several hours thereafter.
• Report breathing difficulty, chest pain, palpitations, activity intolerance, swelling of feet/ankles.

AVAILABLE FORMS

Parenteral for IV use • Capsules • Tablets (sustained release) • Capsules (controlled dose)

diphenhydramine HCl
(dye-fen-hye′dra-meen)
Benadryl, Benahist, Benoject, Benylin, Diphenacen, Diphenadryl, Diphenhist, Genahist, Hydramine, Hyrexin, Wehdryl

Classifications: Antihistamine, antitussive

USUAL DOSE

PO, adults: 25-50 mg 3-4 times daily • Do not exceed 300 mg/day.
P PO, children: 1-2 mg/kg/dose up to 5 mg/kg/day; given in divided doses 3-4 times daily
IV/IM, adults: 10-50 mg; up to 100 mg may be used. • Do not exceed 400 mg/day.
P IV/IM, children: 5 mg/kg/day in divided doses q6-8h • Do not exceed 300 mg/day.

---

italic = common side effects   **bold** = life-threatening reactions

ADMINISTRATION

IM: Inject deeply into large muscle. • Local irritation possible • Effects delayed, unpredictable in emergencies

▼ **Direct IV:** Emergencies: inject ≤25 mg over ≥1 min. • **Nonemergency situations:** Inject each dose over 4-5 min. May be given undiluted

IV, intermit inf: Infuse over 10-20 min.

PREPARATION

IV, intermit inf: Dilute in 50 ml compatible solution; larger or smaller volumes may be used.

Compatible fluids: D_5W, $D_{10}W$, 0.45% NaCl, 0.9% NaCl, LR, prepared combinations of these solutions

ACTIONS

H_1 receptor antagonist; blocks histamine activity at receptor sites • The following histamine-mediated effects are blocked: bronchial constriction; bronchial, salivary, lacrimal, gastric hypersecretion; small vessel dilation; excessive capillary permeability; hypotension; edema; pruritus • Causes CNS depression, drowsiness • Has antiemetic, central anticholinergic effects • Antagonizes opiate-induced contractions of biliary smooth muscle • No effect on gastric acid secretion, which is mediated by H_2 receptors

PHARMACOKINETICS

ROUTE	ONSET	PEAK	DURATION
PO	15 min	1-4 hr	To 7 hr
IV	Rapid	<1 hr	To 7 hr

DISTRIBUTION
Widely distributed; 80%-85% protein bound

ELIMINATION
Substantial first-pass metabolism in liver, excreted by kidneys; half-life 2.4-9.3 hr

INDICATIONS

Relief of allergy symptoms • Adjunct to epinephrine in managing anaphylactic reactions • Drug-induced extrapyramidal symptoms • Cough relief • Prevention/treatment of nausea, vomiting, vertigo associated with motion sickness • Short-term management of insomnia • Symptomatic treatment of parkinsonian syndrome in older adults unable to tolerate more potent agents • Topically for temporary relief of pruritus/pain associated with sunburn, insect bites, minor skin irritations

PRECAUTIONS/ CONTRAINDICATIONS

Precautions: Commercial preparations may contain sulfites, which can cause serious allergic reactions.

Use caution with: Asthma, COPD; thickening of bronchial secretions may cause obstruction. • Angle-closure glaucoma, increased intraocular pressure, prostatic hypertrophy, stenosing peptic ulcer, pyloroduodenal obstruction, bladder neck obstruction; anticholinergic effects may worsen condition. • Hyperthyroidism, CV disease, hypertension • Young children: More susceptible to toxic, CNS stimulant effects • Older adults: Diz-

ziness, sedation, hypotension
more likely
B **Pregnancy category:** Safety
not clearly established
Contraindications: Hypersensitivity to diphenhydramine
P • Acute asthma • Newborns,
premature infants

ADVERSE EFFECTS

CNS: *Drowsiness, dizziness, impaired coordination,* weakness, paradoxical excitation, restlessness, insomnia, tremors, **seizures** (rare)
Resp: *Nose/throat dryness, thickening of bronchial secretions,* wheezing, nasal stuffiness
CV: Palpitations, hypo/hypertension, tachycardia, extrasystoles
GI: *Mouth dryness, epigastric distress,* anorexia, nausea, vomiting, diarrhea, constipation
GU: Urinary retention, dysuria
Misc: Autonomic effects—dry mouth, blurred vision, urinary retention, visual disturbances; hypersensitivity reactions; photosensitivity

TOXICITY/OVERDOSE

Symptoms: Marked drowsiness, sedation, coma, hypotension, respiratory depression/apnea • CNS stimulation, hallucinations, tremors/convulsions; stimulation occurs more frequently in children, older adults.
P
G • **Anticholinergic symptoms:**
Fixed dilated pupils, flushing, dry mouth, fever/hyperthermia
P (particularly in children) • ECG changes, including torsades de pointes • Cerebral edema, nephrosis, cardiopulmonary collapse

Management: After recent ingestion, implement guidelines for management of acute overdose (Appendix I). • Ipecac effective if given early before full sedative, antiemetic effects • If ipecac unsuccessful or gag reflex absent, initiate gastric lavage followed by instillation of activated charcoal. • Protect airway by ET intubation, keeping cuff inflated. • Saline cathartics (e.g., magnesium sulfate) may be used. • Maintain airway/support ventilation. • **Hypotension:** Elevate legs, administer IV fluids; use dopamine, norepinephrine, or phenylephrine if unresponsive to volume replacement. Avoid epinephrine, which may lead to further lowering of BP (see Interactions). • Avoid stimulants, which may cause seizures. • Physostigmine sometimes given to counteract CNS anticholinergic effects • Diazepam used for seizures not responsive to physostigmine
• Propranolol may be used for ventricular dysrhythmias.

INTERACTIONS

alcohol ↑ CNS depression
anesthetics ↑ CNS depression
barbiturates ↑ CNS depression
benzodiazepines ↑ CNS depression
epinephrine Blocked alpha effects; unopposed beta activity; profound hypotension
hypnotics ↑ CNS depression
MAO inhibitors ↑ Anticholinergic effects
opioid analgesics ↑ CNS depression
phenothiazines Hypotension, extrapyramidal reactions, additive CNS depression

---

italic = common side effects   **bold** = life-threatening reactions

sedatives ↑ CNS depression
tranquilizers ↑ CNS depression

Y-SITE COMPATIBILITIES

Acyclovir, ciprofloxacin, heparin, meperidine, ondansetron, piperacillin-tazobactam, potassium chloride

IN-SYRINGE COMPATIBILITIES

Atropine, chlorpromazine, droperidol, fentanyl, glycopyrrolate, hydromorphone, hydroxyzine, meperidine, metoclopramide, midazolam, morphine, nalbuphine, pentazocine, prochlorperazine, promethazine

Y-SITE INCOMPATIBILITIES

Cefepime, phenytoin

PATIENT CARE IMPLICATIONS

• May cause drowsiness, dizziness; use appropriate safety precautions according to patient condition.
• Administer 20-30 min before desired onset of effects.
• Reserve parenteral therapy for urgent/emergent situations or when PO route unacceptable (e.g., vomiting, NPO status). Convert to PO therapy as soon as possible.
• Administer PO doses with meals or milk to prevent GI side effects.
Vital signs/hemodynamics: Monitor VS frequently and use continuous pulse oximetry in heavily sedated patients (e.g., those also receiving opiates). IV: Monitor HR, BP immediately before and after administration.
• As available, monitor ECG for tachycardia, dysrhythmias.
Physical assessment: Assess neurologic status for excessive

sedation, dizziness, impaired physical coordination; ↓ dose as necessary. • Assess the following parameters according to indication for use: Allergic rhinitis: Relief from nasal stuffiness, rhinorrhea, sneezing • Anaphylaxis: Airway patency, breath sounds, HR, BP, resolution of urticaria • Cough suppression: Nature/frequency of cough, sputum production • Extrapyramidal reactions: Relief from restlessness, uncontrolled motor movement, parkinsonian symptoms • Insomnia: Sleep patterns, quality • Nausea: Relief from nausea, vomiting episodes • Pruritus: Resolution of itching, rash, inflammation
Laboratory tests: May suppress reaction to antigen skin testing; when possible, discontinue diphenhydramine for 4 days before skin testing.

PATIENT/FAMILY TEACHING

Purpose of medication is to relieve itching or other allergic symptoms, suppress coughing, reduce nausea, promote sleep.
• May cause dizziness, drowsiness; call for assistance when getting out of bed until response to drug established. • Take with meals or milk to avoid GI upset. • Frequent oral hygiene and use of hard candy or gum may relieve dry mouth.
Outpatient: Avoid concurrent use of alcohol or other drugs that cause sedation while taking this medication • Avoid driving and other activities requiring mental alertness or physical coordination. • May cause sensitivity to sunlight; avoid prolonged exposure, use sunblock.
• Contact physician about rash, fever, easy bruising, unusual

bleeding, difficulty urinating, excessive sedation.

AVAILABLE FORMS

Parenteral for IV/IM injection • Capsules, tablets, elixir, syrup for PO use

dipyridamole
(dye-peer-id'a-mole)
Persantine

Classification: Platelet inhibitor

USUAL DOSE

PO, adults: 75-100 mg 4 times daily
IV, intermit inf: 0.57 mg/kg of diluted solution over 4 min.

PREPARATION

IV: Dilute each ml (5 mg) in at least 2 ml of compatible solution. Total volume should be 20-50 ml. Failure to dilute dipyridamole could cause vein irritation.
Compatible fluids: 0.45% NaCl, 0.9% NaCl, D_5W

ACTIONS

Reduces platelet aggregation • Lengthens platelet survival time in patients with prosthetic heart valves • Increases coronary blood flow, coronary sinus O_2 saturation by selective coronary vasodilation • IV causes ↑ HR/slight ↓ BP

PHARMACOKINETICS

ROUTE	ONSET	PEAK	DURATION
PO	<45 min	45-150 min	6-8 hr
IV	immed	6-7 min	30 min

DISTRIBUTION
91%-99% bound to plasma protein
ELIMINATION
Metabolized in liver, excreted mainly in feces

D

INDICATIONS

Adjunct to PO anticoagulants in prevention of postop thromboembolic complications after cardiac valve replacement • IV used during thallium myocardial perfusion imaging
Unlabeled/investigational:
Alone and with aspirin to prevent myocardial reinfarction, reduce mortality after MI; maintenance of graft patency after cardiac surgery

PRECAUTIONS/ CONTRAINDICATIONS

Use caution with: Hypotension
B Pregnancy category: Safety not clearly established
Contraindications: Hypersensitivity to dipyridamole • Children: Safety/effectiveness not established

ADVERSE EFFECTS

CNS: Headache, dizziness, weakness
CV: Peripheral vasodilation, hypotension, flushing
IV: Chest pain, S-T segment changes
GI: Nausea
Derm: Rash, pruritus

TOXICITY/OVERDOSE

Symptoms: Hypotension, usually of short duration

---

italic = common side effects   **bold** = life-threatening reactions

Management: After recent ingestion, implement guidelines for management of acute overdose (Appendix I). • **Hypotension:** Elevate legs, administer fluids; use vasopressors (e.g., dopamine, norepinephrine) for prolonged hypotension. • Dialysis is not likely to be beneficial.

INTERACTIONS

alcohol Dizziness, hypotension

anticoagulants, oral; aspirin; heparin; NSAIDs, thrombolytics ↑ Risk of bleeding complications

cefamandole, cefoperazone, cefotetan ↑ Risk of bleeding complications

PATIENT CARE IMPLICATIONS

• Not indicated for relief of acute anginal pain

Vital signs/hemodynamics: Measure BP routinely; use caution when administering to hypotensive patients. • IV: Monitor BP/ECG frequently

PATIENT/FAMILY TEACHING

Purpose of medication is to decrease clot formation or assist in diagnostic testing. • Change position slowly to prevent dizziness, fainting. • Use of alcohol increases risk of low BP, dizziness, fainting. • Avoid aspirin, NSAIDs (e.g., ibuprofen) unless specifically prescribed.

AVAILABLE FORMS

Tablets • IV solution

---

disopyramide
(dye-soe-peer'a-mide)
Rhythmodan

disopyramide phosphate
Napamide, Norpace, Norpace CR

Classification: Antidysrhythmic membrane stabilizer, Vaughan-Williams Class IA

USUAL DOSE

Individually adjust each dose according to CV status, patient response; use lowest effective dose.

PO, adults: Loading, initially 300 mg; if dysrhythmia not controlled within 6 hr, give 200 mg q6h until controlled; if no response within 48 hr, increase to 250-300 mg q6h with careful monitoring; discontinue for signs of toxicity. • Maintenance, 150 mg q6h • **Cardiomyopathy, possible cardiac decompensation:** Initially 100 mg q6-8h, adjust cautiously; do not give loading dose. • **Renal/hepatic impairment or weight <50 kg:** 100 mg q6h; use 200-mg loading dose.

PO controlled rel, adults: 300 mg q12h; not used for initial or loading therapy • **Renal/hepatic impairment or weight <50 kg:** 200 mg q12h

ACTIONS

Decreases cardiac excitability by increasing threshold for electrical excitation • PR interval, slightly prolonged; widens QRS/prolongs QT interval • Blocks fast sodium channels to suppress automaticity in His-Purkinje system, ectopic atrial/

---

ventricular pacemakers • Decreases conduction velocity in accessory pathways • AV nodal, His-Purkinje conduction velocity unaffected • Prolongs effective refractory period in atria, ventricles • Sinus pacing rate unaffected • Direct negative inotropic effect may ↓ CO up to 15%. • Increases peripheral vascular resistance average of 20% • Principal metabolite, MND (mono-*N*-dealkyldisopyramide), exhibits antidysrhythmic, anticholinergic properties.

PHARMACOKINETICS

ROUTE	ONSET	PEAK	DURATION
PO	30 min	≤2 hr	1.5-8.5 hr

DISTRIBUTION
Wide; throughout extracellular fluid; 50%-65% protein bound

ELIMINATION
Metabolized in liver, excreted by kidneys; half-life 4-10 hr

Therapeutic range: 2-8 µg/ml

INDICATIONS

Suppression/prevention of symptomatic life-threatening ventricular dysrhythmias, atrial fibrillation, PAT • Use only as alternative therapy after failure of lidocaine, procainamide, quinidine in conversion of dysrhythmias.

PRECAUTIONS/ CONTRAINDICATIONS

Precautions: May cause profound hypotension • Worsens heart block in patients with pre-existing AV block • May widen QRS/prolong PR, QT intervals in patients with ventricular dysrhythmias • Hypokalemia renders drug ineffective; hyperkalemia enhances drug effects.
• Improved survival has not been demonstrated with antidysrhythmic therapy.

Use caution with: CHF, cardiomyopathy, acute MI, possible cardiac decompensation, especially if receiving other negative inotropes • Conduction abnormalities (WPW, sick sinus syndrome); effects not well established • Renal/hepatic insufficiency; reduce dose.
• Benign prostatic hypertrophy.

c Pregnancy category: Use only if safer alternative unavailable.

Contraindications: Hypersensitivity to disopyramide • Prolonged QT syndrome • Urinary retention, myasthenia gravis; potent anticholinergic activity

ADVERSE EFFECTS

CNS: *Dizziness, fatigue, headache, nervousness*
EENT: *Dry nose/throat, blurred vision*
Resp: Dyspnea, **apnea** (rare)
CV: **hypotension, CHF, new/ exacerbated heart block,** syncope, chest pain, conduction disturbances, peripheral edema
GI: *Dry mouth, constipation, nausea,* abdominal discomfort, vomiting
GU: *Urinary hesitancy, retention, frequency, urgency;* elevated creatinine
Endo: Hypoglycemia
Derm: Rash, itching
Syst: *Muscle aches, malaise,* weakness, hypokalemia

TOXICITY/OVERDOSE

Symptoms: Excessive widening of QRS prolonged QT interval, torsades de pointes, hypotension, exacerbated CHF, anticholinergic effects, bradycardia, asystole, apnea

---

italic = common side effects   **bold** = life-threatening reactions

Management: After recent ingestion, implement guidelines for management of acute overdose (Appendix I). • **Heart failure:** Use positive inotropic agents (e.g., dopamine, dobutamine, digitalis), diuretics.
• **Hypotension:** Elevate legs; use inotropic agents. If unresponsive to dopamine/other positive inotropes, use norepinephrine; phenylephrine used if hypotension fails to respond to other agents. • **Symptomatic bradycardia:** Use ACLS guidelines (Appendix P). • Reverse anticholinergic effects with neostigmine. • Hemodialysis or charcoal hemoperfusion may be helpful.

Toxic serum level: >9 µg/ml

INTERACTIONS

antidysrhythmics, Type I (quinidine, procainamide) ↑ Risk of hypotension, heart failure, heart block, QT prolongation leading to torsades de pointes.

beta-blockers ↑ Risk of hypotension, heart failure

calcium channel blockers ↑ Risk of hypotension, heart failure

potassium Slowed conduction; ↑ risk of disopyramide toxicity

PATIENT CARE IMPLICATIONS

• Not indicated for immediate stabilization of ventricular dysrhythmias; use synchronized or unsynchronized cardioversion for emergency stabilization of patients with ventricular dysrhythmias (ACLS guidelines, Appendix P).
• Digitalize patients in atrial fibrillation or flutter before receiving disopyramide to avoid anticholinergic-mediated tachycardia.

• Correct hypokalemia before initiating therapy.
• Avoid administering disopyramide within 48 hr before or 24 hr after verapamil therapy; concurrent therapy likely to cause profound cardiac depression.
• Never crush or break sustained-release capsules; dangerous overdose could result.

Vital signs/hemodynamics: Monitor BP, HR, RR hourly during initial loading and with dose adjustments; thereafter assess routinely. Consult physician of symptomatic bradycardia, unusual or rapid tachycardia.
• Monitor ECG for new dysrhythmias, excessive prolongation of PR/QT intervals, QRS complex. If QT, QRS increase by ≥ 25%, withhold next dose, notify physician. • Monitor ECG for heartblock: reduce dose for 1° heart block; discontinue for 2°, 3° heart block or uni/bi/trifascicular block unless ventricular pacemaker in place.
• Measure I&O, observing for low UO, possible urinary retention.

Physical assessment: Assess for perfusion/oxygenation deficit: ↓ level of consciousness, chest pain, activity intolerance, hypotension, dizziness. • Assess for CHF/pulmonary edema: bibasilar crackles (rales), neck vein distention, edema, S_3 gallop. • Assess for urinary retention: palpable bladder, pain, abdominal distention. Elderly males with benign prostatic hypertrophy require careful assessment because of anticholinergic effects.

Laboratory tests: Monitor: Electrolytes, especially potassium • Disopyramide levels; therapeutic level, 2-8 µg/ml

PATIENT/FAMILY TEACHING

Purpose of medication is to control irregular heartbeats. • Take medication on time, exactly as directed. Do not skip, double doses. • Side effects often occur: dry eyes, nose, mouth, throat; urinary hesitancy, retention; constipation. • Drink plenty of fluids, consume high-fiber diet for prevention of constipation. • Report chest pain, dizziness, fainting, breathing difficulty, activity intolerance. • Extended-release capsules should never be broken, chewed, or crushed.

AVAILABLE FORMS

Capsules • Extended-release capsules

---

dobutamine HCl
(doe-byoo'ta-meen)
Dobutrex

Classifications: Sympathomimetic, adrenergic agent, inotropic agent

USUAL DOSE

IV, cont inf, adults: Initially 2.5 µg/kg/min (e.g., approx 11 ml/hr of 250 mg/250 ml solution for 70-kg adult); increase as needed to improve CO.
• Maintenance, 2.5-15 µg/kg/min • Maximum dose, 40 µg/kg/min; ↑ risk of tachycardia, dysrhythmias with high-dose therapy

ⓟIV, cont inf, children (unlabeled/investigational): Initially 2.5 µg/kg/min; increase as needed to improve CO. • Maximum dose, 20 µg/kg/min; ↑ risk of tachycardia, dysrhythmias with high-dose therapy

ADMINISTRATION

IV, cont inf: Titration schedule: Increase by 2-3 µg/kg/min q10min; titrate to optimal CO.
• Use lowest effective dose. • Infusion pump necessary • See Infusion Rate table Appendix Q. **D**

PREPARATION

DILUTION	CONCENTRATION
250 mg/250 ml	1,000 µg/ml
500 mg/250 ml	2,000 µg/ml
1,000 mg/250 ml	4,000 µg/ml

More concentrated solutions may be used if necessary to limit fluid volume intake but should not exceed 250 mg/50 ml.

Compatible fluids: D₅W, 0.9% NaCl, LR, prepared combinations of these solutions **Peritoneal dialysis solution compatibility:** Dianeal PD—1 with 1.5, 4.25% dextrose **Stability:** Stable for 24 hr at room temp; pink discoloration indicates oxidation but not loss of potency; do not use yellow, brown, or cloudy solutions.

ACTIONS

Beta-1-adrenergic receptor agonist; results in cardiac stimulation, positive inotropic effects • Mild stimulation of beta-2, alpha-1 receptors; minimal effects on BP • **Hemodynamic effects:** ↑ Myocardial contractility, ↑ SV; ↑ CO; ↑ HR at higher doses; ↓ PVR; BP unchanged or slightly ↑ ; PAP ↓ or unchanged; generally decreases ↑ LVEDP • Likelihood of dysrhythmias < with dopamine, isoproterenol • Amrinone has inotropic, vasodilatory effects but less likely than dobutamine to cause dysrhythmias. • Does not affect dopaminergic receptors; causes no renal or

---

italic = common side effects   **bold** = life-threatening reactions

mesenteric vasodilation • UO usually ↑ as CO improves.

PHARMACOKINETICS

ROUTE	ONSET	PEAK	DURATION
IV	1-2 min	2-10 min	<10 min

DISTRIBUTION

Unknown

ELIMINATION

Metabolized in liver, other tissues; half-life 2 min

INDICATIONS

To improve CO in patients with depressed contractility when little effect on peripheral vasculature desired • Preferable to dopamine immediately after cardiopulmonary bypass surgery because of mild lowering of PVR and lack of dependence on release of endogenous catecholamines • Used concurrently with afterload-reducing agents such as sodium nitroprusside in severe left ventricular failure • Useful along with volume loading in patients with hemodynamically significant right ventricular infarction • Used concurrently with dopamine in stabilized cardiogenic shock to reduce dopamine requirements. *Unlabeled/investigational:* ❶ Cardiogenic shock in children, but without clear advantage over dopamine

PRECAUTIONS/ CONTRAINDICATIONS

Precautions: Not indicated for BP support in severe hypotension • May increase intrapulmonary shunt because improved CO increases perfusion to poorly ventilated lung segments • May increase myocardial workload, resulting in imbalance of myocardial O_2 supply/demand • Digitalize patients with atrial fibrillation before dobutamine administration. • May exacerbate ventricular ectopy • May ↓ serum potassium levels • Commercial preparations may contain sulfites, which can cause serious allergic reactions.

Use caution with: Preexisting hypertension; sudden hypertension possible

c Pregnancy category: Use only if safer alternative unavailable.

Contraindications: Hypersensitivity to dobutamine • IHSS or marked mechanical obstruction (e.g., severe valvular aortic stenosis) • Safety not established for use in pregnancy, lactation, ❶ children

ADVERSE EFFECTS

CNS: Headache
Resp: Dyspnea
CV: ↑ *HR,* ↑ *BP, exacerbation of ventricular ectopy, angina, palpitations,* hypotension (rare)
Derm: Inflammation/pain with extravasation
Syst: Allergic reactions, especially in patients with sulfite sensitivity
Misc: Hypokalemia

TOXICITY/OVERDOSE

Symptoms: Hypertension, increased vascular resistance • Dysrhythmias • Hypotension
Management: Reduce rate or discontinue until condition stabilizes. Because of short duration of action, other treatment usually unnecessary • **Dysrhythmias:** Manage according to ACLS guidelines (Appendix P).

INTERACTIONS

anesthetics ↑ Dysrhythmias

beta-blockers Antagonism of beta effects; predominance of pressor response

bretylium ↑ Dysrhythmias

phenytoin Bradycardia, hypotension

sympathomimetics ↑ Dysrhythmias

TCAs Potentiation of pressor effects

Y-SITE COMPATIBILITIES

Amiodarone, amrinone, atracurium, bretylium, calcium chloride, calcium gluconade, ciprofloxacin, diltiazem, dopamine, enalaprilat, famotidine, haloperidol, insulin, lidocaine, magnesium sulfate, meperidine, nitroglycerin, nitroprusside, pancuronium, potassium chloride, ranitidine, vecuronium, verapamil, zidovudine

Y-SITE INCOMPATIBILITIES

Acyclovir, alteplase, alkaline solutions, aminophylline, furosemide, heparin, piperacillin-tazobactam, **sodium bicarbonate**

PATIENT CARE IMPLICATIONS

• Correct hypovolemia before initiating therapy; in emergencies, may be administered to patient in hypovolemic state with simultaneous fluid replacement.

• Do not initiate dobutamine therapy in patients with atrial fibrillation until digitalized; because of possible ventricular response, CV decompensation.

• Do not administer sodium bicarbonate or other alkaline solution through same IV line.

Vital signs/hemodynamics: Initially, monitor BP, HR q5-15min; progressively advance according to titration schedule, hemodynamic stability. Anticipate 5-15 bpm ↑ in HR. Consider dosage reduction if HR ↑ >10% above baseline. • Establish clear parameters for titration (e.g., desired CO, BP). Always use lowest possible dose to achieve desired effect.

• Monitor ECG for dysrhythmias, ischemic changes, especially during initial therapy. Stable patients without titration may not require continuous ECG monitoring. • As available, monitor PCWP, CVP, CO; immediately correct hypovolemia.

• Monitor UO, consult physician if ≤5 ml/kg/hr or ≤30 ml/hr.

Physical assessment: Assess for evidence of heart failure: bibasilar crackles (rales), neck vein distention, S_3 gallop, breathing difficulty, especially in patients with CHF, cardiomyopathy. • Assess for perfusion/oxygenation deficit: changes in mentation, ↓ BP, activity intolerance, chest discomfort.

Laboratory tests: Monitor: Electrolytes, particularly potassium; promptly correct hypokalemia.

PATIENT/FAMILY TEACHING

Purpose of medication is to improve heart's blood-pumping ability. • Immediately report chest pain or discomfort, palpitations, pain at infusion site.

AVAILABLE FORMS

Parenteral concentrate for IV admixture

---

italic = common side effects   **bold** = life-threatening reactions

dopamine HCl
(doe'pa-meen)
Dopastat, Intropin,
Revimine ✦

Classifications: Sympathomimetic, adrenergic, vasopressor, inotropic agent

USUAL DOSE

IV, cont inf, adults: ↑ Renal perfusion: 0.5-2 µg/kg/min • ↑ Myocardial contractility: 2-10 µg/kg/min • Hypotension: 10-20 µg/kg/min • Maximum dose, 50 µg/kg/min

Ⓟ **IV, cont inf, children (unlabeled/investigational):** ↑ Renal perfusion: 1-5 µg/kg/min • ↑ Myocardial contractility: 5-10 µg/kg/min • Hypotension: 10-20 µg/kg/min

ADMINISTRATION

IV, cont inf: ↑ Renal perfusion/CO: Increase by 1-4 µg/kg/min q10-30min; titrate to optimal CO, UO. • Serious hypotension: Increase by 5-10 µg/kg/min q5-10min; titrate to optimal BP, CO. • Always use lowest effective dose. • Infusion pump necessary • Administer via central, antecubital, or other large vein. Avoid using veins in hands, ankles, legs. • See Infusion Rate table Appendix Q.

PREPARATION

DILUTION	CONCENTRATION
200 mg/250 ml	800 µg/ml
400 mg/250 ml	1,600 µg/ml
800 mg/250 ml	3,200 µg/ml

More concentrated solutions may be used if necessary to limit volume intake.

Compatible fluids: D_5W, 0.9% NaCl, LR, prepared combinations of these solutions
Stability: Stable for 24 hr at room temperature; yellow, brown, or pink to purple discoloration indicates decomposition; do not use discolored or cloudy solutions.

ACTIONS

Endogenous catecholamine and precursor of norepinephrine that stimulates dopaminergic, beta-1-adrenergic, alpha-adrenergic receptors with variable dose-related effects • Indirectly causes release of norepinephrine stores • Low (renal) dose (0.5-2 µg/kg/min): Stimulates dopaminergic receptors; results in renal, mesenteric, coronary cerebral vasodilation; renal blood flow/UO ↑ • Intermediate dose (2-10 µg/kg/min): Stimulates dopaminergic, beta-1-adrenergic receptors. Myocardial contractility/SV increase, improving CO. Minimal to mild effects on BP; SBP may increase slightly. Peripheral vasodilation, decreased vascular resistance result in unchanged or slightly decreased MAP. • High dose (>10-20 µg/kg/min): Stimulation of alpha-adrenergic receptors causes increased peripheral/renal vascular resistance. Stimulation of myocardial contractility continues. UO usually decreases; SBP, DBP increase. Increase in afterload may increase cardiac workload; resulting imbalance in myocardial O_2 supply/demand may worsen ischemic heart disease, CHF, cardiogenic shock. • Very high dose (>20 µg/kg/min): predominant alpha stimulation with profound vasoconstriction and compromised peripheral/renal perfusion.

PHARMACOKINETICS

ROUTE	ONSET	PEAK	DURATION
IV	2-5 min	Rapid	10 min

DISTRIBUTION

Wide; very little crosses blood-brain barrier

ELIMINATION

Metabolized in liver, kidneys, plasma; excreted in urine; half-life 2 min

INDICATIONS

Low dose (0.5-2 µg/kg/min): To improve renal blood flow • **Intermediate to high dose** (≥2 µg/kg/min): To increase CO, BP, UO in nonhypovolemic shock states • If doses <20 µg/kg/min are not effective, a strong alpha agent (e.g., norepinephrine) usually indicated. Dopamine is then ↓ to renal dose (0.5-2 µg/kg/min) to salvage kidneys. • Low CO syndrome after open heart surgery; however, dobutamine may be preferable because of ability to ↓ PVR over wide dose range. • Severe CHF; frequently administered concurrently with an afterload reducer (e.g., sodium nitroprusside) • Treatment of hepatorenal syndrome; cirrhosis; acute renal failure; barbiturate, meprobamate, salicylate intoxication • Infants/children (unlabeled/investigational) • Low to moderate doses for management of nonhypovolemic shock

PRECAUTIONS/ CONTRAINDICATIONS

Precautions: Drug-related increases in myocardial workload may lead to imbalance between myocardial O_2 supply and demand. • May increase intrapulmonary shunt as improved CO increases perfusion to poorly ventilated lung segments • Hypoxia, hypercapnia, acidosis reduce drug effectiveness, increase incidence of adverse effects. • Extravasation may lead to necrosis, sloughing of tissue (Appendixes K and L). • Commercial preparations may contain sulfites, which can cause serious allergic reactions. **Use caution with:** Arteriosclerosis, Raynaud's disease, cold injury, diabetic enarteritis, other occlusive vascular disease; closely monitor peripheral perfusion. • Cardiogenic shock, CHF, cardiomyopathy, any condition associated with severely compromised myocardial function; high doses may cause paradoxical hypotension because of ↑ afterload. • Children: Safety not established peripheral gangrene reported **Pregnancy category:** Use only if safer alternative unavailable.

Contraindications: Hypersensitivity to dopamine • Pheochromocytoma with hypertension • Uncorrected tachydysrhythmias • Ventricular fibrillation

ADVERSE EFFECTS

CNS: Headache, anxiety
Resp: Dyspnea, ventilatory depression in patients dependent on hypoxic drive
CV: *Tachycardia,* **dysrhythmias, ventricular dysrhythmias;** bradycardia, widened QRS complex, palpitations, **hypotension,** hypertension, vasoconstriction, angina, gangrene of extremities
GI: *Nausea, vomiting*
GU: Azotemia
Endo: ↑ Serum glucose

---

italic = common side effects   **bold** = life-threatening reactions

Derm: Pain, inflammation, tissue necrosis, skin sloughing with extravasation

TOXICITY/OVERDOSE

Symptoms: Hypertension, increased SVR • Dysrhythmias
Management: Reduce infusion rate or discontinue until condition stabilizes. • Because of short duration of action, other treatment is usually unnecessary. • If hypertension persists, use short-acting alpha-adrenergic blockers (e.g., phentolamine).

INTERACTIONS

anesthetics ↑ Pressor effects; dysrhythmias more likely
beta-blockers Antagonism of pressor/cardiac-stimulating effects
bretylium ↑ Dysrhythmias
MAO inhibitors ↑ Pressor effects
phenytoin Bradycardia, hypotension; risk of seizures
prazosin Antagonism of pressor effects
sympathomimetics ↑ Dysrhythmias
tricyclics Antagonism of pressor effects

Y-SITE COMPATIBILITIES

Amiodarone, amrinone, atracurium, ciprofloxacin, diltiazem, dobutamine, enalaprilat, esmolol, famotidine, haloperidol, heparin (in 0.9% NaCl), labetalol, lidocaine, meperidine, morphine, nitroglycerin, nitroprusside, pancuronium, pipercillian-tazobactam, potassium chloride, ranitidine, vecuronium, verapamil, zidovudine

Y-SITE INCOMPATIBILITIES

Acyclovir, alkaline solutions, alteplase, heparin (in D₅W), **sodium bicarbonate**

PATIENT CARE IMPLICATIONS

• Correct hypovolemia before initiating therapy; in emergencies, may be administered to patient in hypovolemic state with simultaneous fluid volume replacement.
• Do not administer sodium bicarbonate, other alkaline solutions through same IV line.
• Monitor for/correct hypoxemia, hypercapnia, acidosis before and during administration.
• If hypotension fails to respond to dosage increase, evaluate fluid volume status, consider addition/use of more potent vasoconstrictors (e.g., norepinephrine).
Vital signs/hemodynamics: Initially, monitor BP, HR q5-15min; progressively advance according to titration schedule, hemodynamic stability. • Establish clear parameters for titration (e.g., desired BP, CO, UO). Use lowest possible dose to achieve desired effect. • Monitor ECG for dysrhythmias, ischemic changes (T wave inversion, ST segment depression/elevation). Continuous ECG monitoring may not be necessary with low-dose therapy.
• Monitor CO, PCWP, CVP, SVR frequently as available; immediately correct hypovolemia. • Monitor UO, consult physician if ≤5 ml/kg/hr or ≤30 ml/hr.
Physical assessment: Assess for evidence of heart failure: bibasilar crackles (rales), neck

vein distention, S_3 gallop, breathing difficulty, especially in patients with CHF, cardiomyopathy. • Assess for perfusion/ oxygenation deficit: changes in mentation, hypotension, chest discomfort. • Assess for evidence of diminished peripheral perfusion: coolness, ↓ pulse intensity, paresthesias, delayed capillary refill. • Check infusion site frequently for signs of extravasation (e.g., blanching along vein pathway, coldness, hardness). If this occurs, change injection site immediately, infiltrate affected area with phentolamine (Appendixes K and L).
Laboratory tests: Monitor: Electrolytes, particularly potassium; promptly correct hypokalemia • ABGs

PATIENT/FAMILY TEACHING

Purpose of medication is to promote blood flow to kidneys, improve heart's blood-pumping ability, increase BP. • Immediately report chest pain or discomfort, palpitations, pain at infusion site.

AVAILABLE FORMS

Parenteral concentrate for IV admixture • Premixed solution for IV infusion

enalaprilat
(en-al-a'prel-at)
Vasotec IV

enalapril maleate
(en-al-a'prel)
Vasotec
enalapril maleate with hydrochlorothiazide
Vaseretic

Classifications: Angiotensin-converting enzyme (ACE) inhibitor, antihypertensive

USUAL DOSE

PO, adults: 5 mg once daily; gradually increase to control BP. • Maximum daily dose, 40 mg
• **Renal impairment/older adults/ diuretic therapy/ CHF:** Initially 2.5 mg; monitor BP closely for 2 hr after initial dose • May increase cautiously to maximum daily dose of 40 mg
Direct IV/intermit inf, adults: 1.25 mg q6h; may increase gradually to control BP; peak effects of first dose may not occur for up to 4 hr. • Maximum dose, 5 mg q6h • **Renal impairment/older adults/ diuretic therapy:** Initial dose, 0.625 mg; may repeat in 1 hr if BP remains elevated

ADMINISTRATION
Direct IV: Inject undiluted solution slowly over at least 5 min
IV, intermit inf: Infuse dilute solution over at least 5 min

PREPARATION
IV, intermit inf: Dilute in 50 ml compatible solution.

italic = common side effects   **bold** = life-threatening reactions

Compatible fluids: D$_5$W, 0.9% NaCl, LR, prepared combinations of these solutions.

ACTIONS

Inhibits ACE and prevents conversion of angiotensin I to angiotensin II, which is a potent vasoconstrictor and stimulator of aldosterone • BP reduced because of ↓ vascular tone, indirectly by ↓ aldosterone secretion with ↓ sodium/water retention • Reduces SBP/DBP by 10%-15% • Little or no effect on HR, contractility (in absence of heart failure) • CHF: Causes ↓ SVR, ↓ CVP, creating reductions in both preload, afterload • Renal blood flow may ↑ slightly, but GFR usually unchanged. • Requires conversion in liver to be activated

PHARMACOKINETICS

ROUTE	ONSET	PEAK	DURATION
PO	<30 min	30-90 min	12-25 hr
IV	<15 min	<4 hr	6 hr

DISTRIBUTION

Not well established; 50%-60% protein bound

ELIMINATION

Metabolized in liver, eliminated in urine/feces; IV half-life 11 hr, PO half-life 3.5-6 hr; half-life prolonged in CHF, hepatic dysfunction

INDICATIONS

Reduction of mild to severe BP; may be used in conjunction with other hypotensive agents, diuretics • BP reduction in renovascular or malignant hypertension • To improve cardiac function, relieve symptoms, improve exercise tolerance in CHF; often in conjunction with cardiac glycosides/diuretics • To delay the development of heart failure in patients with asymptomatic left ventricular dysfunction (ejection fraction ≤35%)

PRECAUTIONS/CONTRAINDICATIONS

Precautions: Initial dose may cause profound hypotension or severe allergic reaction.
Use caution with: Renal impairment; reduce dose, monitor renal function. • Collagen vascular disease, immunosuppression; risk of bone marrow depression • Concurrent diuretic therapy, hypovolemia, hyponatremia, surgery/anesthesia; severe hypotension possible • *CHF, diuretic therapy, dehydration;* risk of severe hypotension, hyperkalemia, renal dysfunction; reduce dose, monitor closely • CAD, cerebrovascular disease, aortic stenosis; hypotensive episodes may worsen condition.
Pregnancy category: Use only if safer alternatives unavailable and risks explained to woman.
Contraindications: Hypersensitivity to enalapril, other ACE inhibitors • Children: Safety/efficacy not established

ADVERSE EFFECTS

CNS: *headache, dizziness, fatigue, vertigo,* somnolence, sleep disturbances, paresthesias
Resp: *Cough*
CV: *Transient or orthostatic hypotension,* **severe hypotension,** tachycardia, bradycardia, chest pain, **cardiac arrest/MI/CVA** (rare; related to ↓ BP)
GI: Diarrhea, nausea, vomiting, abdominal pain
GU: ↓ **Renal function,** proteinuria, glycosuria

Hema: Anemia, leukopenia, agranulocytosis, thrombocytopenia, eosinophilia

Derm: Maculopapular rash, wheals, itching, excessive sweating, **exfoliative dermatitis** (rare)

Misc: Hypersensitivity reactions, including anaphylaxis, muscle cramps, hyponatremia, hyperkalemia

TOXICITY/OVERDOSE

Symptoms: Hypotension • ↓ Level of consciousness • Renal insufficiency, renal failure, hyperkalemia, hyponatremia, • MI, CVA, or cardiac arrest from severe hypotension in high-risk patients

Management: After recent ingestion, implement guidelines for management of acute overdose (Appendix I). • Support respiration as needed with O_2 and/or mechanical ventilation. • Hypotension: Elevate legs; usually responsive to intravascular volume expansion using 0.9% NaCl or LR • Hemodialysis facilitates drug removal.

INTERACTIONS

alcohol ↑ Risk of hypotension

calcium channel blockers Profound hypotension

digoxin ↑ Digoxin levels

diuretics Additive hypotensive effects

diuretics, potassium-sparing Hyperkalemia

indomethacin, other NSAIDs ↓ Enalapril effectiveness

potassium supplements Hyperkalemia

sympathetic blockers Additive hypotensive effects with risk of profound hypotension

PATIENT CARE IMPLICATIONS

• Correct hypovolemia, evaluate renal function before initiating therapy.

• Protect patients from injury associated with orthostatic hypotension, especially when initiating therapy.

• Vomiting, diarrhea, excessive perspiration, dehydration could cause excessive decrease in BP.

• Do not attempt to crush and reconstitute tablets; PO formulation not stable in solution.

Vital signs/hemodynamics: Monitor BP, HR frequently when initiating therapy and in high-risk situations (hypertensive crisis, acute CHF, use of hypotensive agents/diuretics)

• Monitor BP, HR q15min during parenteral therapy. • For transient hypotension during initial therapy, use IV 0.9% NaCl.

• As available, continuously monitor ECG for PVCs, ST segment elevation/depression, especially when initiating therapy in patients with CHF or CAD or with IV use

Physical assessment: Assess for perfusion/oxygenation deficit: chest discomfort, changes in mentation, activity intolerance, hypotension, dizziness. • Assess neurologic status q2-4h after initiation of therapy until BP controlled. • Assess for fluid volume overload: bibasilar crackles, dyspnea, peripheral edema, neck vein distention, weight gain. • Assess for progressive edema, proteinuria, other evidence of ↓ renal function. • Monitor fluid balance; weigh daily.

Laboratory tests: Monitor: BUN, creatinine, bilirubin, liver

E

---

italic = common side effects   **bold** = life-threatening reactions

enzymes, CBC with differential • Blood glucose levels in patients with diabetes • Digoxin/lithium levels as appropriate • Be alert for hyperkalemia, hyponatremia. Renal impairment, CHF, diabetes mellitus, or use of potassium-sparing diuretics, potassium supplements, or salt substitutes increases risk of hyperkalemia.

PATIENT/FAMILY TEACHING

Purpose of drug is to lower BP and/or relieve symptoms of heart failure. • May cause serious allergic reaction. Immediately report swelling of eye, lips, tongue or face; difficulty swallowing or breathing; rash, itching • May cause dizziness, fainting, especially during initiation of therapy; use caution when changing positions, walking. Alcohol use, hot weather, vigorous activity, vomiting, diarrhea, dehydration, prolonged standing make these symptoms more likely. • Lie down immediately if lightheaded or dizzy. • Medication is not a cure for high BP; other therapies, including life-style modifications, must be continued. • Report fever, sore throat, infection; chest pain. • May interfere with taste perception or cause persistent coughing; notify health care provider if these effects bothersome.

Outpatient: Take medication exactly as prescribed. Do not stop taking medicine even if you feel better. If medication abruptly discontinued, you may develop dangerously high BP. • Avoid driving and other activities requiring mental alertness until individual response to drug known. • Avoid salt substitutes or other foods high in potassium. • Weigh twice/wk; report weight gain or edema. • Consult physician or pharmacist before taking cough, cold, or allergy preparations.

AVAILABLE FORMS

Parenteral for IV injection • Tablets • Tablets with hydrochlorothiazide

enoxaparin sodium
(in-ox′a-par-in)
Lovenox

Classification: Anticoagulant, low-molecular-weight heparin

USUAL DOSE

SC, adult: 30 mg bid • Initiate therapy immediately after surgery; must start within 24 hr postoperatively; continue for 7-14 days until deep vein thrombosis no longer a risk • Dose adjustments for renal **G** impairment, advanced age have not been established

ADMINISTRATION

SC: Administer deep into subcutaneous tissue by grasping abdominal skin between thumb and forefinger and inserting entire length of needle into subcutaneous pocket of skinfold. • Patient should be lying down. • Use 25–27-gauge ⅝-inch needle; do not aspirate or massage when giving injection. • Rotate injection sites from left to right anteriolateral, then left to right posterolateral abdominal wall. • *Do not administer IM.*

ACTION

Augments the inhibitory effects of antithrombin III, thereby preventing the conversion of fibrinogen to fibrin and prothrombin to thrombin • Less effect on thrombin than unfractionated heparin • At usual doses does not significantly affect platelet aggregation, PT, APTT, fibrinogen level • Derived from porcine tissue

PHARMACOKINETICS

ROUTE	ONSET	PEAK	DURATION
SC	Rapid	3-5 hr	12 hr

DISTRIBUTION
Throughout plasma
ELIMINATION
Half-life 4.5 hr

INDICATIONS

Prevention of deep vein thrombosis (DVT), which could lead to pulmonary embolism, after hip replacement surgery
Unlabeled/investigational:
Prevention of DVT after knee replacement, certain other orthopedic surgeries.

PRECAUTIONS/ CONTRAINDICATIONS

Precautions: Not for IM use • Cannot be used interchangeably with heparin, other low-molecular-weight heparin • May cause moderate thrombocytopenia; monitor closely
Use caution with: History of heparin-induced thrombocytopenia • Any condition associated with increased risk of hemorrhage: congenital or acquired bleeding disorder, severe hepatic or renal dysfunction, recent GI ulceration or bleeding, hemorrhagic CVA, severe hypertension, subacute bacterial endocarditis; recent brain, spinal or opthalmologic surgery • Advanced age; delayed elimination is possible
Pregnancy category: Use only if safer alternative not available.
Contraindications: Hypersensitivity to enoxaparin or pork • Active major bleeding • Thrombocytopenia with positive antiplatelet antibody test • Safe and effective use in children has not been established.

ADVERSE EFFECTS

CNS: Confusion
CV: Edema
GI: Nausea, ↑ AST/ALT
Hema: Thrombocytopenia, **bleeding**
Local: Irritation, redness, pain, hematoma
Misc: Fever, bruising

TOXICITY/OVERDOSE

Symptoms: Hemorrhage, related complications
Management: Antidote is protamine sulfate, 1 mg for each mg of enoxaparin. Protamine can cause severe hypotension and anaphylaxis; use only if necessary; emergency medications and equipment must be readily available • For acute allergic reaction, see Appendix N.

INTERACTIONS

anticoagulants, incl. other heparins, thrombolytics, warfarin ↑ Risk of bleeding
antiplatelet agents, incl. NSAIDs, dipyridamole, ticlopidine ↑ Risk of bleeding

---

italic = common side effects   **bold** = life-threatening reactions

PATIENT CARE IMPLICATIONS

• Review history for contraindi-cations. Do not administer if bleeding disorder is present.
• Inform all personnel caring for patient of anticoagulant ther-apy. Place highly visible written notice in patient's room.
• If unexplained decrease in Hct/Hgb, hypotension, or other evidence of hemorrhage, look for a bleeding site.
• Avoid unnecessary arterial and venous punctures, IM injec-tions. If possible, use saline or heparin lock for blood drawing. If venipuncture necessary, hold manual pressure over site until bleeding stops.
• Avoid arterial/venous invasive procedures in areas where direct pressure is difficult to apply: subclavian, jugular veins.
Vital signs/hemodynamics: Immediately consult physician of severe or uncontrolled hyper-tension: SBP >180 or DBP >110 mm Hg. Prepare to initi-ate hypotensive therapy.
Physical assessment: Assess for unusual bleeding: petechiae, ecchymosis, bleeding from gums/mucous membranes, ex-cessive bleeding from superfi-cial injury. • Assess for occult bleeding: headache, altered mentation, paralysis, joint pain, shortness of breath, unexplained swelling, hypotension, shock.
• Note blood in urine, other body fluids.
Laboratory tests: Monitor: Platelet count; Hgb/Hct; stools, gastric drainage/emesis for oc-cult blood • AST/ALT • **May cause:** Moderate thrombocyto-penia, reversible elevations in AST/ALT • Discontinue for platelet count <100,000/mm³

PATIENT/FAMILY TEACHING

Purpose of medication is to pre-vent clots from forming in leg veins. • Report unusual bruising or bleeding from IV sites, nose, mouth, or in urine/stools. • Re-main on bed rest throughout therapy. • Avoid possible tissue damage from shaving, tooth-brushing; avoid activities that may cause injury. • Inform lab-oratory personnel, other health care workers of anticoagulant therapy.

AVAILABLE FORMS

Parenteral for SC injection
Storage: Store prefilled syrin-ges at or below 25° C.

ephedrine sulfate
(e-fed′rin)
Efedrin

Classifications: Sympathomi-metic, adrenergic agent—mixed, vasopressor, bronchodilator, CNS stimulant

USUAL DOSE

PO, adults: 12.5-50 mg q4h
🄿 **PO, children:** 2-3 mg/kg/24 hr in evenly divided doses q4-6h
IM/SC, adults: 25-50 mg q4-6h • Maximum dose, 150 mg/24 hr
Direct IV, adults: 5-25 mg q5-10min as needed to maintain SBP • Maximum dose, 150 mg/24 hr
🄿 **Direct IV/SC, children:** 3 mg/kg/24 hr in evenly divided doses q4-6h

---

ADMINISTRATION

▼**Direct IV:** Slowly inject at rate not >10 mg/min. • May be given undiluted • Administration via central vein preferable; avoid using small veins. Verify labeling; must use specific solution for IV injection • Not usually added to IV solutions

ACTIONS

Potent sympathomimetic; stimulates both alpha, beta receptors • Releases endogenous norepinephrine; hemodynamic response variable because of mixed alpha, beta-2 activity • Promotes relaxation of bronchial smooth muscle • Strong CNS stimulant • Less potent but longer acting than epinephrine • Depletion of norepinephrine stores results in refractoriness with prolonged use. • **CV/ hemodynamic:** Strong alpha effects produce arteriolar vasoconstriction, ↑ PVR, ↑ SBP/DBP; beta-1 effects stimulate myocardium, ↑ CO; chronotropic stimulation may ↑ HR, but effects usually countered by reflex vagal activity as BP rises; causes ↑ cardiac workload/myocardial O_2 consumption; may constrict or dilate pulmonary vessels; usually increases PAP. • **Resp:** Beta-2 stimulation relaxes bronchial smooth muscle, relieves bronchospasm, improves air exchange, causes ↑ vital capacity, ↓ residual volume. • **CNS:** Stimulates cerebral cortex, subcortical centers; effects similar to amphetamines; increases cerebral blood flow

PHARMACOKINETICS

ROUTE	ONSET	PEAK	DURATION
PO	15-60 min		4 hr
IM	10-20 min		60 min
IV	Immed	Rapid	60 min

DISTRIBUTION
Wide; crosses blood-brain barrier

ELIMINATION
Metabolized slowly by liver, excreted in urine; half-life 6 hr

INDICATIONS

Acute hypotensive states, especially those associated with spinal anesthesia; sympathectomy, other hypotension that fails to respond to volume repletion, positioning • Stokes-Adams syndrome with complete heart block; isoproterenol usually more effective • Urinary incontinence, myasthenia gravis • Occasionally as bronchodilator • Nasal decongestant (topical)

PRECAUTIONS/ CONTRAINDICATIONS

Precautions: Depletes norepinephrine stores and tachyphylaxis to pressor effects may develop • Increases Cardiac workload/O_2 consumption; may precipitate angina • ↑ Ventricular irritability may cause dysrhythmias • May cause hypertension, resulting in intracranial hemorrhage • Renal vasoconstriction may ↓ urine formation • Postcapillary vasoconstriction may cause fluid shift from vascular compartment, reducing circulating blood volume, resulting in perpetuation of shock or hypotension when drug discontinued. • Prolonged use may produce anxiety syndrome • Administration through small veins may cause severe vasoconstriction, tissue sloughing

E

---

italic = common side effects   **bold** = life-threatening reactions

Use caution with: Heart disease, particularly when myocardium sensitized (e.g., digitalization, ischemic electrolyte abnormalities); risk of dysrhythmias • Hypertension, hyperthyroidism; severe hypertension may cause intracranial hemorrhage. • Diabetes, peripheral vascular disease • Prostatic hypertrophy

c Pregnancy category: Use only if safer alternative unavailable.

Contraindications: Hypersensitivity to ephedrine, other sympathomimetics • Substantial organic heart disease, including angina (some manufacturers) • Narrow-angle glaucoma • Cyclopropane or halothane anesthesia • Thyrotoxicosis • Uncontrolled hypertension • Phenothiazine (e.g., chlorpromazine) overdose; profound hypotension possible • Obstetrics when maternal BP >130/80 • Commercial preparations may contain sulfites, which can cause serious allergic reactions.

ADVERSE EFFECTS

CNS: *Anxiety, tremors,* headache, insomnia, restlessness, nervousness, dizziness, confusion, delirium, **seizures**
EENT: Dilated pupils, nose/throat dryness
Resp: **Dyspnea**
CV: Palpitations, tachycardia, precordial pain, **dysrhythmias**
GI: *Nausea, vomiting, anorexia*
GU: Dysuria, urinary retention
Endo: Hyperglycemia in diabetic patients
Misc: Tolerance may develop.

TOXICITY/OVERDOSE

Symptoms: Initial hypertension, followed by hypotension

• Tachycardia, dysrhythmias
• Pulmonary edema, respiratory failure • Convulsions, coma
Management: After recent ingestion, implement guidelines for management of acute overdose (Appendix I). • Maintain airway/support ventilation as necessary. • Initiate seizure precautions. • **Hypertension:** Administer phentolamine. • **Hypotension:** Elevate legs, administer IV fluids; avoid vasopressors. • **Seizures:** Administer diazepam. • **Tachydysrhythmias:** Use beta-blockers (e.g., propranolol).

INTERACTIONS

aminophylline Dysrhythmias; risk of theophylline toxicity
anesthetics ↑ Pressor effects; dysrhythmias
atropine ↑ Pressor effects
beta-blockers ↓ Pressor/cardiac-stimulating effects
digoxin Dysrhythmias
furosemide, other diuretics ↓ Pressor effects
MAO inhibitors ↑ **Pressor effects;** avoid concurrent use
phentolamine ↓ Pressor effects
sympathomimetics Additive effects; dysrhythmias; avoid concurrent use

Y-SITE COMPATIBILITIES

Data not available

Y-SITE INCOMPATIBILITIES

Aminophylline, phenobarbital

PATIENT CARE IMPLICATIONS

• Correct hypovolemia before initiating therapy; in emergencies, may be administered to patient in hypovolemic state with simultaneous fluid replacement.

• Infuse via central, antecubital, or other large vein. Avoid using veins in hands, ankles, legs.
• Administer with sedative or tranquilizer to minimize CNS stimulation.

Vital signs/hemodynamics: Initially, monitor BP, HR q5-15min; progressively advance according to hemodynamic stability. • Continuously monitor ECG for dysrhythmias, ischemic changes. • Monitor central hemodynamics, CO frequently as available. Be alert for/immediately correct hypovolemia.

Physical assessment: Assess for evidence of heart failure: bibasilar crackles (rales), neck vein distention, S_3 gallop, breathing difficulty, especially in patients with CHF, cardiomyopathy. • Assess for perfusion/oxygenation deficit: changes in mentation, ↓ BP, activity intolerance, chest discomfort. • Assess for evidence of diminished peripheral perfusion: coolness, ↓ pulse intensity, paresthesias, delayed capillary refill. • Check infusion site frequently for signs of extravasation (e.g., blanching along vein pathway, coldness, hardness). If this occurs, change injection site immediately, infiltrate affected area with phentolamine (Appendixes K and L).
• Monitor UO, consult physician if ≤5 ml/kg/hr or ≤30 ml/hr.
• Monitor for voiding difficulty, urinary retention.

Laboratory tests: Monitor: Electrolytes • Blood glucose in patients with diabetes

PATIENT/FAMILY TEACHING

Purpose of medication is to increase BP, improve heart's blood-pumping ability. • Immediately report chest pain or discomfort, palpitations, pain at infusion site.

AVAILABLE FORMS

50-mg ampules for IV/IM/SC use • Oral capsules • Nasal solution

E

epinephrine
(ep-i-nef'rin)
adrenalin
EpiPen; Sus-Phrine
Primatine, Bronkaid,
Medihaler-Epi

Classifications: Sympathomimetic, vasopressor, bronchodilator

USUAL DOSE

Cardiac arrest, adults: Direct IV: 1 mg (10 ml of 1:10,000); may repeat q3-5min. If ineffective, consider other ACLS regimens:
Intermediate: 2-5 mg q3-5min
Escalating: 1 mg, 3 mg, 5 mg, 3 min apart
High: 0.1 mg/kg (0.1 ml/kg of 1:1,000) q3-5min
ET: Use 2-2.5 times usual IV dose diluted in 10 ml sterile 0.9% NaCl
Children: Direct IV/intraosseous: 0.01 mg/kg (0.1 ml/kg of 1:10,000); may repeat q3-5min • Repeat doses of 0.1 mg/kg may be used • ET: 0.1 mg/kg (0.1 ml/kg of 1:1,000) diluted in 2-5 ml sterile 0.9% NaCl • Minimum dose, 1 mg (1 ml of 1:10,000)
Hypotension/bradycardia: IV, cont inf, adults: Initially, 1 μg/min; titrate for desired effect. Usual range, 2-10 μg/min • Doses >10 μg/min sometimes

---

italic = common side effects   **bold** = life-threatening reactions

used in severe hypotension • IV, ℗ **cont inf, children:** Initially, 0.1 µg/kg/min; titrate for desired effect. Usual range, 0.1-1.0 µg/kg/min

Sensitivity reactions: SC/IM, adults: 0.1-0.5 mg (0.1-0.5 ml of 1:1,000); repeat at 10–15-min intervals as needed. • SC/ ℗ IM, children: 0.01 mg/kg (0.01 ml/kg of 1:1,000), not to exceed 0.5 mg; repeat at 20-min intervals as needed.

Anaphylactic shock: Direct IV, adults: 0.1-0.25 mg (1-2.5 ml of 1:10,000) given over 5-10 min; repeat as needed at 5-15 min intervals or follow with continuous IV infusion of 1-4 ℗ µg/min. • Direct IV, children: 0.1 mg (10 ml of 1:100,000) given over 5-10 min; may follow with continuous IV infusion of 0.1-1.5 µg/kg/min

Asthma/bronchospasm: Metered dose inhaler, adults/ ℗ children >4 yr: 1-2 inhal; wait 1-5 min between inhal. • May repeat after 3 hr, up to 4-6 times/day • Nebulization/ ℗ IPPB, adults/children >4 yr: 0.3 mg (0.03 ml 1% solution) in solution as needed for delivery • **Suspension SC, adults:** 0.5-1.5 mg (0.1-0.3 ml of 1:200) • Use for prolonged effects. ℗ • **Suspension SC, children:** 0.02-0.025 mg/kg (0.004-0.005 ml/kg of 1:200), not to exceed single dose of 0.75 mg in children ≤30 kg • Use for prolonged effects.

ADMINISTRATION

Carefully check strength, verify dose before administering; medication errors may be fatal.
SC/IM: Check dose, route, type (solution vs suspension) before administration. • Use tuberculin syringe to ensure accurate measurement. • Shake suspension immediately before withdrawing; administer promptly. • Rotate injection sites. • Massage site after administration to enhance absorption. • Avoid IM injections into gluteal muscle.

V Direct IV, cardiac arrest: Administer rapidly via largest available vein. • Flush with 20 ml bolus IV fluid.

V Direct IV: Dilute in at least 10 ml; administer slowly over 5-10 min. • Administer via central, antecubital, or other large vein.
• *Too rapid injection may be fatal; IV route limited to shock states when impaired absorption of SC/IM injections likely.*
IV, cont inf: Start at 1 µg/min (15 ml/hr of 1 mg/250 ml solution); increase by 1 µg/min q5min until desired BP, HR achieved. • Infusion pump is necessary. • Administer via central (preferable), antecubital, or other large vein. • See Infusion Rate table, Appendix Q.

℗ **ET, adults/children:** Dilute desired dose in 10 ml sterile 0.9% NaCl for adults; use 2-5 ml for children. Provide several quick ventilations, then expel via catheter passed just beyond ETT. Follow with several quick ventilations.

PREPARATION

Direct IV: Carefully check concentration. • To control administration of small doses, dilute 0.1 ml of 1:1,000 solution with 10 ml 0.9% NaCl for concentration of 0.01 mg/ml (1:100,000 solution).

IV, cont inf

DILUTION	CONCENTRATION
1 mg/250 ml	4 µg/ml
3 mg/250 ml	12 µg/ml

More concentrated solutions may be used if necessary to limit fluid intake. Do not use cloudy or discolored solutions.

Compatible fluids: D_5W, 0.9% NaCl, LR

ACTIONS

Endogenous catecholamine with mixed alpha- and beta-adrenergic activity • Beta effects (bronchodilation, ↑ HR/contractility) predominate at low doses • Alpha effects (potent peripheral/renal vasoconstriction) predominate at higher doses used during resuscitation, shock; variable effect on CO dependent on increases in afterload. • **CV/hemodynamic:** Stimulates SA node, causes ↑ AV conduction, ↑ HR, ↑ left ventricular stroke work, ↑ cardiac workload/myocardial O_2 consumption; usually causes ↑ SV, CO unless greatly ↑ afterload. Causes ventricular irritability, promotes dysrhythmias, especially when myocardium sensitized by digitalis, anesthetics, electrolyte abnormalities, acute MI. During asystolic cardiac arrest, may restore electrical activity ↑ SVR/myocardial contractility improve BP; high doses increase cerebral, brainstem, coronary blood flow. • **Resp:** Relaxes bronchial smooth muscle; constricts bronchial arterioles; increases tidal volume, vital capacity; transiently increases RR; inhibits histamine release; antagonizes histamine-induced bronchiolar constriction, vasodilation, edema; increased left atrial pressure, redistribution of blood to pulmonary circulation may result in pulmonary arterial hypertension, pulmonary edema. • **Renal:** Causes renal vasoconstriction, ↑ renal vascular resistance; ↓ renal blood flow, UO; if substantial ↑ in CO will ↑ renal blood flow, UO • **Metabolic:** Increases glycogenolysis, reduces peripheral glucose uptake, inhibits insulin release, resulting in hyperglycemia; may cause transient hyperkalemia, followed by hypokalemia.

PHARMACOKINETICS

ROUTE	ONSET	PEAK	DURATION
SC	5-10 min	20 min	*
IM	5-10 min	20 min	20-30 min
IV	Immed	Rapid	5-30 min
ET	Rapid	Rapid	†
Inhal‡	1 min	20 min	1-3 hr

DISTRIBUTION

Crosses placenta, not blood-brain barrier

ELIMINATION

Metabolized in liver, other tissues

*20-30 min (solution); 6 hr (suspension).
†Somewhat more sustained than IV.
‡Limited systemic absorption.

INDICATIONS

Shock/symptomatic bradycardia: To promote vasoconstriction, increase HR/contractility; especially useful in shock associated with norepinephrine depletion (e.g., after CABG, extended critical illness) • **Cardiac arrest:** Potent alpha effects improve coronary, cerebral perfusion; restores electrical mechanical activity; may facilitate defibrillation • **Sensitivity reactions/anaphylaxis:** ↑ BP, antagonize histamine-induced bronchospasm, angioedema, vasodilation, parenteral administration preferred if hemodynamic

---

italic = common side effects

bold = life-threatening reactions

E

instability; antihistamines, corticosteroids used concurrently for sustained relief of allergic symptoms • **Asthma/bronchospasm:** To relieve bronchospasm associated with asthma, bronchitis, emphysema, other causes; administer SC/IV when inhal therapy likely to be ineffective (e.g., low tidal volume, profound tachypnea); refractoriness to effects may occur with status asthmaticus, severe bronchial constriction, metabolic acidosis; rebound bronchospasm may occur; tolerance develops with prolonged use. • **Hemostasis:** Applied topically to control superficial bleeding from small vessels
Unlabeled/investigational:
Selective intraarterial administration to control GI or renal arterial bleeding

PRECAUTIONS/ CONTRAINDICATIONS

Precautions: Increases in myocardial workload may lead to imbalance of myocardial O_2 supply/demand, resulting in ischemia, infarction. • Asthmatic patients who show paradoxical worsening of respiratory function after use may be experiencing adverse reactions to sulfites contained in commercial preparations.
Use caution with: General anesthesia, digoxin, acid-base imbalance; tachycardia, ventricular dysrhythmias more likely **G** • CV disease • Older adults • Parkinsonian syndrome; increases rigidity, tremors • Diabetes; insulin requirements may increase. • Psychiatric disorders • Hypertension, hyperthyroidism, coronary insufficiency; extreme caution indicated

c **Pregnancy category:** Use only if safer alternative unavailable.
Contraindications: Hypersensitivity to epinephrine • Cardiogenic shock, organic heart disease • Inhalant anesthetics (e.g., trichloroethylene, cyclopropane) • Organic brain damage, cerebral atherosclerosis • Angleclosure glaucoma • Overdose of adrenergic blocking agents, phenothiazines; unopposed beta effects may lead to profound hypotension. • Use in fingers, toes, ears, nose, genitalia (in conjunction with local anesthetics). • Labor/delivery if maternal BP >130/80 • Commercial preparations may contain sulfites, which can cause serious allergic reactions.

ADVERSE EFFECTS

CNS: Restlessness, apprehension, headache, tremor, **cerebrovascular hemorrhage**
Resp: *Transient tachypnea,* bronchial irritation, rebound bronchospasm, pulmonary edema
CV: *Tachycardia; ↓ T wave amplitude;* palpitations, **dysrhythmias, ventricular fibrillation,** hypertension, angina
GI: Nausea, vomiting
GU: ↓ UO
Derm: *Pallor, coldness of skin;* tissue necrosis at injection site
Metabolic: Acidosis (prolonged/ high-dose therapy)
Misc: Refractoriness, tolerance (prolonged use), syncope in **P** children

TOXICITY/OVERDOSE

Symptoms: Hypertension, dysrhythmias, pulmonary edema • Cerebrovascular, other hemor- **G** rhage, especially in older adults

Management: Reduce infusion rate or discontinue until condition stabilizes; because of short duration of action, other treatment usually unnecessary. • Persistent hypertension: Use short-acting alpha-adrenergic blockers (e.g., phentolamine). • Dysrhythmias: Use beta-adrenergic blocker (e.g., propranolol). • Pulmonary edema: Usually results from pulmonary arterial hypertension; manage with alpha-adrenergic blockers, positive-pressure ventilation.

INTERACTIONS

alpha blockers ↓ **Effectiveness; profound hypotension**
anesthetics Dysrhythmias
beta-blockers (noncardioselective) Hypertension, bradycardia
bretylium Dysrhythmias
chlorpromazine Blocked alpha effects; profound hypotension
digoxin Dysrhythmias
esmolol Mutual antagonism; profound bradycardia
hypoglycemics, oral; insulin Hyperglycemia, ↑ insulin requirements
phenothiazines Blocked alpha effects; profound hypotension
propranolol Reduced effectiveness in anaphalyxis
sympathomimetics Dysrhythmias
TCAs Hypertension, dysrhythmias

Y-SITE COMPATIBILITIES

Amrinone, atracurium, calcium chloride, calcium gluconate, diltiazem, famotidine, heparin, hydrocortisone sodium succinate, pancuronium, potassium chloride, vercuronium

Y-SITE INCOMPATIBILITIES

Aminophylline, ampicillin, cephapirin, **sodium bicarbonate**/other alkaline solutions

PATIENT CARE IMPLICATIONS

• Correct hypovolemia before initiating therapy; in emergencies, may be administered to patient in hypovolemic state with simultaneous fluid volume replacement.
• Carefully check concentration, route before administration.
• Avoid repeated injections in same site because necrosis possible.
• Avoid IM injections into gluteal muscle; infection has been reported.
IV
• Use central vein if available; may use antecubital or other large vein. Avoid using veins in hands, ankles, legs.
• Monitor for/correct hypoxemia, hypercapnia, acidosis before and during drug administration.
• Do not administer sodium bicarbonate or other alkaline solutions through same IV line.
Vital signs/hemodynamics: Initially, monitor BP, HR, RR at 5–15-min intervals depending on stability, route; progressively advance according to stability.
• For patients with bronchospasm/anaphalyxis, continuously monitor O_2 saturation by pulse oximetry • IV inf: Establish clear parameters for titration (e.g., desired BP, HR, CO, UO). Use lowest possible dose to achieve desired effect. • Monitor ECG for dysrhythmias, ischemic changes (e.g., T wave inversion, ST depression/

E

---

italic = common side effects   **bold** = life-threatening reactions

elevation). • Monitor CO, PCWP, CVP, SVR frequently as available; immediately correct hypovolemia. • Monitor UO, consult physician if ≤5 ml/kg/hr or ≤30 ml/hr.

Physical assessment: Monitor breathing patterns, breath sounds for evidence of improved air exchange. Consult physician of deterioration or failure to improve. • Monitor character, amount of respiratory secretions. • Assess for evidence of diminished peripheral perfusion: pallor, coolness, ↓ pulse intensity, paresthesias, delayed capillary refill. • Assess for perfusion/oxygenation deficit: changes in mentation, hypotension, chest discomfort. • **IV inf:** In addition to above assess for MODS. Assess for pulmonary edema: bibasilar fluid crackles (rales), breathing difficulty, S_3 gallop. • Assess abdomen: size, bowel sounds, pain, tenderness. • Check IV infusion site frequently for signs of extravasation (e.g., blanching along vein pathway, coldness, hardness). If this occurs, change site immediately, infiltrate affected area with phentolamine (Appendixes K and L).

Laboratory tests: Monitor: Electrolytes, particularly potassium • Blood glucose, especially in patients with diabetes • ABGs

PATIENT/FAMILY TEACHING

Purpose of medication is to relieve breathing difficulty, improve BP, improve cardiac performance. • Immediately report chest pain or discomfort, palpitations, pain at infusion site. • With inhalation therapy, report failure to improve, palpitations,

angina. • Consult health care professional before taking any over-the-counter medications.

AVAILABLE FORMS

Parenteral solution for IV/IM/SC • SUSPENSION ONLY FOR SC USE • Inhal • Aerosol/solution for nebulization

---

erythromycin PO/ophth
(er-ith-roe-mye'sin)

erythromycin base, delayed-release
E-Base, E-Mycin, ERYC, Ery-Tab, PCE, Robimycin
erythromycin estolate
Ilosone
erythromycin ethylsuccinate
E.E.S., EryPed
erythromycin ethylsuccinate with sulfisoxazole acetyl
Eryzole, E.S.P, Pediazole, Sulfimycin
erythromycin stearate
Erythrocin, Wyamycin-S
erythromycin ophthalmic
Ak-Mycin, Ilotycin, Ocu-Mycin

Classification: Macrolide antibiotic

USUAL DOSE

PO, adults: 250-500 mg q6h or 333-666 mg q8h • **Severe infection:** 500 mg-1 g q6h • **Bacterial endocarditis prophylaxis:** 1 g 1 hr before procedure, 500 mg 6 hr later **❷ PO, children:** 30-50 mg/kg/24 hr in equally divided doses q6h

• **Severe infection:** 60-100 mg/kg/24 hr in equally divided doses q6h • **Bacterial endocarditis prophylaxis:** 20 mg/kg 1 hr before procedure, 10 mg/kg 6 hr later
Ophth: 0.5-2 cm 0.5% ointment in lower conjunctival sac once or twice daily

ACTIONS

Usually bacteriostatic but may be bactericidal in high doses and against particularly susceptible organisms; penetrates bacterial cell wall, inhibits protein synthesis; greatest effect with gram-positive bacteria • Active against gram-positive cocci/bacilli, including *Staphylococcus, Streptococcus pyogenes, S. pneumoniae, S. viridans*
• Gram-negative activity includes *Neisseria, Legionella pneumophila, Haemophilus influenzae* (unpredictable), *Bordetella pertussis* (whooping cough) • *Chlamydia, Mycoplasma* usually susceptible
• Not active against Enterobacteriaceae, *Pseudomonas* species

PHARMACOKINETICS

ROUTE	ONSET	PEAK	DURATION
PO	Rapid*	1-4 hr	Approx 6-8 hr

DISTRIBUTION
Widely distributed; low CSF levels

ELIMINATION
Most excreted unchanged in bile; half-life 1.5-2 hr

*Partially inactivated by gastric acid.

INDICATIONS

Alternative treatment for patients allergic to penicillin, cephalosporins • Mild to moderately severe respiratory tract, soft tissue infections • Choice agent for legionnaires' disease

(with rifampin), mycoplasma pneumonia, whooping cough
• Alternative agent for chlamydial infections when doxycycline, tetracycline cannot be used • Treatment of early syphilis when penicillin, tetracycline cannot be used, except estolate formulation in pregnancy
• Ophth preparation used for conjunctivitis, superficial corneal infections; concomitant systemic therapy required except for very superficial infections
Unlabeled/investigational:
Choice agent for chancroid genital ulcers; early Lyme disease when penicillin, tetracycline cannot be used

PRECAUTIONS/CONTRAINDICATIONS

Precautions: Bacterial or fungal overgrowth may occur.
Use caution with: Hepatic impairment, preexisting liver disease, impaired biliary excretion because of hepatotoxicity
C Pregnancy category: Safety not established; avoid using estolate preparation during pregnancy.
Contraindications: Hypersensitivity to erythromycins • Hepatic dysfunction (estolate salt)
• Concurrent astemizole, terfenadine therapy

ADVERSE EFFECTS

EENT: Hearing loss, tinnitus, vertigo
GI: *Abdominal pain/cramping, nausea, vomiting, diarrhea;* ↑ AST, ALT, alkaline phosphatase, bilirubin; **pseudomembraneous colitis, hepatic dysfunction** (rare)
Derm: Rash, wheals, itching

---

italic = common side effects   **bold** = life-threatening reactions

Misc: *Hypersensitivity;* **anaphylaxis** (rare); superinfection, colonization

TOXICITY/OVERDOSE

Symptoms: Extension of side effects/adverse reactions
Management: Discontinue drug; initiate symptomatic/supportive measures. • After recent ingestion, implement guidelines for management of acute overdose (Appendix I). • For acute allergic reaction, see Appendix N. • Hemodialysis or peritoneal dialysis is not effective in drug removal.

INTERACTIONS

anticoagulants, PO Excessive
G anticoagulation, esp. in elders
astemizole Prolonged QT, serious dysrhythmias; avoid concurrent use
carbamazepine ↑ Carbamazepine levels; risk of toxicity
cyclosporine ↑ Cyclosporine levels; risk of nephrotoxicity
digoxin ↑ Digoxin levels, risk of toxicity
disopyramide QT prolongation, ventricular tachycardia
midazolam ↑ Sedation
phenytoin ↑ Phenytoin levels; risk of toxicity
terfenadine Prolonged QT, serious dysrhythmias; avoid concurrent use
theophylline ↑ Theophylline levels; risk of toxicity
triazolam ↑ Sedation

PATIENT CARE IMPLICATIONS

• Obtain specimens for culture and sensitivity before initiating antibiotic therapy. Initiate therapy before results received.
• Absorption in presence of food variable according to spe-cific formulation; generally, optimal absorption occurs if given on empty stomach; however, enteric-coated tablets, capsules containing enteric-coated particles may be given with meals if GI irritation occurs. Do not administer with citrus juices.
• Contents of capsules containing enteric-coated pellets may be sprinkled on applesauce immediately before administration. Pellets should not be crushed or chewed. • **Ophth:** Use new tube for each patient.
Vital signs: Monitor VS for indicators of infection, complications.
Physical assessment: Assess for improvement in primary infection or symptoms of super/suprainfection: appearance of sputum, urine, stool, wound drainage; presence of fever, candidiasis, vaginitis, WBC. • Assess for hepatotoxicity: right upper quadrant abdominal pain, excessive fatigue, jaundice, pale stools, dark urine.
Laboratory tests: Monitor: Liver enzymes, bilirubin with high-dose/prolonged therapy or hepatic/biliary impairment
• **May cause:** False elevation of urinary catecholamines; falsely ↑ AST, ALT

PATIENT/FAMILY TEACHING

Purpose of drug is to limit growth of infection-causing bacteria. • Report diarrhea, fever, vaginal itching or discharge, furry growth on tongue. • Report abdominal pain, dark urine, light stools, excessive tiredness, yellowish tint to skin or whites of eyes.
Outpatient: Take at evenly spaced intervals over each 24-hr period. • Take on empty stom-

ach; may take with food for
stomach upset. Do not take with
orange or other citrus juices.
• Do not crush, chew, or divide
capsules; must be swallowed
whole, if indicated, contents of
capsule may be sprinkled on applesauce. • Use calibrated measuring device for liquid preparations. • Take all of medication
exactly as prescribed. Do not
stop taking medicine even if
you feel better. Failure to take
all of antibiotic may result in
recurrence or additional infection. Do not save or share unused medicine.

AVAILABLE FORMS

Capsules • Chewable tablets
• PO suspension

**erythromycin
parenteral**
(er-ith-roe-mye'sin)

**erythromycin
gluceptate**
Ilotycin
**erythromycin
lactobionate**
Erythrocin

Classification: Macrolide antibiotic

USUAL DOSE

IV, adults/children: 15-20 mg/
kg/24 hr in divided doses q6h
or as continuous infusion • Severe infections: Up to 4 g/24
hr

ADMINISTRATION

IV, intermit inf: Infuse prepared solution over 20-60 min.
• ↓ Infusion rate if injection
site painful. • *Do not adminis-*

*ter initial dilution by direct IV
push.*
IV, cont inf: Administer continuously at prescribed rate.

PREPARATION

IV, intermit inf: Reconstitute
250-500 mg vial with 10 ml
sterile water for injection without preservatives; use 20 ml for
1 g vial. Shake until dissolved.
MUST FURTHER DILUTE by
adding to ≥100 ml 0.9% NaCl
or other compatible IV solution
for concentration not >5 mg/ml
(e.g., 500 mg/100 ml); do not
dilute single dose in <100 ml.
Shake well to ensure complete
dilution.
IV, cont inf: Reconstitute as
just directed. Further dilute concentrated solution by adding to
sufficient volume of 0.9% NaCl
or other compatible solution for
concentration of 1-2 mg/ml
(e.g., 1-2 g/1,000 ml). Shake
well to ensure complete dilution.
Compatible solutions: D_5W
(to improve admixture stability,
buffer with sodium bicarbonate),
0.9% NaCl, LR, prepared combinations of these solutions
Stability: Greatest stability in
0.9% NaCl or LR; to improve
stability in D_5W, buffer with 1
ml 4% sodium bicarbonate
(neutral) for each 100 ml before
adding erythromycin.

ACTIONS

Usually bacteriostatic but may
be bactericidal in high doses
and against particularly susceptible organisms; penetrates bacterial cell wall, inhibits protein
synthesis; greatest effect with
gram-positive bacteria • Active
against gram-positive cocci/
bacilli, including *Staphylococ-*

cus, *Streptococcus pyogenes, S. pneumoniae, S. viridans* • Gram-negative activity includes *Neisseria, Legionella pneumophila, Haemophilus influenzae* (unpredictable), *Bordetella pertussis* (whooping cough) • *Chlamydia, Mycoplasma* usually susceptible • Not active against Enterobacteriaceae, *Pseudomonas* species

PHARMACOKINETICS

ROUTE	ONSET	PEAK	DURATION
IV	Immed	End infusion	Approx 6 hr

DISTRIBUTION
Widely distributed; low CSF levels

ELIMINATION
Most excreted unchanged in bile; half-life 1.5-2 hr

INDICATIONS

Alternative treatment for patients allergic to penicillin, cephalosporins • Mild to moderately severe respiratory tract, soft tissue infections • Choice agent for legionnaires' disease (with rifampin), mycoplasma pneumonia, whooping cough • Treatment of early syphilis when penicillin, tetracycline cannot be used
Unlabeled/investigational:
Early Lyme disease when penicillin, tetracycline cannot be used

PRECAUTIONS/ CONTRAINDICATIONS

Precautions: Bacterial or fungal overgrowth may occur.
Use caution with: Hepatic impairment, preexisting liver disease, impaired biliary excretion because of hepatotoxicity
c **Pregnancy category:** Safety not established; use only if clearly needed.

Contraindications: Hypersensitivity to erythromycins • Concurrent therapy with astemizole, terfenadine

ADVERSE EFFECTS

EENT: Hearing loss, tinnitus, vertigo
CV: Rarely—prolonged QT, ventricular ectopy, atypical **ventricular tachycardia**
GI: *Abdominal pain/cramping, nausea, vomiting, diarrhea;* ↑ AST, ALT, alkaline phosphatase, bilirubin; hepatic dysfunction (rare) pseudomembranous colitis
Derm: Rash, urticaria, pruritus
Local: *Pain, phlebitis*
Misc: *Hypersensitivity;* **anaphylaxis** (rare); superinfection, colonization

TOXICITY/OVERDOSE

Symptoms: Extension of side effects/adverse reactions
Management: Discontinue drug; initiate symptomatic/supportive measures. • For acute allergic reaction, see Appendix N. • Hemodialysis or peritoneal dialysis is not effective in drug removal.

INTERACTIONS

anticoagulants, PO Excessive
G anticoagulation esp. in elders
astemizole Prolonged QT, serious dysrhythmias; avoid concurrent use
carbamazepine ↑ Carbamazepine levels; risk of toxicity
cyclosporine ↑ Cyclosporine levels; risk of nephrotoxicity
digoxin ↑ Digoxin levels; risk of toxicity
disopyramide QT prolongation, ventricular tachycardia
midazolam ↑ Sedation

phenytoin ↑ Phenytoin levels; risk of toxicity

terfenadine Prolonged QT, serious dysrhythmias; avoid concurrent use

theophylline ↑ Theophylline levels; risk of toxicity

triazolam ↑ Sedative effects

Y-SITE COMPATIBILITIES

Lactobionate formula: Acyclovir, amiodarone, diltiazem, enalaprilate, esmolol, famotidine, hydromorphone, labetalol, magnesium sulfate, meperidine, morphine, multivitamins, zidovudine

Y-SITE INCOMPATIBILITIES

Lactobionate formula: Fluconazole

PATIENT CARE IMPLICATIONS

• Obtain specimens for culture and sensitivity before initiating antibiotic therapy. Initiate therapy before results received.

• Initiate PO therapy as soon as possible.

Vital signs: Monitor VS for indicators of infection, complications.

Physical assessment: Assess for improvement in primary infection or symptoms of super/suprainfection: appearance of sputum, urine, stool, wound drainage; presence of fever, candidiasis, vaginitis; WBC. • Assess for hepatotoxicity: right upper quadrant abdominal pain, excessive fatigue, jaundice, pale stools, dark urine. • Frequently assess IV site for patency, complications.

Laboratory tests: Monitor: Liver enzymes, bilirubin with high-dose/prolonged therapy, hepatic/biliary impairment.

• **May cause:** False elevation of urinary catecholamines; falsely ↑ AST, ALT

PATIENT/FAMILY TEACHING

Purpose of drug is to limit growth of infection-causing bacteria. • Report diarrhea, fever, vaginal itching or discharge, furry growth on tongue. • Report abdominal pain, dark urine, light stools, excessive tiredness, yellowish tint to skin or whites of eyes.

AVAILABLE FORMS

Parenteral for IV infusion

---

erythropoietin (recombinant)
(er-ith-row-poe′ee-tin)

epoetin alfa, EPO
Epogen, Procrit

Classification: Erythrocyte stimulator

USUAL DOSE

Chronic renal failure (CRF) IV/SC injection, adults: Initially 50-100 U/kg (e.g., 3,000-6,000 u for 60-kg patient) 3 times/wk • Maintenance: Reduce or increase dose by 25 U/kg to maintain Hct of 30%-33%. Reduce if Hct increases more than 4 points in 2 wk because ↑ Hct may exacerbate hypertension. Withhold if Hct approaches or exceeds 36%; restart as Hct reaches target levels. Increase dose if Hct fails to increase by 5-6 points after 8 wk of therapy. • Median maintenance dose, dialysis patients: 75 U/kg 3 times/wk; usual maintenance dose for nondialysis patients: 75-150 U/kg/wk

---

italic = common side effects   **bold** = life-threatening reactions

• Usually given IV; SC used for nondialysis patients

Malignancy: 100-150 U/kg 3 times a week; 200-300 U/kg 5 times a week has been used

HIV-infected patients: IV/SC injection, adults: Initially 100 U/kg IV or SC 3 times/wk for 8 wk • Maintenance: Adjust dose by 50-100 U/kg 3 times/wk at 4–8-wk intervals to maintain Hct ≥36%. • Patients who fail to respond to 300 U/kg 3 times/wk unlikely to respond to higher doses

ADMINISTRATION

V Direct IV: Administer undiluted over at least 1 min; give directly into vein, IV line, or venous line after hemodialysis.

PREPARATION

Avoid shaking, which may inactivate drug. • Use only 1 dose per vial; do not reenter vial. • Discard unused portion. • Contains no preservatives; administer immediately after withdrawal. • Store Procrit in refrigerator.

ACTIONS

Recombinant glycoprotein with same effects as endogenous erythropoietin • Stimulates RBC production in patients with anemia caused by deficient erythropoietin levels • Adequate iron stores necessary for effectiveness • Reticulocyte count increases within 10 days • RBC count, Hct, Hgb increase within 2-6 wk.

INDICATIONS

To elevate/maintain RBC levels, decrease need for transfusions in anemic patients with CRF, HIV infection malignancy/ antineoplastic therapy, perisurgical blood loss; autologous blood donors • Not effective for iron-deficient or folate-deficient anemia, hemolytic anemias

Unlabeled/investigational:
Low hematocrit associated with acute/chronic blood loss, preoperatively to minimize transfusion requirements

PRECAUTIONS/CONTRAINDICATIONS

Precautions: May increase BP, especially during initial therapy • Rapid rises in Hct exacerbate hypertension • ↑ risk of seizures in dialysis patients • Diminished response to therapy may occur with iron deficiency; occult blood loss; hematologic disorder; folic acid or vitamin B_{12} deficiency; hemolysis; high-dose AZT therapy; underlying infectious, inflammatory, or malignant process.

Use caution with: Preexisting vascular disease; risk of thromboembolic events (MI, CVA, TIA) • Porphyria

c Pregnancy category: Use only if safer alternative unavailable.

Contraindications: Hypersensitivity to mammalian cell-derived products or human albumin • Uncontrolled hypertension • Children: Safety/effectiveness not established

ADVERSE EFFECTS

CNS: *headache,* fatigue, euphoria, hypertensive encephalopathy, **seizures**
CV: *Hypertension, tachycardia,* edema, chest pain
Resp: *Shortness of breath,* cough, respiratory congestion
GI: *Nausea,* vomiting, diarrhea
MS: Arthralgia

Hema: Thrombosis at vascular access, clotting during dialysis
Misc: *Pyrexia in AZT-treated, HIV-infected patients;* hyperkalemia in CRF patients

TOXICITY/OVERDOSE

Symptoms: Up to 1,500 U/kg 3 times/wk given without toxicity • Polycythemia may develop if Hct not closely monitored.
Management: For Hct exceeding target range, temporarily withhold therapy. • If polycythemia develops, may use phlebotomy to ↓ Hct

INTERACTIONS

iron supplements ↑ Effectiveness

INCOMPATIBILITIES

Consider incompatible with other agents.

PATIENT CARE IMPLICATIONS

• Control hypertension before initiating therapy.
• Initiate seizure precautions for dialysis patients.
• Supplemental iron therapy is necessary for most patients.
Vital signs/hemodynamics: Monitor BP regularly; aggressively control hypertension. Withhold therapy, consult physician of severe hypertension.
Physical assessment: Increased risk of seizures in dialysis patients, especially during first 90 days of therapy. Assess for premonitory neurologic symptoms.
Laboratory tests: Monitor: Hct twice/wk until stabilized, then regularly; with dosage change, check Hct twice/wk for 2-6 wk until stabilized. • CBC with differential • Electrolytes,

particularly potassium • Blood chemistries • Iron concentration, total iron-binding capacity, transferrin saturation, serum ferritin.

PATIENT/FAMILY TEACHING

Purpose of medication is to relieve anemia by increasing RBCs. • Frequent blood work, BP monitoring are necessary to prevent dangerous complications. • **Dialysis patients:** Increased risk of seizures during first 90 days of therapy; immediately report premonitory symptoms. Outpatients must report any seizure activity. Avoid potentially hazardous activity (e.g., driving, operating heavy machinery). • Medication greatly improves how you feel but still necessary to take medications as prescribed, continue dialysis, follow dietary recommendations.

AVAILABLE FORMS

Vials for IV/SC use

esmolol HCl
(ess'moe-lol)
Brevibloc

Classifications: Antidysrhythmic, cardioselective beta-adrenergic blocker, antihypertensive, Vaughan-Williams Class II

USUAL DOSE

IV, adults: Initial loading dose of 500 µg/kg over 1 min; follow with infusion of 50 µg/kg/min over 4 min. If SVT not controlled, repeat same loading dose, follow with infusion of 100 µg/kg/min. Continue to repeat initial loading dose fol-

---

italic = common side effects   **bold** = life-threatening reactions

lowed by 4-min infusions increased at increments of 50 µg/kg/min (see table) until desired effects achieved. Do not exceed maximum of 200 µg/kg/min
• **Maintenance:** Infusion of 25-200 µg/kg/min initiated when desired HR, BP achieved

Esmolol: progressive loading doses

1 MIN LOADING BOLUS (µg/kg)	4 MIN LOADING INFUSION (µg/kg/min)
500	50
500	100
500	150
500	200

ADMINISTRATION

▼ IV, adults: Using 10 mg/ml solution, inject loading dose over 1 min, followed by loading infusion over 4 min. When HR/BP controlled, initiate maintenance infusion (see table). Closely monitor during loading. Slow or stop infusion for symptomatic bradycardia, HR <45 bpm, hypotension, 2nd/3rd degree heart block, CHF. Infusion pump is necessary. Administer via central, antecubital, or other large vein; extravasation may cause necrosis.

Dosage/infusion rate (ml/hr)
Esmolol concentration 10 mg/ml

kg*	50	60	70	80	90	100
50	15	18	21	24	27	30
75	23	27	32	36	41	45
100	30	36	42	48	54	60
125	38	45	53	60	68	75
150	45	54	63	72	81	90
175	53	63	74	84	95	105
200	60	72	84	96	108	120

Desired dose (µg/kg/min)

*Weight (kg)

PREPARATION

Esmolol HCl for loading injection (10 mg/ml) does not require dilution. Concentrate (250 mg/ml) must be diluted before use. To prepare infusion, remove 20 ml from 500-ml bag/bottle, then add 5 g (20 ml) esmolol. Resulting concentration is 10 mg/ml. Concentrations exceeding 10 mg/ml not recommended.
Compatible fluids: D_5W, 0.9% NaCl, LR, prepared combinations of these solutions

ACTIONS

Blocks sympathetic stimulation of beta-1-adrenergic receptors in myocardium • In usual doses has little effect on beta-2 receptors of vasculature, bronchial smooth muscle • Decreases HR, BP, force of contraction, myocardial O_2 consumption • Depresses AV conduction, myocardial automaticity, particularly in SA node; prolongs refractory period • Cardioselectivity lost at doses >300 µg/kg/min; may ↑ airway resistance

PHARMACOKINETICS

ROUTE	ONSET	PEAK	DURATION
IV	Immed	5-30 min	Approx 30 min after end of infusion

DISTRIBUTION
Widely distributed into most tissue; 55% protein bound

ELIMINATION
Primarily metabolized by erythrocytes, excreted in urine; half-life 5-23 min

INDICATIONS

Rapid, temporary control of SVTs (e.g., PAT, atrial flutter/fibrillation, sinus tachycardia), including those associated with acute MI, cardiac surgery, other

surgery associated with cardiac impairment • Similar in efficacy to verapamil but may be preferred because of ease of control • Rapid onset, short duration of action especially useful in patients at risk for adverse effects of beta-blockers (e.g., mild CHF, mild COPD, asthma, diabetes mellitus, older adults)
Unlabeled/investigational: Control of hypertension associated with surgery, especially in CAD; to limit myocardial ischemia associated with acute MI, unstable angina

PRECAUTIONS/ CONTRAINDICATIONS

Precautions: May cause profound bradycardia, hypotension, CHF, particularly if preexisting cardiac impairment • Abrupt cessation may induce angina, ventricular dysrhythmias, acute MI. • Children: Safety/efficacy not established

Use caution with: COPD, asthma • Preexisting heart disease • Renal insufficiency • Diabetes mellitus

c Pregnancy category: Use only if safer alternative unavailable.

Contraindications: Hypersensitivity to esmolol • Severe sinus bradycardia, 2nd/3rd degree heart block • CHF (unless resulting from tachycardia) • Cardiogenic shock • Severe asthma

ADVERSE EFFECTS

CNS: Dizziness, drowsiness, confusion, headache, anxiety, **seizures** (rare)
Resp: Dyspnea, wheezing, **bronchospasm**
CV: *Hypotension, diaphoresis* **bradycardia, heart failure, worsened AV heart block**

GI: *Nausea,* vomiting,
GU: Urinary retention
Endo: Blocked symptoms of hypoglycemia/hyperthyroidism
Derm: *Pain/inflammation at injection site,* tissue necrosis (with extravasation)

TOXICITY/OVERDOSE

Symptoms: Symptomatic bradycardia, HR <45, profound hypotension, heart failure, advanced heart block, hypoglycemia, possible seizures
Management: Discontinue infusion. • **Bradycardia, heart block:** Administer atropine, epinephrine, isoproterenol according to ACLS guidelines (Appendix P). • **Bronchospasm:** Use aminophylline, isoproterenol. • **Heart failure:** Provide inotropic support (e.g., dobutamine, dopamine), diuretics, possibly cardiac glycosides (e.g., digoxin). • **Hypotension:** Elevate legs, administer IV fluids; use vasopressors (e.g., dopamine, norepinephrine) for severe hypotension refractory to inotropic agents. • **Hypoglycemia:** Administer IV glucose. • Hemodialysis is generally ineffective.

INTERACTIONS

antidiabetic agents Masked symptoms and prolonged recovery from hypoglycemic episodes
calcium channel blockers Extreme bradycardia; hypotension
digoxin ↑ Digoxin levels
disopyramide ↑ Negative inotropy; heart failure
epinephrine, Unopposed alpha stimulation (hypertension, bradycardia, dysrhythmias); reduced effectiveness in anaphylaxis

---

italic = common side effects   **bold** = life-threatening reactions

isoproterenol ↓ Bronchodilatory effectiveness

lidocaine Lidocaine toxicity; negative inotropy; heart failure

morphine ↑ Esmolol levels

NMBAs Prolonged effects of NMBAs

quinidine Additive cardiac depression

theophylline ↓ Bronchodilation

vasoconstrictors/
sympathomimetics (dopamine, norepinephrine) Blocked ß₁ receptors and ↓ cardiac contractility. If ↑ SVR may cause profound CV decompensation.

Y-SITE COMPATIBILITIES

Amikacin, aminophylline, ampicillin, at racurium, butorphanol, calcium chloride, cefazolin, cefoperazone, ceftazidime, ceftizoxime, chloramphenicol, cimetidine, clindamycin, dopmaine, diltiazem, enalaprilat, famotidine, fentanyl, gentamicin, heparin, magnesium sulfate, morphine, nafcillin, pancuronium, penicillin G potassium, phenytoin, piperacillin potassium chloride, potassium phosphate, rantidine, streptomycin, tobramycin, trimethoprim-sulfamethoxazole, vancomycin, vecuronium

Y-SITE INCOMPATIBILITIES

Diazepam, furosemide, sodium bicarbonate, thiopental sodium

PATIENT CARE IMPLICATIONS

• Identify patients with asthma or COPD. Monitor closely; use lowest effective dose to avoid bronchospasm.

• Gradually withdraw therapy to avoid rebound hypertension, angina, possible acute MI.

Vital signs/hemodynamics:
Monitor ECG continuously for development/advancement of heart block, bradycardia, prolongation of PR interval, widening of QRS complex. If present, slow or stop infusion, consult physician. • Measure BP q2-5 min throughout initial administration; progress to q15min during maintenance infusion, q30min for 2 hr after infusion complete. • Measure CVP, PCWP, CO as available. Report CO, ↑ filling pressure, or other symptoms of heart failure.
• Monitor closely if other antidysrhythmics or antihypertensives used concurrently.

Physical assessment: Assess for perfusion/oxygenation deficit: ↓ level of consciousness, hypotension, chest discomfort, dizziness. • Assess for CHF, pulmonary edema: bibasilar crackles (rales), S₃ gallop, neck vein distention, breathing difficulty, peripheral edema. • Assess for bronchoconstriction, respiratory distress in patients with history of asthma or COPD. • Assess diabetic patients for sweating, because tachycardia/tremors associated with hypoglycemia may be blocked by therapy.

Laboratory tests: Monitor: Electrolytes • Blood sugar, particularly in patients with diabetes

PATIENT/FAMILY TEACHING

Purpose of medication is to slow rapid heart rate; frequent monitoring is required. Remain in bed during initial therapy and for at least 2 hr after medication discontinued. Call for assistance before getting out of bed. • Report breathing difficulty, dizzi-

---

P pediatric   **G** geriatric   **V** Direct IV

ness, palpitations, chest pain, sweating.

AVAILABLE FORMS

Single-dose vials for IV injection • Ampules with concentrate for IV infusion

---

ethacrynic acid
(eth-a-kri'nik)
Edecrin
ethacrynate sodium
(eth-a-kri'nate)

Classification: Loop diuretic

USUAL DOSE

PO, adults: 25-50 mg once daily in AM or bid with meals; may be gradually increased by 25 mg/day. • Maximum daily dose, 400 mg
IV, adults: 50 mg or 0.5-1.0 mg/kg; may repeat once if necessary. Single dose of 100 mg has been used in critically ill patients • Initiate PO therapy as soon as possible.

ADMINISTRATION

▼**Direct IV, adults:** Infusion preferred • Inject each 10 mg or less over at least 1 min. Too-rapid injection may cause tinnitus. • If additional dose necessary, use different IV site to prevent thrombophlebitis.
IV, intermit inf, adults: Infuse entire dose over 20-30 min. • If additional dose necessary, use different IV site to prevent thrombophlebitis.

PREPARATION

IV: Reconstitute powder with 10 ml 0.9% NaCl; further dilute in 40 ml 0.9% NaCl or D_5W for concentration of 1 mg/ml.

• 0.9% NaCl recommended because some D_5W solutions (with pH <5) result in hazy solution. • Use within 24 hr.
Compatible fluids: D_5W, 0.9% NaCl, LR, prepared combinations of these solutions

ACTIONS

Potent, rapid-acting diuretic • inhibits reabsorption of chloride in ascending limb of loop of Henle; ↓ sodium, chloride reabsorption in distal renal tubule; ↑ excretion of sodium, chloride, potassium, calcium, magnesium, hydrogen, water • Reduced plasma volume results in hypotension in some patients. • May cause mildly ↑ blood glucose • May cause paradoxical ↓ in UO with nephrogenic diabetes insipidus

PHARMACOKINETICS

ROUTE	ONSET	PEAK	DURATION
PO	30 min	2 hr	6-12 hr
IV	5 min	15-30 min	2 hr

DISTRIBUTION
90% protein bound
ELIMINATION
Excreted in urine, bile; half-life 60 min

INDICATIONS

Reduce edema associated with cardiac, renal, or hepatic impairment • Often effective in patients refractory to other diuretics • Used cautiously when pulmonary edema is complication of cardiogenic shock, because overaggressive diuresis may result in hypovolemia ↓ CO • Also used in short-term management of ascites associated with malignancy, for lymphedema and undiagnosed edema.

Unlabeled/investigational:
To reduce edema in hospitalized
children with congenital heart
defects or nephrotic syndrome.
To increase renal excretion of
calcium in hypercalcemia; concomitantly with mannitol in ethylene glycol poisoning

PRECAUTIONS/
CONTRAINDICATIONS

Precautions: Excessive diuresis may cause hypovolemia,
electrolyte imbalance, especially
in older adults, chronic cardiac
disease. • Fluid/electrolyte depletion may lead to severe hypotension, thrombus formation,
malignant dysrhythmias, sudden
death. • May cause reversible
elevation of BUN, creatinine,
particularly in renal impairment
• Moderate to severe hearing
impairment and/or tinnitus may
occur, especially with very high
doses, rapid IV administration,
use with other ototoxic agents
B Pregnancy category: Safety
not clearly established; use only
if potential benefits justify risk.
Use caution with: Renal impairment; ↓ plasma volume may
↓ GFR. • Cirrhosis, nephrotic
syndrome, digitalized patients;
may cause profound hypokalemia • Cirrhosis, hepatic failure;
rapid fluctuations in fluids/elec-
trolytes may cause hepatic coma
• Children: Safe use not well
established
Contraindications: Hypersensitivity to ethacrynic acid. Increasing azotemia and/or oliguria • Untreated severe hepatic
coma • uncorrected fluid/
electrolyte depletion; • severe
watery diarrhea • Do not use in
infants.

ADVERSE EFFECTS

CNS: Dizziness, fatigue, confusion, headache, **seizures** (rare)
EENT: Tinnitus, hearing impairment, deafness, ear pain/
fullness
Resp: Alkalosis, compensatory
respiratory depression
CV: *Orthostatic hypotension,*
hypotension, dysrhythmias
(PACs, PVCs), **ventricular
fibrillation**
GI: Nausea, vomiting, anorexia,
severe diarrhea, GI bleeding,
↑ liver enzymes, **hepatic
coma** (with preexisting liver
disease)
GU: Elevated BUN/creatinine
Endo: Hypoglycemia, hyperglycemia, glycosuria
F&E: *Hypokalemia, hypochloremia, hyponatremia, metabolic
alkalosis,* hypophosphatemia,
hypocalcemia, dehydration,
hemoconcentration
Hema: Neutropenia, agranulocytosis, thrombocytopenia
Derm: Rash; local irritation,
pain, thrombophlebitis at IV
site
Misc: hyperuricemia, gout

TOXICITY/OVERDOSE

Symptoms: Hypotension, circulatory collapse • Dehydration,
thromboembolic complications
• Electrolyte loss, metabolic al-
kalosis/associated weakness,
dizziness, mental confusion,
vomiting, cramping
Management: After recent ingestion, implement guidelines
for management of acute overdose (Appendix I). • Administer
IV fluids, replace electrolytes
based on laboratory results;
closely monitor sodium/potas-
sium balance. • Support respiration as needed with O_2 and/or

---

mechanical ventilation. • **Hypotension:** Elevate legs, administer fluids; if unresponsive to fluid replacement, use vasopressors (dopamine, epinephrine).

INTERACTIONS

aminoglycosides ↑ Risk or ototoxicity

amphotericin B Severe potassium depletion

antidiabetic agents, PO Interference with glucose-lowering effects

beta-blockers Hypotension

calcium channel blockers Hypotension

corticosteroids Severe potassium depletion

coumarin anticoagulants ↑ Anticoagulation, bleeding

digoxin Digoxin toxicity, potentially fatal cardiac dysrhythmias

diuretics Enhanced diuretic effects; ↑ potassium depletion; severe hypokalemia

diuretics potassium sparing ↑ Diuretic effects with less potassium loss

hypotensives Profound hypotension

indomethacin, other NSAIDs ↓ Diuretic effectiveness

insulin Interference with hypoglycemic effects

nondepolarizing NMBAs Prolonged neuromuscular blockade

phenytoin ↓ Diuresis

Y-SITE COMPATIBILITIES

Heparin, potassium chloride, vitamin B complex with C

Y-SITE INCOMPATIBILITIES

Solutions/drugs with pH <5

PATIENT CARE IMPLICATIONS

• Evaluate response to therapy, considering diuretic response, fluid balance, weight, electrolytes. Strict I&O and daily weights recommended

• Severe watery diarrhea occurs in some patients; drug should be discontinued.

• Potassium supplements are frequently necessary, especially in digitalized patients.

• Consider use of a potassium-sparing diuretic if other diuretics used concomitantly.

Vital signs/hemodynamics: Monitor BP frequently, especially with high-dose/IV therapy. • As available, continuously monitor ECG. Note presence of PVCs, dysrhythmias, hypokalemic ECG changes (flattened ST interval, T wave inversion, U wave). Digitalized patients should be carefully monitored for these and other dysrhythmias associated with digitalis toxicity.

• Hemodynamic monitoring strongly recommended for patients with severe CHF, cardiac failure associated with acute MI, cardiogenic shock, hemodynamic instability; monitor closely for overaggressive diuresis, excessive lowering of preload resulting in ↓ CO

Physical assessment: Assess extremities, face, sacrum for improvement in edema. • Assess for signs/symptoms of electrolyte imbalance: dysrhythmias, confusion, dizziness, weakness, muscle cramps, faintness, headache, paresthesias, thirst, anorexia, vomiting. • Assess for perfusion/oxygenation deficit caused by hypovolemia: chest discomfort, ↓ level of consciousness, activity intolerance, hypotension, dizziness. • Assess patients with CHF, cardiomyopathy for symptoms of pul-

E

---

monary edema: bibasilar crackles (rales), S_3 gallop, neck vein distention, breathing difficulty.
• Assess hearing, particularly in older adults, with parenteral/high-dose therapy, with use of other ototoxic agents **G**
Laboratory tests: Monitor: Electrolytes • CBC • BUN, creatinine • Bilirubin, liver enzymes • Blood glucose, particularly in patients with diabetes • If present, hypokalemia may lead to serious or fatal complications, including severe dysrhythmias, digoxin toxicity.

PATIENT/FAMILY TEACHING

Purpose of medication is to encourage elimination of excess body fluid. • If IV route used, stay in bed during and for at least 3 hr after end of infusion. Call for assistance when getting out of bed. • May cause low BP, dizziness, especially when starting therapy. Use caution when changing positions, walking. Alcohol, hot weather, vigorous activity, prolonged standing make these symptoms more likely.
• Report symptoms of heart failure: breathing difficulty, palpitations, dizziness, activity intolerance, chest pain. • Report symptoms of electrolyte imbalance: confusion, weakness, dizziness, fatigue, faintness, headache, tingling sensations, muscle cramps, persistent thirst, anorexia, nausea, vomiting.
Outpatient: Take medication in morning. Never double doses.
• Continue taking medication as prescribed even if feeling better. Drug controls but does not cure hypertension/CHF. • If GI irritation occurs, take with food or milk. • Take potassium supplements as prescribed, particularly

if also taking digoxin. See dietician for high-potassium diet (as indicated). • Use sunscreen, wear protective clothing to prevent photosensitivity reactions.
• Weigh twice/wk; notify physician of weight gain, edema.

AVAILABLE FORMS

Tablets • Powder to be reconstituted for IV use

famciclovir
(fam-sye′kloe-ver)
Famvir

Classification: Antiviral

USUAL DOSE

PO, adults: 500 mg, q8h for 7 days • **Renal insufficiency:** Use reduced dose

ADMINISTRATION

PO: May be given without regard to meals

ACTION

Inhibits viral DNA synthesis; has selective activity against herpes simplex virus, varicella-zoster virus

PHARMACOKINETICS

ROUTE	ONSET	PEAK	DURATION
PO	rapid	60 min	Approx 8 hr

DISTRIBUTION
Wide; <20% plasma protein bound

ELIMINATION
Metabolized to penciclovir and renally excreted. Half-life = 2.3 hr.

INDICATIONS

Acute herpes zoster (shingles)

PRECAUTIONS/ CONTRAINDICATIONS

Precautions: Dosage reduction necessary for creat. cl. <60 ml/min; data not available to support use with creat. cl. <20 ml/min

Contraindications: Hypersensitivity to famciclovir • Safe and effective use in children not established

B Pregnancy category: Use only if safer alternative not available

ADVERSE EFFECTS

CNS: *Headache, fatigue*
GI: *Nausea,* diarrhea

TOXICITY/OVERDOSE

Symptoms: Data not reported.
Management: After recent ingestion, implement guidelines for management of acute overdosage (Appendix I). • Treat symptomatically • Effectiveness of hemodialysis unknown

INTERACTIONS

probenecid ↑ Famciclovir levels

PATIENT CARE IMPLICATIONS

Initiate therapy as soon as possible after initial symptoms occur, preferably within 48 hr of rash onset; must be within 72 hr
Physical assessment: Evaluate resolution of infection: diminished pain, itching, lesions

PATIENT/FAMILY TEACHING

Purpose of medication is to treat shingles. It controls symptoms, but does not cure the infection. Medicine may be taken with meals to reduce stomach upset.

AVAILABLE FORMS

Tablets

---

famotidine
(fam-o'te-dine)
Pepcid

Classification: Histamine H_2 antagonist

USUAL DOSE

PO, adults: Initially 40 mg once daily hs or 20 mg bid • Maintenance: 20 mg once daily hs • **Pathologic hypersecretory conditions:** 20-160 mg q6h • **Renal impairment:** 20 mg once daily hs or 40 mg q3-4d hs; drug levels not affected by hemodialysis
IV, adults: 20 mg q12h • Increase frequency of administration rather than dose if necessary to relieve symptoms.

ADMINISTRATION

G-tube: Use oral suspension.
▼Direct IV, adults: Dilute, then inject each 20 mg dose over at least 2 min.
IV, intermit inf, adults: Infuse prepared solution over 15-30 min.

PREPARATION

Direct IV, adults: Dilute 20 mg in 5-10 ml sterile water or 0.9% NaCl.
IV, intermit inf, adults: Dilute 20 mg in 100 ml compatible solutions.
Compatible fluids: D_5W, $D_{10}W$, 0.9% NaCl, LR, prepared combinations of these solutions

ACTIONS

Inhibits action of histamine on H_2 receptors of parietal cells,

---

thus reducing gastric acid secretion • Reduces basal, nocturnal, stimulated gastric acid secretion • 20-150 times potency of cimetidine in controlling gastric acid hypersecretion • Little if any hormonal effects • Not anticholinergic

PHARMACOKINETICS

ROUTE	ONSET	PEAK	DURATION*
PO	≤1 hr	1-4 hr	8-12 hr
IV	Immed	20 min	10-15 hr

DISTRIBUTION

Wide; 15%-20% protein bound

ELIMINATION

Renal excretion; half-life 2.5-4 hr, prolonged with renal impairment

*Dose dependent.

INDICATIONS

Reduce pain, promote healing in short-term treatment of active benign gastric, duodenal ulcers • In reduced doses to prevent ulcer recurrence • Management of hypersecretory conditions (Zollinger-Ellison syndrome, postop hypersecretion) • Short-term management of gastroesophageal reflux, esophagitis *Unlabeled/investigational:* Control of gastric pH and stress-related upper GI bleeding in critically ill patients

PRECAUTIONS/ CONTRAINDICATIONS

Use caution with: Renal dysfunction; reduced dose indi-Ⓟcated • Children: Safety not established

Ⓑ**Pregnancy category:** Safety not clearly established

Contraindications: Hypersensitivity to famotidine, other histamine H₂ antagonists

ADVERSE EFFECTS

CNS: *Headache,* dizziness, paresthesias, insomnia, sleepiness, hallucinations, **seizures** (rare)

CV: Rarely—dysrhythmias, palpitations, AV block

GI: *Constipation, diarrhea,* nausea, vomiting, bilirubin/liver enzymes

Hema: Blood dyscrasias (rare)

Derm: Acne, pruritus, urticaria, dry skin, rash

Misc: Fever, flushing, muscle cramps, tinnitus, irritation at IV injection site, **anaphylaxis** (rare)

TOXICITY/OVERDOSE

Symptoms: No data available on overdose in humans

Management: After recent ingestion, implement guidelines for management of acute overdose (Appendix I). • Initiate appropriate symptomatic/supportive measures. • Hemodialysis is not helpful.

INTERACTIONS

Caffeine, smoking ↓ Famotidine effectiveness

Y-SITE COMPATIBILITIES

Aminophylline, ampicillin, ampicillin-sulbactam, amrinone, atropine, bretylium, calcium gluconate, cephalosporins (most), dexamethasone, digoxin, dobutamine, dopamine, enalaprilat, epinephrine, erythromycin, esmolol, fluconazole, furosemide, gentamicin, haloperidol, heparin, insulin, isoproterenol, labetalol, lidocaine, magnesium, meperidine, metoclopramide, midazolam, morphine, nafcillin, nitroglycerin, norepinephrine, ondansetron, penicillins (most), phenylephrine, piperacillin potassium chloride, potassium phosphate, procainamide, sodium bicarbonate, sodium nitroprusside theophylline, ticarcillin, ticarcillin-clavulanate, verapamil

Y-SITE INCOMPATIBILITIES

Cefepime, piperacillin-tazobactam

PATIENT CARE IMPLICATIONS

• May be administered with antacids
Physical assessment: Assess for epigastric or abdominal pain. Consult physician for persistent or severe pain. • Monitor for evidence of GI bleeding (e.g., occult blood in emesis or stool, orthostatic changes).
Laboratory tests: Monitor: Liver enzymes, bilirubin • BUN, creatinine • CBC

PATIENT/FAMILY TEACHING

Purpose of medication is to reduce stomach acid, relieve pain. • Smoking decreases effectiveness of famotidine, increases stomach acidity; smoking cessation programs/therapy recommended. • Report black tarry stools, blood in stools or emesis, dizziness, changes in mentation. • May cause drowsiness, dizziness, or mental confusion; avoid activities requiring mental alertness until response to drug known. • Avoid coffee, caffeine, alcohol, aspirin, ibuprofen, other food or drugs that may cause gastric irritation.
• Take all doses as prescribed, even if feeling better. • Increase fluid intake, exercise regularly, increase dietary fiber to reduce risk of constipation.

AVAILABLE FORMS

Tablets • Powder for PO suspension • Single-use/multidose vials

---

felodipine
(fell-ode'i-peen)
Plendil

Classification: Calcium channel blocker, antihypertensive

USUAL DOSE

PO, adults: 5-10 mg once daily; maximum dose 20 mg/day • **Advanced age/hepatic insufficiency:** Use lower dose; do not exceed 10 mg/day.

ADMINISTRATION

PO: Tablets are extended release and must be swallowed whole; do not crush or chew. May be given without regard to meals

ACTION

Inhibits movement of calcium ions across myocardium and vascular smooth muscle with greater effect on vascular smooth muscle • Dilates peripheral arteries, decreases peripheral vascular resistance, reduces BP • Renal vascular resistance decreased; mild diuresis, especially during initial therapy • Reflex increase in HR, especially when initiating therapy; no significant effect on cardiac conduction • Serum calcium levels not affected

---

italic = common side effects   **bold** = life-threatening reactions

PHARMACOKINETICS

ROUTE	ONSET	PEAK	DURATION
PO	2-5 hr	5-11 hr	≥24 hr

DISTRIBUTION
>99% protein bound

ELIMINATION
Eliminated in urine, feces. Terminal half-life = 11-16 hr

INDICATIONS

Hypertension; used alone or with other agents.

PRECAUTIONS/CONTRAINDICATIONS

Precautions: May cause hypotension 2-5 hr after dosing • Reflex tachycardia may precipitate angina.
Use caution with: CHF, beta-blocker therapy; possibility of negative inotropy—may worsen/precipitate heart failure **G** • Hepatic insufficiency, advanced age; use lower dose, **P** monitor closely • Children: safe use not established
c **Pregnancy category:** Use only if safer alternative not available
Contraindications: Hypersensitivity to felodipine • Hypertensive emergencies due to slow onset of action

ADVERSE EFFECTS

CNS: *headache,* dizziness, weakness, paresthesia
EENT: *gingival hyperplasia*
RESP: cough, dyspnea
CV: *peripheral edema,* flushing, hypotension, chest pain
GI: nausea, abdominal pain

TOXICITY/OVERDOSE

Symptoms: Hypotension, reflex tachycardia; possible bradycardia

Management: After recent ingestion, implement guidelines for management of acute overdosage (Appendix I) • For hypotension, elevate legs, administer IV fluids; consider dopamine or other vasopressors if necessary. Use atropine for symptomatic bradycardia. IV calcium gluconate may reverse hemodynamic effects of calcium channel blockade • Hemodialysis is not likely to be helpful

INTERACTIONS

antihypertensives Profound hypotension
beta-blockers Profound hypotension
calcium ↓ Felodipine effectiveness
digoxin Transient increase in digoxin levels
phenytoin ↓ Felodipine levels
theophylline Theophylline levels

PATIENT CARE IMPLICATIONS

• Discontinue slowly to avoid angina symptoms in susceptible individuals.
G • Older adults more likely to experience hypotension. Use lowest effective dose; monitor closely.
Vital signs/hemodynamics: Monitor BP to insure effective therapy; hypotension rare because of gradual onset of vasodilation.
Physical assessment: Assess for perfusion/oxygenation deficit: ↓ level of consciousness, hypotension, activity intolerance, chest discomfort. • Assess for dysrhythmias

PATIENT/FAMILY TEACHING

Purpose of medication is to control high BP.

Outpatient: Take exactly as prescribed. Do not stop taking medicine even if you feel better. If medication is abruptly discontinued, you may develop dangerously high BP, chest pain. • Swallow whole; do not break, crush, or chew tablets. • May cause gum swelling; good oral hygiene is necessary • Medication is not a cure for high BP; other therapies, including lifestyle modifications, must be continued. • Consult health care professional before taking non-prescription preparations.

AVAILABLE FORMS

Tablets

---

fentanyl
(fen′ta-nil)
Duragesic (transdermal)
fentanyl citrate
Sublimaze
fentanyl citrate with droperidol
Innovar

Classifications: Opiate agonist, narcotic analgesic
Schedule II controlled substance

USUAL DOSE

Always use lowest effective dose; response varies, each patient requires individual dose. *Use caution, reduced dose in* elderly or debilitated patients. Reduce to ¼-⅓ usual dose when used within 24 hr of other CNS depressants (e.g., opiate analgesics, general anesthetics, alcohol, antihistamines, barbiturates, hypnotics, sedatives, neuroleptics).

IM, adults: Preop: 50-100 μg 30-60 min before surgery
• Postop: 50-100 μg q1-2h
Epidural injection, adults: 25-50 μg/hr as needed for pain control
Transdermal, adults: Initially 25 μg/hr system q72h, usually with supplemental analgesic
• Increase dose by 25 μg as needed, q3-6d, depending on supplemental opiate requirements. Replace system 48-72 hr. • Do not use for acute or postoperative pain management. Fever increases medication absorption; use reduced dose, observe carefully for toxicity/respiratory depression.

ADMINISTRATION

Direct IV, adults: Inject ≤100 μg over 1-2 min with continuous ECG monitoring; bradycardia requiring atropine may occur. • Too-rapid IV injection may cause muscle rigidity, seizures, laryngospasm, apnea. Assisted ventilation/neuromuscular blockers (e.g., succinylcholine) may be required. • May be administered via PCA system.
Epidural, adults: Often administered via PCA pump • ↑ Basal rate as necessary to relieve pain without excessive sedation.
Transdermal, adults: Apply to dry, nonirritated, hairless (clip if necessary) skin on flat surface of upper torso; do not use soaps, oils, lotions, or alcohol before application. • Press firmly into place, hold for 10-20 sec; complete contact with skin essential. • Remove used system before applying new one. • Rotate application sites.

---

italic = common side effects   **bold** = life-threatening reactions

PREPARATION

Direct IV, adults: Dilute each dose in ≥5 ml sterile water or 0.9% NaCl.

ACTIONS

Opium derivative that acts at receptor sites in CNS, other tissue to inhibit pain perception, produce analgesia • Analgesic action more prompt, less prolonged than with morphine, meperidine • Approx 80 times more potent than morphine mg for mg • Causes CNS/respiratory depression; *respiratory depressant effects outlast analgesic action.* • Less likely to cause nausea, vomiting than other opiate agonists • Minimal hypnotic activity • Rarely causes histamine release • Residual activity potentiates effects of subsequent doses resulting in ↑ analgesia, possible respiratory depression.

PHARMACOKINETICS

ROUTE	ONSET	PEAK	DURATION*
IM	7-15 min	20-30 min	1-2 hr
IV	Rapid	Minutes	30-60 min
Transderm		12-24 hr	48-72 hr

DISTRIBUTION

Wide; readily crosses placenta

ELIMINATION

Metabolized in liver, excreted in urine; half-life 1.5-6 hr, transderm 30-40 hr

*Duration of analgesia. Respiratory depressant effects outlast analgesic effects. All effects cumulative with repeat doses.

INDICATIONS

Perioperatively, during surgery, immediate preop/postop periods when potent analgesia required • Relief of postop tachypnea, delirium • Supplement to general or regional anesthesia • Alone for minor surgical procedures, as anesthetic agent with O_2, skeletal muscle relaxant when minimal stress surgery important (e.g., open heart, neurosurgery) • Transdermal for management of chronic moderate to severe pain that requires continuous opioid administration

PRECAUTIONS/ CONTRAINDICATIONS

Precautions: Severe respiratory depression possible, especially with IV use • *Respiratory depression lasts longer than analgesia; effects potentiated by other opiates/sedatives.* • IV administration may cause muscle rigidity, bronchospasm, apnea. • May cause profound bradycardia, hypotension • 50, 75, 100 μg/hr Duragesic systems should only be used in patients with established opioid tolerance.

Use caution with: Meperidine hypersensitivity; chemical structure similar • Asthma, COPD, other pulmonary disease • Head injury, CNS depression, seizure disorder; respiratory depression may cause CO_2 retention, cerebral vasodilation • Alcoholism • Shock • Bradycardia • Adrenal insufficiency • Children • Hepatic/renal dysfunction, older adults, debilitation; reduced dose necessary

c Pregnancy category: Use only if safer alternative unavailable.

Contraindications: Hypersensitivity to fentanyl • Respiratory depression without mechanical ventilation • Undiagnosed acute abdominal conditions • Ulcerative colitis • Concurrent use of MAO inhibitors • Benign prostatic hypertrophy • IM route contraindicated with hypothermia, shock, hypotension, impaired circulation • Infants, labor/delivery: safety not established

ADVERSE EFFECTS

CNS: *Sedation, confusion,* dizziness, weakness, agitation, **seizures**

EENT: Constricted pupils, visual disturbances

Resp: **Respiratory depression, apnea, laryngospasm**

CV: *Orthostatic hypotension, bradycardia,* hypertension, profound hypotension, reflex tachycardia, sweating, flushing

GI: *Nausea, vomiting, constipation*

GU: Urinary retention

Derm: Pruritus, urticaria

Local: IV injection site phlebitis, pain; transdermal site *erythema*

Misc: Muscular rigidity, hypothermia, tolerance, physical/psychologic dependence

TOXICITY/OVERDOSE

Acute symptoms: Profound CNS, respiratory depression • Bradycardia, hypotension • Hypothermia • Cool, clammy skin • Risk of apnea, circulatory collapse, cardiopulmonary arrest • Potentially fatal complications, including pneumonia, shock, pulmonary edema

Management: Establish/maintain airway, administer O$_2$. • Naloxone (opiate antagonist) reverses effects; repeat doses may be necessary because fentanyl effects may be sustained. • **Hypotension:** Elevate legs, administer IV fluids; use vasopressors (e.g., dopamine, norepinephrine) for circulatory collapse. • **Bradycardia:** Use atropine. • If assisted ventilation hindered by muscular rigidity, use IV muscle relaxants, NMBA • Remove transdermal system if present.

INTERACTIONS

alcohol, ethyl ↑ CNS depression

Antihistamines ↑ CNS depression; enhanced analgesia

Anesthetics, general ↑ CNS depression

Naloxone Acute withdrawal in opiate-dependent patients

Opiate agonist-antagonists (e.g., buprenorphine, butorphanol, nalbuphine, pentazocine) Acute withdrawal in opiate-dependent patients

opiate analgesics ↑ CNS depression

phenothiazines ↑ or ↓ Analgesia; additive CNS depression

sedatives ↑ CNS depression

tranquilizers ↑ CNS depression; enhanced analgesia

Y-SITE COMPATIBILITIES

Atracurium, enalaprilat, esmolol, heparin, hydrocortisone sodium succinate, labetalol, nafcillin, pancuronium, potassium chloride, vecuronium

Y-SITE INCOMPATIBILITIES

Pentobarbital, thiopental

PATIENT CARE IMPLICATIONS

• Dose must be individualized for each patient (see Usual Dose).
• Administer before pain becomes severe.
• Frequently used combination product (Innovar) contains fentanyl, droperidol; analgesic/respiratory depressant effects potentiated

---

• Patients receiving fentanyl for pain control do not develop psychologic dependence. As tolerance develops, progressively higher doses may be necessary to relieve pain during long-term therapy.

Transdermal
• See Administration for many implications.
• Supplement with other opiate analgesics until pain controlled with transdermal system. Gradually discontinue drug after long-term use to prevent withdrawal symptoms.

IV/epidural
• Have atropine, naloxone, NMBA, resuscitation equipment immediately available.

Vital signs/hemodynamics: Assess BP, pulse, RR before and frequently during initial administration; withhold for bradycardia, hypotension, respiratory depression. With IV use, monitor q5min for first 15 min and frequently thereafter. During transdermal use, monitor q2-4h until stable. • Continuous pulse oximetry recommended with IV use.

Physical assessment: Assess type, location, intensity of pain before and after administration. • Assess ventilation: note rate, depth of respirations; auscultate breath sounds. • Assess bowel function: bowel sounds, abdominal distention, elimination patterns. • Monitor I&O. Assess for urinary retention or bladder distention.

PATIENT/FAMILY TEACHING

Purpose of medication is to relieve pain. Request medication/trigger PCA before pain becomes severe • Change positions slowly to avoid dizziness.

• Change position, cough, deep breathe every 2 hr to prevent atelectasis. • Do not perform hazardous tasks requiring mental alertness or physical coordination. Call for assistance when ambulating.

Transdermal: See Administration. Use different site for each application. Fold used systems so that adhesive adheres to itself; discard safely. Fever may cause more rapid absorption of transdermal systems; dose may need reduction; consult nurse or physician. Keep out of reach of ⓟchildren.

Outpatient: Avoid concurrent use of alcohol or other CNS depressants while taking this medication.

AVAILABLE FORMS

Ampules, vials for IV/IM injection • Transdermal systems

flecainide acetate
(fle-kay′nide)
Tambocor

Classifications: Antidysrhythmic, membrane-stabilizer, Vaughan-Williams Class IC

USUAL DOSE:

PO, adults: Initially 50-100 mg q12h; if dysrhythmia not controlled in 4 days, increase dose by 50 mg q12h. • Continue to increase slowly as necessary for dysrhythmia control; too rapid or excessive doses increase possibility of life-threatening dysrhythmias. • Plasma levels used to facilitate dose adjustments • Maximum dose, 400 mg/24 hr

---

ⓟ pediatric   ⓖ geriatric   ▼ Direct IV

ACTIONS

Decreases cardiac excitability by increasing threshold level for electrical excitation • Blocks fast sodium channels; decreases conduction velocity in His-Purkinje system, atrium, AV node • Prolongs effective refractory period of ventricles, accessory conduction pathways • Increases sinus node recovery time, which may adversely affect patients with preexisting sinus node dysfunction • May prolong PR/QT intervals, QRS complex • Negative inotropic effects may decrease CO.

PHARMACOKINETICS

ROUTE	ONSET	PEAK	DURATION
PO	In 30 min	2-3 hr	Up to 30 hr

DISTRIBUTION

Wide; 40%-50% bound to plasma proteins

ELIMINATION

Metabolized in liver, excreted by kidneys; acid urine increases excretion; half-life 12-27 hr

Therapeutic level: 0.2-1.0 μg/ml

INDICATIONS

Suppression/prevention of severe refractory ventricular tachycardia, SVTs, including AV nodal reentrant tachycardia, WPW, paroxysmal atrial fibrillation/flutter • Serious, potentially fatal drug-induced dysrhythmias limit use.

PRECAUTIONS/ CONTRAINDICATIONS

Precautions: May worsen heart failure or dysrhythmias, especially with preexisting heart disease • May worsen or precipitate heart block, prolong QRS complex, QT interval • May cause sinus bradycardia, pauses,

arrest • Increases cardiac pacing thresholds; may suppress ability of artificial pacemaker to achieve capture • Potassium imbalances antagonize antidysrhythmic effects.

Use caution with: CHF • History of MI • Sick sinus syndrome • Renal/hepatic insufficiency

C Pregnancy category: Use only if safer alternative unavailable.

Contraindications: Hypersensitivity to flecainide • 2nd/3rd degree heart block unless functional ventricular pacemaker in place or readily available • Nonsustained asymptomatic dysrhythmias • Cardiogenic shock • Severe cardiac/hepatic disease

ADVERSE EFFECTS

CNS: *Dizziness, faintness, visual disturbances, headache,* weakness, tremors, confusion

Resp: *Dyspnea*

CV: *Palpitations,* **exacerbation of heart failure, new/worsened ventricular dysrhythmias,** bradycardia, hypotension, chest pain, peripheral edema, **sinus pause/arrest**

GI: *Nausea, constipation, abdominal discomfort,* vomiting

Syst: Leukopenia, thrombocytopenia, fever

TOXICITY/OVERDOSE

Symptoms: Hypotension • Ventricular dysrhythmias, profound bradycardia, asystole • Heart failure • Prolongation of PR/QT intervals, QRS complex • Respiratory failure

Management: After recent ingestion, implement guidelines for management of acute overdose (Appendix I). • **Respira-**

F

---

italic = common side effects   **bold** = life-threatening reactions

tory failure: Establish/maintain airway; initiate mechanical ventilation as necessary. • **Hypotension:** Elevate legs, administer IV fluids; use vasopressors (e.g., dopamine, norepinephrine) if necessary. • **Heart failure:** Use positive inotropic agents (e.g., dobutamine, dopamine). • Manage symptomatic bradycardia, ventricular dysrhythmias according to ACLS guidelines (Appendix P). • Hemodialysis cannot remove drug.
Toxic level: >1 µg/ml

INTERACTIONS

amiodarone ↑ Antidysrhythmic effects; ↑ flecainide levels
antihypertensives Excessive hypotension
cimetidine ↑ Flecainide levels
digoxin ↑ Digoxin levels
disopyramide ↑ Negative inotropy; heart failure
propranolol ↑ Flecainide levels
verapamil ↑ Negative inotropy; heart failure

PATIENT CARE IMPLICATIONS

• *May cause serious or fatal dysrhythmias; use reserved for life-threatening dysrhythmias*
• Continuous clinical, ECG monitoring necessary during initiation of therapy
• Gradual dosage increments reduce incidence of malignant dysrhythmias. Always use lowest effective dose.
• Correct hypoxemia, hypercapnia, hypokalemia, other fluid/electrolyte imbalance before initiating therapy.
Vital signs/hemodynamics: Continuously monitor ECG during initiation of therapy. Note signs of toxicity, including profound bradycardia, heart block, ventricular dysrhythmias. Consult physician immediately.
• Monitor BP frequently during initiation of therapy, when dosage increased. • Observe patients with artificial pacemakers for failure to sense or capture.
Physical assessment: Assess for perfusion/oxygenation deficit: chest discomfort, changes in mentation, activity intolerance, hypotension, dizziness. • Assess for fluid volume overload: bibasilar crackles, dyspnea, peripheral edema, neck vein distention, weight gain.
Laboratory tests: Monitor: Electrolytes, particularly potassium • Plasma levels of flecainide; therapeutic levels, 0.2-1.0 µg/ml

PATIENT/FAMILY TEACHING

Purpose of medication is to control abnormal heartbeats.
• Report chest discomfort, activity intolerance, dizziness, breathing difficulty, swelling of extremities, rapid weight gain.
• Dizziness, blurred vision may occur; use caution, avoid driving until individual effects of therapy established.

AVAILABLE FORMS

Tablets

fluconazole
(floo-con′a-zole)
Diflucan

Classifications: Antifungal antibiotic, triazole derivative

USUAL DOSE

PO/IV, adults: 100-400 mg/day depending on severity of infection. Loading dose usually

>daily dose. • **Vaginal candidiasis:** Single dose of 150 mg po. • **Renal impairment:** Initially 50-400 mg, followed by reduced dose according to creatinine clearance

P PO/IV, children 3-19 yr: 3-6 mg/kg/24 hr in single dose • Experience limited

ADMINISTRATION

G-tube: Use oral suspension
IV, intermit inf: Infuse each 200 mg over 60 min.

PREPARATION

IV inf: All preparations prediluted, ready for use; do not mix with other medications or IV fluids.

ACTIONS

Broad-spectrum antifungal agent; fungistatic effects from disruption of fungal cell membranes • Unlike ketoconazole, does not significantly affect human steroid/cholesterol synthesis • Active against variety of fungi, including *Candida albicans, Cryptococcus neoformans, Histoplasma capsulatum, Blastomyces dermatitidis* • Not active against bacteria, rickettsiae, viruses

PHARMACOKINETICS

ROUTE	ONSET	PEAK	DURATION
PO	Rapid	1-2 hr	Usual dosing results in steady state by day 2 of therapy
IV	Immed	End infusion	

DISTRIBUTION

Widely distributed; readily crosses blood-brain barrier

ELIMINATION

Renal excretion; half-life 30 hr

INDICATIONS

Treatment of serious candidal infections of urinary tract, lower respiratory tract, peritoneum, other sites • Oral/esophageal candidiasis, particularly in immunocompromised adults • Vaginal candidiasis • Acute cryptococcal meningitis when amphotericin B cannot be used • Maintenance therapy for prevention of relapse of cryptococcal meningitis in AIDS patients

PRECAUTIONS/ CONTRAINDICATIONS

Precautions: Serious hepatotoxicity possible
Use caution with: Hypersensitivity to other triazole or imidazole antifungal agents • AIDS, malignancy, immunocompromised patients; increased risk of
P exfoliative skin disorders • Children: Safety not established for those ≤13 yr
c Pregnancy category: Risk of fetal damage unknown; use only if safer alternative unavailable.
Contraindications: Hypersensitivity to fluconazole

ADVERSE EFFECTS

CNS: *Headache,* dizziness, somnolence, fatigue, paresthesias, **seizures** (rare)
GI: *Nausea, vomiting, diarrhea, abdominal discomfort;* ↑ liver enzymes/bilirubin **hepatic necrosis** (rare)
Derm: *Rash,* pruritus
Misc: Hypersensitivity, **anaphylaxis**

TOXICITY/OVERDOSE

Symptoms: Limited information available • Very high doses in animals cause hypoventilation, cyanosis, seizures, death.

F

---

italic = common side effects   **bold** = life-threatening reactions

Management: After recent ingestion, implement guidelines for management of acute overdose (Appendix I) • Initiate symptomatic/supportive measures, including airway management/ventilation. • Hemodialysis or peritoneal dialysis removes drug.

INTERACTIONS

anticoagulants, PO ↑ Anticoagulation

astemizole Prolonged QT, serious dysrhythmias; avoid current use

cyclosporine ↑ Cyclosporine levels

phenytoin ↑ Phenytoin levels; risk of toxicity

rifampin ↓ Fluconazole levels

sulfonylurea PO antidiabetic agents (e.g., tolbutamide) ↓ Metabolism of antidiabetic agent; hypoglycemia

terfenadine Prolonged QT, serious dysrhythmias; avoid current use

theophylline ↑ Theophylline levels; monitor closely

Y-SITE COMPATIBILITIES

Acyclovir, amikacin, aminophylline, cefazolin, cefotetan, cefoxitin, chlorpromazine, cimetidine, dexamethasone, diltiazem, diphenhydramine, droperidol, famotidine, gancyclovir, gentamicin, heparin, meperidine, metoclopramide, metronidazole, midazolam, morphine, nafcillin, odansetron, oxacillin, penicillin G potassium, prochlorperazine edisylate, promethazine, tobramycin, vancomycin, zidovudine

Y-SITE INCOMPATIBILITIES

Amphotericin B, ampicillin, calcium gluconate, cefotaxime, ceftazidime, ceftriaxone, cefuroxime, chloramphenicol, clindamycin, diazepam, digoxin, erythromycin, furosemide, haloperidol, hydroxyzine, imipenem-cilastatin, pentamidine, piperacillin, ticarcillin, trimethoprimsul famethaxazole

PATIENT CARE IMPLICATIONS

• As indicated, obtain specimens for culture and sensitivity before initiating antifungal therapy. Initiate therapy before results received.

• Serious hepatotoxicity possible; if liver enzymes or bilirubin become elevated, monitor closely, discontinue if clinical signs of liver disease (anorexia, jaundice, abdominal pain, dark urine, light stools).

IV

• Reduce risk of thrombophlebitis by using large veins and small catheters/needles, rotating infusion sites.

Vital signs: Monitor VS for indicators of infection, complications.

Physical assessment: Assess for improvement in primary infection or resistance to fluconazole therapy, as evidenced by recurrent infection, failure to respond to therapy. • Observe for symptoms of hypersensitivity: rash, pruritus, wheezing, laryngeal edema, hypotension. • If rash develops, monitor closely; discontinue fluconazole if rash worsens. Use particular caution with immunocompromised patients, because serious dermatologic reactions possible.

Laboratory tests: Monitor: CBC with differential • Liver enzymes, bilirubin • Initially, BUN, creatinine

---

PATIENT/FAMILY TEACHING

Purpose of drug is to limit growth of infection-causing fungal organisms. • Report diarrhea, rash, itching, wheezing. • May cause dizziness, drowsiness; until effects known, use caution when performing hazardous tasks requiring mental alertness or physical coordination. • Take all medication exactly as prescribed. Do not stop taking medicine even if you feel better. Failure to take entire prescription may result in recurrence or additional infection. Do not save or share unused medicine.

AVAILABLE FORMS

Tablets • PO suspension • Parenteral for IV use

---

flumazenil
(floo-maz′een-ill)
Romazicon

Classification: Benzodiazepine antagonist/antidote

USUAL DOSE

Direct IV, adults: Reversal of sedation: 0.2 mg; repeat q60sec as needed. If sedation recurs, after 20 min, may repeat initial dose. Do not exceed total dose of 1 mg (0.2 mg repeated 5 times) or 3 mg/hr. • **Benzodiazepine overdose:** 0.2 mg; if after 30 sec desired level of consciousness not achieved, give additional dose of 0.3 mg. Single doses up to 0.5 mg may be given at 1-min intervals. Do not exceed cumulative dose of 3 mg without response or 5 mg if partial response to lower doses. Small, frequent doses (e.g., 0.2

mg q1min) may be used for more gradual arousal. *Resedation is likely, particularly with long-acting benzodiazepines (e.g., diazepam); close monitoring necessary.* If sedation recurs, give 0.5 mg q1min up to 1 mg q20min. Do not exceed cumulative dose of 3 mg/hr.

Direct IV, older adults: Even though reduced doses of benzodiazepines used, recommended doses of flumazenil are unchanged

ADMINISTRATION

Direct IV, adults: Inject each dose rapidly over 15-30 sec through freely flowing IV solution. • Dilution not necessary. • Use large vein, rapidly flowing IV solution to minimize injection site pain. • Avoid extravasation, which causes local irritation. • Do not mix or administer with other agents. **Compatible fluids:** D_5W, 0.9% NaCl, LR

ACTIONS

Antagonizes CNS effects of benzodiazepines by competitive activity at gamma-aminobutyric acid (GABA)/benzodiazepine receptor site • Reverses sedation/other benzodiazepine effects; amnesia may not be completely reversed • Resedation is possible, particularly in patients who have received large or long-acting benzodiazepine doses • Rapid reversal of sedation in benzodiazepine overdose may result in CNS excitation. • Does not reverse effects of ethanol, barbiturates, general anesthetics, opioid analgesics

---

PHARMACOKINETICS

ROUTE	ONSET	PEAK	DURATION
IV	1-2 min	6-10 min	15-60 min

DISTRIBUTION
Wide; 50% protein bound

ELIMINATION
Metabolized by liver, eliminated by kidneys; half-life 41-79 min

INDICATIONS

Complete or partial reversal of sedation associated with benzodiazepine use • Management of acute benzodiazepine overdose

PRECAUTIONS/ CONTRAINDICATIONS

Precautions: Benzodiazepine-dependent patients may experience dose-dependent withdrawal symptoms, including seizures • Benzodiazepine-related hypoventilation may not be completely reversed or may recur as flumazenil effects wear off; monitor closely for hypoventilation • May trigger seizures, particularly with benzodiazepine physical dependence, long-term use of benzodiazepines, cyclic antidepressant overdose, major sedative-hypnotic drug withdrawal, recent therapy with repeated doses of parenteral benzodiazepines, previous myoclonic jerking, other seizure activity • Use of flumazenil may complicate management of alcohol, barbiturate, sedative withdrawal. • Do not use with NMBAs until effects of NMBAs no longer present. **Use caution with:** Emergency, other patients who may have unrecognized benzodiazepine dependence • Critically ill patients with high-dose sedation over brief period may develop unrecognized benzodiazepine dependence; withdrawal symptoms, seizures may be precipitated by flumazenil. • Head injury, seizure disorder, elevated ICP; ↑ risk of seizures/altered cerebral perfusion • Hepatic dysfunction; give usual initial dose, but reduce dosage/frequency of repeat doses.

c Pregnancy category: Risk unknown; use only if safer alternative unavailable.

Contraindications: Hypersensitivity to flumazenil, benzodiazepines • History of panic disorder; may cause panic attack • Use of benzodiazepines for control of potentially life-threatening conditions (e.g., status epilepticus) • Serious cyclic antidepressant overdose • Diagnosis of unknown coma or sedation because of possible undiagnosed benzodiazepine dependence, risk of seizures **P** • Children: Safety/efficacy unknown

ADVERSE EFFECTS

CNS: *Dizziness,* headache, agitation, blurred vision, paresthesias, **seizures**
Resp: Dyspnea, hyperventilation
CV: *Sweating,* palpitations, flushing, PVCs, bradycardia, tachycardia, hypertension, chest pain
GI: *Nausea, vomiting*
Local: *Pain,* thrombophlebitis, rash

TOXICITY/OVERDOSE

Symptoms: Too rapid or excessive reversal of benzodiazepine sedation may cause anxiety, agitation, increased muscle tone, seizures. • No serious adverse effects when administered in absence of benzodiazepines

---

P pediatric   **G** geriatric   **V** Direct IV

Management: Maintain airway/support ventilation as necessary. • Administer IV fluids. • **Seizures:** Have diazepam/lorazapam (Ativan), phenytoin, barbiturates readily available; greater than usual doses of diazepam may be required.

INTERACTIONS

cyclic antidepressants; mixed drug overdose Seizures, dysrhythmias when benzodiazepine effects are reversed

INCOMPATIBILITIES

Numerous; do not mix in syringe or solution or administer at Y site with other agents.

PATIENT CARE IMPLICATIONS

• Administer in increments, use smallest effective dose; especially important if physical dependence on benzodiazepines or benzodiazepines used for seizure suppression or with mixed drug overdosage, esp TCA.
• Hospitalized patients receiving benzodiazepine therapy for sedation may have unrecognized benzodiazepine dependence; withdrawal symptoms, convulsions may be precipitated by flumazenil (e.g., when used for reversal of conscious sedation).
• Stabilize airway/support ventilation before flumazenil administration in patients with significant respiratory depression/severe respiratory disease.
• On awakening, patients may become agitated, confused, and attempt to withdraw ETTs or IV lines.
• Be prepared to manage seizures, especially in patients with long-term benzodiazepine therapy, brief high-dose parenteral

therapy, physical dependence, cyclic antidepressant overdose.
Vital signs/hemodynamics: Monitor HR, RR, BP frequently for 2 hr or until stable. • Monitor ECG for dysrhythmias, esp. with mixed or unknown drug overdosage.
Physical assessment: Assess for twitching, rigidity, focal seizures, myoclonic jerking, other seizure activity. Avoid further flumazenil administration; be prepared to protect airway, support ventilation, manage seizures. • Assess for resedation, monitor breathing patterns q15-30 min for at least 2 hr after flumazenil administration, because benzodiazepine-related hypoventilation may not be completely reversed or may recur. Longer periods of observation required if diazepam (Valium)/other long-acting benzodiazepines or large doses of short-acting agents (e.g., >10 mg midazolam [Versed]) are used. Use continuous pulse oximetry to detect decreasing O_2 saturation related to hypoventilation.

PATIENT/FAMILY TEACHING

Benzodiazepine-induced amnesia not completely reversed; instructions need written/verbal reinforcement. • Purpose of medication is to reverse effects of certain sedative medications. • Effects of flumazenil wear off in 1-2 hr; sedation, drowsiness may recur. Call for assistance when getting out of bed, walking. • Avoid driving and other activities requiring mental alertness or physical coordination for 24 hr (or longer, depending on dose, type of benzodiazepine). • Avoid use of alcohol or

F

---

italic = common side effects   **bold** = life-threatening reactions

other drugs that cause sedation for 24 hr (or longer, depending on dose, type of benzodiazepine).

AVAILABLE FORMS

5-, 10-ml ampules for parenteral use

---

furosemide
(fur-oh'se-mide)
Lasix, Furomide ✤,
Norosemide, Uritol ✤

Classification: Sulfonamide-type loop diuretic

USUAL DOSE

PO, adults: Edema: 20-80 mg qAM; may repeat 20–40-mg dose q6-8h until desired diuresis • Maximum dose, 600 mg/day with severe edema • **Hypertension:** 10-40 mg bid

PO, children: 2 mg/kg as single dose; may increase in 1–2-mg/kg increments q6-8h until desired diuresis • Maximum dose, 6 mg/kg

IV/IM, adults: Initially 20-40 mg once to induce diuresis; may repeat ≥20 mg q2h until desired diuresis • Acute pulmonary edema: 0.5-1.0 mg/kg • Initiate PO therapy as soon as possible.
Unlabeled/investigational: Up to 4 g/24 hr for severe CHF; use caution/monitor closely • **Cont IV inf:** Sometimes used for brief period; rate: 0.5-4 mg/min

IV/IM, children: 1 mg/kg once to induce diuresis; may be increased by 1 mg/kg q2h until desired diuresis • Maximum dose, 6 mg/kg • Initiate PO therapy as soon as possible.

ADMINISTRATION

Direct IV: Inject each 20 mg undiluted solution slowly over 1-2 min. • IV infusion recommended for high-dose therapy
IV, intermit inf: Infuse diluted solution over 10-30 min. Do not exceed rate of 10 mg/min.
IV inf, adults: Titrate infusion of 0.5-4.0 mg/min to desired diuresis, preload reduction. • Use rate-controlling device.

PREPARATION

IV inf: Mix desired dose in ≥50-100 ml compatible solution. Concentrated solutions (e.g., 500 mg/dl for concentration of 5 mg/ml) are used to limit total fluid intake. • Do not use yellow or discolored solutions.
Compatible fluids: D_5W, 0.9% NaCl, LR, prepared combinations of these solutions; unstable in acidic solutions (pH <5.5)

ACTIONS

Produces rapid diuresis, venous vasodilation • Venodilation increases peripheral venous capacitance, reduces preload. • Decreases renal vascular resistance, increases renal blood flow • Results in excretion of sodium, chloride, potassium, hydrogen, calcium, magnesium, ammonium, bicarbonate, phosphate, water • Excessive losses of potassium, hydrogen, chloride may induce metabolic alkalosis.
• Beneficial effects in CHF include reduced plasma volume, increased Hct, decreased peripheral resistance, increased CO.
• Reduced plasma volume results in hypotensive effects in some patients. • Affects glucose

---

metabolism, may cause mild elevations of blood glucose

PHARMACOKINETICS

ROUTE	ONSET	PEAK*	DURATION
PO	30-60 min	1-2 hr	6-8 hr
IV	5-10 min	60-70 min	4 hr

DISTRIBUTION

Wide; 95% protein bound; crosses placenta

ELIMINATION

Metabolized in liver, eliminated in urine/feces; half-life ≤2 hrs; prolonged in renal failure

---

*Peak diuretic effects. Venodilation, peak reduction of left ventricular filling pressure occur 15 min after IV administration.

INDICATIONS

Edema associated with CHF, hepatic cirrhosis, nephrotic syndrome, renal insufficiency • IV route recommended for uremic patients, because diuretic response greater, more predictable • Adjunct in treatment of acute pulmonary edema • Used cautiously when pulmonary edema is complication of cardiogenic shock; overaggressive diuresis, ↓ CO possible • Hypertension, especially with CHF, renal insufficiency

Unlabeled/investigational:
Hypertensive crises; enhances hypotensive action of other agents, counteracts sodium retention caused by some antihypertensives • Alone or with NaCl to increase calcium excretion in hyperparathyroidism and serious hypercalcemia

PRECAUTIONS/ CONTRAINDICATIONS

Precautions: Excessive diuresis may cause hypovolemia, severe electrolyte imbalance, including hypokalemia, metabolic alkalosis • May cause interstitial nephritis, lead to acute renal failure • Hearing impairment may occur with high doses, rapid IV administration, concurrent use with other ototoxic agents • Uric acid elevation may lead to gout.

G **Use caution with:** Older adults, CHF; fluid/electrolyte imbalance more likely • Sulfonamide sensitivity; allergic reactions possible • Renal impairment; diuresis, reduced plasma volume may decrease GFR. • Cirrhosis/hepatic failure, rapid changes in fluids/electrolytes can prompt hepatic coma. • Digitalized patients; hypokalemia may trigger digitalis toxicity. • Nephrotic syndrome; profound hypokalemia possible

C **Pregnancy category:** Animal reproduction studies show evidence of fetal risk; use only if potential benefits justify risk.

Contraindications: Hypersensitivity to furosemide • Anuria • Untreated electrolyte depletion or hepatic coma

ADVERSE EFFECTS

CNS: Dizziness, headache, blurred vision, paresthesias, tinnitus, hearing loss
Resp: Alkalosis with compensatory respiratory depression
CV: *Orthostatic hypotension;* **hypotension;** PACs, PVCs, **ventricular fibrillation**
GI: Nausea, vomiting, anorexia, diarrhea, ↑ liver enzymes, jaundice, **hepatic coma** (preexisting liver disease)
GU: ↑ BUN/creatinine, bladder spasms, urinary frequency
Endo: Hyperglycemia, glycosuria
F&E: *Hypokalemia, hypochloremia,* hypovolemia, metabolic alkalosis, hypocalcemia, mag-

---

nesium depletion, ↑ ammonia, dehydration, hemoconcentration

Hema: Anemia, leukopenia, neutropenia, thrombocytopenia

Derm: Photosensitivity, rash, pruritus, urticaria, **exfoliative dermatitis**

Local: Injection site pain, thrombophlebitis

Misc: Exacerbation/precipitation of SLE, hyperuricemia, gout (rare)

TOXICITY/OVERDOSE

Symptoms: Hypotension, hypovolemia, circulatory collapse • Electrolyte loss: weakness, dizziness, confusion, vomiting, cramps • Dysrhythmias

Management: After recent ingestion, implement guidelines for management of acute overdose (Appendix I). • Support respiration as needed with O_2 and/or mechanical ventilation. • Administer IV fluids/replace electrolytes based on laboratory results; closely monitor sodium/potassium balance. • **Hypotension:** Elevate legs, administer IV fluids; if unresponsive to fluid replacement, use vasopressors (e.g., dopamine, norepinephrine). • Hemodialysis is ineffective.

INTERACTIONS

aminoglycosides ↑ Risk of ototoxicity; avoid concurrent use in renal dysfunction

amphotericin B Severe potassium depletion

antidiabetic agents Interference with glucose-lowering effects

beta-blockers Profound hypotension

calcium channel blockers Profound hypotension

corticosteroids Severe potassium depletion

digoxin Hypokalemia, hypomagnesemia, predisposition to digoxin toxicity, potentially fatal cardiac dysrhythmias

diuretics ↑ Diuretic effects; severe hypokalemia

hypotensive agents Synergistic effect with risk of hypotension

insulin Interference with glucose-lowering effects

lithium ↓ Renal clearance; lithium toxicity

NMBAs (e.g., pancuronium) Prolonged neuromuscular blockade

NSAIDs ↓ Furosemide effectiveness, ↓ renal function

phenytoin ↓ Diuresis

probenecid ↓ Uricosuric effects

sucralfate ↓ Furosemide effectiveness; separate administration by ≥2 hr

Y-SITE COMPATIBILITIES

Amikacin, famotidine, heparin, hydrocortisone sodium succinate, kanamycin, piperacillin-tazobactam, potassium chloride, tobramycin, vitamin B complex with C

Y-SITE INCOMPATIBILITIES

Diltiazem, dobutamine, dopamine, droperidol, epinephrine, esmolol, gentamicin, hydralazine, labetalol, meperidine, metoclopramide, milrinone, morphine, netilmicin, norepinephrine, ondansetron, any highly acidic (pH <5.5) solution

PATIENT CARE IMPLICATIONS

• Correct electrolyte/acid-base imbalance before initiating therapy.

 P pediatric   **G** geriatric   **V** Direct IV

- Potassium supplements are frequently necessary, especially in digitalized patients.
- Consider use of potassium-sparing sparing diuretic if other diuretics will be used concomitantly (e.g., spironolactone, amiloride).
- Adjust dose according to response to therapy, consider diuretic response, fluid balance, weight, electrolytes.
- If prerenal patients become progressively more oliguric or azotemic, discontinue use.
- Excessive diuresis may cause dehydration, vascular thrombosis, embolism, esp in older adults.
- Exposure to light may cause yellow discoloration. Do not administer discolored tablets or solutions.

IV • Precipitation is likely with all catecholamines (e.g., dopamine, dobutamine, epinephrine); avoid simultaneous infusion/injection via same IV line.

Vital signs/hemodynamics: **PO:** Monitor BP, UO carefully, especially with initial or high-dose therapy. • **IV:** Monitor VS, UO hourly. Consult physician for hypotension or oliguria. Monitor ECG as available. Note presence of PVCs, dysrhythmias, hypokalemic changes (i.e., flattened ST, T wave inversion, U wave). If present, check potassium level, correct as necessary. Digitalized patients should be carefully monitored for these and other dysrhythmias associated with digitalis toxicity.
- Hemodynamic monitoring is recommended for patients with severe CHF, cardiac failure associated with acute MI, cardiogenic shock, hemodynamic instability. Anticipate mild

reduction of left ventricular filling pressures/PCWP BEFORE onset of diuresis (usually within 5-15 min of IV administration). Monitor closely for overaggressive diuresis, excessive lowering of preload, resulting in reduced CO.

Physical assessment: Assess for improvement in pulmonary edema: clear breath sounds, reduced neck vein distention, unlabored breathing. • Assess for signs/symptoms of electrolyte imbalance: dysrhythmias, lethargy, headache, confusion, dizziness, weakness, muscle cramps, paresthesias, thirst, anorexia, vomiting. • Assess for perfusion/oxygenation deficit caused by hypovolemia: chest discomfort, decreased level of consciousness, activity intolerance, hypotension, dizziness.
- Assess hearing, particularly in older adults, with parenteral or high-dose therapy, with concurrent use of other ototoxic agents (e.g., aminoglycosides). • Weigh patient daily.

Laboratory tests: Monitor: Electrolytes (e.g., sodium, potassium, chloride, calcium, magnesium) especially important with IV/high-dose therapy
- BUN, creatinine • Bilirubin, liver enzymes • CBC • Blood glucose, especially in diabetic patients • Promptly correct imbalances. • **May cause:** Severe hypokalemia with dysrhythmias, ↑ ↓ effects of other drugs, including cardiac glycosides, antidiabetic agents

PATIENT/FAMILY TEACHING

Purpose of drug is to eliminate excess body fluid. • May cause dizziness, especially during initiation of therapy; use caution when changing positions, walking. IV/IM: Call for assistance before getting out of bed. • Report signs/symptoms of heart failure: breathing difficulty, palpitations, dizziness, activity intolerance, chest pain. • Report signs/symptoms of electrolyte imbalance: confusion, weakness, dizziness, fatigue, faintness, headache, paresthesias, muscle cramps, persistent thirst, nausea, vomiting.

Outpatient: Take medication in morning. Never double doses. • Continue taking medication as prescribed even if feeling better. Drug controls but does not cure hypertension/CHF. • If GI upset occurs, take with food or milk. Dosage may need adjustment because effectiveness of drug reduced when taken with food. • Take potassium supplements as prescribed, particularly if also taking digoxin. • Use sunscreen, wear protective clothing to prevent photosensitivity reactions. • Weigh twice/wk; report weight gain, edema. • **Diabetic patients:** Insulin dose may need adjustment.

AVAILABLE FORMS

Parenteral for IV/IM use. • Tablets • PO solution • Store all preparations in light-resistant containers.

gentamicin sulfate
(jen-ta-mye′sin)
Alcomicin ✤,
Cidomycin ✤, Garamycin,
Jenamicin, Storz-G

Classification: aminoglycoside antibiotic

USUAL DOSE

IV/IM, adults: 1 mg/kg q8h • **Severe infections:** Up to 5 mg/kg/24 hr q6-8h • **Extensive burns:** Altered pharmacokinetics may reduce serum levels; adjust dose to therapeutic levels. • **Renal insufficiency:** Reduce dose and/or frequency; adjust to therapeutic levels.
Unlabeled/investigational: 5-7 mg/kg once daily. Obtain random serum level 12 hr after initial dose; adjust subsequent dose as necessary
IV/IM, children >1 mo: 6-7.5 mg/kg/24 hr q8h
Intrathecal/intraventricular, adults: 4-8 mg as single daily dose in conjunction with parenteral therapy
Intrathecal/intraventricular, children >3 mo: 1-2 mg as single daily dose in conjunction with parenteral therapy

ADMINISTRATION

IM: Inject deep into large muscle mass (e.g., gluteus maximus, lateral thigh).
IV, intermit inf: Infuse prepared solution over 30 min.

PREPARATION

IV: Dilute single dose in 50-100 ml D₅W or 0.9% NaCl.
Compatible fluids: D₅W, 0.9% NaCl, LR, 1.5%/4.25% dextrose peritoneal dialysis solutions, 1.5% peritoneal dialysis solution with heparin 1,000 U/L
Stability: Reconstituted solution stable for 24 hr at room temperature

ACTIONS

Bactericidal; inhibits bacterial cell protein synthesis, causing cellular death • Active against

P pediatric   G geriatric   V Direct IV

many aerobic gram-negative bacteria, including *Pseudomonas aeruginosa, Escherichia coli, Enterobacter, Klebsiella, Proteus, Salmonella, Serratia, Shigella* • Active against some aerobic gram-positive bacteria, including *Staphylococcus aureus, S. epidermidis*

PHARMACOKINETICS

ROUTE	ONSET	PEAK	DURATION
IM	Rapid	30-90 min	Approx
IV	Immed	End infusion	6-8 hr

DISTRIBUTION

Widely distributed into extravascular fluids; CSF levels low

ELIMINATION

Filtered through glomeruli and excreted; half-life 2-3 hr, greatly prolonged with renal impairment

Therapeutic levels: Peak levels, 4-10 μg/ml; trough levels, 1-2 μg/ml

INDICATIONS

Treatment of serious gram-negative bacterial infections such as skin infections in burn patients; septicemia; bone, respiratory tract, complicated urinary tract, postop intraabdominal infections • Useful with strains resistant to other antibiotics • Frequently combined with extended-spectrum penicillin (e.g., piperacillin, ticarcillin) or other antibiotic for treatment of serious *Pseudomonas* infections, particularly in immunosuppressed patients • With penicillins for treatment of enterococcal endocarditis • Not indicated for gram-positive bacterial infections if other, less toxic antibiotics could be used

PRECAUTIONS/ CONTRAINDICATIONS

Precautions: Bacterial or fungal overgrowth possible • Systemic absorption with toxicity possible when used in irrigating solutions or for intrapleural/ peritoneal instillation • Some preparations contain sulfites, which can cause serious allergic reactions in susceptible individuals.

Use caution with: Renal impairment, older adults, preexisting hearing disorder, high-dose/ prolonged therapy, dehydration; ototoxicity/nephrotoxicity more likely • Preexisting neuromuscular disease, hypocalcemia, massive transfusions, general anesthesia, NMBAs; neurotoxicity more likely • Concurrent use of other ototoxic, neurotoxic, nephrotoxic agents

C Pregnancy category: Other aminoglycosides have caused fetal damage; use only if safer alternative unavailable and risks explained to woman.

Contraindications: Hypersensitivity to gentamicin, possibly other aminoglycosides

ADVERSE EFFECTS

CNS: 8th cranial nerve damage, *ototoxicity,* **permanent hearing loss** (rare), vertigo, dizziness, peripheral numbness/ twitching, weakness, neuromuscular blockade

Resp: **Respiratory paralysis/ apnea** (rare)

GI: Nausea, vomiting, ↑ liver enzymes

GU: *Nephrotoxicity,* tubular necrosis, **renal failure**

Local: Injection site irritation, pain

---

italic = common side effects   **bold** = life-threatening reactions

Misc: Hypersensitivity; superinfection, colonization

TOXICITY/OVERDOSE

Symptoms: Ototoxicity, nephrotoxicity • Neurotoxicity with neuromuscular blockade, possible respiratory paralysis, seizures

Management: Discontinue drug. • Initiate symptomatic/supportive measures, including airway management/ventilation. • Hemodialysis or peritoneal dialysis may be helpful.

INTERACTIONS

amphotericin B ↑ Risk of nephrotoxicity

anticoagulants, PO Additive prolongation of PT

cephalosporins (e.g., cephalothin) ↑ Risk of nephrotoxicity; synergistic antibacterial activity

diuretics ↑ Risk of ototoxicity, nephrotoxicity

ethacrynic acid ↑ Risk of ototoxicity, nephrotoxicity; avoid concurrent use

NMBAs ↑ Risk of respiratory paralysis

NSAIDs ↑ Risk of nephrotoxicity

penicillins Synergistic antibacterial activity

Y-SITE COMPATIBILITIES

Acyclovir, amiodarone, atracurium, diltiazem, enalaprilat, esmolol, famotidine, fluconazole, hydromorphone, insulin, labetalol, magnesium sulfate, meperidine, morphine, multivitamins, ondansetron, pancuronium, vecuronium

Y-SITE INCOMPATIBILITIES

Cephalosporins, furosemide, heparin, hetastarch, penicillins

PATIENT CARE IMPLICATIONS

• Obtain specimens for culture and sensitivity before initiating antibiotic therapy.
• To avoid drug incompatibility/interaction, administer at separate site; stagger schedules when penicillins, cephalosporins also prescribed.
• IV route necessary for severe infections or when shock present.

Vital signs/hemodynamics: Monitor VS for indicators of infection, complications. • Carefully monitor UO; evaluate I&O ratio. Decreasing volume, cloudy or pink urine may indicate nephrotoxicity. Keep patient well hydrated by oral or parenteral fluids of sufficient volume to produce adequate **G** UO. Older, debilitated, seriously ill, or renal-impaired patients are at greatest risk. • As available, monitor CVP, PCWP, central hemodynamics to optimize fluid volume balance.

Physical assessment: Assess for improvement in primary infection or symptoms of super/suprainfection: appearance of sputum, urine, stool, wound drainage; presence of fever, candidiasis, vaginitis; WBC. • Assess for evidence of neurotoxicity: numbness, tingling, muscle twitching, weakness; respiratory depression. • Assess hearing before initiating therapy. Monitor at intervals for symptoms of ototoxicity: tinnitus, roaring in ears, hearing loss, dizziness, vertigo, nausea; particularly important with advanced age, preexisting hearing disorder, renal impairment, high-dose/prolonged therapy.

P pediatric   **G** geriatric   **V** Direct IV

Laboratory tests: Peak/ trough levels: Draw peak levels 30 min after administration complete; draw trough levels just before next dose. Therapeutic peak levels, 4-10 µg/ml; trough levels, 1-2 µg/ml • Narrow therapeutic range requires close monitoring, particularly **G** with advanced age, high-dose therapy, renal insufficiency.
Monitor: Electrolytes, liver enzymes, PT, PTT, CBC with differential. • Urinalysis, BUN, creatinine, creat. cl. Increase hydration if signs of renal irritation (e.g., casts, proteinuria); reduce dose or discontinue if evidence of renal dysfunction.

PATIENT/FAMILY TEACHING

Purpose of drug is to limit growth of infection-causing bacteria. • Report rash, itching, diarrhea, fever, vaginal itching or discharge, dizziness, hearing difficulties.

AVAILABLE FORMS

Parenteral for IV/IM use • Parenteral for IV/IM use in children • Preservative-free preparation for intrathecal use • Premixed solution for IV infusion • Ophthalmic ointment, solution • Topical cream, ointment

---

glucagon HCl
(gloo'kah-gon)

Classification: Hormone

USUAL DOSE

1 U = 1 mg
IV/IM/SC, adults: Hypoglycemia: 0.5-1 mg; may administer 1-2 additional doses at 5–20-min intervals if needed; give IV dextrose for failure to respond to glucagon. • **Diagnostic aid to GI radiography:** 1-2 mg IM or 0.25-2 mg IV
P IV/IM/SC, children: Hypoglycemia: 0.025 mg/kg; may administer 1-2 additional doses q5-20min if needed; give IV dextrose for failure to respond to glucagon.

ADMINISTRATION

▼ Direct IV: Inject at rate of 1 mg/min.

PREPARATION

IV/IM/SC: Dilute each unit (mg) with 1 ml of diluent provided by manufacturer. • For dilution of doses >2 mg, use sterile water. • Use immediately after preparation.
Compatible fluid: D_5W

ACTIONS

Pancreatic hormones extracted from alpha cells of islets of Langerhans • Raises blood glucose by stimulating rapid conversion of hepatic glycogen to glucose • Enhances peripheral utilization of glucose • Relaxes GI smooth muscle, inhibits pancreatic/gastric secretions • Positive inotropic, chronotropic effects similar to epinephrine

PHARMACOKINETICS

ROUTE	ONSET	PEAK	DURATION
IV	Rapid	<30 min	1-2 hr
ELIMINATION			

Metabolized in liver; half-life 3-10 min

INDICATIONS

Acute hypoglycemia, particularly when IV dextrose cannot be administered • Ineffective if hepatic glycogen stores depleted (e.g., chronic hypoglycemia,

---

starvation, adrenal insufficiency)
• Diagnostic aid in radiographic exams of GI tract when hypotonic state desired
Unlabeled/investigational: Cardiac stimulation to counter myocardial depressant effects associated with beta-blocker overdose

PRECAUTIONS/ CONTRAINDICATIONS

Precautions: *Not a substitute for IV dextrose in emergency situations when hypoglycemia suspected* • Prolonged hypoglycemia may cause profound, permanent cortical damage; IV dextrose required for deep coma, failure to respond to glucagon. • Not as effective in children with diabetes; administer carbohydrate as soon as condition allows.
Use caution with: Insulinoma • Pheochromocytoma
C Pregnancy category: Use only if safer alternative unavailable.
Contraindications: Hypersensitivity to beef or pork proteins • Hypersensitivity to glycerin/phenol contained in diluent

ADVERSE EFFECTS

GI: *Nausea, vomiting*
Misc: Hypersensitivity reactions

INTERACTIONS

anticoagulants, PO Potentiates anticoagulant effects
ß-blockers Transient ↑ in BP/HR; ↓ glucagon effectiveness

Y-SITE INCOMPATIBILITIES

Solutions containing sodium chloride, potassium chloride, calcium chloride

PATIENT CARE IMPLICATIONS

• Not substitute for IV dextrose, which must be used for deep coma or failure to respond to glucagon.
• When used for acute hypoglycemia, anticipate return to consciousness within 5-20 min. Follow administration with supplemental carbohydrates as soon as condition allows.
• Vomiting may occur on awakening; position patient on side, have suction immediately available.
• When used as smooth muscle relaxant, as effective as anticholingergics but with fewer side effects.
Vital signs/hemodynamics: Monitor VS q5-15min until fully awake/stable.
Physical assessment: Monitor level of consciousness; expect awakening within 5-20 min.
• Assess nutritional, metabolic status; ineffective if hepatic glycogen stores depleted (e.g., chronic hypoglycemia, starvation, adrenal insufficiency); glucose indicated if glycogen stores depleted.

PATIENT/FAMILY TEACHING

Purpose of medication is to cause increase in blood sugar.
Home glucagon therapy: Take oral glucose as soon as symptoms of hypoglycemia occur. Use glucagon only if patient unable to swallow because of decrease in mental status.
• Be sure to use correct technique when preparing/administering injection. (Have family member return demonstration of correct technique.) • Keep patient turned on side until fully

awake; vomiting, aspiration possible. • Give patient oral glucose as soon as fully awake, able to swallow. • Check expiration date regularly; replace outdated medication. • Wear Medic-Alert ID bracelet; carry sugar source at all times.

AVAILABLE FORMS

Parenteral for IV/IM/SC injection

---

haloperidol
(ha-loe-per′idole)
haloperidol decanoate
Haldol

Classifications: Antipsychotic, tranquilizer, butyrophenone

USUAL DOSE

Dose requires individual adjustment; use lowest effective dose; lower dose if other CNS depressants also used.
PO tablets/solution, adults: 0.5-2.0 mg bid-tid • Severe symptoms/resistance: 3.0-5.0 mg bid-tid • Up to 100 mg/day sometimes necessary
PO tablets/solution, older adults: 0.5-2.0 mg bid-tid; adjust gradually.
PO tablets/solution, children 3-12 yr: 0.05-0.15 mg/kg/ 24 hr in 2-3 evenly divided doses; adjust gradually.
IM lactate, adults: 2-5 mg q4-8h; may repeat q1h if necessary • Use lower dose range for older adults. • Convert to PO therapy as soon as possible.
IM decanoate (long-acting), adults: 10-15 times PO daily dose q4wk • Maximum dose, 100 mg

IV, adults (unlabeled/investigational): Use haloperidol lactate. • Mild agitation: 0.5-2 mg • Moderate agitation: 2-10 mg • Severe agitation: ≥10-20 mg • May repeat q30min or more often until acute agitation relieved • Repeat effective dose q1-4h as needed for onset of agitation. • Continuous infusion of 3-25 mg/hr has been used • Concurrent IV lorazepam enhances effects. • Convert to PO therapy as soon as possible.

ADMINISTRATION

Check label carefully—for IV administration use haloperidol lactate only; haloperidol decanoate contains oil, must never be given IV.
Direct IV, adults (unlabeled/investigational): Inject each dose of ≤5 mg over 1 min • Dilution not necessary • If heparin lock used, flush with ≥2 ml 0.9% NaCl to clear heparin solution before and after injection.
IV inf, adults (unlabeled/investigational): Infuse over 30 min. If heparin lock used, flush with ≥2 ml 0.9% NaCl to clear heparin solution before and after infusion. • Cont inf has been used.

PREPARATION

IV inf, adults (unlabeled/investigational): Dilute in 50-100 ml compatible solution • Avoid direct skin contact with parenteral solution.
Compatible fluids: D_5W, 0.9% NaCl

ACTIONS

Potent dopamine receptor antagonist; blocks central effects of dopamine • Causes tranquiliza-

---

tion, sedation; has antiemetic and weak central anticholinergic effects • Does not block dopamine-mediated increases in renal blood flow • Less likely to cause marked sedation, hypotension, hypothermia than chlorpromazine • When IV route used in critically ill patients, has fewer effects on BP, HR, RR, SVR, PAP than benzodiazepines (e.g., diazepam)

PHARMACOKINETICS

ROUTE	ONSET	PEAK	DURATION
PO	30-60 min	2-6 hr	Days-wk
IM*	10 min	30-45 min	Days-wk
IV	Immed	Rapid	Days-wk

DISTRIBUTION

Distributed to many body tissues, highest concentration in liver; 92% protein bound

ELIMINATION

Metabolized mainly by liver, slowly excreted by kidneys

*Haloperidol lactate.

INDICATIONS

Reduce hallucinations, autonomic hyperactivity, other symptoms in schizophrenia, psychotic disorders • Symptomatic control of tics, vocalizations associated with Tourette's disorder • Severe behavioral **P** problems in children manifested by extreme hyperexcitability or hyperactivity
Unlabeled/investigational:
Prevention/control of nausea/vomiting associated with cancer chemotherapy; relief of intractable hiccups; IV route widely used to control acute agitation or delirium in medically ill patients • Useful in critically ill patients because of relative potency but mild cardiopulmonary effects; IV preferred over IM route because of more predicta-

ble absorption, lack of interference with muscle enzyme studies, fewer extrapyramidal side effects.

PRECAUTIONS/ CONTRAINDICATIONS

Precautions: Risk of serious adverse CNS effects, including irreversible tardive dyskinesia, potentially fatal neuroleptic malignant syndrome • Antiemetic effects may complicate diagnosis of disorders when vomiting a prominent feature (e.g., intestinal obstruction, Reye's syndrome). • Tablets may contain tartrazine dye (FD&C yellow no. 5), which can cause allergic reactions, especially in patients with aspirin sensitivity.
Use caution with: Seizure disorders; may precipitate seizures • CNS depressants, severe CV disease, hepatic/renal dis- **G** ease, older adults, debilitation, glaucoma, prostatic hypertrophy, exposure to organophosphate insecticides, temperature extremes, thermoregulatory failure; reduced dose indicated • COPD, asthma, acute respiratory infections, limited ventilatory reserve; may depress ventilatory drive • Thyrotoxicosis; severe neurotoxicity possible
c Pregnancy category: Animal studies show fetal damage at high doses; human risk not established; use only if safer alternative unavailable.
Contraindications: Hypersensitivity to haloperidol • Severe CNS depression, coma • Parkinsonian syndrome • Reye's syn- **P** drome • Children <3 yr

ADVERSE EFFECTS

CNS: *Drowsiness,* insomnia, anxiety, euphoria, paradoxical

P pediatric   **G** geriatric   **V** Direct IV

excitation, weakness, cata-
tonic-like state, **seizures,** extrapyramidal reactions: *parkinsonian signs/symptoms* (e.g.,
drooling, tremors, fixed stare);
dystonia (e.g., neck/back muscle rigidity, hyperreflexia, difficulty swallowing/talking);
feelings of motor restlessness;
tardive dyskinesia (e.g.,
tongue protrusion, involuntary
chewing motions); **neuroleptic
malignant syndrome** (rare)
characterized by hyperthermia,
severe hypertonicity, decreased
level of consciousness, autonomic instability (tachycardia,
dysrhythmias, BP instability)
Resp: Laryngospasm, bronchospasm, hyperventilation
CV: Hypotension, tachycardia,
dizziness, ECG changes including QT interval and **torsades de pointes**
GI: Anorexia, constipation, diarrhea, nausea, vomiting
Endo: Gynecomastia, hyper/
hypoglycemia, hyponatremia
Hema: Transient mild leukocy-
tosis, leukopenia, anemia
Derm: Rash, hair loss, photosensitivity, contact dermatitis
(parenteral formulation, PO
concentrate)
Misc: Autonomic effects, including dry mouth, blurred vision, urinary retention, diaphoresis, priapism; visual
disturbances; hyperpyrexia

TOXICITY/OVERDOSE
Symptoms (acute toxicity):
Severe extrapyramidal symptoms • Hypotension • Sedation,
respiratory depression, coma
• QT interval prolongation, torsade de pointes (atypical ventricular tachycardia) • Toxicity
more likely with concurrent in-

gestion of alcohol, other CNS
depressants
Management: After recent ingestion, implement guidelines
for management of acute overdose (Appendix I). • Maintain
airway/support ventilation; administer IV fluids. • Hypotension: Elevate legs, administer
IV fluids, use vasopressor (dopamine, norepinephrine) as necessary for hypotension unresponsive to volume replacement. Do not use epinephrine
because haloperidol antagonizes
alpha-adrenergic effects, unopposed beta activity causes profound hypotension. • **Extrapyramidal reactions:** Use
diphenhydramine or benztropine
mesylate (Cogentin).

INTERACTIONS
alcohol ↑ CNS depression
anticholinergics ↑ Intraocular
pressure
anticoagulants ↓ Anticoagulation
barbiturates ↑ CNS depression
benzodiazepines Synergistic sedation
epinephrine Profound hypotension
lithium Acute encephalopathic
syndrome
opioid analgesics ↑ CNS depression
propranolol Bradycardia, hypotension
sedatives CNS depression

Y-SITE COMPATIBILITIES
Cimetidine, dobutamine, dopamine, famotidine, lidocaine, nitroglycerine, norepinephrine, ondansetron, phenylephrine,
theophylline

H

---

italic = common side effects   **bold** = life-threatening reactions

Y-SITE INCOMPATIBILITIES

Buprenorphine, cefepime, fluconazole, foscarnet, heparin, piperacillin-tazobactam

PATIENT CARE IMPLICATIONS

• Risk of serious adverse CNS effects increase with high doses/long-term use; use smallest effective dose, shortest possible duration.

G • Older adults more likely to develop extrapyramidal reactions, paradoxical excitation, other adverse reactions; monitor frequently.

• Skin contact with PO concentrate/solution for injection may cause contact dermatitis.

• May cause drowsiness, mild hypotension, especially during first week of therapy; use appropriate safety precautions according to patient condition; when possible, administer hs.

• Large quantities should not be prescribed for patients with severe depression, suicidal tendencies, history of substance abuse.

• Use IM route only in urgent/emergency situations or when PO route unacceptable (e.g., vomiting, NPO status); convert to PO therapy as soon as possible.

Direct IV (unlabeled/investigational)

• IV preferred route for critically ill patients because of more predictable absorption, lack of interference with muscle enzyme studies, fewer extrapyramidal side effects; minimal cardiopulmonary effects relative to many other sedatives.

• Monitor closely during injection for adverse effects (hypotension, tachycardia, ECG changes). Titrate dose for relief of acute agitation. Once effective dose established, administer as soon as patient begins to show signs of anxiety/agitation. Patient should remain in bed for at least 1 hr, requires assistance with initial ambulation.

• Have resuscitation equipment immediately available.

• Administer with lorazepam for synergistic sedative effects.

G **Older adults** • Closely monitor for adverse effects, including lethargy, ↓ thirst sensation. Complications include: dehydration, impaired ventilation, bronchopneumonia; periodically assess need for continued therapy.

Vital signs/hemodynamics: Monitor VS frequently in heavily sedated patients (e.g., those also receiving opiates).

Direct IV: Monitor BP, HR, RR during and frequently after administration. • Monitor ECG for tachycardia, prolongation of QT interval, dysrhythmias. • Stop injection, consult physician for widening of QRS or prolonged QT interval. • Use continuous pulse oximetry for heavily sedated patients.

Physical assessment: Assess neurologic status for excessive sedation, dizziness, impaired physical coordination. Reduce dose as necessary. • Assess for hypoventilation in patients with history of COPD, cardiopulmonary disease.

Laboratory tests: Monitor: Liver enzymes • BUN/creatinine • CBC

PATIENT/FAMILY TEACHING

Purpose of medication is to reduce agitation or hallucinations. • May cause dizziness, drowsiness; call for assistance when

---

P pediatric   **G** geriatric   **V** Direct IV

getting out of bed, walking; change positions slowly. These reactions are less likely to occur after first week of therapy. • Encourage frequent oral hygiene, use of sugarless hard candy or gum to relieve dry mouth. • Immediately report muscle twitching, tremors, involuntary muscle movement.

Outpatient: Full effects may not be apparent for several weeks. Do not increase dose or stop taking medicine without consulting physician. • Avoid driving and other activities requiring mental alertness or physical coordination until individual response to medication apparent. • May contribute to development of heatstroke; avoid hot weather, seek air conditioning. • Avoid using alcohol or other drugs that cause sedation while taking this medication. • Inform nurse or physician if you may be pregnant or are considering pregnancy. • Avoid prolonged exposure to sunlight; wear protective clothing, use sunscreen.

AVAILABLE FORMS

Tablets • PO concentrate • Parenteral solution (haloperidol lactate) for IM/IV use • Oil-based parenteral solution (haloperidol decanoate) for IM use only

---

heparin sodium
(hep'a-rin)
Liquaemin

Classification: Anticoagulant

USUAL DOSE

Thrombotic disorders/full-dose therapy: Continuous IV infusion preferred to minimize complications; dose adjusted to maintain APTT at 1.5-2 times control value • Weight-based dosing may be used.

IV, cont inf, adults: Initial loading dose of 5,000 U, then continuous infusion of 800-1,600 U/hr (Appendix Q)

IV, intermit inf, adults: Initial loading dose of 10,000 U, then 5,000-10,000 U q4-6h

SC, adults: Initial loading dose of 5,000 U IV and 10,000-20,000 U, SC, then 8,000-10,000 q8h or 15,000-20,000 U q12h

IV, cont inf, children: Initial loading dose of 50 U/kg, then continuous infusion of 25 U/kg/hr

IV, intermit inf, children: Initial loading dose of 100 U/kg, then 50-100 U/kg q4h

Prophylaxis of postop thromboembolism: SC, adults: Preop, 5,000 U 2 hr before surgery • Postop, 5,000 U q8-12h for ≥5-7 days until full mobility

DIC: IV, adults 50-100 U/kg q4h • Discontinue after 4-8 hr if no improvement.

IV, children: 25-50 U/kg q4h • Discontinue after 4-8 hr if no improvement.

ADMINISTRATION

SC: Use concentrated solution and 25–27-gauge ⅜–⅝-inch needle. • Check dose for accuracy with another licensed nurse. • Administer deeply into fatty tissue of abdomen but not within 2 inches of umbilicus or above iliac crest. • Do not aspirate or massage. • Rotate sites frequently.

Direct IV: Inject initial dose slowly at rate of 1,000 U over 1 min (in event of allergic reac-

H

tion). • Inject subsequent doses at rate of ≤5,000 U over 1 min. • Check dose for accuracy with another licensed nurse.

IV, intermit inf: Administer initial dose no more rapidly than 1,000 U/min (in event of allergic reaction). • Infuse subsequent doses over 10-20 min.

IV, cont inf: Use infusion pump or other rate-controlling device.

PREPARATION

IV, intermit: Dilute in 50-100 ml 0.9% NaCl or D₅W.

IV, cont inf: Dilute in compatible solution for usual concentration of 10-50 U/ml. • Mix thoroughly by inverting at least 6 times.

DILUTION (U/1,000 ml)	CONCENTRATION (U/ml)
10,000	10
20,000	20
40,000	40
50,000	50

Compatible fluids: 0.9% NaCl, 0.45% NaCl, LR, D₅W
Stability: Slight yellow discoloration does not affect potency. Avoid exposure to heat.

ACTIONS

Promotes rapid anticoagulation by combining with antithrombin III to prevent conversion of prothrombin to thrombin • Higher doses inactivate thrombin, prevent conversion of fibrinogen to fibrin. • Low doses inhibit thrombus formation; higher doses prevent extension of existing thrombi. • Does not dissolve established clots

PHARMACOKINETICS

ROUTE	ONSET	PEAK	DURATION
SC	20-60 min	2-4 hr	
IV	Immed	Rapid	2-5 days

DISTRIBUTION
Extensively plasma bound

ELIMINATION
Metabolized in liver, RE system, kidneys; excreted in urine; half-life 1-2 hr

INDICATIONS

Prevention/treatment of venous thrombosis and its extension, pulmonary embolism; embolism related to atrial fibrillation/mitral valve disease; peripheral arterial embolism • Diagnosis/treatment of DIC • Adjunct in treatment of coronary occlusion associated with acute MI • Prevention of clotting during hemodialysis, vascular/cardiac surgery • Maintenance of IV, arterial catheter patency • Several days of concurrent therapy necessary when converting from heparin to PO anticoagulant (e.g., warfarin) therapy

Unlabeled/investigational:
Adjunct with antiplatelet therapy (e.g., aspirin) in prevention of reocclusion after thrombolytic therapy during acute MI; prophylaxis of left ventricular thrombi immediately after MI; with coumarin therapy in patients with TIAs to reduce risk of recurrent TIA, CVA

PRECAUTIONS/CONTRAINDICATIONS

Precautions: Many strengths available; read label, check dose carefully. • Potentially fatal bleeding complications possible • May cause "white clot syndrome"—heparin-induced thrombosis (HIT), thrombocytopenia • Derived from animal tis-

---

sue; hypersensitivity reactions, anaphylaxis possible • Avoid any IM injections; bleeding, hematomas possible. • Commercial preparations may contain sulfites, which can cause serious allergic reactions.

Use caution with: Bleeding disorders or when bleeding likely: hemophilia, thrombocytopenia, subacute bacterial endocarditis, dissecting aneurysm, GI bleeding or ulcer disease, ulcerative colitis, tube drainage of stomach/intestines, visceral carcinoma, diverticulitis, menstruation, threatened abortion, severe renal/hepatic disease, uncontrolled hypertension, after spinal tap/spinal anesthesia, surgery of eye, brain, spinal cord • Older adults; ↑ risk of bleeding

c Pregnancy category: Use with caution and only if safer alternative unavailable.

Contraindications: Hypersensitivity to heparin, specific animal protein in preparation; check labeling. • Uncontrollable bleeding, except DIC • Severe thrombocytopenia • Severe hepatic disease with hypoprothrombinemia • Inability to obtain blood coagulation tests regularly, except with low-dose therapy.

ADVERSE EFFECTS

EENT: *Gingival bleeding, nosebleeds*
CV: Vasospastic reactions, local/generalized; **arterial thromboses** (rare)
Endo: **Adrenal hemorrhage, ovarian hemorrhage**
Hema: **Hemorrhage,** *bruising, ecchymosis, hematoma,* **thrombocytopenia**
Derm: Cutaneous necrosis; hematoma (SC)

Local: SC injection site irritation, hematoma
Misc: Hypersensitivity reactions, including chills, fever, urticaria, bronchospasm, shock, anaphylaxis

TOXICITY/OVERDOSE

Symptoms: Hematuria, melena, petechiae, ecchymoses • Gum/mucous membrane bleeding • Intracranial, GI, other bleeding
Management: Discontinue drug • Short half-life; no other treatment may be necessary. • **Severe bleeding:** Administer protamine sulfate to neutralize heparin immediately. • Packed RBCs used to replace significant blood loss

INTERACTIONS

alcohol ↑ Risk of gastric bleeding; additive prolongation of bleeding time
anticoagulants, oral ↑ Risk of bleeding
aspirin ↑ Anticoagulation
nitroglycerin ↓ Anticoagulation; check APTT when initiating/discontinuing IV nitroglycerin
NSAIDs ↑ Risk of bleeding
streptokinase Partial resistance to anticoagulation; ↑ doses may be necessary

Y-SITE COMPATIBILITIES

Aminophylline, ampicillin, atracurium, atropine, calcium gluconate, cephalothin, cephapirin, cimetidine, digoxin, dobutamine (in 0.9% NaCl), dopamine, enalaprilat, epinephrine, esmolol, famotidine, fentanyl, furosemide, hydralazine, insulin (regular), isoproterenol, labetalol, lidocaine, magnesium sulfate, meperidine, methacillin, metoclopramide, morphine, nitroglycerin, norepinephrine, ondansetron, oxacillin, pancuroniam, penicillin G potassium, pentazocine, piperacillin, tazobactam, prednisolone, procainamide, prochlorperazine, propranolol, ranitidine, sodium bicarbonate, streptokinase, vecuronium

Y-SITE INCOMPATIBILITIES

Alteplase, amiodarone, ciprofloxacin, codeine, diazepam, dobutamine (in D_5W), gentamicin, haloperidol, phenytoin, promethazine, tobramycin, vancomycin

PATIENT CARE IMPLICATIONS

• Inform all personnel caring for patient of anticoagulant therapy. Place highly visible written notice in patient's room.
• Administer initial IV dose slowly (see Administration); monitor for hypersensitivity reaction: fever, chills, urticaria, wheezing, hypotension. If symptoms develop, stop injection; consult physician.
• Avoid unnecessary venipuncture, invasive procedures, IM injections. Apply manual pressure to venipuncture sites until bleeding stops.
• Monitor for heparin-induced thrombosis (HIT), thrombocytopenia. Discontinue immediately for thrombocytopenia or evidence of new thrombosis.
• Avoid arterial/venous invasive procedures in areas inaccessible to manual compression (e.g., internal jugular, subclavian).
• IV nitroglycerin may bind with heparin and ↓ anticoagulant activity. Exaggerated heparin effects may occur when nitroglycerin is discontinued. Monitor closely and check APTT 6 hr after significant change or discontinuation of nitroglycerin.
• To minimize heparin incompatibility reactions, flush heparin locks with 0.9% NaCl before and after any drug administration.

PHYSICAL ASSESSMENT

Assess for unusual bleeding: petechiae, ecchymosis, bleeding from gums/mucous membranes, excessive bleeding from superficial injury. • Assess for occult bleeding: altered mentation, paralysis, headache, joint pain, shortness of breath, unexplained swelling, hypotension, shock.
• Note blood in urine, other body fluids. Check emesis, stool for occult blood. Discontinue heparin if bleeding complications occur. • Assess for thromboembolic complications of HIT —skin necrosis, impaired perfusion of extremity, acute MI, pulmonary embolism, TIA/CVA symptoms.

LABORATORY TESTS

Monitor: APTT before initiating therapy, at 4–6 hr intervals until stable, then daily; maintain range of 1.5-2 times control value • CBC, particularly platelet count, Hct
May cause: Prolonged PT • Elevated AST, ALT

PATIENT/FAMILY TEACHING

Purpose of medication is to prevent unwanted clots from forming. • Immediately report unusual bruising, skin discoloration, blood in urine/stools, vomiting of blood, bleeding from venipunctures, nose, mouth, gums. • Use soft toothbrush, electric razor; avoid activities that may cause injury.
• Inform laboratory personnel,

---

other health care workers of anti-coagulant therapy.

AVAILABLE FORMS

Single-use prefilled syringes • Vials for multidose use or IV admixture • Premixed flush solution • Prepared solution for IV infusion

hepatitis B immune globulin (HBIG)
H-BIG, Hep-B-Gammagee, Hyperhep

Classifications: Serum, immune globulin

USUAL DOSE

P IM, adults/children: 0.06 ml/kg (3-5 ml in adults) as soon as possible after exposure preferably within 24 hr; initiate hepatitis B virus (HBV) vaccine series at same time; administer at separate site.

P IM, neonates: Perinatal exposure: 0.5 ml within 12 hr of birth; initiate HBV vaccine at same time; administer at separate site.

ADMINISTRATION

FOR IM USE ONLY; DO NOT ADMINISTER SC, INTRADERMALLY, IV.

P IM, adults/older children: Inject deeply into deltoid or anterolateral thigh muscle. Use gluteal muscle for large volumes in adults or when multiple injections required.

P IM, neonates/small children: Inject into anterolateral thigh muscle.

ACTIONS

Sterile solution of antibody-containing globulins prepared from plasma of donors with high titers of antibody to HBV • Provides passive immunity by increasing antibody titer, neutralizing HBV

PHARMACOKINETICS

ROUTE	ONSET	PEAK	DURATION
IM	1-6 days	3-11 days	2-6 mo

DISTRIBUTION
Probably crosses placenta
ELIMINATION
Half-life 21 days

INDICATIONS

Passive immunity, prevention of infection after known exposure to HBV or hepatitis B surface antigen (HBsAg)–positive body fluids • Provides rapid, temporary immunity • NOT indicated for acute HBV or chronic active HBV infections

PRECAUTIONS/ CONTRAINDICATIONS

Precautions: Inadvertent IV administration may cause serious allergic reaction. Aspirate before injecting to verify IM injection.
Use caution with: Bleeding disorders; IM injection may cause bleeding.
C **Pregnancy category:** Specific effects on fetus unknown; use only if clearly indicated.
Contraindications: Hypersensitivity to immune globulin, thimerosal • Selective IgA deficiencies; may cause severe anaphylaxis • Clinical manifestations of HBV; is ineffective

ADVERSE EFFECTS

MS: Arthralgia
Derm: Urticaria, rash, pruritus
Misc: Fever; pain, tenderness, swelling, redness at injection site; repeated injections may

H

cause allergic response; **ana-phylaxis** (rare)

INTERACTIONS

HBV vaccine Avoid administration in same syringe or at same site

vaccines, live (measles, mumps, rubella, oral polio) May interfere with immune response to live vaccines; may need to defer administration for 3 mo after H-BIG

PATIENT CARE IMPLICATIONS

• Determine time of exposure to infection. Administer as soon as possible after exposure to HBV.
• Have epinephrine, antihistamine, resuscitation equipment immediately available at time of injection.
• *Do not mix in same syringe or administer in same site as HBV vaccine.*
• Record lot number of immune globulin according to institutional guidelines.
Vital signs/hemodynamics: Monitor BP, HR, RR, temperature before and 30 min after injection.
Physical assessment: Assess for allergic/anaphylactic reaction: chills, fever, sweating, rash, itching, laryngeal edema, wheezing. • **Outpatients:** Observe for at least 30 min after injection.
Laboratory tests: Source of exposure may be tested for HBsAg if status unknown.
• Previously vaccinated, exposed individuals may be tested for antibody to HBsAg (anti-HBs). If inadequate, immune globulin is indicated. • Exposed sexual contacts may be tested

for antibody to hepatitis B core antigen (anti-HBc). If negative, immune globulin is indicated.

PATIENT/FAMILY TEACHING

Provides rapid temporary protection from HBV infection; for long-term protection, HBV vaccination series is necessary.
• Pain, tenderness, redness, swelling at injection site may occur. • Immediately report chills, fever, sweating, itching, difficulty breathing.

AVAILABLE FORMS

Vials for single-dose/multidose IM use • Prefilled syringes for single-dose IM use
Storage: Refrigerate at 2°-8° C (35°-46° F); do not freeze.

hepatitis B virus vaccine, recombinant
Engerix-B, Recombivax HB, Recombivax HB Dialysis Formulation

Classification: Vaccine

USUAL DOSE
Preexposure prophylaxis:
Total of 3 doses. • Follow initial dose with 2nd dose 1 mo later; give 3rd dose 6 mo after initial dose. • 4-dose series may be used for dialysis/immunocompromised patients.
Postexposure prophylaxis:
Total of 3 doses • Give initial dose within 7 days of exposure.
• Administer 1st dose with hepatitis B immune globulin (HBIG) but at separate sites. • Follow with 2nd dose 1 mo later; give 3rd dose 6 mo after initial dose.
Recombivax HB: IM, adults: 10 µg

IM, adults, dialysis/immuno-compromise: 40 µg
Ⓟ IM, children 11-19 yr: 5 µg
Ⓟ IM, neonates/children <11 yr: 2.5 µg
Engerix-B: IM, adults ≥20 yr: 20 µg.
IM, adults, dialysis/immuno-compromise: Two 20 µg doses in separate sites
Ⓟ IM, neonates/children ≤19 yr: 10 µg

ADMINISTRATION

Ⓟ **IM, adults/children:** Shake vigorously before withdrawing.
• Inject into deltoid; vaccine may fail if inadvertently injected into fatty tissue of buttocks.
Ⓟ **IM, infants:** Shake vigorously before withdrawing. • Inject into anterolateral thigh muscle.
• May be administered SC with bleeding disorders (e.g., thrombocytopenia, hemophilia) • DO NOT ADMINISTER IV.

ACTIONS

Vaccine prepared from yeast cultures using recombinant methods • Produces active immunity by stimulating production of serum antibodies to hepatitis B surface antigen (anti-HBs) • Anti-HBs neutralizes hepatitis B virus (HBV), prevents infection with HBV and delta virus (dependent on HBV). • Protective levels of anti-HBs seen in 89%-96% of
Ⓟ healthy children/adults who complete immunization series
• Seroconversion rates lower with hemodialysis, immunosuppression

PHARMACOKINETICS

ROUTE	ONSET	PEAK	DURATION
IM	2 wk	6 mo	>3 yr

INDICATIONS

In high-risk individuals to provide active immunity against infection with HBV, delta virus
• Partial list of individuals at risk includes recipients of multiple blood transfusions; immunosuppressed/cancer patients; organ transplant recipients; residents/staff of institutions for developmentally disabled; health care personnel with potential contact with blood, body secretions; prehospital emergency personnel; injecting drug users; male homosexuals; heterosexuals with multiple sex partners; male/female prostitutes; individuals traveling to areas endemic for HBV; neonates born to HBsAg-positive women (consult CDC guidelines or other specialized reference for complete listing of high-risk categories)
• With HBIG for postexposure prophylaxis • Not indicated for HBsAg carriers.

PRECAUTIONS/CONTRAINDICATIONS

Precautions: May cause serious allergic reaction, including anaphylaxis • Hemodialysis, immunosuppressed patients require higher doses, may not have optimal response to immunization.
Use caution with: Thrombocytopenia, hemophilia, other bleeding disorder; IM injection may cause bleeding. • Febrile or severely ill patients; defer immunization, because febrile or adverse reaction may pose significant risk.

H

---

c Pregnancy category: Not contraindicated, but fetal risk unknown; may be used if clearly needed
Contraindications: Hypersensitivity to HBV vaccine, yeast, other vaccine components

ADVERSE EFFECTS

CNS: *Headache, dizziness,* somnolence, irritability
Resp: Upper respiratory symptoms, pharyngitis
GI: Nausea, vomiting, diarrhea
MS: Arthralgia; myalgia; pain/stiffness in back, neck, shoulder
Local: *Soreness, tenderness, erythema,* induration, pruritus, ecchymosis, swelling, burning, nodule formation at injection site
Misc: *Fatigue, malaise, weakness, fever,* delayed hypersensitivity reaction, **anaphylaxis** (rare)

INTERACTIONS

chemotherapy, ↓ Immune response; ↑ dose of vaccine required
corticosteroids ↓ Immune response; ↑ dose of vaccine required
HBV immune globulin Avoid administration in same syringe at same site

PATIENT CARE IMPLICATIONS

• Determine previous vaccination history, reactions.
• Have epinephrine, antihistamine, resuscitation equipment immediately available at time of injection.
Vital signs/hemodynamics: Monitor BP, HR, RR, temperature before and 30 min after injection.

Physical assessment: Assess for allergic/anaphylactic reaction: chills, fever, sweating, rash, itching, laryngeal edema, wheezing. Observe outpatients for 30 min after injection.

PATIENT/FAMILY TEACHING

Vaccination provides long-term protection from HBV, delta virus. Vaccine does not protect against other forms of hepatitis.
• Low-grade fever and/or pain, tenderness, redness, muscle stiffness at injection site may occur. • Immediately report symptoms of allergic reaction: chills, fever, sweating, itching, difficulty breathing. • Titers to confirm full protection may be drawn after vaccination series, especially in dialysis/immunosuppressed patients. • Recommendations for booster doses not established

AVAILABLE FORMS

Suspension in various strengths for IM use • Suspension for IM use in dialysis patients
Storage: Refrigerate at 2°-8° C (35°-46° F); do not freeze.

hetastarch, hydroxyethyl starch
(het′a-starch)
HES, Hespan

Classification: Plasma volume expander

USUAL DOSE

Dose, rate variable according to clinical condition, estimated fluid loss, hemodynamics, presence of pulmonary congestion, plasma oncotic pressure

IV inf, adults: Shock, hypovolemia: 500 ml initial dose; infuse additional doses as needed. Maximum dose, 20 ml/kg/24 hr or approx 1,500 ml/24 hr; higher doses have been used. • **Leukapheresis:** 250-700 ml infused at constant fixed ratio, usually 1:8, to venous whole blood

ADMINISTRATION

IV inf, adults: Infuse each 500 ml over 30 min to 4 hr. • For hypovolemic shock more rapid infusion over 15-20 min may be necessary. • For rapid administration, use 20-gauge or larger needle/catheter. • Complete infusion within 4 hr of opening.

PREPARATION

Solution should be transparent. • Do not use if solution appears turbid or brown, contains crystals.

ACTIONS

Maintains/restores plasma volume by encouraging fluid shift from interstitial to intravascular space by colloidal osmotic effects; similar to human albumin in colloidal effects • Plasma volume expansion slightly greater than volume infused • Increases plasma volume, BP, CO, PCWP for 24-36 hr • Hemodilution may cause a ↓ in total serum protein/hematocrit levels. • Increases erythrocyte sedimentation rate, resulting in improved efficiency of centrifugal granulocyte collection

PHARMACOKINETICS

ROUTE	ONSET	PEAK	DURATION
IV	Rapid	End infusion	Usually 24-36 hr; dose dependent

DISTRIBUTION

Throughout plasma

ELIMINATION

40% of smaller molecules excreted in urine within 24 hr, larger molecules are degraded and excreted more slowly.

INDICATIONS

Plasma volume expansion, in hypovolemic shock or serious hypovolemia caused by hemorrhage, trauma, burns, surgery, other conditions resulting in fluid volume deficit, especially when blood not immediately available • Comparable to albumin as volume expander • Unlike dextrans, has little or no antigenic properties • Leukapheresis for more efficient granulocyte harvesting
Unlabeled/investigational:
Priming fluid for pump oxygenators; plasma volume expansion during cardiopulmonary bypass

PRECAUTIONS/CONTRAINDICATIONS

Precautions: Rapid or excessive infusion may cause circulatory overload • Not blood substitute; whole blood or packed cells indicated for bleeding or anemic patients • Restoration of volume/vascular pressure in surgery, trauma, with other acute bleeding may increase rate of bleeding
Use caution in: Heart failure, cardiac decompensation, pulmonary edema • Older adults • Renal/hepatic disease • Thrombocytopenia, bleeding disorders • Cerebrovascular disease, head trauma, neurosurgery

italic = common side effects   **bold** = life-threatening reactions

c **Pregnancy category:** Risk to fetus unknown; use only if safer alternative not available.
Contraindications: Hypersensitivity to hetastarch • Nonhypovolemic shock • Severe CHF • Severe renal failure • Serious bleeding disorders • Subarachnoid hemorrhage • Children: safety/effectiveness unknown

ADVERSE EFFECTS

CNS: Headache
Resp: Dyspnea, **pulmonary edema**
CV: Elevated CVP, PCWP; **circulatory overload**
GI: Vomiting, ↑ indirect bilirubin
Hema: Prolonged PT, PTT, bleeding, clotting times; hemodilution
Misc: Fever, chills, itching, **anaphylaxis**

TOXICITY/OVERDOSE

Symptoms: Circulatory overload; ↑ CVP, PCWP • Dyspnea, pulmonary edema • ↑ bleeding time, bleeding complications
Management: Stop infusion. • Treat bleeding complications symptomatically. • For management of allergic reactions, see Appendix N.

INTERACTIONS

anticoagulants ↑ Risk of bleeding

Y-SITE COMPATIBILITIES

Cimetidine, diltiazem, enalaprilat

Y-SITE INCOMPATIBILITIES

Amikacin, ampicillin, cefamandole, cefazolin, cefoperazone, cefotaxime, cefoxitin, cephalothin, gentamicin, ranitidine, theophylline, tobramycin

PATIENT CARE IMPLICATIONS

• Not replacement for transfusion therapy; for actively bleeding or anemic patients, use as adjunct to whole blood or packed cells.
Vital signs/hemodynamics: Monitor BP, HR q15-60 min depending on indication, rate of administration. • Monitor CVP, PAPs, CO as available. Administer at rate, dosage to restore intravascular fluid volume, avoid overload. Stop or slow infusion, consult physician for CVP >6 mm Hg or PCWP > 12 mm Hg or established range. • Monitor UO; note patient response before and after therapy.
Physical assessment: Assess for circulatory overload, especially with rapid infusion: crackles (rales), S_3 gallop, dyspnea, neck vein distention. • Assess for bleeding complications, especially if patient is receiving concurrent anticoagulants, has undergone neurosurgery. • **Surgery, trauma, other acute bleeding:** As intravascular volume/pressure restored, assess for ↑ bleeding.
Laboratory tests: Monitor: Hgb, Hct • Electrolytes • Bilirubin • With leukapheresis, monitor CBC, total leukocyte/platelet counts, leukocyte differential count, Hgb/Hct, PT, PTT.

PATIENT/FAMILY TEACHING

Purpose of medication is to expand blood volume or facilitate leukapheresis. • Immediately report fever, chills, breathing difficulty, unusual bleeding.

P pediatric   G geriatric   V Direct IV

AVAILABLE FORMS

6% solution in 500-ml bottle of 0.9% NaCl

---

hydralazine
(hye′dral′a-zeen)
Alazine, Apresoline, Novo-Hylazin ✹, Nw Hydral ✹
hydralazine with hydrochlorothiazide
Apresazide, Apresoline-Esidrix, Hydra-zide, Hy-Zide
hydralazine with reserpine
Serpasil-Apresoline

Classifications: Antihypertensive, peripheral vasodilator

USUAL DOSE

PO, adults: Initially 10 mg 4 times daily for 2-4 days, then increase to 25 mg 4 times daily for next 4-6 days. • Gradually increase dose until BP controlled. • Up to 300-400 mg/day may be necessary.
IM, adults: 10-50 mg; start with lower dose, repeat dose gradually increase until BP controlled.
Direct IV, adults: 5-20 mg; start with lower dose, repeat dose gradually increase until BP controlled.

ADMINISTRATION

▼**Direct IV inj:** Inject undiluted solution over 60 sec. • Avoid contact with metal parts, which may cause discoloration; prepare syringe just before injection.
Compatible fluids: 0.9% NaCl, LR, prepared combina-
tions of these solutions; decomposition possible with D_5W

ACTIONS

Relaxes vascular smooth muscle, reducing BP/total peripheral resistance • Arteriolar dilation >venodilation • DBP usually reduced more than SBP • HR, CO, SV ↑ along with slight ↑ in coronary, cerebral, renal blood flow.
• PAPs may ↑ . • Increases in renin activity stimulate angiotensin/aldosterone, resulting in sodium/water retention, especially with prolonged therapy.
• Generally does not cause postural hypotension.

PHARMACOKINETICS

ROUTE	ONSET	PEAK	DURATION
PO	20-30 min	30-120 min	6-8 hr
IM	10-30 min	60 min	2-6 hr
IV	5-20 min	10-80 min	2-6 hr

DISTRIBUTION
Widely distributed; 85% protein bound
ELIMINATION
Metabolized by GI mucosa, liver; eliminated in urine; half-life 2-4 hr

INDICATIONS

Reduction of moderate to severe hypertension; generally reserved for patients resistant to more conventional therapy (e.g., diuretics, beta-blockers, angiotensin-converting enzyme inhibitors, calcium channel blockers) • Parenteral route used for severe hypertension • Choice agent for pregnancy-associated hypertensive emergencies
Unlabeled/investigational:
Adjunct in short-term management of severe CHF, including that associated with mitral/aortic regurgitation or ventricular septal defect

---

italic = common side effects   **bold** = life-threatening reactions

PRECAUTIONS/ CONTRAINDICATIONS

Precautions: Sodium/water retention may cause refractoriness to hypotensive effects. • Increased risk of drug-induced SLE in slow acetylators (50% of white/black Americans) • Marked decrease in BP may cause psychotic reaction in severely hypertensive uremic patients.

Use caution with: CHF, cardiac impairment; fluid retention may worsen condition. • Myocardial ischemia; tachycardia may be detrimental. • Renal failure; lower dose indicated

c Pregnancy category: Safety not established; use only if safer alternative unavailable.

Contraindications: Hypersensitivity to hydralazine, sulfites • Tablets may contain tartrazine dye (FD&C yellow no. 5); contraindicated if allergic to tartrazine • Mitral valve disease • Parenteral use in CVA, cerebral edema, encephalopathy, increased ICP • Children: Safety/ efficacy not established

ADVERSE EFFECTS

CNS: *Headache,* dizziness, **cerebral ischemia**

CV: *Palpitations, tachycardia,* orthostatic hypotension, *sodium/fluid retention,* edema, weight gain, angina, **myocardial ischemia**

GI: Nausea, vomiting, diarrhea, constipation, adynamic ileus

Hema: Blood dyscrasias

Derm: Rash, urticaria, pruritus

Misc: Hypersensitivity reactions including SLE-like or rheumatoid arthritis–like syndrome

TOXICITY/OVERDOSE

Symptoms: Hypotension, shock • Tachycardia, dysrhythmias, myocardial ischemia

Management: After recent ingestion, implement guidelines for management of acute overdose (Appendix I). • Stabilize hypotension before inducing emesis or gastric lavage. • Maintain airway/support breathing as needed; administer O_2. • **Hypotension:** Elevate legs; administer crystalloid or colloid plasma volume expanders. Avoid vasopressors; if necessary for profound hypotension, use agent least likely to precipitate dysrhythmias (e.g., Neosynephrine, phenylephrine). • **Tachycardia:** Use beta-adrenergic blockers. • Experience with dialysis not reported

INTERACTIONS

antihypertensives   Additive hypotension

diazoxide   Profound hypotension

diuretics   Potentiation of hypotensive effects

epinephrine   Reduced pressor effects

indomethacin; possibly other NSAIDs   Decreased effectiveness of hydralazine

MAO inhibitors   Hypotension

Y-SITE COMPATIBILITIES

Dobutamine, heparin, potassium chloride, verapamil, vitamin B complex with C

Y-SITE INCOMPATIBILITIES

Aminophylline, ampicillin, furosemide, nitroglycerin, phenobarbital

---

PATIENT CARE IMPLICATIONS

• Parenteral/PO doses not equivalent; 20-25 mg IV approx equal to 75-100 mg PO
• Usually used with diuretic, another hypotensive agent; concurrent use of beta-adrenergic blocker minimizes tachycardia, risk of angina in coronary artery disease.

Parenteral

• Patient must remain in bed with appropriate safety precautions during and for at least 1 hr after parenteral administration; caution, assistance required with initial ambulation.
• Do not discontinue until BP controlled by other (preferably PO) agent.

Vital signs/hemodynamics: IV: Closely monitor BP, HR during initial use, until stable.
• As available, monitor ECG, noting tachycardia, dysrhythmias, ischemic ECG changes (ST depression/elevation, T wave inversion).

Physical assessment: Assess for perfusion/oxygenation deficit: chest discomfort, shortness of breath, ↓ level of consciousness, confusion, dizziness. • Assess for CHF: dyspnea, bibasilar crackles (rales), peripheral edema, weight gain, S_3 gallop, neck vein distention. • Assess for SLE-type or rheumatoid arthritis–type syndrome: fever, arthralgia, splenomegaly, malaise, edema. • Monitor fluid balance; weigh daily.

Laboratory Tests: Monitor: BUN, creatinine • Electrolytes • CBC with differential • Bilirubin, liver enzymes • If symptoms of SLE-type or rheumatoid arthritis–type syndrome, check for elevated ANA titer, presence of LE cells, positive direct Coombs' test.

PATIENT/FAMILY TEACHING

Purpose of drug is to lower BP and/or relieve heart failure.
• May cause dizziness; change position slowly. • **IV/IM:** Do not attempt to get out of bed without assistance • Immediately report dizziness, chest discomfort, confusion, breathing difficulty.
• Report unexplained fever, malaise, edema, muscle/joint pain.

Outpatient: Medicine is not cure for high BP; Other therapies, including life-style modifications, must be continued.
• Take medication exactly as prescribed; often taken with at least other antihypertensives (e.g., diuretic, beta-blocker). Do not stop taking medicine even if you feel better. If medication abruptly discontinued, you may develop dangerously high BP.
• Use caution in performing hazardous tasks requiring mental alertness or physical coordination until individual effects of drug known. • Weigh twice/wk; notify physician of weight gain, edema. • Consult physician or pharmacist before taking cold, cough, or allergy preparations.

AVAILABLE FORMS

Tablets, capsules • Parenteral for IM/IV injection

hydrochlorothiazide
(hye-droe-klor-oh-thye'a-zide)
Diaqua, Esidrix, Hydrodiuril, Hydrozide ✹, Mictrin, Thiuretic Urozide ✹

Classifications: Thiazide diuretic, antihypertensive

USUAL DOSE
PO, adults: 25-100 mg 1-2 times daily; 25-50 mg 1-2 times daily when used with other antihypertensives • Maximum dose, 200 mg/day
Ⓟ PO, children 6 mo-12 yr: 2.2 mg/kg daily, given in two doses
Ⓟ PO, children <6 mo: 3.3 mg/kg/day bid

ACTIONS
Interferes with sodium transport across distal renal tubule; causes ↑ excretion of sodium, chloride, water • Also ↑ excretion of potassium, bicarbonate, magnesium, phosphate • Reduces calcium, ammonia, uric acid excretion • Increases plasma renin activity, causing slightly ↑ aldosterone secretion • In hypertensive patients, reduces BP, augments action of the antihypertensives • May ↑ blood glucose • Paradoxically reduces UO in diabetes insipidus

PHARMACOKINETICS

ROUTE	ONSET	PEAK	DURATION
PO	2 hr	4-6 hr	6-12 hr

DISTRIBUTION
Wide; crosses placenta

ELIMINATION
Excreted unchanged in urine; delayed excretion with CHF, renal impairment; half-life 5.6-14.8 hr

INDICATIONS
Edema associated with right-sided/mild left-sided heart failure, liver cirrhosis, nephrotic syndrome, other factors • To ↓ BP in hypertensive patients; used alone or with other agents early in course of antihypertensive therapy • May not be effective in long-term management of edema associated with significant renal impairment
Unlabeled/investigational:
To reduce excessive UO associated with diabetes insipidus; treatment of electrolyte disturbances associated with renal tubular acidosis; prophylaxis of renal calculi associated with hypercalciuria

PRECAUTIONS/ CONTRAINDICATIONS
Precautions: May cause hypokalemia, hypochloremic alkalosis • Digitalis toxicity more likely in hypokalemic patients; potassium supplements indicated • Dilutional hyponatremia may slowly develop in patients receiving chronic therapy. • Parathyroid dysfunction associated with hypercalcemia/hypophosphatemia possible with long-term therapy • Uric acid elevation, gout possible •Some preparations contain sulfites, which may trigger serious allergic reactions. • Some preparations contain tartrazine dye (FD&C yellow no. 5), which may cause allergic reactions.
Ⓖ Use caution with: Older adults; fluid/electrolyte imbalance more likely • Renal impairment; reduced plasma volume may decrease GFR, and precipitate azotemia. • Cirrhosis, hepatic failure; rapid fluctua-

---

Ⓟ pediatric   Ⓖ geriatric   Ⅴ Direct IV

tions in fluids/electrolytes may prompt hepatic coma. • Diabetic patients; hyperglycemia possible
B Pregnancy category: Safety not clearly established
Contraindications: Hypersensitivity to hydrochlorothiazide, other thiazides, sulfonamides • Anuria • Severe uncorrected electrolyte depletion or hepatic **P** coma • Children: Safety not clearly established

ADVERSE EFFECTS

CNS: Dizziness, headache, paresthesias, weakness, restlessness
Resp: Alkalosis/compensatory respiratory depression
CV: Orthostatic hypotension, **hypotension,** dysrhythmias (PACs, PVCs), **ventricular fibrillation, pulmonary edema** (rare)
GI: Nausea, vomiting, diarrhea, abdominal pain, **hepatic coma** (preexisting liver disease)
GU: ↑ BUN/creatinine, progressive azotemia, hematuria
Endo: Hyperglycemia, glycosuria
F&E: *Hypokalemia, hypochloremia,* hyponatremia, metabolic alkalosis, hypercalcemia, elevated ammonia/total cholesterol
Derm: Photosensitivity, rash, urticaria, purpura, **toxic epidermal necrolysis** (rare)
Misc: Exacerbation/precipitation of SLE, fever, hyperuricemia, gout

TOXICITY/OVERDOSE

Symptoms: Hypotension, dehydration, circulatory collapse • Electrolyte loss with weakness, dizziness, mental confusion, vomiting, muscle cramps

Management: After recent ingestion, implement guidelines for management of acute overdose (Appendix I). • Support respiration as needed with O_2 and/or mechanical ventilation. • Replace electrolytes; closely monitor sodium/potassium balance. • **Hypotension:** Elevate legs, administer IV fluids; if unresponsive to fluid replacement, use vasopressors (e.g., dopamine, norepinephrine). • Avoid administration of cathartics, which could contribute to fluid/electrolyte imbalance.

INTERACTIONS

alcohol Hypotension
amphotericin B Severe potassium depletion
antidiabetic agents Interference with glucose-lowering effects
antihypertensives Hypotension
beta-blockers Hypotension
calcium channel blockers Hypotension
corticosteroids Severe hypokalemia
digoxin Hypokalemia, hypomagnesemia, digoxin toxicity, dysrhythmias
diuretics Enhanced diuresis; potassium depletion
insulin Interference with glucose-lowering effects
lithium Reduced renal clearance; lithium toxicity
NSAIDs Fluid retention; ↓ diuresis; renal failure
nondepolarizing (NMBAs (e.g., pancuronium) Prolonged neuromuscular blockade
opiates Hypotension
probenecid Blocked thiazide-related uric acid retention
quinidine Quinidine toxicity

---

italic = common side effects   **bold** = life-threatening reactions

PATIENT CARE IMPLICATIONS

• Evaluate response to therapy, considering diuretic response, fluid balance, weight, electrolytes. Adjust dose accordingly.
• Potassium supplements frequently necessary, especially in digitalized patients
• Consider use of potassium-sparing sparing diuretic (e.g., spironolactone, amiloride) if other diuretics used concomitantly.
• Combination formulas inappropriate for initial therapy, may cause profound hypotension.

Vital signs/hemodynamics: Monitor BP, HR, UO. • As available, continuously monitor ECG. Note presence of PVCs, dysrhythmias, hypokalemic ECG changes (i.e., flattened ST, T wave inversion, U wave). If present, check potassium level, correct as necessary. Carefully monitor digitalized patients for these and other dysrhythmias associated with digitalis toxicity.

Physical assessment: Assess extremities, face, sacrum for improvement in edema. • Assess for signs/symptoms of electrolyte imbalance: dysrhythmias, lethargy, headache, confusion, dizziness, weakness, muscle cramps, paresthesias, thirst, anorexia, vomiting. • Assess for perfusion/oxygenation deficit caused by hypovolemia: chest discomfort, ↓ level of consciousness, activity intolerance, hypotension, dizziness. • Assess hyperuricemic patients for toe or foot pain, suggesting gout.
• Weigh patient daily. • CHF: Assess for improvement: clear breath sounds, reduced neck vein distention, resolution of edema.

Laboratory tests: Monitor: Electrolytes, particularly sodium, potassium, chloride, calcium, magnesium • BUN, creatinine • CBC • Blood glucose levels, especially in patients with diabetes • **May cause:** Hypokalemia resulting in severe dysrhythmias, increased/decreased effects of other drugs, including cardiac glycosides, antidiabetic agents. Likelihood of digitalis toxicity increases with hypokalemia. Correct promptly.

PATIENT/FAMILY TEACHING

Purpose of drug is to encourage elimination of excess body fluid and lower BP. • May cause dizziness, especially when starting therapy; use caution when changing positions, walking.
• Report breathing difficulty, palpitations, dizziness, activity intolerance, chest pain, confusion, weakness, faintness, muscle cramps, persistent thirst, vomiting.

Outpatient: Alcohol, hot weather, vigorous activity, prolonged standing may cause dizziness, faintness. • Take potassium supplements as prescribed, particularly if also taking digitalis derivatives. • Take medication in morning. Never double doses. • Continue taking medication as prescribed even if feeling better. Drug controls but does not cure hypertension.
• Take with food or milk for stomach upset. • Do not take ibuprofen, other nonprescription drugs without consulting health care professional. • Use sunscreen, wear protective clothing to prevent photosensitivity reac-

tions. • Routine follow-up exams are important to detect/prevent serious side effects.
• **Patients with diabetes:** Blood glucose levels may increase. Insulin dose may need adjustment.

AVAILABLE FORMS

Tablets • PO solution

---

hydrocortisone, cortisol
(hye-droe-kor'ti-sone)
Cortef, Hydrocortone
hydrocortisone sodium succinate
Solu-Cortef, A-Hydrocort
hydrocortisone sodium phosphate
Hydrocortone Phosphate

Classifications: Adrenocortical steroid, corticosteroid, glucocorticoid, antiinflammatory agent

USUAL DOSE

All doses individually based on severity of condition, patient response
PO, adult: 10-320 mg daily in 3-4 equally divided doses
P PO, children: 0.5-0.8 mg/kg daily in 3-4 equally divided doses
Sodium succinate
IV/IM, adult: 100-500 mg q2-10h • Doses as high as 2 g q2-6h may be used in profound shock until condition stabilizes.
P IV/IM, children: 0-15-1.0 mg/kg in divided doses q12h until condition stabilizes
Sodium phosphate
IV/IM/SC, adult: Initially 15-240 mg/day, usually q12h

P IM, children: 0.15-1.0 mg/kg in divided doses q12h until condition stabilizes

ADMINISTRATION

PO: When possible, administer with meals to minimize gastric irritation.
V Direct IV: Sodium succinate: Inject each 500 mg over at least 1 min. • Injection is preferred route but may be administered by intermit or cont inf
Sodium phosphate: Inject each 25 mg over at least 1 min; slow rate of injection for injection site burning. • May be administered by intermit or cont inf over 30 min

PREPARATION

IV: Sodium succinate: Reconstitute from Mix-O-Vial by removing outer cap, turning rubber stopper ¼ turn, pressing down on stopper; diluent released into lower chamber to mix with powdered medication. Shake or twirl gently to mix solution. Withdraw solution from vial using sterile technique.
• Alternately, solution may be reconstituted using 2 ml bacteriostatic water for injection for each 250 mg. For cont or intermit inf, add reconstituted solution to volume of compatible solution to yield concentration of 0.1-1 mg/ml. • **Sodium phosphate:** May be administered without dilution • For intermit inf, add to 50-100 ml compatible solution.
Compatible fluids: D_5W, 0.9% NaCl

ACTIONS

Potent, fast-acting adrenocortical steroid that reduces inflammation (glucocorticoid effect), pro-

---

motes renal sodium retention (mineralocorticoid effect) • Stabilizes lysosomal membranes in leukocytes, prevents release of acid hydrolases, thus reducing inflammation • Inhibits macrophage accumulation in inflamed tissues • Reduces leukocyte adhesion to capillary walls, decreases capillary permeability/ edema • Antagonizes histamine, kinin release • Suppresses immune response by producing lymphocytopenia, ↓ Ig/ complement, ↓ volume/activity of lymphatic system • Mineralocorticoid effects may result in edema, hypertension

PHARMACOKINETICS

ROUTE	ONSET	PEAK	DURATION
PO	<60 min	4-6 hr	Dose dependent approx 8-12 hr
IM	<60 min	4-6 hr	
IV	Rapid	4-6 hr	

DISTRIBUTION

Widely distributed throughout body tissue

ELIMINATION

Metabolized in liver, eliminated by kidneys; biologic half-life 8-12 hr

INDICATIONS

Replacement of cortisol in established/suspected adrenal insufficiency, including adrenal crisis, stress, trauma, critical illness • Allergic reactions, including hypersensitivity, asthma, anaphylaxis, serum sickness • Short-term adjunctive therapy in rheumatic disorders • Autoimmune conditions (e.g., SLE, polymyositis) • Inflammatory respiratory, GI, neuromuscular disorders refractory to other therapies • Acute idiopathic thrombocytopenic purpura (ITP), hemolytic anemia • Palliative management of leukemias, lymphomas • To prevent rejection of transplanted organs • Intraarticular or soft tissue injection for arthritis, bursitis, gout, tendonitis

PRECAUTIONS/ CONTRAINDICATIONS

Precautions: Prolonged therapy suppresses adrenal synthesis of glucocorticoids/mineralocorticoids, resulting in withdrawal symptoms with abrupt discontinuation. • May mask signs of infection, ↓ resistance to infection • May cause edema, particularly in renal impairment • Peptic ulceration possible in high-risk patients (e.g., history of peptic ulcer, liver-intestinal disease, nephrotic syndrome, critical illness) • Excessive sodium/water retention possible; may contribute to hypertension • Renal excretion of potassium/ calcium may cause electrolyte imbalance.

Use caution with: Diabetes; insulin requirements may increase. • Renal insufficiency, chronic nephritis, acute glomerulonephritis; may cause fluid retention/electrolyte imbalance • Osteoporosis • Seizure disorder • CHF • Concurrent anticholinesterase therapy • Acute MI • Recent CVA • Phlebitis • Active tuberculosis; use only in severe cases and as adjunct to chemotherapy. • Chronic active hepatitis; may promote liver failure

C Pregnancy category: Use only if safer alternative unavailable.

Contraindications: Hypersensitivity to hydrocortisone, any corticosteroid • Systemic fungal infections; indicated if reaction to amphotericin B • Recent administration of live viral vaccine (e.g., smallpox)

ADVERSE EFFECTS

CNS: *Euphoria, insomnia, mood swings, depression,* psychosis, headache, paresthesias, **seizures, ↑ ICP**

CV: *Hypertension,* hypokalemic ECG changes fluid retention/ CHF, thrombophlebitis

GI: *Nausea,* vomiting, weight gain, **peptic ulceration, GI bleeding, pancreatitis**

Endo: *Adrenal suppression, menstrual irregularities,* hyperglycemia, growth suppression in children, "steroid-induced" diabetes mellitus

F&E: Hypokalemia, hypokalemic alkalosis, sodium/fluid, fluid retention

MS: *Muscle wasting, osteoporosis,* aseptic joint necrosis

Derm: *Diminished wound healing, petechiae, ecchymosis, hirsutism, acne, thinning of skin,* hypo-hyperpigmentation

Misc: *Cushingoid appearance, susceptibility to infection, symptoms of infection*

TOXICITY/OVERDOSE

Symptoms: Cushingoid: Moon face, central obesity, hirsutism, acne, hypertension, osteoporosis, diabetes mellitus, hyperlipidemia, peptic ulcers, myopathy, immunosuppression, fluid/electrolyte imbalance • Acute adrenal insufficiency: Fever, anorexia, malaise, nausea, dizziness, fainting, dyspnea, hypoglycemia, myalgia, arthalgia; follows rapid withdrawal of therapy **Management:** After recent ingestion, implement guidelines for management of acute overdose (Appendix J). • Hypoten-

sion: Elevate legs, administer IV fluids; use vasopressor (e.g., dopamine, norepinephrine) or inotrope (e.g., dopamine, dobutamine) as appropriate. • Severe fluid overload: Administer diuretics; replace potassium as necessary. • Adrenal insufficiency: Supplement with additional corticosteroid; taper dose gradually before withdrawal.

INTERACTIONS

amphotericin B Profound hypokalemia

antidiabetic agents (PO, insulin) ↑ Antidiabetic drug requirements

carbamazepine ↓ Corticoid effects

cholestyramine ↓ Corticoid effects; stagger administration

diuretics, potassium losing Profound hypokalemia

oral contraceptives Excessive corticosteroid effects

phenytoin ↓ Corticoid effects

rifampin ↓ Corticoid effects

Y-SITE COMPATIBILITIES

Hydrocortisone sodium phosphate: Cefepime, fluconazole, ondansetron, piperacillin-tazobactam

Hydrocortisone sodium succinate: Aminophylline, ampicillin, amrinone, atracurium, atropine, calcium gluconate, cephalothin, cephapirin, chlorpromazine, digoxin, diphenhydramine, dopamine, droperidol, enalaprilat, epinephrine, esmolol, famotidine, fentanyl, furosemide, hydralazine, insulin, isoproterenol, lidocaine, magnesium sulfate, meperidine, methicillin morphine, neostigmine, norepinephrine, ondansetron, oxacillin, pancuronium, penicillin G potassium, pentazocine, piperacillin-tazobactam, procain-

H

---

italic = common side effects   **bold** = life-threatening reactions

amide, propranolol, sodium bicarbonate, vercuronium

Y-SITE INCOMPATIBILITIES

Hydrocortisone sodium succinate: Ciprofloxacine, diazepam, phenytoin, promazine, promethazine, vancomycin

PATIENT CARE IMPLICATIONS

• Administer daily dose in AM to coincide with physiologic peak in cortisol levels.
• Administer PO dose with meals to avoid gastric irritation.
• Dosage should be gradually tapered to avoid adrenal insufficiency.
• Dosage increases are necessary when patients subjected to severe emotional, physical stress
• Prolonged therapy (≥1 wk) suppresses hypothalamic-pituitary-adrenal axis, may lead to suppression of adrenal synthesis of glucocorticoids/mineralocorticoids. Abrupt discontinuation may cause withdrawal symptoms: fatigue, anorexia, nausea, hypotension, hypoglycemia, depression, fever, dizziness, joint pain, malaise, fainting.
• Drug-related immunosuppression may mask signs of infection. Monitor closely; initiate antibiotic therapy as soon as infection is suspected.

Vital signs/hemodynamics: Frequency of VS monitoring depends on patient condition rather than drug effects. Hypovolemic shock possible with adrenal crisis; VS should be monitored q15min or more often until condition stabilizes.

Physical assessment: Assess for adrenal insufficiency: fever, anorexia, malaise, nausea, dizziness, fainting, dyspnea, hypoglycemia, myalgia, arthralgia. Presence of these symptoms indicates insufficient dosage or too rapid withdrawal of therapy. • Assess for cushingoid symptoms: moon face, central obesity, hirsutism, acne, hypertension, osteoporosis, diabetes mellitus, hyperlipidemia, peptic ulcers, myopathy, immunosuppression, fluid/electrolyte imbalance. Presence of these symptoms indicates excessive dosage.
• Assess for weight gain, peripheral edema, dyspnea, crackles (rales). Sodium/water retention more likely in patients with renal impairment. • Check stools and emesis for occult blood. • Monitor I&O; weigh daily.

Laboratory tests: Monitor: Electrolytes, especially sodium, potassium, calcium • Blood glucose • CBC with differential

PATIENT/FAMILY TEACHING

Purpose of medication is to reduce inflammation of affected area or body system. • Take exactly as prescribed. Do not double dose if missed. Sudden cessation of therapy may cause adrenal insufficiency: weakness, fatigue, nausea, low BP, low blood sugar. • Take with meals to minimize stomach upset.
• Drug causes suppression of immune system, may mask signs of infection. Avoid individuals with contagious illnesses. Report fever, prolonged malaise, any symptom of infection immediately. • Report rapid weight gain, unusual swelling, very dark or bloody stools, vomiting of blood, sores slow to heal significant behavior changes. • Inform health care providers of medication regimen before treatment. • Carry

---

P pediatric   **G** geriatric   **V** Direct IV

Medic-Alert ID describing medication regimen.

AVAILABLE FORMS

Parenteral solution for IV/IM injection • Tablets • PO suspension

hydromorphone
(hye-droe-mor'fone)
Dilaudid

Classifications: Opiate agonist, narcotic analgesic Schedule II controlled substance

USUAL DOSE

Use smallest effective dose to minimize CNS depression, tolerance. *Use caution, reduced dose in* elderly/debilitated patients.

PO, adults: Moderate pain: 1-2 mg q4-6h • Severe pain: 4-6 mg q4-6h • Severe pain/opiate tolerance: ≥10 mg q4-6h

Rectal, adults: 3 mg q6-8h

IM/SC, adults: Moderate pain: 2 mg q4-6h • Severe pain: 4-6 mg q4-6h • Severe pain/opiate tolerance: ≥10 mg q4-6h; use 10 mg/ml formulation (Dilaudid-HP) to limit volume of injection.

Direct IV, adults: 1-2 mg q1-4h • Higher doses may be used with severe pain/opiate tolerance, but cont inf generally preferred for these patients.

IV, cont inf, adults: 1-3 mg/hr for severe chronic pain in opiate-dependent patients. PCA pump may be used.

ADMINISTRATION

Direct IV, adults: Inject dilute solution slowly at rate of ≤2 mg over 3-5 min. • Too-rapid administration may cause apnea and/or hypotension. • Have naloxone, resuscitation equipment nearby.

IV, cont inf, adults: Titrate to relieve pain without depressing RR, BP. • May be administered via PCA pump ↑ basal rate as necessary to relieve pain without excessive sedation • Have naloxone, resuscitation equipment nearby.

PREPARATION

IM/SC: READ LABELS CAREFULLY; MULTIPLE STRENGTHS AVAILABLE. • Concentrated solution (Dilaudid-HP, 10 mg/ml) for use only in patients with opiate tolerance, severe chronic pain

Direct IV, adults: Dilute in 4-5 ml sterile water or 0.9% NaCl.

IV, cont inf: Prepare solution with concentration of 1 mg/10 ml (e.g., 25 mg hydromorphone in 250 ml D_5W). • More concentrated solutions may be used. • Infusion pump necessary

Compatible fluids: D_5W, 0.9% NaCl, LR

ACTIONS

Potent, semisynthetic, morphine-like opiate agonist • Acts at specific receptor sites in CNS, other tissue to inhibit pain perception, produce analgesia • Reduces apprehension associated with pain • Causes sedation, CNS depression • Suppresses coughing, depresses respiratory centers in brainstem • Causes peripheral vasodilation, reduced SVR; may lead to hypotension • 1.5 mg IM or 7.5 mg PO similar in analgesic effectiveness to morphine, 10 mg IM

italic = common side effects   **bold** = life-threatening reactions

PHARMACOKINETICS

ROUTE	ONSET	PEAK	DURATION
PO	15-30 min	60 min	4-6 hr
IM	15-30 min	30-60 min	4-5 hr
IV	Immed	30 min	3-4 hr

DISTRIBUTION

Wide; readily crosses placenta

ELIMINATION

Metabolized in liver, excreted in urine; half-life 2-3 hr

INDICATIONS

Relief of moderate to severe acute/chronic pain, apprehension associated with trauma, malignancies, surgery, other painful conditions • Highly concentrated injection containing 10 mg/ml especially useful for IM/SQ injections in opiate-tolerant patients and when small-volume injections indicated (e.g., cachexia, small muscle mass)

PRECAUTIONS/ CONTRAINDICATIONS

Precautions: HIGH-POTENCY PARENTERAL FORMULATION (10 mg/ml) AVAILABLE; READ LABEL CAREFULLY WHEN PREPARING. • Severe respiratory depression possible, especially with IV use • May cause hypotension, especially with rapid IV administration, in hypovolemia, with other CNS depressants • Commercial preparations may contain sulfites, which can cause serious allergic reactions.

G **Use caution with:** Older adults, hepatic/renal dysfunction, debilitation; use reduced dose. • COPD • CNS depression • Prostatic hypertrophy, urethral stricture • Acute MI ↑ ICP; respiratory depression/CO_2 retention may further ↑ ICP • Seizure disorder; may precipitate seizures

c **Pregnancy category:** Use only if safer alternative unavailable.

Contraindications: Hypersensitivity to hydromorphone • Status asthmaticus • Respiratory depression • Undiagnosed acute abdominal conditions • Ulcerative colitis • Diarrhea caused by poisoning • Labor/delivery • IM route contraindicated with hypothermia, shock, hypotension, impaired circulation • IM/IV route used only for patients with established opiate **P** tolerance • Children/infants: Safety not established

ADVERSE EFFECTS

CNS: *Sedation, confusion,* dizziness, mental clouding, weakness, somnolence, coma
EENT: Pupillary constriction, visual disturbances, nystagmus
Resp: *Suppression of cough reflex,* **respiratory depression, apnea**
CV: *Orthostatic hypotension,* hypotension, reflex tachycardia, SVT
GI: Constipation, anorexia, nausea, vomiting
GU: Urinary retention
Derm: Pruritus, urticaria
Misc: Tolerance, physical/psychologic dependence

TOXICITY/OVERDOSE

Acute toxicity/overdose: Profound CNS depression, coma • Pupillary constriction • Hypothermia/cool, clammy skin • Respiratory depression, apnea • Hypotension, circulatory collapse, cardiopulmonary arrest
Chronic toxicity: Tolerance, psychologic/physical dependence • Physical dependence results in withdrawal symptoms

when drug abruptly discontinued.

Management: After recent ingestion, implement guidelines for management of acute overdose (Appendix I). Gastric lavage may be effective even hours after ingestion, because pylorospasms may cause much of drug to remain in stomach. • **Hypoventilation:** Establish/maintain airway; administer O$_2$; if ventilatory efforts hindered by muscular rigidity, administer IV muscle relaxants, NMBAs.
• **Hypotension:** Elevate legs, administer IV fluids; use vasopressors (e.g., dopamine, norepinephrine) for circulatory collapse. • **Antidote:** naloxone, opiate antagonist used to reverse respiratory depression, other symptoms

INTERACTIONS

alcohol, ethyl ↑ CNS depression
anesthetics, general ↑ CNS depression
opiate agonist-antagonists(e.g., buprenorphine, butorphanol, nalbuphine, pentazocine) Acute withdrawal in opiate-dependent patients
naloxone Reversal of effects; acute withdrawal in opiate-dependent patients
opiate analgesics ↑ CNS depression
phenothiazines Enhanced/antagonized analgesia; additive CNS depression
procarbazine ↑ CNS depression
sedatives ↑ CNS depression
tranquilizers ↑ CNS depression; enhanced analgesia
TCAs ↑ CNS depression

Y-SITE COMPATIBILITIES

Amikacin, ampicillin, cefamandole, cefoperazone, cefotaxime, cefoxitin, ceftazidime, ceftizoxime, cefuroxime, cephalothin, cephapirin, chloramphenicol, clindamycin, doxycycline, erythromycin, gentamicin, magnesium sulfate, nafcillin, ondansetron, oxacillin, piperacillin, piperacillin-tazobactam, ticarcillin, tobramycin, vancomycin

Y-SITE INCOMPATIBILITIES

Cloxacillin, diazepam, phenobarbital, phenytoin, sodium bicarbonate, tetracycline, thiopental

PATIENT CARE IMPLICATIONS

• Administer prn doses before pain becomes severe; regularly scheduled, continuous, or PCA dosing more effective than prn scheduling.
• Administer with peripherally acting nonnarcotic analgesics (e.g., acetaminophen, ibuprofen) for additive analgesia.
• Administer with antihistamines (e.g., hydroxyzine) or tranquilizers (e.g., prochlorperazine) to potentiate effects.
• Have naloxone, resuscitation equipment immediately available, particularly with IV/IM/SC use.
• Tolerance develops in patients receiving opiate analgesics for long-term pain control; progressively higher doses necessary.
• Use concentrated solution (Dilaudid-HD, 10 mg/ml) for IM/SC injection in patients with limited muscle mass or opiate tolerance/severe pain.

---

italic = common side effects   **bold** = life-threatening reactions

• Gradually discontinue drug after long-term use to prevent withdrawal symptoms.
• Administer with food or milk to enhance PO absorption.

Vital signs/hemodynamics: Assess BP, pulse, RR before and frequently during initial administration; withhold for hypotension, respiratory depression. With IV use, monitor q5min for first 15 min and frequently thereafter according to patient condition.

Physical assessment: Assess type, location, intensity of pain before and after administration.
• Assess ventilation: note rate, depth of respirations; auscultate breath sounds. • Assess bowel function: bowel sounds, abdominal distention, elimination patterns. • Monitor I&O. Assess for urinary retention, bladder distention.

PATIENT/FAMILY TEACHING

Purpose of medication is to relieve pain. • Request/use medication before pain becomes severe • Change positions slowly to avoid dizziness. • Change position, cough, deep breathe every 2 hr to prevent lung problems. • Do not perform hazardous tasks requiring mental alertness or physical coordination. Call for assistance when ambulating (initial therapy). • Drink plenty of fluids; eat high-fiber foods. Use stool softeners if necessary to minimize constipation.
Outpatient: Avoid using alcohol or other sedatives while taking this medication.

AVAILABLE FORMS

Parenteral concentrate (10 mg/ml) for IM/SC use with opi-

ate tolerance • Parenteral concentrate for IV admixture • Tablets • Suppositories • Parenteral for IV/IM/SC use.

hydroxyzine HCl/hydroxyzine pamoate
(hye-drox'i-zeen)
Anxanil, Atarax, E-Vista, Hydroxacen, Hyzine, Neucalm, Quiess, Vistacon, Vistaril, Vistazine

Classifications: Antihistamine, sedative

USUAL DOSE

Strongly potentiates opiate analgesics, other CNS depressants; reduce opiate, CNS depressant dose by ½ when used with hydroxyzine; use caution. Always use lowest effective dose; adjust to individual response.

PO, adults: 50-100 mg tid-qid
Ⓟ PO, children: 0.6 mg/kg tid-qid • Pruritus/anxiety: See table

AGE (yr)	TOTAL DAILY DOSE (mg)
<6	50 in 3-4 divided
>6	50-100 in 3-4 divided

IM, adults: Nausea/vomiting: 25-100 mg q4-6h • Preop/analgesia adjunct/anxiety: 50-100 mg q4-6h
Ⓟ IM, children: Preop/analgesia adjunct: 0.5-1.1 mg/kg

ADMINISTRATION

IM: Use Z-track method
• Avoid IV/SC injection.
• Adults: Inject deeply into gluteus maximus or other large

P muscle. • Children: Inject deeply into midlateral thigh.

ACTIONS

Multiple effects: antihistamine, CNS depressant, anticholinergic, antispasmodic, antiemetic, sedative, local anesthetic • Blocks histamine at H_1-receptor sites • Reduces bronchial constriction/hypersecretion, blocks following histamine-mediated effects: small vessel dilation, increased capillary permeability, edema, pruritus • Suppresses subcortical CNS activity, producing sedation, skeletal muscle relaxation • Antiemetic effects from central anticholinergic, CNS depressant activity • Antispasmodic effects mediated through interference with endogenous spasmogenic agents (e.g., serotonin, acetylcholine, histamine)

PHARMACOKINETICS

ROUTE	ONSET	PEAK	DURATION
PO	15-30 min	2-4 hr	4-6 hr
IM	15 min	<2 hr	4-6 hr

DISTRIBUTION
Widely distributed

ELIMINATION
Metabolized in liver; biliary elimination

---

*Sedative effects. Suppression of inflammatory response may last up to 4 days.

INDICATIONS

To potentiate action/reduce dosage requirements of opiate analgesics • Periop for sedative/antiemetic effects, to potentiate action of opiate analgesics • Anxiety, tension, agitation, including that associated with acute alcohol withdrawal • Nausea, vomiting • Pruritus associated with chronic urticaria, contact dermatoses, allergic reactions, other conditions

PRECAUTIONS/ CONTRAINDICATIONS

Precautions: See usual dose warning. • Inadvertent SC/IV/intraarterial administration may lead to thrombosis, gangrene.
Use caution with: Because of anticholinergic effects, use caution with: Increased intraocular pressure, prostatic hypertrophy, stenosing peptic ulcer, pyloroduodenal obstuction, bladder neck obstruction • Asthma, COPD; anticholinergic effects thicken bronchial secretions/cause obstruction. • Hyperthyroidism • CV disease • Patients at risk for respiratory depression • Hypotension • Heavy sedation
C **Pregnancy category:** Fetal damage in animal studies; risk not established in humans; avoid use in early pregnancy; use later only if safer alternative unavailable.
Contraindications: Hypersensitivity to hydroxyzine • Early pregnancy • IV/SC Route

ADVERSE EFFECTS

CNS: *Drowsiness,* excessive sedation, dizziness, weakness, slurred speech, headache, tremors, **seizures,** paradoxical agitation/anxiety
Resp: Wheezing
CV: Hypotension, hypertension, chest tightness, flushing
GI: *Mouth dryness,* bitter taste, constipation
Local: *Pain,* erythema, irritation, tissue necrosis at injection site

TOXICITY/OVERDOSE

Symptoms: Excessive sedation • Hypotension • Involuntary

H

---

italic = common side effects   **bold** = life-threatening reactions

motor activity, tremors, seizures

Management: After recent ingestion, implement guidelines for management of acute overdose (Appendix I). • Ipecac may be given early before sedative/antiemetic effects appear. If ipecac unsuccessful or gag reflex absent, initiate gastric lavage followed by instillation of activated charcoal. Protect airway by ET intubation, keeping cuff inflated. • **Hypotension:** Elevate legs, administer IV fluids; use vasopressor (e.g., dopamine, norepinephrine) if unresponsive to volume replacement. Avoid epinephrine, which may lead to further lowering of BP. • Avoid stimulants (e.g., caffeine), which may cause seizures. • Dialysis is not likely to be helpful.

INTERACTIONS

alcohol Profound CNS depression
anesthetics ↑ CNS depression
anticholinergics ↑ Anticholinergic effects
barbiturates Profound CNS depression
benzodiazepines ↑ CNS depression
epinephrine Blocked alpha effects; unopposed beta activity; profound hypotension
hypnotics ↑ CNS depression
opioid analgesics (e.g., morphine, hydromorphone) Profound CNS depression; cardiac arrest has occurred
tranquilizers ↑ CNS depression

COMPATIBILITIES

In syringe: atropine, chlorpromazine, cimetidine, codeine, diphenhydramine, doxapram, droperidol, fentanyl, glycopyrrolate, hydromorphone, meperidine, metoclopramide, midazolam, morphine, ondansetron, oxymorphone, pentazocine, prochlorperazine, promazine, promethazine, scopolamine

INCOMPATIBILITIES

In syringe: pentobarbital, ranitidine

PATIENT CARE IMPLICATIONS

• May cause drowsiness, dizziness; use appropriate safety precautions according to patient condition.
• Large quantities should not be prescribed for patients with severe depression, suicidal tendencies, history of substance abuse.
• Use IM route only when PO route unacceptable (e.g., vomiting, NPO status). Convert to PO therapy as soon as possible. See Administration for special instructions with IM use.
Vital signs/hemodynamics: Monitor VS frequently in heavily sedated patients (e.g., those also receiving opiates), during immediate postop period. Use continuous pulse oximetry for heavily sedated patients.
Physical assessment: Assess neurologic status for excessive sedation, dizziness, impaired physical coordination. Reduce dose as necessary. • Assess following parameters according to indication for use: Anxiety: Mental status, mood, presence of agitation/restlessness
Nausea, vomiting: Relief from nausea, vomiting; bowel sounds
Pruritus: Resolution of itching, rash, inflammation
Laboratory tests: May cause: suppressed reaction to antigen skin testing; when possible, discontinue for 4 days before skin testing. • Falsely ele-

vated urinary concentrations of 17-hydroxycorticosteroids

PATIENT/FAMILY TEACHING

Hydroxyzine has multiple uses: to relieve anxiety, reduce symptoms of allergic reaction, increase effectiveness of pain medicine. • May cause dizziness, drowsiness; call for assistance when getting out of bed until response to drug established. • As appropriate for patient condition, encourage frequent oral hygiene and use of hard candy or gum to relieve dry mouth.

Outpatient: Avoid using alcohol or other drugs that cause sedation while taking this medication and for several days after last dose. • Consult with physician or pharmacist before taking any cold, allergy, or sleeping preparations. These may contain antihistamines and cause excessive sedation. • Avoid driving and other activities requiring mental alertness or physical coordination until response to medication well established. • May interfere with allergy skin testing; inform health care provider

AVAILABLE FORMS

Tablets • Capsules • Syrup • PO • Parenteral solution for IM injection.

---

ibuprofen
(eye-byoo′proe′fen)
Advil, Medipren ✷,
Motrin, Nuprin,
PediaProfen, Rufen

Classifications: Nonsteroidal antiinflammatory agent, analgesic, antipyretic

USUAL DOSE/ADMINISTRATION

PO, adult: Mild pain: 200-400 mg q4-6h • **Inflammatory disorders:** 300-800 mg 3-4 times daily • Do not exceed 3200 mg/day. • Older adults: Use lower doses; ↑ risk of adverse reactions.
PO, children >6 mo: Fever <102.5° F: 5mg/kg q6-8h • Fever >102.5° F: 10 mg/kg q6-8h: Do not exceed 40 mg/kg/24 hr.

ADMINISTRATION

PO: Administer with food or milk to ↓ gastric irritation.
G-tube: Use PO suspension.
PO suspension: Shake well before administration.

ACTIONS

Inactivates enzyme necessary for prostaglandin synthesis, thus inhibiting prostaglandin release, reducing pain/inflammation • Analgesic effects primarily peripheral, but hypothalamic or other central mechanisms possibly involved • Reduces fever by hypothalamic action, which causes vasodilation, increased peripheral blood flow, heat dissipation • Inhibits platelet aggregation; prolongs bleeding time

---

italic = common side effects   **bold** = life-threatening reactions

PHARMACOKINETICS

ROUTE	ONSET	PEAK	DURATION*
PO	30 min	1-2 hr	4-8 hr

DISTRIBUTION
90%-99% plasma protein bound

ELIMINATION
Hepatically metabolized, renally excreted; half-life 2-4 hr, longer in older adults

---

*Dose related.

INDICATIONS

Mild to moderate pain, dysmenorrhea • Fever reduction • Pain, inflammation associated with rheumatoid arthritis, osteoarthritis, musculoskeletal injury, other disorders • Used with opiate analgesics (e.g., codeine, meperidine) to augment analgesia, ↓ opiate requirements

PRECAUTIONS/ CONTRAINDICATIONS

Precautions: Chronic use may cause GI ulceration, bleeding, perforation. • May cause dose-dependent reduction in renal prostaglandins, causing fluid retention/possible renal failure, especially with renal/hepatic impairment, heart failure, advanced age, concurrent diuretic therapy • Inhibits platelet aggregation, may prolong bleeding time
Use caution with: Peptic ulcer disease, alcoholism, smoking, ↑ risk of GI bleeding • Older adults; ↑ risk of GI bleeding, renal toxicity • Renal/hepatic impairment, hypertension, heart failure; fluid retention may worsen condition
c Pregnancy category: Safety not established; use only if safer alternative unavailable. NSAIDs associated with fetal closure of ductus arteriosus; avoid use in last trimester.

Contraindications: Hypersensitivity to ibuprofen • Severe allergic reaction to aspirin, other NSAIDs • Active GI bleeding, ulcer disease • Last trimester of pregnancy • Children <12 yr unless specifically prescribed by physician

ADVERSE EFFECTS

CNS: *Dizziness, headache, nervousness,* confusion, drowsiness
EENT: Tinnitus, ↓ hearing, blurred vision
CV: Peripheral edema, fluid retention, **CHF** (preexisting heart disease), ↑ BP, palpitations
GI: *Epigastric pain, nausea, heartburn,* vomiting, diarrhea, constipation, jaundice, hepatitis, **GI bleeding, peptic ulceration/perforation**
GU: ↓ Creat. cl., acute renal failure
Hema: ↓ Hgb, ↑ bleeding time, neutropenia, thrombocytopenia
Derm: *Rash, pruritus,* urticaria
Misc: Allergic reactions, including bronchospasm, **anaphylaxis**

TOXICITY/OVERDOSE

Symptoms: Drowsiness, dizziness, nystagmus • Metabolic acidosis, coma • Hypoventilation, cyanosis, apnea
Management: After recent ingestion, implement guidelines for management of acute overdose (Appendix I). • **Respiratory depression:** Establish/maintain airway; administer O_2, provide ventilatory support as needed. • Ibuprofen is acidic, excreted in urine; forced alkaline diuresis may be helpful. • NSAIDs strongly protein bound; dialysis not helpful

---

INTERACTIONS

alcohol Gastric mucosal damage; ↑ bleeding time

anticoagulants, PO Bleeding complications

digoxin ↑ Digoxin levels

diuretics, ↓ Diuretic effect; nephrotoxicity

heparin Bleeding complications

thrombolytics Bleeding complications

PATIENT CARE IMPLICATIONS

• Administer prn doses at onset of pain.
• Relief of arthritis pain may take 1-2 wk of continuous therapy.

Vital signs/hemodynamics: Antipyretic effects may mask fever associated with infection.
• Monitor temperature before and 1-2 hr after administration when used as antipyretic.
• Measure/record UO. Be alert for evidence of renal insufficiency, especially in older adults, patients with renal, hepatic, CV disease.

Physical assessment: Assess for level of pain, range of motion (as indicated) before and after administration. • Carefully observe for unusual bleeding, bruising. Be especially careful in patients who have coagulation disorders or are receiving anticoagulants. • Assess for GI bleeding. Test stools, emesis for occult blood. Consult physician of positive results. • Assess for fluid retention, edema.

Laboratory tests: Monitor: Hgb/Hct • BUN, creatinine • Electrolytes • Bilirubin, liver enzymes

PATIENT/FAMILY TEACHING

Purpose of medication is to relieve pain/inflammation and reduce fever. • Ask for/take medicine before pain becomes severe. • Immediately report dark tarry stools, blood in stool, vomiting of blood.

Outpatient: Take with food, milk, or antacids to reduce stomach upset. • Consult with physician before using alcohol or taking aspirin, acetaminophen, other over-the-counter (OTC) medications. • Inform dentist or physician of medication regimen before treatment or surgery. • Do not take OTC ibuprofen preparations for more than 10 days for pain or 3 days for fever; consult health care provider if pain or fever persists or worsens. • Report rash, itching, visual disturbances, rapid weight gain, swelling/fluid retention, black stools, unusual bruising/bleeding, severe/persistent headache.

AVAILABLE FORMS

Tablets • PO suspension

---

imipenem/cilastatin sodium
(i-me-pen'em/sye-la-stat'in)
Primaxin

Classification: Carbapenem (penicillin-like) antibiotic/renal dehydropeptidase inhibitor

USUAL DOSE

IM, adults: 500-750 mg q12h
• Maximum dose, 1.5 g/24 hr
IV, adults/children >12 yr: 250-500 mg q6-8h • **Severe infections:** 500 mg-1 g q6-8h
• Maximum dose, 50 mg/kg/24

---

hr or 4 g/24 hr, whichever lower • **Renal insufficiency:** Reduce dose/frequency for creatinine clearance ≤70 ml/min; for creatinine clearance ≤5 ml/min, use only if hemodialysis within 48 hr.

ADMINISTRATION

IM: Inject deep into large muscle mass (e.g., gluteus maximus, lateral thigh). Avoid intravascular injection. • Must use specific preparation labeled for IM use
IV, intermit inf: Infuse each 250-500 mg or less over 20-30 min. • Infuse 1 g dose over 40-60 min. • Slow infusion rate for nausea, vomiting, hypotension.

PREPARATION

IM SUSPENSION NOT FOR IV USE
IM: Use specifically labeled product. Reconstitute with 2-3 ml 1% lidocaine HCl for injection. • Shake well to form suspension. • Prepare immediately before use.
IV, cont inf: Initially dilute with 10 ml 0.9% NaCl; further dilute with 100 ml 0.9% NaCl. Final concentration will be 2.5 mg/ml when 250-mg dose used, 5 mg/ml when 500-mg dose used. Do not exceed final concentration of 5 mg/ml. • Shake well to dissolve. • To transfer all contents of vial into infusion container, return 10 ml prepared solution to vial, shake, withdraw, return to infusion container.
Compatible fluids: 0.9% NaCl, D_5W (for approx 4 hr)
Stability: Reconstituted IV solution stable for 10 hr at room temperature if prepared with

0.9% NaCl • Stable for 4 hr if other solutions used

ACTIONS

Very broad-spectrum bactericidal antibiotic that interferes with bacterial cell wall synthesis/division, thus causing cellular death. Cilastatin, which has no antibacterial activity alone, added in equal amounts to prevent rapid metabolism of imipenem • Excellent activity against most gram-positive organisms, including *Enterococcus faecalis,* gram-negative/anaerobic organisms • More active against *Pseudomonas aeruginosa, Bacteroides fragilis* than 3rd generation cephalosporins

PHARMACOKINETICS

ROUTE	ONSET	PEAK	DURATION
IM	Rapid	2 hr	Up to 12 hr
IV	Immed	End infusion	6-8 hr

DISTRIBUTION
Widely distributed; low CSF levels

ELIMINATION
75% excreted unchanged in urine within 10 hr; half-life 1.3 hr, longer with renal dysfunction

INDICATIONS

Treatment of serious bacterial infections caused by multiple or antibiotic-resistant organisms • Often used for hospital-acquired infections or respiratory tract, skin/soft tissue, GU tract, bone/joint infections; also for septicemia, endocarditis, intraabdominal infections • Preferred over 3rd generation cephalosporins for intraabdominal infections because of activity against *B. fragilis* • Choice agent for serious infections involving *Enterobacter, Acinetobacter,* sometimes in combination with aminoglycoside

• When used for *Pseudomonas* infections, concurrent aminoglycoside therapy recommended to prevent resistance • Useful in patients with impaired renal function as alternative to aminoglycoside therapy

PRECAUTIONS/ CONTRAINDICATIONS

Precautions: IM suspension not for IV use; read label carefully when preparing. • IM route not indicated for severe infections • Bacterial or fungal overgrowth possible

Use caution with: Renal impairment, advanced age, preexisting CNS disorder, high-dose/prolonged therapy; adverse CNS effects more likely • Hypersensitivity to penicillins, cephalosporins; hypersensitivity more likely • Children ≤12 yr: Safety not established

Pregnancy category: Fetal risk unknown; use only if safer alternative unavailable.

Contraindications: Hypersensitivity to imipenem, cilastatin • IM injection (reconstituted with lidocaine), with lidocaine hypersensitivity, heart block, severe shock • Meningitis • Severe renal impairment with creatinine clearance ≤5 ml/min, unless hemodialysis performed within 48 hr

ADVERSE EFFECTS

CNS: Dizziness, somnolence, confusion, headache, tremor, **seizures**

GI: *Nausea, vomiting, diarrhea;* ↑ liver enzymes; pseudomembranous colitis

Hema: Leukopenia, neutropenia, agranulocytosis, thrombocytopenia, positive direct Coombs' test

Derm: Rash, pruritus, urticaria

Local: Painful injection, phlebitis (IV)

Misc: Hypersensitivity, **anaphylaxis;** superinfection, colonization

TOXICITY/OVERDOSE

Symptoms: Neuromuscular excitability/seizures, particularly in renal impairment, high-dose therapy, preexisting CNS disease • Acute allergic reaction • Pseudomembranous colitis with abdominal pain, diarrhea

Management: Discontinue drug. • Initiate symptomatic/supportive measures, including airway protection/anticonvulsant therapy, as needed. • For acute allergic reaction, see Appendix N. • Treat severe pseudomembranous colitis, with PO vancomycin or metronidazole. • Hemodialysis may be useful.

INTERACTIONS

cephalosporins Antagonistic antibacterial activity

cyclosporine CNS toxicity

ganciclovir Seizures

penicillins, extended spectrum Antagonistic antibacterial activity

theophylline CNS toxicity

Y-SITE COMPATIBILITIES

Acyclovir, cefepime, diltiazem, famotidine, insulin, ondansetron, zidovudine

Y-SITE INCOMPATIBILITIES

Aminoglycosides, fluconazole, meperidine

PATIENT CARE IMPLICATIONS

• Obtain specimens for culture and sensitivity before initiating

---

italic = common side effects   **bold** = life-threatening reactions

antibiotic therapy. Initiate therapy before results received.
• Determine previous antibiotic use, including reactions to penicillins, cephalosporins. Cross-reactivity may occur; monitor closely.
• Have epinephrine, antihistamine, resuscitation equipment readily available for use with severe allergic reaction.
• Seizure precautions indicated for patients with preexisting CNS disease or receiving hemodialysis.
• If focal tremors, myoclonus, seizures develop, reduce dose or discontinue therapy.
• Do not discharge patient for at least 30 min after antibiotic administration.

IV
• Reduce risk of thrombophlebitis by using large veins and small catheters/needles, rotating infusion sites.
• IV preferred over IM route and must be used for severe infections or when shock present.
Vital signs: Monitor VS for indicators of infection, complications.
Physical assessment: Assess for improvement in primary infection or symptoms of super/suprainfection: appearance of sputum, urine, stool, wound drainage; presence of fever, candidiasis, vaginitis. • Observe for symptoms of hypersensitivity: rash, pruritus, wheezing, laryngeal edema, hypotension. • Assess for evidence of CNS toxicity: confusion, muscle twitching, focal tumors, seizures. Monitor closely if preexisting CNS disorder, severe renal failure, high-dose therapy.
Laboratory tests: Monitor: Electrolytes • ALT, AST, alka-

line phosphatase • CBC with differential • Urinalysis, BUN, creatinine • **May cause:** Positive direct antiglobulin (Coombs') test

PATIENT/FAMILY TEACHING
Purpose of drug is to limit growth of infection-causing bacteria. • Immediately report rash, swelling, intense itching, difficulty breathing, other signs of allergic reaction. • Report diarrhea, blood/mucus in stool, fever, abdominal pain, vaginal discharge, furry growth on tongue, muscle twitching, mental confusion.

AVAILABLE FORMS
Suspension for IM use • Solution for IV use

---

immune globulin (Ig), immune gamma globulin (IgG), immune serum globulin (ISG)
Gamastan, Gamimune N, Gammar, Sandoglobulin

Classification: Serum, immune globulin

USUAL DOSE
🅟 **IM, adults/children:** Hepatitis A virus (HAV) exposure: Single dose of 0.02 ml/kg as soon as possible after exposure • HAV prevention: Single dose of 0.02 ml/kg when anticipated exposure ≤3 mo; use 0.06 ml/kg q4-6mo when exposure >3 mo • Hepatitis C percutaneous exposure: Single dose of 0.06 ml/kg as soon as possible after exposure • Measles (rubeola) exposure: Single

dose of 0.25 ml/kg within 6 days of exposure; not to exceed 15 ml; if >15 mo; follow with measles vaccine in 3 mo.
• **Measles (rubeola) exposure, immunosuppressed individuals:** Single dose of 0.5 ml/kg; not to exceed 15 ml
• **Immunodeficiency disease:** Initially 1.2 ml/kg; maintenance, 0.6 ml/kg q2-4wk or more often; maximum dose, adults, 30-50 ml; children, 20-30 ml
IV, intermit inf: Dosing regimens vary according to specific preparation, indication. Consult individual manufacturer's literature for details • **Immunodeficiency syndrome:** 100-400 mg/kg q3-4 wk; dose individualized to achieve/maintain IgG levels, therapeutic response • Loading dose of 200-400 mg/kg may be given. • **Idiopathic thrombocytopenic purpura (ITP):** 400-1,000 mg/kg for 2-5 days and intermittently to maintain platelet count

ADMINISTRATION

IM AND IV PREPARATIONS NOT INTERCHANGEABLE; CHECK LABEL BEFORE USE. Solution is transparent to opalescent, colorless to brown; do not use if cloudy or discolored.
IM: Inject deep into large muscle mass. Multiple injection sites necessary for volumes >10 ml. Use anterolateral thigh for injections in young children. Draw back on plunger to verify IM placement before injection; inadvertent IV administration may cause serious hypersensitivity reaction.
IV, intermit inf: Administration recommendations vary according to specific preparation; consult individual manufacturer's literature. In all cases, use slow infusion rate initially and monitor closely for hypersensitivity, other adverse effects. Too-rapid infusion may cause profound hypotension. Stop or slow infusion for ↓ BP, other reactions. Do not mix or infuse with other solutions • **Sandoglobulin:** First infusion: 0.5-1.0 ml/min for first 15-30 min; may increase to 1.5-2.5 ml/min if no adverse effects. Subsequent infusions: 2-2.5 ml/min • **Gamimune N:** 0.01 to 0.02 ml/kg/min for first 30 min (0.8-1.6 ml/min for 80-kg person); may increase to 0.08 ml/kg/min if no adverse effects

PREPARATION

Strict sterile technique required throughout preparation. In-line filter or filtration via filter needle (usually provided by manufacturer) is necessary for all preparations. Specific equipment and technique required for each brand; check manufacturer's literature.

ACTIONS

Sterile solution of antibody-containing globulins prepared from plasma of pooled donors • Provides immediate passive immunity by temporarily increasing antibody titer. • Aids in prevention of or modifies response to some infectious diseases, including HAV, measles (rubeola) • Improves immunologic response of patients with immunosuppressive disorders

---

PHARMACOKINETICS

ROUTE	ONSET	PEAK	DURATION
IM	Rapid	2 days	1-3 mo
IV	Immed.	End inf.	21 days

INDICATIONS

IM: To provide passive immunity after exposure to measles (rubeola), hepatitis A virus (HAV), certain infectious diseases, esp. in patients with immunoglobin deficiency • Prevention of HAV infection in travelers to foreign countries with high risk of exposure • Replacement therapy to prevent infection in individuals with IgG, certain other antibody-deficiency diseases
IV: To rapidly increase gamma globulin levels in individuals with immunosupression, ↑ risk of infection. Includes those with symptomatic HIV infection, organ transplants, hematologic malignancies, extensive burns, severe collagen-vascular disease

PRECAUTIONS/ CONTRAINDICATIONS

Precautions: IM, IV formulations not interchangeable • Not for SC use; do not skin test
Use caution with: History of systemic hypersensitivity reactions; anaphylaxis more likely, especially with repeated doses • **IM:** Thrombocytopenia, hemophillia—injection may cause bleeding; avoid use with severe bleeding disorder
c Pregnancy category: Safety not established; use only when clearly needed.
Contraindications: Hypersensitivity to immune globulin, thimerosal (preservative) • Selective IgA deficiencies; may cause severe anaphylaxis

ADVERSE EFFECTS

CNS: Headache, malaise
MS: Arthralgia, myalgia
Derm: Itching
Local: *Pain, tenderness, muscle stiffness,* inflammation at injection site
Misc: Fever, repeated injections may cause allergic response with chills, fever, sweating, hypotension, **anaphylaxis**

INTERACTIONS

Vaccines, live (measles, mumps, rubella, oral polio) May interfere with immune response to live vaccines; may need to defer administration for 3 mo after immune globulin

PATIENT CARE IMPLICATIONS

• Have epinephrine, antihistamine, resuscitation equipment immediately available at time of injection.
IM: Determine date of exposure to infection. Administer within 2 wk of HAV exposure, within 6 days of measles (rubeola) exposure.
Vital signs: Monitor VS before and 30 min after IM injection. Monitor VS closely during first 60 min of IV inf.
Physical assessment: Assess for allergic reaction (e.g., chills, fever, sweating, itching, rash, laryngeal edema, wheezing), especially with repeated injections. Outpatients should be observed for at least 30 min after injection.
Laboratory tests: Testing for anti-HAV antibodies recommended for individuals requiring repeat prophylaxis

PATIENT/FAMILY TEACHING

Purpose of medication is to provide temporary immunity against hepatitis, measles, other infectious diseases. • Pain, tenderness, muscle stiffness at injection site may occur. • Immediately report allergic reaction such as chills, fever, sweating, itching, breathing difficulty.
• HAV prophylaxis: To minimize risk of infection, travelers should avoid potentially contaminated water, food. Hepatitis A vaccine recommended.

AVAILABLE FORMS

Parenteral for IM use • Store refrigerated at 2°-8° C (35°-46° F); do not freeze.

---

insulin
(in'su-lin)

regular, crystalline zinc
Humulin R, Novolin R, Velosulin Human
isophane, NPH
Humulin N, NPH, Novolin N
lente, insulin zinc
Humulin L, Lente, Novolin L
ultralente, extended insulin zinc
Humulin U, Ultralente U
isophane 70% with regular 30%
Humulin 70/30, Novolin 70/30
isophane 50% with regular 50%
Humulin 50/50

Classifications: Hormone, insulin

USUAL DOSE

Regular insulin: IV inj/inf, adults/children: Highly variable, according to condition/individual response; often formula based; usual range, 2-12 U/hr; much higher doses may be required in severe diabetic ketoacidosis (DKA). • Each unit regular insulin decreases blood glucose level by approx 10 mg/dl. • Formula-based dose, suggested formula:

Blood glucose level − 100 ÷ 40
    = Dose of regular insulin (U)

DKA: 1-2 U/kg in 2 equally divided doses: 1 SC, 1 IV; then formula-based dosing used; continuous IV inf facilitates once daily administration. • **SC, adults:** Total daily dose of 0.5-1.5 U/kg administered in 2-4 divided doses, usually before meals and hs • May be administered by SC infusion using external or internal controlled-infusion device • **SC, children:** total daily dose of 1-2 U/kg administered in 2-4 divided doses, usually 15-30 min before meals and hs
Semilente insulin: SC, adults/children: 10-20 U 30 min before breakfast and repeated 30 min before dinner
• Dose adjusted to blood glucose level
Isophane (NPH)/lente insulin: SC, adults/children: Initially, total daily dose of 0.1-0.4 U/kg once daily 30 min before breakfast • Maintenance, gradually ↑ as needed to 0.5-1.2 U/kg once daily 30 min before breakfast. When dose exceeds 30 U/day, administer in two divided doses, usually 30 min be-

---

fore breakfast and 30 min before dinner

Ultralente insulin: SC, adults: Initially, 7-26 U q24-48h 30-60 min before breakfast • Maintenance, gradually increase as needed according to blood glucose.

Isophane (NPH) 70% with regular 30% insulin: SC, adults/children: Initially, total daily dose of 0.5-0.6 U/kg; give ⅔ of total daily dose 30-60 min before breakfast. Give remaining ½ 30-60 min before dinner • Maintenance, gradually increase as needed according to blood glucose levels.

ADMINISTRATION

All insulins: SC inj: Inject deep into subcutaneous tissue; 90° angle generally used for all but very thin individuals, for whom 45° angle may be necessary; Rotate injection sites

Regular insulin only:

IV inj: Inject ≤50 units over 1 min. • May be diluted to facilitate administration • Use only clear, colorless insulin.

IV, cont inf: Usually 2-12 U/hr. • Titrate according to blood glucose levels, which must be checked q1-4h • Partial absorption of insulin by IV infusion set may cause variability in amount of insulin delivered to patient (see Preparation). *Careful monitoring with appropriate adjustment of insulin dose is essential.*

PREPARATION

SC: To promote even suspension/accurate dose, roll vial between palms to mix before withdrawing insulin. • When mixing in syringe, ensure compatibility (see table); withdraw regular insulin first. • Never mix various sources of insulin (e.g., beef, pork, biosynthetic).

Syringe compatibility of insulins

TYPE	COMPATIBLE
Regular	All insulins
Isophane	Regular only
Lente	Regular, semilente
Ultralente	Regular, semilente
Isophane with regular combinations	Premixed; do not mix with other insulins

IV: To promote even suspension/accurate dose, roll vial between palms to mix before withdrawing insulin. • Dilute in 100-1,000 ml compatible solution, usually 0.9% or 0.45% NaCl. • Concentrated solutions may be used if necessary to limit fluid intake. • Standard filters, bottles, bags, infusion sets absorb up to 80% of insulin, although 20%-30% loss typical. DO NOT USE IV FILTER. Most absorption occurs within first 30-60 min; actual dose delivered may be highly variable, especially with initial infusion/subsequent IV tubing changes. Methods to reduce insulin absorption include addition of albumin to infusion solution, flushing administration set before use, use of syringe pump with short IV tubing.

DILUTION	CONCENTRATION
125 U/500 ml	0.25 U/ml
125 U/250 ml	0.50 U/ml
100 U/100 ml	1.0 U/ml
200 U/100 ml	2.0 U/ml

More concentrated solutions may be used.

Compatible fluids: D_5W, 0.4%/0.9% NaCl, LR, prepared combinations of these solutions

ACTIONS

Facilitates transport of glucose from bloodstream across cell membranes into cells; provides subtrates for energy production, lowers blood glucose levels • Facilitates glycogen production/storage • Promotes conversion of amino acids to proteins in muscle, stimulates formation of triglycerides • Promotes intracellular shift of potassium, magnesium • Effects antagonized by epinephrine, growth hormone, estrogens, adrenocorticoids, thyroid hormones • Beef, pork traditional insulin sources; porcine most similar to human insulin; Humulin/Novolin of recombinant DNA origin

PHARMACOKINETICS

SC administration

TYPE*	ONSET	PEAK	DURATION
R	30-60 min	2-4 hr	4-8 hr
I	1-2 hr	4-12 hr	18-24 hr
L	1-3 hr	6-16 hr	18-24 hr
U	4-8 hr	8-20 hr	24-36 hr
I/R	30-60 min	2-12 hr	18-24 hr

DISTRIBUTION

Widely distributed throughout extracellular fluids

ELIMINATION

Metabolized by liver; 80% reabsorbed by kidneys

*R, Regular; I, isophane; L. lente; U, ultralente; IR, Isophane 70% with regular 30%.

INDICATIONS

To supplement deficient/absent endogenous insulin, thus facilitating carbohydrate, fat, protein metabolism/storage • Management of hyperglycemia, prevention of DKA • Management of hyperglycemia, hyperglycemic hyperosmolar nonketotic coma (HHNK, HHNC) DM unresponsive to diet and/or PO agents

• As additive in hyperalimentation solutions to assist in appropriate utilization of glucose, prevent hyperglycemia • In combination with dextrose to reduce serum potassium levels in hyperkalemia

PRECAUTIONS/CONTRAINDICATIONS

Precautions: Many different preparations available; check label carefully before administration. • Changes in insulin regimen require close monitoring for 3-21 days • Resistance to insulin possible; doses ≥ 200 U/day may be required. • Changes in insulin source (e.g., beef, pork, biosynthetic) may lower dosage requirements. • Excessive dosage causes hypoglycemia, coma, irreversible neurologic damage • Breakdown of fatty tissue at injection site (lipoatrophy) may leave skin depressions, particularly with nonbiosynthetic insulin. • Accumulation of fatty tissue at injection site (lipohypertrophy) occurs with repeated injection into one site; decreased insulin absorption results.

Use caution with: Stress, severe illness/injury, pregnancy, surgery; ↑ dosage may be necessary.

C Pregnancy category: Use only if safer alternative unavailable.

Contraindications: Hypersensitivity to insulin source (beef, pork), additives/preservatives in particular insulin product

ADVERSE EFFECTS

Endo: **Hypoglycemia,** rebound hyperglycemia

---

italic = common side effects   **bold** = life-threatening reactions

Local: *Lipoatrophy, lipohyper-trophy,* redness, itching, pain, swelling at injection site
Misc: Allergic reactions, **anaphylaxis**

TOXICITY/OVERDOSE

Symptoms: Hypoglycemia: Anxiety, nervousness, confusion, cool pale skin, cold sweats, irritability, headache, nausea, shakiness, weakness, altered mental status, progressing comma

Management: Obtain blood glucose via venipuncture or arterial line; fingerstick samples may be falsely low. In severe cases, do not delay treatment pending laboratory results.
• Mild hypoglycemia: Administer rapidly absorbed PO carbohydrate (e.g., 120-180 ml fruit juice, 2-3 tsp granulated sugar, 2-4 glucose tablets). • Severe hypoglycemia: Requires immediate treatment with 50% dextrose, 25-50 ml IV push for adults; glucagon used if unable to obtain IV access • Failure to readily detect/correct hypoglycemia may lead to irreversible, severe neurologic impairment/death. • Continue to monitor closely blood glucose levels q30-60min to detect recurrence of hypoglycemia, rebound hyperglycemia.

INTERACTIONS

alcohol, aspirin, beta-blockers, haloperidol Hypoglycemia corticosteroids; diltiazem; diuretics, thiazide; glucagon; oral contraceptives; sympathomimetics (e.g., epinephrine, dopamine, norepinephrine) ↓ Insulin effectiveness

Y-SITE COMPATIBILITIES

Regular insulin only—ampicillin, ampicillin-sulbactam, cefazolin, cefotetan, digoxin, dobutamine, famotidine, gentamicin, heparin, imipenem cilastatin, magnesium sulfate, meperidine, morphine, pentobarbital, potassium chloride, sodium bicarbonate, ticarcillin, ticarcillin-clavulanate, tobramycin, vancomycin

INCOMPATIBILITIES

Regular insulin only—aminophylline, dobutamine, nafcillin

PATIENT CARE IMPLICATIONS

• Split-dose (twice daily) regimen may be necessary for optimal control of blood glucose. Multidose therapy (3-4 injections daily) sometimes necessary to achieve control; portable insulin pump indicated if not controlled with multidose therapy
• Resistance to insulin possible; doses ≥ 200 U/day may be required. Changes in insulin source (e.g., beef, pork, biosynthetic) may result in lower dosage requirements; this effect may be used to therapeutic advantage.
• Many implications during preparation/administration; see previous sections.

Vital signs/hemodynamics: Monitor VS according to patient condition. • Hypoglycemia, DKA, HHNK: Frequent monitoring of BP, PR; continuous ECG monitoring necessary
• DKA, HHNK: PAP monitoring necessary for optimal management of fluid volume status; initial PCWP, CVP readings

---

usually < 5 mm Hg, reflecting hypovolemic status; profound hypovolemia usually results in CI < 2.5 L/min/m². Replace fluids, monitoring closely as PCWP, CVP, CI improve. Avoid overaggressive fluid resuscitation; hourly measurements usually necessary until condition stabilizes. Hourly UO measurement necessary to manage fluid status

Physical assessment: Assess for hypoglycemia: anxiety, nervousness, confusion, cool pale skin, cold sweats, irritability, headache, nausea, shakiness, weakness, altered mental status progressing to coma; must be readily detected/managed with rapidly absorbed oral carbohydrates, glucagon, IV dextrose, as appropriate. Failure to detect/correct may lead to irreversible, severe neurologic impairment. • Assess for hyperglycemia: drowsiness, tiredness, hot dry skin, fruity breath odor, urinary frequency, thirst. • **Type I DM:** Extended period of inadequate insulin maintenance or inadequate replacement during times of stress (e.g., infection, trauma, surgery, severe illness) may result in DKA, life-threatening condition manifested by profound hyperglycemia, ketoacidosis, tachypnea, tachycardia, hypovolemic shock. • **Type II DM:** Inadequate oral hypoglycemic or inadequate supplemental insulin therapy may result in HHNK, life-threatening condition manifested by profound hyperglycemic/hypovolemic shock. • Assess for local reactions such as redness, itching, swelling, pain at injection sites; may result from improper injection technique, sensitivity to type of insulin, skin cleaning solution, preservatives. • Assess visual acuity in patients preparing for home insulin preparation. Devices (e.g., magnifiers, pens) are available for patients with poor vision.

Laboratory tests: Monitor: Blood glucose • Serum potassium • Glycohemoglobin • Discontinue continuous insulin infusion when blood glucose reaches 250 mg/dl. • **Severe DKA, HHNK:** Monitor blood glucose q1h until condition stabilizes; insulin requirements widely variable; as much as 20,000 U may be required in first 24 hr. Frequent (e.g., q2h) potassium monitoring necessary because insulin will accelerate intracellular potassium shift after correction of acidosis; serious hypokalemia may develop.

PATIENT/FAMILY TEACHING

Purpose of medication is to lower blood sugar. • Medication controls blood sugar but does not cure DM. Compliance with dietary, activity, insulin administration regimen is essential to control blood sugar, prevent serious complications. • Symptoms of hypoglycemia (low blood sugar) include anxiety, nervousness, confusion, cool pale skin, cold sweats, irritability, headache, nausea, shakiness, weakness. Take rapid-acting sugar such as hard candy, fruit juice, or sugar and report to health care provider. • Symptoms of hyperglycemia (high blood sugar) include drowsiness, tiredness, hot dry skin, fruity breath odor, frequent urination, thirst. Measure blood sugar using home device (if prescribed). • Verify correct use

---

italic = common side effects   **bold** = life-threatening reactions

of home blood sugar monitor. Monitor closely during illness or stress. • Report nausea, vomiting, loss of appetite, fever or uncontrolled blood sugar levels. • Weigh periodically; report substantial changes in body weight, because dose adjustment may be necessary. • Carry source of sugar (hard candy, sugar packets), Medic-Alert ID at all times. • Avoid alcohol use; can contribute to hypoglycemia. Do not use any other medications without consulting primary health care provider. • Notify all health care providers of insulin therapy. • Verify appropriate injection technique; include system for rotation of injection sites and mixing instructions (see Preparation).

AVAILABLE FORMS

Regular insulin in parenteral suspension for IV/IM/SC injection • Other insulins in suspension for IM/SC use only
Storage: Store opened insulin at room temperature. Store unopened insulin in refrigerator. Avoid exposure to direct sunlight or extreme heat.

ipecac syrup
(ip'e-kak)
Ipecacuanha syrup

Classification: Emetic

USUAL DOSE

Check label carefully; use ipecac syrup, not ipecac fluid extract (fluid extract not available in US)
P PO, adults/children: Dose according to age (see below)

• Clear carbonated beverages
P may be used with children who refuse water; fluids may be given before ipecac. • Repeat dose once in 30 min if vomiting has not occurred. If vomiting does not occur within 30 min of 2nd dose, perform gastric lavage and/or administer activated charcoal. • When activated charcoal also prescribed, give ipecac first; wait for completion of vomiting before administering charcoal. Alternatively, charcoal may be given at least 10 min after ipecac and readministered after vomiting.
P PO, adults/children >12 yr: 30 ml followed by 200-300 ml water
P PO, children 1-11 yr: 15 ml followed by 100-200 ml water
• Activity may induce emesis sooner.
P PO, children 6 mo-1 yr: 5-10 ml followed by 60-100 ml water; Do not administer with milk. • Gentle bouncing may induce emesis sooner.

ACTIONS

Produces vomiting by stimulating CTZ in medulla, irritating gastric mucosa • Contents of stomach, upper intestine regurgitated • Emptying may be incomplete.

PHARMACOKINETICS

ROUTE	ONSET	PEAK/DURATION
PO	<20 min	90% of patients vomit within 30 min

INDICATIONS

Oral drug overdose/poisonings except strychnine, caustic/corrosive agents, volatile oils
• Sometimes used after ingestion of petroleum distillates, de-

pending on amount ingested, risk of systemic toxicity • Most effective when administered shortly after ingestion of poison • When used after acute overdose of cardiac glycosides, may potentiate high-degree AV block, strong vagal activity

PRECAUTIONS/ CONTRAINDICATIONS

Use caution with: Cardiac glycoside overdose, impaired cardiac function; may potentiate high-degree AV block • Cerebrovascular disease, hypertension; vomiting may increase BP, lead to hemorrhage. • History of seizure disorder, ingestion of toxins likely to cause seizures • Ingestion of sedatives; use only if ingestion recent, patient fully alert.

c Pregnancy category: Use in pregnancy only when clearly needed and benefits outweigh risk.

Contraindications: Hypersensitivity to ipecac • Ingestion of caustic/corrosive substances • Ingestion of petroleum distillates when risk of toxicity low, risk of aspiration high • CNS depression, ↓ level of consciousness, severe inebriation, seizures, absent gag reflex

ADVERSE EFFECTS

Side effects more likely if vomiting does not occur and ipecac systemically absorbed
CNS: Sedation, **seizures**
CV: Tachycardia, **dysrhythmias, hypotension**
GI: *Protracted vomiting,* diarrhea

TOXICITY/OVERDOSE

Symptoms, acute toxicity:
Usually associated with inadver-

tent substitution of ipecac fluid extract (14 times potency of ipecac syrup) for ipecac syrup • Cardiac conduction disturbances, bradycardia, atrial fibrillation, tachycardia • Diminished myocardial contractility, hypotension, potentially fatal myocarditis • Bloody diarrhea, protracted emesis • Dyspnea, shock • Seizures, coma

Symptoms, chronic toxicity:
Potentially fatal cardiotoxicity, myopathy associated with chronic abuse by individuals with eating disorders • Cardiotoxic effects: chest pain, dyspnea, hypotension, cardiac failure, SVT, ventricular tachycardia/fibrillation, cardiac arrest • Myopathy manifested by weakness, muscle aching, hyporeflexia, stiffness, dysphagia, slurred speech, difficulty with motor tasks

Management: Initiate symptomatic/supportive care. • Use gastric lavage and/or activated charcoal if vomiting does not occur. • Cardiac glycosides/ pacemakers used to counter cardiotoxicity

INTERACTIONS

antiemetics Depression of CTZ; ineffective response to ipecac
charcoal Absorption of ipecac; reduced effectiveness
digoxin With digoxin overdose, vagal activity may trigger high-degree AV block

PATIENT CARE IMPLICATIONS

• Obtain history; do not administer to patients who have ingested caustic/corrosive substances, volatile oils, petroleum distillates when risk of toxicity low, risk of aspiration high

---

italic = common side effects   **bold** = life-threatening reactions

• Assess neurologic status; avoid administration to patients with CNS depression, diminished level of consciousness, severe inebriation, seizures, absent gag reflex.
• Have airway management/resuscitation equipment immediately available.
• Always administer with appropriate amount of water or clear carbonated beverages (see Usual Dose). Do not administer with milk.
• When possible, keep patient active, moving after administration to facilitate emesis. Gentle ⓟ bouncing of young children may induce emesis sooner.
• If vomiting does not occur within 30 min of 2nd dose, perform gastric lavage and/or administer activated charcoal to absorb ipecac.
Vital signs/hemodynamics: Monitor VS frequently according to substance ingested, patient condition. • Monitor ECG if cardiotoxic substance ingested, history of cardiac disease, if vomiting not induced.
Physical assessment: Assess for CNS depression. Be prepared to protect airway if patient becomes lethargic, unresponsive, or lacks gag reflex.
• After administration, monitor amount, consistency, frequency of emesis.

PATIENT/FAMILY TEACHING

Vomiting is desired effect, occurs within 20-30 min. • **Home use:** Contact poison control center or physician before administration. Avoid inducing ⓟ vomiting if child has ingested caustic/corrosive substance, volatile oil, petroleum distillate or ⓟ if child unconscious, drowsy,

convulsing. Check expiration date annually and before use.

AVAILABLE FORMS

Syrup

isoetharine HCl
isoetharine mesylate
(eye-soe-eth'-a-reen)
Bronkosol, Bronkometer

Classification: Beta-2-adrenergic agonist

USUAL DOSE

Metered dose inhaler, adults: 1-2 puffs q4-6h
Nebulizer/IPPB, adults: 4 ml of 0.125% solution • 2.5 ml of 0.2% solution • 2 ml of 0.25% solution • 0.5 ml of 1% solution, diluted with NaCl

ADMINISTRATION

Nebulization/IPPB: Dilute 1% solution with 0.9% NaCl in 1:3 ratio. • Adjust flow rate of nebulizer to deliver entire dose over 15-20 min.

ACTIONS

Stimulates beta-adrenergic receptors; predominant effects on beta-2 (bronchial, uterine, vascular smooth muscle) receptors at usual doses; cardiac, CNS stimulatory effects more likely at higher doses • Results in bronchodilation, mild vasodilation, slight decreases in BP; may cause reflex tachycardia, especially at higher doses • Little or no effect on alpha-adrenergic receptors

PHARMACOKINETICS

ROUTE	ONSET	PEAK	DURATION
Inhal	Rapid	5-15 min	1-4 hr

DISTRIBUTION
Not clearly established

ELIMINATION
Metabolized in lungs, liver; excreted in urine; half-life 3-5 hr

INDICATIONS

Relief of bronchospasm in asthma, chronic bronchitis, emphysema • Longer duration, less likely to cause cardiac stimulation than isoproterenol

PRECAUTIONS/ CONTRAINDICATIONS

Precautions: Acidosis ↓ effectiveness, ↑ adverse effects • Tolerance may develop with prolonged use. • Repeated/excessive use may lead to paradoxical bronchoconstriction. • Commercial preparations may contain sulfites, which may cause serious allergic reactions.

Use caution with: Cardiac disorders • Hypertension • Hyperthyroidism • Diabetes mellitus • Cerebral arteriosclerosis

c **Pregnancy category:** Use only if safer alternative unavailable.

Contraindications: Hypersensitivity to isoetharine

ADVERSE EFFECTS

CNS: *Tremors, nervousness,* insomnia, headache, dizziness, restlessness, irritability
Resp: Cough, bronchial irritation, paradoxical bronchospasm
CV: Palpitations, tachycardia, ↑ ↓ BP, dysrhythmias
GI: Nausea, vomiting
Misc: Tolerance

INTERACTIONS

beta-blockers ↓ Isoetharine effectiveness
sympathomimetics Tachycardia, dysrhythmias, ↑ ↓ BP

PATIENT CARE IMPLICATIONS

• For optimal benefits in controlling bronchospasm, schedule doses at regular intervals.
• Acidosis decreases effectiveness, increases risk of dysrhythmias, other adverse effects; when possible correct before initiating therapy.

Vital signs/hemodynamics: Monitor ECG for tachycardia, dysrhythmias. • Monitor VS for hypo/hypertension, improved RR. • Use pulse oximeter to evaluate O_2 saturation before and after administration.

Physical assessment: Assess work of breathing, ventilatory excursion, breath sounds. • As available, check peak flow before and after treatment until stable.

Laboratory tests: Monitor: ABGs

PATIENT/FAMILY TEACHING

Purpose of medication is to relieve bronchospasm, improve breathing. • Report increased breathing difficulty, chest pain, palpitations. • Sips of water or sugarless gum may help dry mouth. • Check with health care professional before taking cold or cough preparations. • Use metered dose inhaler as demonstrated. Be certain to exhale completely before use, close lips firmly around mouthpiece, inhale deeply while activating the inhaler. Hold breath for as long as possible, exhale slowly.

---

italic = common side effects **bold** = life-threatening reactions

• Use exactly as directed. If ineffective, do not increase dose or frequency of use; consult primary health care provider.

AVAILABLE FORMS

Solution for oral inhalation therapy • Metered dose inhaler

isoproterenol HCl/isoproterenol sulfate

(eye-soe-proe-ter′e-nole)
Isopro, Isuprel, Medihaler-Iso, Norisodrine

Classifications: Sympathomimetic, inotropic agent, beta-adrenergic agonist, bronchodilator, antidysrhythmic

USUAL DOSE

Direct IV, adults: Heart block/bradycardia/shock: Initially 0.02-0.06 mg (1-3 ml 1:50,000 *dilute* solution); thereafter 0.01-0.2 mg (0.5-10 ml 1:50,000 *dilute* solution) according to patient's response • **Asthma, bronchospasm:** 0.01-0.02 mg (0.5-1 ml 1:50,000 *dilute* solution), may be administered IM/SC, but will delay onset of action.
IV, cont inf, adults: 0.5-2.0 μg/min (8 ml/hr of 4 μg/ml solution) maximum recommended dose, 30 μg/min; >rates used with advanced shock
P IV, cont inf, children: 0.1-1.0 μg/kg/min • Maximum recommended dose, 1.6 μg/kg/min
Metered-dose inhal: 1-2 inhal 3-6 times/day
Nebulization/IPPB, adults: 0.5 ml 0.5% solution in 2-2.5 ml sterile water or 0.9% NaCl up to 5 times/day • Adjust flow rate to deliver dose over 10-20 min. • Do not exceed 2 doses/hr.
P Nebulization/IPPB, children: 0.25 ml 0.5% solution in 2-2.5 ml sterile water or 0.9% NaCl up to 5 times/day. • Adjust flow rate to deliver dose over 10-20 min. • Do not exceed 2 doses/hr.

ADMINISTRATION

V Direct IV: Inject each 0.02 mg (1 ml 1:50,000 *dilute* solution) or smaller dose over at least 1 min. • SOLUTION MUST BE DILUTED BEFORE INJECTION.
IV, cont inf: Infuse via central, antecubital, or other large vein. • Use infusion pump. • Start at 0.5 μg/min for adults or increase by 0.5-2 μg/min q5-15min until desired HR/CO achieved (Infusion Rate table, Appendix Q). • Always use lowest effective dose.

PREPARATION

Direct IV: Dilute 0.2 mg (1 ml 1:5,000 solution) with 0.9% NaCl for total volume of 10 ml to yield 0.02 mg/ml or 20 μg/ml (1:50,000 solution).
IV, cont inf:

DILUTION	CONCENTRATION
1 mg/250 ml	4μg/ml
2 mg/250 ml	8μg/ml

More concentrated solutions may be used if necessary to limit fluid intake.

P IV, cont inf, children: 0.6x weight (kg) = mg of drug to be added to IV solution for total volume of 100 ml. Rate of 1 ml/hr = 0.1 mcg/kg/min. Alternately, standard dilutions of 1-2 mg/250 ml may be used.

Compatible solutions: D$_5$W, 0.9% NaCl, LR
Stability: Stable for >48 hr at room temperature; do not use pink or discolored solutions.

ACTIONS

Stimulates beta-adrenergic receptors, resulting in positive inotropic/chronotropic cardiac stimulation (beta-1 effects), ↑ CO; relaxes bronchial, vascular smooth muscle (beta-2 effects), resulting in bronchodilation, ↓ vascular resistance • **CV/hemodynamic:** Increases strength of ventricular contraction, stimulates SA node, shortens AV conduction time; increases HR/ejection velocity; SV usually unchanged; myocardial O$_2$ requirements greatly ↑ ; arterial dilation, reduces peripheral/pulmonary vascular resistance; SBP usually ↑ because of ↑ CO, DBP usually ↓ because of vasodilation, mean BP unchanged; does not usually affect PAPs, but ↑ PAP associated with pulmonary embolism may be slightly ↓ ; does not usually ↑, may ↓ renal blood flow. • **Metabolic:** Stimulates glycogenolysis but also stimulates insulin production; does not usually cause significant hyperglycemia

PHARMACOKINETICS

ROUTE	ONSET	PEAK	DURATION
IV	Immed	<15 min	8-50 min
Inhal	Immed	Rapid	1 hr

DISTRIBUTION
Throughout body tissue

ELIMINATION
Metabolized in liver, other organs; half-life 2 min

INDICATIONS

Heart block/bradycardia: Temporary control of hemodynamically significant, atropine-refractory bradycardia/heart block when epinephrine not appropriate; epinephrine preferred over isoproterenol for bradycardia associated with hypotension; isoproterenol used only until pacing available because ↑ myocardial O$_2$ requirements may induce or exacerbate ischemia
• **Asthma/bronchospasm:** Dilation of bronchial smooth muscle in patients with asthma, bronchitis, emphysema, COPD, other forms of bronchospasm; SC/IV routes used when low tidal volume, tachypnea prevent effective inhal therapy; dysrhythmias associated with use in 🅟 adults less likely in children
• **Shock:** To improve CO, reduce afterload in shock states characterized by low CO, vaso🅟 constriction in children/young adults without evidence of CAD; dopamine increases SV, renal blood flow more effectively; generally preferred over isoproterenol.
Unlabeled/investigational:
Temporary reduction of pulmonary arterial hypertension during pulmonary embolism

PRECAUTIONS/CONTRAINDICATIONS

Precautions: Increases in myocardial workload result in imbalance between myocardial O$_2$ supply/demand; may cause/extend ischemia. • Profound hypotension possible, particularly with hypovolemia • Relaxation of pulmonary vasculature may increase intrapulmonary shunt, reduce arterial O$_2$ tension.
• Tachycardia, dysrhythmias may occur; more likely with high-dose therapy, general anesthesia, hypokalemia, hypoxia,

---

italic = common side effects   **bold** = life-threatening reactions

acidosis, cardiogenic shock, concurrent digoxin use. • Excessive inhalation may result in loss of effectiveness; do not increase dose; alternative therapy required. • Commercial preparations may contain sulfites, which could cause serious allergic reactions.

G Use caution with: Older adults • Diabetes • Hypertension • CV disease • Renal disease • Hyperthyroidism

c Pregnancy category: Safety not established; use only if safer alternatives unavailable.

Contraindications: Hypersensitivity to isoproterenol • Digitalis toxicity • Tachycardia, ventricular dysrhythmias

ADVERSE EFFECTS

CNS: *Headache, tremor, anxiety,* sweating, dizziness, weakness

Resp: Bronchial irritation, pulmonary edema

CV: *Palpitations, tachycardia,* ↑ ↓ BP, angina, **ventricular tachycardia/fibrillation**

GI: Nausea, vomiting

Endo: Mild hyperglycemia

TOXICITY/OVERDOSE

Symptoms: Tachycardia • Dysrhythmias • Angina • Hypo/hypertension • Shock if inotropic effects diminished due to ischemia/myocardial depression

Management: Reduce rate or discontinue. • Short duration of action; other treatment usually unnecessary • Hypotension: Elevate legs, administer IV fluids. • Tachycardia: Propranolol reduces HR but should not be used with asthma, COPD because it increases bronchoconstriction.

INTERACTIONS

aminophylline Dysrhythmias
anesthetics Dysrhythmias
beta-blockers (noncardioselective) Blocked beta effects; ↓ bronchodilation
antidysrhythmics Dysrhythmias
digoxin Dysrhythmias
diuretics Dysrhythmias
epinephrine Excessive cardiac stimulation; dysrhythmias; avoid concurrent use
sympathomimetics Dysrhythmias
TCAs Hypertension, dysrhythmias

Y-SITE COMPATIBILITIES

Amiodarone, amrinone, bretylium, famotidine, heparin, hydrocortisone sodium succinate, pancuronium, potassium chloride, vecuronium

Y-SITE INCOMPATIBILITIES

Aminophylline, lidocaine, sodium bicarbonate

PATIENT CARE IMPLICATIONS

• Correct hypovolemia before initiating therapy.
• Monitor for/correct hypoxemia, hypercapnia, acidosis before and during drug administration.
• Do not administer sodium bicarbonate through same IV line.
• Monitor for significant dysrhythmias, hypertension, chest pain or other anginal symptoms, ECG evidence of ischemia.
• Effectiveness for patients with heart block or shock is evaluated by observing HR/rhythm, measuring hemodynamic parameters, urine flow. Effectiveness for patients with bronchospasm is evaluated by assessment for improved air exchange.

P pediatric   **G** geriatric   **V** Direct IV

Vital signs/hemodynamics:
Monitor BP, HR, RR before and after each dose. • Continuous monitoring of ECG necessary. Observe for dysrhythmias, ST depression (ischemia). Reduce dose or discontinue for excessive tachycardia. • For patients with bronchospasm, closely monitor O_2 saturation by pulse oximetry.
IV: Establish clear parameters for titration (e.g., desired HR, BP, CO, UO). Use lowest possible dose to achieve desired effect. • Initially, monitor BP, HR, RR q5-15min; progressively advance according to stability. • Monitor CO, PCWP, CVP, SVR frequently as available; immediately correct hypovolemia. • Monitor UO; consult physician if ≤5 ml/kg/hr or ≤30 ml/hr.
Physical assessment: Monitor breathing patterns, lung sounds for evidence of improved air exchange. • Assess for evidence of inadequate CO: changes in mentation, activity intolerance, bibasilar fluid crackles, S_3 gallop.
Laboratory tests: Monitor: Electrolytes, particularly potassium • Blood glucose, especially in patients with diabetes • ABGs

PATIENT/FAMILY TEACHING

Purpose of medication is to relieve breathing difficulty, improve BP, improve cardiac performance. • Immediately report chest pain, breathing difficulty, palpitations. • Inhal: Demonstrate use of inhaler/other device. Drug turns red when exposed to air; saliva/sputum may appear pink or red

AVAILABLE FORMS

Parenteral for IV injection/infusion • Tablets for SL use • Aerosol/nebulizer solution • Metered-dose inhaler

isosorbide dinitrate
(eye-soe-sor′bide)
Coronex ✹, Isordil, Sorbitrate

isorbide dinitrate, extended release
Cedocard SR ✹, Coradur ✹, Coronex ✹, Dilatrate, Iso-Bid, Isordil Tembids, Isotrate Timecelles, Sorbitrate SA

Classifications: Antianginal, vasodilator, nitrate

USUAL DOSE

SL/intrabuccal/chewable tablets, adults: Angina prevention: 2.5-10 mg q2-3h • Acute angina: 1 tablet (2.5-10 mg) at onset of angina; if symptoms not relieved, may repeat in 5-10 min up to total of 3 tablets in 15-30 min • Do not exceed initial dose of 5 mg with chewable tablet
PO: 10-20 mg 3-4 times daily
PO, ext rel: 20-40 mg q6-8h or 80 mg q8-12h

ADMINISTRATION

SL/intrabuccal: Place tablet under tongue or between cheek and gum (as appropriate) until completely dissolved.
Chewable tablets: Chew thoroughly before swallowing.
PO: Administer on empty stomach, 1 hr before or 2 hr after meals.

ACTIONS

Relaxes vascular smooth muscle, causing vasodilation; venous dilation > arteriolar dilation • Venodilation encourages peripheral pooling of blood volume, thus reducing right (CVP)/left (PCWP) ventricular filling pressures. • Arteriolar dilation decreases SVR/PVR, reduces resistance to ventricular ejection (afterload). • Relief of ischemic chest pain attributed to ↓ myocardial O_2 consumption, ↑ coronary arterial perfusion • Causes slight reduction in SBP, DBP

PHARMACOKINETICS

ROUTE	ONSET	PEAK	DURATION
SL	3 min	<60 min	2 hr
Chewable	3 min	<60 min	0.5-2 hr
PO, std	60 min	<3hr	5-6 hr
PO, ext rls	30 min	2-4 hr	6-8 hr

DISTRIBUTION

Widely distributed throughout body tissue

ELIMINATION

Metabolized in liver, eliminated in urine

INDICATIONS

Relief of acute angina pectoris in patients intolerant of or resistant to nitroglycerin, which is faster in relieving angina • Prevention of anginal attacks when administered before likely precipitating events

PRECAUTIONS/ CONTRAINDICATIONS

Precautions: ↓ SBP, DBP possible • Orthostatic hypotension, transient cerebral hypoperfusion common • >15% reduction in DBP may precipitate myocardial ischemia, angina pectoris. • Angina associated with hypertrophic cardiomyopathy may be worsened by nitrates. • Tolerance to drug effects, cross-tolerance to other nitrates may develop with long-term repeated use; short-acting preparations less likely to cause tolerance. • Abrupt cessation of therapy may exacerbate angina.
Use caution with: Hypovolemia • Hypotension • Ethanol intoxication
C Pregnancy category: Safety not established; use only if safer alternative unavailable.
Contraindications: Hypersensitivity to isosorbide • Increased ICP, inadequate cerebral perfusion • Rapid-acting forms with acute MI • Severe hypotension **P** • Severe anemia • Children: Safety/efficacy not established

ADVERSE EFFECTS

CNS: *Headache,* dizziness, weakness, restlessness, nervousness
CV: *Hypotension, orthostatic hypotension,* ↑ chest pain, tachycardia, paradoxical bradycardia, dysrhythmias
GI: Nausea, vomiting
Derm: Sweating, flushing, rash
Misc: Tolerance/cross-tolerance to other nitrates

TOXICITY/OVERDOSE

Symptoms: Hypotension, tachycardia, heart block, diaphoresis • Circulatory collapse, dyspnea, bradypnea • ↑ ICP with confusion, fever • Nausea, vomiting
Management: After recent ingestion, implement guidelines for management of acute overdose (Appendix I). • Support breathing as needed with O_2 and/or mechanical ventilation. • **Hypotension:** Elevate legs, administer IV fluids; if unresponsive to fluid replacement, use vasopressors (e.g., dopa-

mine, norepinephrine). Inotropic agents (e.g., dobutamine, dopamine) may be used to stimulate contractility. Avoid epinephrine, which may not be effective in correcting hypotension.

INTERACTIONS

alcohol Severe hypotension; CV collapse

aspirin Nitrate accumulation, ↑ effects

calcium channel blockers Orthostatic hypotension, profound hypotension

epinephrine Blocked alpha-adrenergic effects with unopposed beta effects (hypotension, tachycardia)

hypotensive agents Profound hypotension

PATIENT CARE IMPLICATIONS

• Have patient supine before administering rapid-onset formulations (SL, intrabuccal, chewable).

• Use appropriate precautions to protect patient from injury associated with falls caused by orthostatic hypotension.

• Correct hypovolemia before administration.

• Use lower dose, extreme caution when administering to patients with ethanol intoxication.

• If headache develops, administer acetaminophen or other prescribed analgesic. Consult physician for severe or persistent headache.

• Use of "rest periods" (6-12 hr/day without drug) may be prescribed to prolong development of tolerance. Nonnitrate therapy may be prescribed during rest periods.

• Gradually reduce dose to avoid rebound hypertension, increased angina.

Vital signs/hemodynamics: Monitor BP, HR frequently during initial therapy or when using for acute angina. • Continuously monitor ECG when used with acute angina. Report new ST segment depression/elevation T wave inversion, serious dysrhythmias.

Physical assessment: Assess for perfusion/oxygenation deficit: chest discomfort, ↓ level of consciousness, activity intolerance, hypotension, dizziness.

PATIENT/FAMILY TEACHING

Purpose of medication is to relieve angina pectoris. • May cause headaches; take acetaminophen or other prescribed analgesic as needed. • May cause dizziness; use caution when changing positions, walking. Alcohol use, hot weather, vigorous activity, and prolonged standing make these symptoms more likely. • **Standard/extended-release tablets:** Take on an empty stomach. Do not break, crush, or chew. • **SL/intrabuccal/chewable tablets:** Place SL tablets under tongue or between cheek and gum only. Chew chewable tablets thoroughly. Do not swallow whole. Dry mouth decreases absorption of drug. Use when seated or lying down.

Outpatient: Do not skip doses even if feeling better. Do not stop taking without notifying your primary health care provider. Sudden cessation may trigger angina, other serious problems. Consult health care professional before using other brands, formulations. • Do not

---

italic = common side effects   **bold** = life-threatening reactions

consume alcohol while taking this drug. • Use SL tablets or chewable tablets to relieve symptoms of acute angina. Immediately contact EMS, notify physician if pain unrelieved by total of 3 tablets taken at 5–10-min intervals.

AVAILABLE FORMS

SL/chewable/PO/extended-release tablets • Extended-release capsules

isosorbide mononitrate
(eye-soe-sor'bide)
ISMO

Classification: antianginal, vasodilator, nitrate

USUAL DOSE

PO, adults: 20 mg bid; 1st dose on awakening, 2nd dose 7 hr later. Drug-free interval of 17 hr necessary to avoid refractory nitrate tolerance • **Advanced age, hepatic/renal insufficiency:** Dose adjustments not necessary

ACTION

Relaxes vascular smooth muscle, causing vasodilation; venous dilation>arteriolar dilation • Venodilation encourages peripheral pooling of blood volume, thus reducing right/left (CVP/PCWP) ventricular filling pressures (preload). • Arteriolar dilation decreases SVR/PVR, reduces resistance to ventricular ejection (afterload). • Slightly reduces systolic/diastolic BP • Relief of ischemic chest pain attributed to reduced myocardial O_2 consumption, improved coronary arterial perfusion

PHARMACOKINETICS

ROUTE	ONSET	PEAK	DURATION
PO	30 min	30-60 min	5-12 hr

ELIMINATION

Denitrated to inactive metabolites. Half-life = 5 hr.

INDICATIONS

Prevention of angina due to coronary artery disease. Because of slow onset of action, not indicated for acute anginal attacks.

PRECAUTIONS/ CONTRAINDICATIONS

Precautions: May cause hypotension/orthostatic hypotension • Severe hypotension and paradoxical bradycardia are possible; increased angina may occur. • Angina associated with hypertrophic cardiomyopathy may be worsened by nitrates. • Tolerance to drug effects, cross-tolerance to other nitrates may develop; daily drug-free intervals help prevent tolerance. • Abrupt cessation of therapy may exacerbate angina.
Use caution with: Hypovolemia, hypotension • Ethanol intoxication
c Pregnancy category: Use only if safer alternative not available
Contraindications: Hypersensitivity to isosorbide • Acute MI; long-acting effects difficult to control; drug-related hypotension, bradycardia may worsen condition • Increased ICP, inadequate cerebral perfusion • Children: Safety/efficacy not established

ADVERSE EFFECTS

CNS: *Headache, dizziness,* weakness, restlessness, nervousness

CV: Orthostatic hypotension, hypotension, increased chest pain, tachycardia, paradoxical bradycardia, **dysrhythmias**

GI: Nausea, vomiting

Misc: Tolerance/cross-tolerance to other nitrates

TOXICITY/OVERDOSE

Symptoms: Vasodilation, hypotension, decreased CO, tachycardia, heart block, diaphoresis, circulatory collapse • Increased ICP, confusion, fever, seizures

Management: After recent ingestion, implement guidelines for management of acute overdosage (Appendix I). • Support breathing with O_2, mechanical ventilation if needed. • For hypotension, elevate legs, administer crystalloids; if unresponsive to fluid resuscitation, use dopamine or norepinephrine. Positive inotropes such as dobutamine may be used to stimulate myocardial contractility. Avoid epinephrine, which may not be effective in correcting hypotension. • Hemodialysis is not likely to be helpful.

INTERACTIONS

alcohol Profound hypotension

calcium channel blockers Orthostatic hypotension

PATIENT CARE IMPLICATIONS

• Correct hypovolemia before administration.

• Use precautions to protect patient from injury associated with orthostatic hypotension.

• If headache develops, administer acetaminophen, other prescribed analgesic. Consult physician for severe or persistent headache.

• Discontinue slowly to avoid rebound hypertension, increased angina.

Vital signs/hemodynamics: Monitor BP, HR frequently during initial therapy.

Physical assessment: Assess for perfusion/oxygenation deficit: ↓ level of consciousness, hypotension, activity intolerance, chest discomfort

PATIENT/FAMILY TEACHING

Purpose of medication is to prevent episodes of angina pectoris

• May cause headache; take acetaminophen or other prescribed mild pain reliever.

• May cause dizziness; use caution when changing positions, walking. Alcohol use, hot weather, vigorous activity, and prolonged standing make these symptoms more likely.

Outpatient: Take exactly as directed; must take second dose 7 hr after first dose. Do not skip doses even if feeling better. Do not stop taking without notifying your primary health care provider. Sudden cessation may trigger angina, other serious problems. • Do not consume alcohol while taking this drug.

• Not intended for the relief of acute chest pain; use nitroglycerin or other prescribed rapid-acting medication for acute angina attacks.

AVAILABLE FORMS

Tablets

ketoconazole
(ke-to-con'a-zol)
Nizoral

Classifications: Antifungal antibiotic, imidazole derivative

USUAL DOSE
PO, adults: 200-400 mg as single dose q24 h • **Severe infection:** 400 mg as single dose q24h • Up to 1,600 mg q24h has been used.
P **PO, children >2 yr:** 3.3-6.6 mg/kg/24 hr in single dose

ADMINISTRATION
PO: Administer with food to reduce GI side effects. Absorption incomplete if gastric pH ≥3; impaired absorption likely with absent/reduced gastric acid; for these patients, administer with 200 ml of 0.1 N hydrochloric acid solution (using glass straw).

ACTIONS
Broad-spectrum antifungal agent; effects result from disruption of fungal cell membranes, growth inhibition. • Directly inhibits synthesis of human cortisol, testosterone • Active against many fungi, including *Cryptococcus neoformans, Histoplasma capsulatum, Blastomyces dermatitidis, Coccidiodes immitis, Trichophyton mentagrophytes* • Not active against rickettsiae, viruses

PHARMACOKINETICS

ROUTE	ONSET	PEAK	DURATION
PO	Rapid	1-4 hr	Approx 24 hr

DISTRIBUTION
Wide; CSF levels unpredictable; highly protein bound

ELIMINATION
Partially metabolized in liver, eliminated via feces; half-life 8 hr

INDICATIONS
Treatment of non–life-threatening, non-CNS fungal infections, including pulmonary or disseminated coccidioidomycosis, histoplasmosis; oral, esophageal candidiasis; chronic mucocutaneous candidiasis • Limited usefulness in treatment of serious or disseminated candidal infections • Not to be used as sole therapy for fungal meningitis • Patients with AIDS or other immunocompromised state may have suboptimal response to therapy.

PRECAUTIONS/ CONTRAINDICATIONS
Precautions: May cause depressed adrenocortical function, reduced testosterone levels • Serious hepatotoxicity leading to death has been reported.
Use caution with: Achlorhydria (absent gastric hydrochloric acid) or acid suppression therapy (e.g., antacids, H_2 antagonists, anticholinergics); absorption reduced • **P** Children: Safety not well established
c Pregnancy category: Risk of fetal damage unknown; use only if safer alternatives unavailable.
Contraindications: Hypersensitivity to ketoconazole

ADVERSE EFFECTS
CNS: Headache, dizziness, somnolence

GI: *Nausea, vomiting,* diarrhea, abdominal discomfort, GI bleeding; **acute hepatic necrosis**

Derm: Pruritus, rash, urticaria

Endo: Gynecomastia, decreased testosterone, **adrenocortical insufficiency** (rare)

Misc: Hypersensitivity, **anaphylaxis**

TOXICITY/OVERDOSE

Symptoms: No reports of toxicity/overdose

Management: After recent ingestion, implement guidelines for management of acute overdose (Appendix I). Gastric lavage with sodium bicarbonate may be helpful. Initiate other symptomatic/supportive measures, including airway management/ventilation.

INTERACTIONS

acid suppression therapy (antacids, anticholinergics, H₂ antagonists), sucralfate ↓ Ketoconazole absorption

anticoagulants, PO Enhanced anticoagulation

astemizole Prolonged QT interval; ventricular dysrhythmias

corticosteroids ↑ Corticosteroid levels; enhanced adrenal suppression

cyclosporine ↑ Cyclosporine levels; renal toxicity

phenytoin ↑ Phenytoin or ketoconazole levels; toxicity

rifampin ↓ Ketoconazole levels

terfenadine Prolonged QT interval; ventricular dysrhythmias

theophylline ↓ Theophylline levels

PATIENT CARE IMPLICATIONS

• Obtain specimens for culture and sensitivity before initiating antifungal therapy. Initiate therapy before results received.

• If antacids, anticholinergics, H₂ antagonists, sucralfate also prescribed, administer at least 2 hr after ketoconazole.

Vital signs: Monitor VS for indicators of infection, complications

Physical assessment: Assess for improvement in primary infection or resistance to ketoconazole therapy, evidenced by recurrent infection or failure to respond to therapy. • Observe for symptoms of hypersensitivity: rash, pruritus, wheezing, laryngeal edema, hypotension.

• Hepatotoxicity possible; if ↑ liver enzymes/bilirubin, monitor closely; discontinue for clinical signs of liver disease (anorexia, jaundice, abdominal pain, dark urine, light stools). • Adrenocortical suppression possible; monitor for hypotension, darkened skin, ↓ Na⁺, ↑ K⁺.

Laboratory tests: Monitor: CBC with differential • Liver enzymes, bilirubin • Electrolytes

May cause: ↓ Testosterone, cortisol levels

PATIENT/FAMILY TEACHING

Purpose of drug is to limit growth of infection-causing fungal organisms. • Report diarrhea, rash, itching, wheezing. • Report signs of liver disease: loss of appetite, yellowish tint to skin or whites of eyes, abdominal pain, dark urine, light stools. Report signs of adrenal insufficiency: fatigue, darkened skin. Follow-up appointments for laboratory studies are essential. • Take with food or milk to avoid stomach upset. • Avoid taking antacids with this drug. Because interactions possible, consult primary health care provider before taking other prescription drugs. • Take all of medication exactly as prescribed. Do not stop taking medicine even if you feel better. Failure to take entire prescription may result in recurrence or additional infection. Do not save or share unused medicine.

AVAILABLE FORMS
Tablets

ketorolac tromethamine
(ke'toe-role-ak)
Acular ✦, Toradol

Classification: NSAID

USUAL DOSE
Duration of PO/IM/IV ketorolac therapy should not exceed 5 days. Convert to oral therapy as soon as possible.

PO, adults: Indicated only as a continuation of ketorolac IV/IM therapy • Patients who received single IM dose of 30 mg or multiple IV/IM doses of 15 mg: 10 mg PO q4-6h. • Patients who received single IM dose of 60 mg or multiple IV/IM doses of 30 mg: First dose, 20 mg PO; thereafter, 10 mg PO q4-6h. • In all cases do not exceed total PO dose of 40 mg/24 hr • Maximum dose, 40 mg/24 hr

IM: Adult <65 yr: Single-dose therapy, 60 mg; multiple-dose therapy, 30 mg q6h; maximum daily dose, 120 mg/day • **Adult** 🅖 **≥65 yr, renal impairment, weight <50 lbs:** Single-dose therapy, 30 mg; multiple-dose therapy, 15 mg q6h; maximum daily dose, 60 mg/day

IV: Adult <65 yr: Single-dose therapy, 30 mg; multiple-dose therapy, 30 mg q6h; maximum daily dose, 120 mg/day • **Adult ≥65 yr, renal impairment, weight <50 lbs:** Single-dose therapy, 15 mg; multiple-dose therapy, 15 mg q6h; maximum daily dose, 60 mg/day

ADMINISTRATION
IM, adult: Inject deep into large muscle mass. Apply pressure for 15-30 sec to minimize ecchymosis, bruising, tingling.
▼**Direct IV, adults:** Administer each dose undiluted over 1-5 min, preferably through freely flowing IV.

ACTIONS
Inactivates enzyme necessary for prostaglandin synthesis, thus inhibiting prostaglandin release, reducing pain/inflammation • Analgesic effects primarily peripheral • Reduces fever by inhibiting prostaglandins that mediate effect of endogenous pyrogen in hypothalamus • No known effects on opiate receptors • 300 times analgesic potency of aspirin; 30 mg IM dose similar in analgesic efficacy to 8-10 mg morphine • GI, renal toxicity attributed to prostaglandin inhibition

PHARMACOKINETICS

ROUTE	ONSET	PEAK	DURATION
PO	30-60 min	2-3 hr	6 hr
IM	10 min	30-60 min	6-8 hr

DISTRIBUTION
Wide; 99% protein bound

ELIMINATION
Metabolized in liver, excreted by kidneys; half-life, young adults, 4-6 hr; older 🅖 adults, 5-8 hr

---

🅟 pediatric   🅖 geriatric   ▼ Direct IV

INDICATIONS

Short-term management of moderate to severe pain especially postoperatively • Used concomitantly with opiate-agonist analgesics (e.g., meperidine, morphine) to reduce requirements for opiate analgesics

PRECAUTIONS/ CONTRAINDICATIONS

Precautions: For short-term (≤5 days) use only; chronic use may cause GI ulceration, bleeding, perforation. • Reduces renal prostaglandin formation; may precipitate renal failure, particularly with preexisting renal impairment, dehydration • Inhibits platelet aggregation; may prolong bleeding time, contribute to bleeding complications
Use caution with: Impaired renal function, heart failure, liver dysfunction, advanced age, diuretic use; risk of renal toxicity • Impaired hepatic function, history of liver disease; may cause ↑ ALT, AST • Older adults; cleared more slowly; ↓ dose indicated • CHF, hypertension, other conditions in which, fluid retention, edema likely • Anticoagulant therapy; ↑ bleeding risk • Postoperative status when impaired hemostasis would ↑ bleeding risk
B **Pregnancy category:** Use only if safer alternatives unavailable.
Contraindications: Hypersensitivity to ketorolac, aspirin, other NSAIDs • Use of other NSAIDs • Bleeding disorders, suspected/confirmed CV hemorrhage • History of/active peptic ulcer disease, GI bleeding • Advanced renal insufficiency, volume depletion • Pregnancy, labor, delivery, nursing mothers • Prophylactically before major surgery, intraoperatively • **P** Probenecid therapy • Children: Safe use not established

ADVERSE EFFECTS

CNS: *Headache,* drowsiness, dizziness, sweating
Resp: Dyspnea
CV: Edema, hypertension, vasodilation, pallor
GI: *Nausea, dyspepsia, GI pain,* diarrhea, constipation, ↑ liver enzymes, **peptic ulcer, GI bleeding,** stomatitis
GU: Increased urinary frequency, oliguria, ARF
Hema: Purpura, postop wound hemorrhage, thrombocytopenia
Derm: Itching, rash, wheals
Misc: IM—pain, ecchymosis, bruising, tingling at injection site; full range of allergic reactions, including anaphylaxis

TOXICITY/OVERDOSE

Symptoms: Renal toxicity: Hematuria, proteinuria, ↑ BUN/creatinine, oliguria, acute renal failure • GI toxicity: Irritation, peptic ulceration, bleeding
Management: After recent ingestion, implement guidelines for management of acute overdose (Appendix I). • Maintain adequate hydration, monitor renal status closely. • Strongly protein bound; dialysis not helpful

INTERACTIONS

alcohol GI mucosal damage; ↑ bleeding time
anticoagulants ↑ Bleeding complications
diuretics, loop ↓ Diuresis; nephrotoxicity
methotrexate Methotrexate toxicity

K

NSAIDs GI/renal toxicity
probenecid ↑ Ketorolac toxicity; avoid concurrent use
thrombolytics ↑ Bleeding complications

SYRINGE INCOMPATIBILITIES

Hydroxyzine, nalbuphine, meperidine, morphine, prochlorperazine, promethazine

PATIENT CARE IMPLICATIONS

Parenteral/PO

• Convert to PO therapy as soon as possible; dosages not interchangeable.

• Administer doses at onset of pain.

• For breakthrough pain between scheduled doses of ketorolac, consider supplemental use of opioid analgesics. Do not ↑ dose or frequency of ketorolac.

• May administer PO doses with food or milk to reduce GI irritation.

• Adverse effects are dose related; always use lowest effective dose.

• Hypersensitivity reactions including anaphylaxis may occur after first IM/IV dose. Have epinephrine, emergency equipment immediately available.

Vital signs/hemodynamics: Antipyretic effects may mask fever associated with infection.

G • Measure/record UO in older adults, patients with renal, hepatic, cardiac disease.

Physical assessment: Assess for level of pain before and 30-60 min after administration.

• Observe for unusual bleeding or bruising. • Assess for edema/fluid retention, renal impairment. • Assess for GI bleeding. Test stools, emesis for occult blood. Closely monitor postoperative patients for incisional bleeding, internal hemorrhage, other bleeding complications.

Laboratory tests: Monitor: Hgb/Hct • BUN, creatinine • Electrolytes • Bilirubin, liver enzymes (ALT, AST)

PATIENT/FAMILY TEACHING

Purpose of medication is to relieve pain, ↓ inflammation.

• Ask for/take medicine before pain becomes severe. • Immediately report dark tarry stools, blood in stool, vomiting of blood. • May cause drowsiness or dizziness; use caution until individual effects recognized.

Outpatient: Take with food, milk, antacids to reduce stomach upset. • Consult with primary health care provider before using alcohol or taking aspirin, ibuprofen, other over-the-counter medications. • Inform dentist or physician of medication regimen before treatment or surgery. • Report rash, itching, rapid weight gain, swelling/fluid retention, unusual bruising or bleeding.

AVAILABLE FORMS

Tablets • Prefilled syringes for parenteral use

---

labetalol
(la-bet'a-lole)
Normodyne, Trandate
labetalol with hydrochlorothiazide
Normozide

Classifications: Nonselective beta-adrenergic blocker, selective alpha₁ adrenergic blocker, antihypertensive

---

USUAL DOSE

PO, adults: 200-400 mg bid; older adults: 100-200 mg bid • Do not exceed 400 mg bid.

Direct IV, adults: Initially 20 mg; may repeat dose of 20-80 mg q10min as needed to control BP • Do not exceed total dose of 300 mg. • Convert to PO therapy as soon as possible.

IV, cont inf, adults: 2 mg/min; increase as needed to control BP.

ADMINISTRATION

G-tube: Crush tablets, dissolve in water; administer immediately.

Direct IV, adults: Inject each 20 mg or less over 2 min. • Discontinue for symptomatic bradycardia, HR <45, hypotension, 2nd/3rd degree heart block.

IV inf: Gradually increase q5-15min as necessary to control BP. • Slow or discontinue for symptomatic bradycardia, HR <45, hypotension, 2nd/3rd degree heart block. Use infusion pump.

PREPARATION

For 1 mg/ml concentration, add 200 mg (40 ml) to 160-ml bag/bottle of compatible IV solution. Remove 90 ml from 250-ml bag to obtain 160-ml bag; then add labetalol.

Compatible fluids: D_5W, 0.9% NaCl, LR, prepared combinations of these solutions

ACTIONS

Blocks sympathetic stimulation of beta-1 receptors of myocardium, beta-2 receptors of vasculature/bronchial smooth muscle, postsynaptic alpha-1 receptors of vasculature • Beta-blocking effects >alpha-blocking effects • At usual doses, decreases BP without significant changes in HR • IV administration in hypertensive patients with acute MI decreases HR, BP, CO, PCWP • AV conduction time decreased at higher doses • Reduces plasma renin levels • Beta-2 blockade may cause bronchial constriction, particularly in asthmatic patients. However, airway effects less than with propranolol, other nonselective beta-blockers

PHARMACOKINETICS

ROUTE	ONSET	PEAK	DURATION
PO	20-120 min	1-4 hr	≥8-24 hr*
IV	2-5 min	5-15 min	2-4 hr

DISTRIBUTION

Wide; 50% protein bound; Minimal crossing of blood-brain barrier

ELIMINATION

Metabolized by liver; excreted in feces, urine; half-life 6-8 hr

*Dose dependent.

INDICATIONS

Control of hypertension, alone and with diuretics; IV especially useful during hypertensive emergencies in patients with ischemic heart disease because of minimal effects on HR, CO *Unlabeled/investigational:* Induction of controlled hypotension to limit bleeding during surgery; management of sympathetic overactivity associated with severe tetanus; management of chronic stable angina pectoris

L

---

italic = common side effects   **bold** = life-threatening reactions

PRECAUTIONS/
CONTRAINDICATIONS

Precautions: May cause severe orthostatic hypotension, loss of consciousness, particularly with IV administration • May cause CHF (rarely), ventricular dysrhythmias, heart block, especially with preexisting cardiac/hepatic disease • Additive impairment of cardiac contractility may occur when used with general anesthesia; drug may be withdrawn before elective surgery. • Abrupt cessation may induce hypertension, angina, acute MI. • May mask symptoms of hypoglycemia

Use caution with: Asthma, COPD; may cause bronchospasm • **Children:** Safety/efficacy not firmly established

c Pregnancy category: Use only if safer alternative unavailable.

Contraindications: Hypersensitivity to labetalol • Symptomatic bradycardia, HR <45, 2nd/3rd degree heart block, CHF, bronchial asthma, severe COPD, cardiogenic shock

ADVERSE EFFECTS

CNS: *Dizziness, fatigue, lethargy,* depression, tremors, insomnia

Resp: Dyspnea, **bronchospasm**

CV: Orthostatic hypotension, **profound hypotension, heart failure, bradycardia, worsened AV heart block**

GI: *Nausea,* vomiting, flatulence, diarrhea, constipation

GU: Impotence, dysuria, urinary retention

Endo: Blocked symptoms of hypoglycemia/hyperthyroidism (e.g., absence of tachycardia, tremors)

Derm: Rash, pruritus

Syst: Muscle cramps, SLE-like syndrome, slight hyperglycemia

TOXICITY/OVERDOSE

Symptoms: Profound hypotension, loss of consciousness • Severe bradycardia, advanced heart block • Heart failure • Bronchospasm

Management: After recent ingestion, implement guidelines for management of acute overdose (Appendix I). • **Bradycardia, heart block:** Administer atropine, epinephrine according to ACLS guidelines (Appendix P). • **Hypotension:** Elevate legs, administer IV fluids; use vasopressors (e.g., dopamine, norepinephrine) for severe hypotension. • **Bronchospasm:** Maintain airway, support ventilation, use aminophylline. • **Heart failure:** Provide inotropic support (e.g., dobutamine, dopamine), diuretics, possibly cardiac glycosides (e.g., digoxin) • Hemodialysis generally ineffective

INTERACTIONS

amiodarone Severe bradycardia; ventricular dysrhythmias

anesthetics, local (e.g., lidocaine) Hypertension, particularly if anesthetic contains epinephrine

antidiabetic agents Masked hypoglycemia-associated tachycardia

barbiturates ↓ Beta-blocker effectiveness

diltiazem Profound bradycardia; hypotension

disopyramide Additive negative inotropy; ↓ CO

epinephrine, possibly other sympathomimetics Blocked

epinephrine beta effects; unopposed alpha stimulation (hypertension, bradycardia, dysrhythmias)

isoproterenol ↓ Bronchodilatory effectiveness

lidocaine ↑ Lidocaine levels; ↓ CO

nicardipine Hypotension

nifedipine Hypotension

phenothiazines Hypotension; enhanced effects of either agent

prazosin Hypotension, especially with initial dose

quinidine ↑ Cardiac depression

rifampin ↑ Beta-blocker metabolism; higher doses required

theophylline ↓ Bronchodilation

verapamil Extreme bradycardia; hypotension

Y-SITE COMPATIBILITIES

Amikacin, aminophylline, ampicillin, butorphanol, calcium gluconate, cefazolin, ceftazidime, ceftizoxime, chloramphenicol, cimetidine, clindamycin, dopamine, enalaprilat, erythromycin, famotidine, fentanyl, gentamicin, heparin, lidocaine, magnesium sulfate, meperidine, morphine, oxacillin, penicillin G potassium, piperacillin, potassium chloride, potassium phosphate, ranitidine, sodium acetate, tobramycin, vancomycin

Y-SITE INCOMPATIBILITIES

Cefoperazone, nafcillin, sodium bicarbonate

PATIENT CARE IMPLICATIONS

• PO/IV doses not interchangeable; carefully check dose, route.
• Tablets may be crushed, dissolved in water to facilitate administration.

• Gradually withdraw therapy to avoid rebound hypertension, angina, acute MI.
• Identify patients with asthma, COPD. Monitor closely; use lowest effective dose to avoid bronchospasm.
• Observe hyperthyroid patients for symptoms of thyrotoxicosis (e.g., tachycardia, hypertension) when withdrawing therapy.

Vital signs/hemodynamics: Monitor BP frequently with parenteral use or when initiating therapy, especially when used with other antihypertensives, antidysrhythmics. • Monitor ECG for significant bradycardia, prolongation of PR interval, widening of QRS complex, advancement of heart block. • Measure CVP, PCWP, CO as available. Consult physician for diminished CO, increasing filling pressures.

IV: Monitor ECG throughout administration. Monitor BP q5-15min during and for 30 min after injection/infusion. Keep patient supine for 3 hr after administration. Slow infusion or discontinue for symptomatic bradycardia, HR <45, hypotension, 2nd/3rd degree heart block. • Establish ability to tolerate upright position; assist with initial ambulation.

Physical assessment: Assess for perfusion/oxygenation deficit: ↓ level of consciousness, activity intolerance, hypotension, chest discomfort, dizziness.
• Assess for CHF, pulmonary edema: bibasilar crackles (rales), S_3 gallop, neck vein distention, breathing difficulty, peripheral edema. • Assess for bronchospasm, respiratory distress in patients with history of asthma,

COPD. • Assess patients with diabetes for confusion, sweating, because tachycardia/tremors associated with hypoglycemia may be blocked by therapy.

Laboratory tests: Monitor: Electrolytes • Blood sugar in diabetic patients

PATIENT/FAMILY TEACHING

Purpose of medication is to control BP. • Change positions slowly to avoid dizziness, low BP. • Report breathing difficulty, palpitations, dizziness, activity intolerance, chest pain, extreme fatigue. • Avoid excessive amounts of coffee, tea, caffeinated soft drinks, which may counteract drug's BP-lowering effects.

Outpatient: Take medication exactly as prescribed. Do not stop taking medicine even if you feel better. If medication is abruptly discontinued, you may develop dangerously high BP, serious heartbeat irregularities, angina. • Check/record resting pulse each day, BP each week. Contact physician for pulse <50 or significant change in BP. • Medication is not cure for high BP; other therapies, including life-style modifications, must be continued. • Medication may cause drowsiness. Avoid driving and other activities requiring mental alertness until individual response to drug known. • Drinking alcohol may cause extreme dizziness, drowsiness, impaired mental alertness. • You may experience increased sensitivity to cold. • Consult physician or pharmacist before taking over-the-counter preparations, particularly cold or allergy preparations. • Carry Medic-Alert ID identifying drug, dosage, specific indication. • Notify physicians and dentists of therapy before treatment. • Therapy blocks tremors, elevated HR, so diabetic/hyperthyroid patients must be aware of other symptoms of crisis.

AVAILABLE FORMS

Parenteral for IV injection/infusion • Tablets

lactulose
(lak'tyoo-lose)
Cephulac, Cholac, Chronulac, Constilac, Constulose, Duphalac, Enulose, Gel-ose ✦, Generlac, Lactulax

Classifications: Ammonia detoxicant, laxative

USUAL DOSE

PO/G-tube, adults: Encephalopathy: For rapid results, give 30-45 ml (20-30 g) qh until laxative effects achieved; alternatively, administer 30-45 ml 3-4 times daily for several days. Maintenance therapy, adjust dose q1-2days to produce 2-3 soft stools daily or until stool acidified with pH of about 5; usual maintenance dose, 30-45 ml 2-4 times daily • Constipation: 15-60 ml once daily

❷ PO/G-tube, children: Encephalopathy: 40-90 ml/day (27-60 g) in divided doses 2-4 times daily; Adjust dose every 1-2 days to produce 2-3 soft stools daily. • Withhold therapy for persistent diarrhea.

Rectal, adults: 300 ml (200 g) with 700 ml water or 0.9% NaCl • Repeat dose every 4-6 hr until encephalopathy improves. • Initiate PO therapy before discontinuing enemas.

ADMINISTRATION

PO: Administer with fruit juice or water to increase palatability.
G-tube: Dilute with water to reduce risk of aspiration pneumonia.
Rectal, adults: Dilute 300 ml (200 g) with 700 ml water or 0.9% NaCl. • Administer via rectal balloon catheter. • Retain for 30-60 min. • Repeat if inadvertently evacuated. • Avoid concomitant use of soap or alkaline cleansing enemas.

ACTIONS

Decreases blood ammonia concentration, reduces encephalopathy associated with cirrhosis and/or portal-systemic bypass • Bacterial action in colon acidifies contents, resulting in diffusion of ammonia, amines into colon. Ammonia, other toxins bound, then expelled by cathartic effects • Osmotic effects increase stool water content, softening stools/increasing frequency of bowel movements.

PHARMACOKINETICS

ROUTE	ONSET	PEAK	DURATION
PO	24-48 hr	var	Var; depends on colonic transit time
Rectal		2hr	

DISTRIBUTION
<3% absorbed

ELIMINATION
Metabolized to lactic, other acids by intestinal bacteria; small amounts excreted unchanged in urine

INDICATIONS

Prevention/treatment of portal-systemic/hepatic encephalopathy • Reduces blood ammonia levels, improves EEG tracings • Relatively nontoxic; preferred over neomycin for long-term therapy • Laxative for chronic constipation

PRECAUTIONS/ CONTRAINDICATIONS

Precautions: Drug-induced diarrhea may cause hypokalemia, electrolyte disturbances, fluid depletion, thus worsening encephalopathy.
Use caution with: Diabetes; solution contains some free lactose, galactose • Children: Limited experience
Pregnancy category: Use only if safer alternative unavailable.
Contraindications: Hypersensitivity to lactulose; diarrhea, low-galactose diet

ADVERSE EFFECTS

GI: *Gaseous distention, belching, flatulence, abdominal cramping, diarrhea,* nausea, vomiting
Endo: Hyperglycemia in diabetic patients

TOXICITY/OVERDOSE

Risks of toxicity minimal • Overdose results in diarrhea, associated fluid/electrolyte disturbances (e.g., dehydration, hypokalemia, hypernatremia). • Reduce dosage; stop therapy if diarrhea persists.

INTERACTIONS

antacids Inhibits desired lowering of fecal pH
antiinfectives Reduce colonic bacteria and interfere with acidifying effects of lactulose
enemas, soap/alkaline Interfere with acidifying effects of lactulose

---

italic = common side effects   **bold** = life-threatening reactions

neomycin Reduces colonic bacteria and interferes with acidifying effects of lactulose

PATIENT CARE IMPLICATIONS

• Do not use other laxatives, because resulting diarrhea may falsely suggest adequate dosage of lactulose.

Physical assessment: Assess for improvement in level of consciousness, mental status. Therapeutic effects may not be apparent for several days. • Assess for abdominal distention. • Note/record frequency, consistency of stools. Adjust dose to maintain 2-3 soft stools each day. Diarrhea indicates excessive dose.

Laboratory tests: Monitor: Electrolytes • Blood sugar • Serum ammonia levels • Anticipate decrease in serum ammonia levels of 25%-50%. • As indicated, measure stool pH using indicator strips. Adjust dose to maintain pH of about 5.

PATIENT/FAMILY TEACHING

Purpose of medicine is to improve mental confusion or relieve constipation. • Mix with water, fruit juice or add to desserts to minimize sweetness. • Distention, burping, gas, abdominal cramping are frequent side effects, especially when starting therapy. • Do not take antacids, laxatives. • Goal of therapy for patients with encephalopathy is 2-3 soft stools daily. Adjust dose accordingly. Report excessive stools, diarrhea.

AVAILABLE FORMS
PO solution

---

lidocaine HCl
(lye′doe-kane)
Xylocaine

Classification: Class IB antidysrhythmic, membrane stabilizer, local anesthetic

USUAL DOSE

IM, adults: 300 mg in deltoid • Use 10% solution (100 mg/ml). • Indicated only when other routes unavailable

Direct IV/ET, adults: 50-100 mg (1 mg/kg), or higher for ET instillation • ET dose must be diluted. • May repeat at dose of 25-50 mg (0.5 mg/kg) q5min • Do not exceed total dose of 150-300 mg (3 mg/kg) in 1 hr. • If successful resolution of ventricular dysrhythmia, immediately follow with cont inf *• Smaller bolus dose may be indicated with CHF, cardiogenic shock, advanced liver disease, advanced age.*

G **Direct IV/intraosseous/ET,**
P **children:** 0.5-1 mg/kg, or higher for ET instillation • ET dose must be diluted. • May repeat in 10-15 min • Do not exceed total dose of 3-5 mg/kg in 1 hr. • If successful resolution of ventricular dysrhythmia, immediately follow with cont inf

IV, cont inf, adults: 1-4 mg/min (15-60 ml/hr of 1 g/250 ml solution) after control of dysrhythmia with lidocaine bolus (Appendix Q). • Use lowest effective dose. • Discontinue for cardiac depression: prolonged PR interval, widened QRS complex aggravation of dysrhythmias. *• Use slower infusion rates with CHF, liver disease,*
G *advanced age.*

IV, cont inf, children: 20-50 µg/kg/min (1.0-2.5 ml/kg/hr of solution containing 120 mg lidocaine/100 ml D₅W) after control of dysrhythmia with lidocaine bolus injection (Appendix Q). • *Use slower infusion rates with shock, liver disease.*

ADMINISTRATION

MULTIPLE PREPARATIONS AVAILABLE; READ LABEL CAREFULLY BEFORE ADMINISTERING. LABEL MUST STATE "FOR IV USE" WITH IV/ET/INTRAOSSEOUS.

Direct IV, adults: Inject single dose of 50-100 mg over 1-2 min. • Given undiluted • Too rapid injection causes seizures.

Direct IV injection/intraosseous, children: Inject single dose of 1 mg/kg over 1-2 min. • May be given undiluted • Too rapid injection causes seizures.

IV, cont inf, adults: Infuse at 1-4 mg/min (15-60 ml/hr of 1 g/250 ml solution); titrate to control ventricular ectopy (Appendix Q). • Use lowest effective dose. • Use infusion pump. • Discontinue for cardiac depression: prolonged PR interval, widened QRS complex, aggravation of dysrhythmias.

IV, cont inf, children: 20-50 µg/kg/min (1-2.5 ml/kg/hr of solution containing 120 mg lidocaine/100 ml D₅W); titrate to control ventricular ectopy (Appendix Q). • Use lowest effective dose. • Use infusion pump or other rate-controlling device. • Discontinue for cardiac depression: prolonged PR interval, widened QRS complex, aggravation of dysrhythmias.

ET, adults/children: Dilute each dose in 10 ml sterile 0.9% NaCl for adults; use 1-2 ml for children. • Provide several quick ventilations, then expel via catheter passed just beyond ETT. • Follow with several quick ventilations

PREPARATION
IV, cont inf, adults:

DILUTION	CONCENTRATION
1,000 mg/250 ml	4 mg/ml
2,000 mg/250 ml	8 mg/ml

More concentrated solutions may be used if necessary to limit fluid intake.

IV, cont inf, children:

DILUTION	CONCENTRATION
120 mg/100 ml	1.2 mg/ml (1,200 µg/ml)

Compatible fluids: D₅W, 0.9% NaCl, LR
Stability: Stable for 24 hr at room temperature

ACTIONS

Decreases cardiac excitability by increasing threshold for electrical excitation • Blocks fast sodium channels, decreases automaticity, decreases action potential duration/effective refractory period in ventricle • Increases ventricular fibrillation threshold • Sinus node recovery time, SA conduction time unaffected • Conduction velocity unchanged in His-Purkinje system; may be slightly reduced or unaffected in AV node • Contractility, BP unchanged with usual dosages • Produces local anesthesia when infiltrated or applied topically; epinephrine added to slow vascular absorption, prolong duration of action

L

---

italic = common side effects   **bold** = life-threatening reactions

PHARMACOKINETICS

ROUTE	ONSET	PEAK	DURATION
IV	Immed	3 min	10-20 min
ET	Immed	3 min	10-20 min

DISTRIBUTION

Wide; crosses placenta

ELIMINATION

Metabolized in liver, eliminated by kidneys.

Therapeutic level: 1.5-6.0 μg/ml

INDICATIONS

Suppression of ventricular tachycardia or sustained, symptomatic ventricular ectopy • In cardiac arrest, used along with defibrillation to control ventricular fibrillation • 1%, 2% solution used to produce local anesthesia via infiltration, nerve block • Jelly, spray used for topical anesthesia

PRECAUTIONS/ CONTRAINDICATIONS

Precautions: May not prevent ventricular fibrillation associated with acute MI • May cause dysrhythmias, including worsened ventricular dysrhythmias, asystole when administered to patients with sinus bradycardia, AV heart block, accelerated ventricular rate in atrial flutter/fibrillation • Hypoxia, electrolyte-acid-base imbalances ↓ drug effectiveness.
Use caution with: Severe respiratory depression • Hypovolemia • Digitalis toxicity • Cardiomyopathy • Preexisting heart **G** block • Older adults, CHF, cardiogenic shock, liver disease; reduced dose indicated
B **Pregnancy category:** Safety not clearly established; use only if necessary.

Contraindications: Hypersensitivity to lidocaine, other amide-type local anesthetics • Sinus bradycardia with ventricular ectopy • 2nd/3rd degree heart block unless functional pacemaker in place or readily available • Stokes-Adams syndrome • WPW (controversial)

ADVERSE EFFECTS

CNS: *Tremors, lightheadedness, confusion, agitation,* **seizures,** visual disturbances, numbness, tinnitus
Resp: **Respiratory depression/ arrest**
CV: Hypotension, **heart block, bradycardia, exacerbation of heart failure**
GI: Nausea, vomiting
Derm: Urticaria, edema

TOXICITY OVERDOSE

Symptoms: Somnolence, paresthesias • Twitching, seizures, coma • Respiratory depression, apnea • CHF, hypotension • Prolonged PR interval, widened QRS complex, heart block • Cardiac arrest
Management: Discontinue infusion. • Initiate seizure precautions. • **Seizures:** Use IV diazepam, lorazepam, or ultra-short-acting barbiturate (e.g., thiopental); short-acting muscle relaxants (e.g., succinylcholine) may be used in anesthetized patients. • **Hypotension:** Elevate legs, administer IV fluids; use inotropic agents (e.g., dobutamine, dopamine), vasopressors (e.g., norepinephrine) if unresponsive to fluids. • Manage dysrhythmias according to ACLS guidelines (Appendix P).
Toxic level: >7 μg/ml

P pediatric   **G** geriatric   **V** Direct IV

INTERACTIONS

beta-blockers Hypotension, bradycardia, toxicity

bretylium Additive cardiac depression

cimetidine ↑ Lidocaine levels risk of toxicity

NMBAs Prolonged neuromuscular blockade

phenytoin Enhanced metabolism; excessive cardiac depression

procainamide Additive cardiac depression

COMPATIBILITIES

Amiodarone, amrinone, cefazolin, ciprofloxacin, diltiazem, dobutamine, dopamine, enalaprilat, famotidine, haloperidol, labetalol, meperidine, morphine, nitroglycerin, nitroprusside, potassium chloride, sodium bicarbonate, verapamil

INCOMPATIBILITIES

Amphotericin B, ampicillin, epinephrine (commercial lidocaine-epinephrine, pH adjusted), isoproterenol, norepinephrine, phenytoin

PATIENT CARE IMPLICATIONS

• Correct hypoxemia, hypokalemia, other fluid/electrolyte imbalance; O_2 therapy usually indicated.

• For continuous infusion, use pump.

• Continuous infusion indicated only if bolus dose suppresses ventricular dysrhythmias.

• Have emergency equipment available to manage seizures, respiratory/cardiac arrest.

Vital signs/hemodynamics: Continuously monitor ECG throughout therapy. Use lowest possible dose for dysrhythmia control. Monitor for toxicity: prolongation of PR interval, widening of QRS complex, bradycardia, heart block, increased ventricular dysrhythmias; if present, reduce or discontinue drip, consult physician immediately. • Monitor BP q5min during IV loading. Thereafter, monitor q15-60min according to titration schedule, patient stability. • As available, measure CO, PCWP q1-4h. Monitor for excessive myocardial depression: ↓ CO, ↑ PCWP, especially with history of heart failure, acute MI, shock, liver disease.

Physical assessment: Assess for perfusion/oxygenation deficit: ↓ level of consciousness, chest pain, breathing difficulty, hypotension, dizziness. • Assess for CNS toxicity: somnolence, paresthesias, twitching, tremors, agitation, confusion, seizures. Stop infusion, consult physician.

Laboratory tests: Monitor: ABGs • Electrolytes • Lidocaine levels; therapeutic level, 1.5-6.0 μg/ml

PATIENT/FAMILY TEACHING

Purpose of medication is to regulate heartbeats. • Call for assistance with position changes. Do not get out of bed until instructed by nurse. • Report chest pain, breathing difficulty, palpitations, dizziness.

AVAILABLE FORMS

Parenteral for IV injection/ET instillation • Parenteral concentrate for IV admixture • Prepared solution for IV infusion • Dilute parenteral solution for local anesthesia • Viscous solution • PO spray • Topical oint-

L

ment • Jelly for topical use
• Topical solution

lisinopril
(lyse-in'oh-pril)
Prinivil, Zestril
**lisinopril with
hydrochlorothiazide**
Prinzide, Zestoretic

Classification: Angiotensin-converting enzyme (ACE) inhibitor, antihypertensive

USUAL DOSE

PO, adults: Initially 10 mg once daily; increase as needed to control BP. • Drug effects more consistent at ≥20 mg/day • Use lower dose with concurrent diuretic therapy. • Maximum dose, 80 mg/day

G PO, older adults/renal impairment: Initially 2.5-5 mg qd; gradually increase as needed to control BP • Maximum dose, 40 mg/day in renal impairment • Observe closely for symptomatic hypotension.

ACTIONS

Inhibits ACE, which prevents conversion of angiotensin I to angiotensin II, a potent vasoconstrictor • BP reduced directly by ↓ vascular tone, indirectly by ↓ in aldosterone secretion and therefore ↓ sodium/water retention; bradykinin accumulation, prostaglandin release may contribute to hypotensive effects; generally reduces SBP/DBP by 15%-20% • Little or no effect on HR, contractility (in absence of heart failure) • Unlike some ACE inhibitors, does not require conversion in liver to be activated

PHARMACOKINETICS

ROUTE	ONSET	PEAK	DURATION
PO	1 hr	6 hr	24 hr

DISTRIBUTION
Widely distributed except into CNS tissue
ELIMINATION
Eliminated in urine; half-life 12 hr, longer with renal impairment

INDICATIONS

Mild to severe hypertension • May be used in conjunction with other hypotensive agents, diuretics • Along with cardiac glycosides/diuretics to improve cardiac function, relieve symptoms, improve exercise tolerance in CHF • Used alone in management of mild to moderate CHF if fluid volume excess not present

PRECAUTIONS/ CONTRAINDICATIONS

Precautions: Initial dose may cause profound hypotension or severe allergic reaction. • Other ACE inhibitors cause agranulocytosis, although risk not well established with lisinopril.
Use caution with: Renal impairment; reduce dose, closely monitor renal function. • Concurrent diuretic use, hypovolemia, hyponatremia, surgery, anesthesia; risk of severe hypotension • CAD, cerebrovascular disease, CHF, aortic stenosis; hypotensive episodes may worsen condition.
D Pregnancy category: Use in pregnancy only if considered life-saving and woman informed of potential hazards to fetus.
Contraindications: Hypersensitivity to lisinopril, other ACE **P** inhibitors • Children: Safety/efficacy not established

---

P pediatric   **G** geriatric   **V** Direct IV

ADVERSE EFFECTS

CNS: *Headache, dizziness, fatigue,* paresthesias, confusion, depression, nervousness

Resp: *Cough,* upper respiratory symptoms, dyspnea

CV: *Transient or orthostatic hypotension,* **profound hypotension,** tachycardia, dysrhythmias, chest pain

GI: *Diarrhea,* vomiting, abdominal pain, altered taste sensation

GU: Proteinuria, urinary tract infection, **acute renal failure** (rare)

F&E: Hyponatremia, hyperkalemia

Derm: Rash, itching, wheals

Misc: Muscle cramps, allergic reactions, **anaphylaxis**

TOXICITY/OVERDOSE

Symptoms: Hypotension, ↓ level of consciousness, possible MI/CVA from severe hypotension in high-risk patients

Management: After recent ingestion, implement guidelines for management of acute overdose (Appendix I). • Support respiration as needed with O_2 and/or mechanical ventilation. • Hypotension usually responsive to IV fluids, 0.9% NaCl, or LR • Hemodialysis facilitates drug removal.

INTERACTIONS

alcohol ↑ Risk of hypotension

antacids ↓ Lisinopril absorption

calcium channel blockers Profound hypotension

digoxin ↑ Digoxin levels

diuretics Additive hypotensive effects

diuretics, potassium sparing Hyperkalemia

lithium Lithium toxicity

indomethacin, other NSAIDs ↓ Lisinopril effectiveness

phenothiazines Hypotension

potassium supplements Hyperkalemia

Sympathetic blockers Profound hypotension

PATIENT CARE IMPLICATIONS

• Correct hypovolemia before administration.

• Evaluate renal function before initiating therapy; use lower dose if renal impairment

• Protect patients from injury associated with orthostatic hypotension, especially when initiating therapy.

• Vomiting, diarrhea, excessive perspiration, dehydration could cause hypotension.

• Tablets may be crushed, dissolved in water to facilitate administration.

Vital signs/hemodynamics: Monitor BP, HR q1-2h until stable when initiating therapy, with following uses: hypertensive crisis, acute CHF, use of additional hypotensive agents, diuretics.

• Use IV 0.9% NaCl for transient hypotensive episodes during initial therapy. • As available, continuously monitor ECG for PVCs, ST segment elevation/depression, especially when initiating therapy in patients with CHF, CAD.

Physical assessment: Assess for perfusion/oxygenation deficit: chest discomfort, ↓ level of consciousness, breathing difficulty, activity intolerance, hypotension, dizziness. • Assess neurologic status q2-4h after initiation of therapy until BP controlled. • Monitor fluid balance, weigh daily.

L

---

italic = common side effects **bold** = life-threatening reactions

Laboratory tests: Monitor: Electrolytes • BUN, creatinine • Bilirubin, liver enzymes • CBC with differential • Hyperkalemia, hyponatremia possible; renal impairment, CHF, diabetes mellitus, use of potassium-sparing diuretics/potassium supplements/salt substitutes ↑ risk of hyperkalemia.

PATIENT/FAMILY TEACHING

Purpose of drug is to lower BP and/or relieve symptoms of heart failure. • May cause orthostatic hypotension/dizziness. Use caution when changing positions, walking. Alcohol, hot weather, vigorous activity, vomiting, diarrhea, prolonged standing make these symptoms more likely. • Lie down immediately if dizzy. • Medication is not cure for high BP; other therapies, including life-style modifications, must be continued. • Immediately report rash; swelling of extremities: fever, sore throat, infection; chest pain; swelling of face, lips, tongue, throat; difficulty breathing. • Medication may interfere with taste perception, cause persistent coughing.
Outpatient: Take medication exactly as prescribed. Do not stop taking medicine even if you feel better. If medication abruptly discontinued, you may develop dangerously high BP. • Avoid driving and other activities requiring mental alertness until individual response to drug is known. • Avoid salt substitutes or other foods high in potassium unless primary health care provider specifies otherwise. • Weigh twice/wk; report sudden weight gain, edema. • Consult health care profes-

sional before taking cough, cold, or allergy preparations.

AVAILABLE FORMS

Tablets

---

lorazepam
(lor-a′ze-pam)
Ativan,
Novo-Lorazem ✦,
NuLoraz ✦

Classifications: Benzodiazepine, sedative-hypnotic, antianxiety agent
Schedule IV controlled substance

USUAL DOSE

Individualize dosage; increase cautiously. Use reduced dose **G** with advanced age, debilitation, low serum albumin, concurrent use of opiate analgesics, hepatic/renal impairment.
PO, adults: 0.5-2 mg bid-tid • May take larger dose (up to 4 mg) hs • Up to 10 mg/day may be required by some individuals.
G PO, older adults: 0.5-1 mg bid-tid • Increase dose cautiously as needed.
SL, adults (unlabeled/investigational): 1 mg as one-time dose when rapid onset of action desired
IM, adults: 0.05 mg/kg; not to exceed single dose of 4 mg
Direct IV, adults: 2 mg or 0.044 mg/kg, whichever smaller • Larger doses may be used for adults ≤50 yr but do not exceed total dose of 4 mg. Continuous IV infusion has been used for critically ill adults on mechanical ventilation.

ADMINISTRATION

PO solution: Mix with semi-solid food (e.g., pudding, applesauce) or liquid; administer immediately. • Discard unused portion.

SL: Use PO tablets. • Hold under tongue until completely dissolved.

IM: Inject deeply into muscle.

▼**Direct IV:** Dilute, inject slowly at 2 mg/min. • Administer directly into vein or through tubing of free-flowing IV line as close as possible to vein insertion. • Use larger vein to avoid irritation/burning; avoid small veins of hand, wrist. Avoid intraarterial administration, which causes arteriospasm, possible gangrene • *Too-rapid administration may result in profound hypotension, respiratory depression.*

PREPARATION

IV: Dilute immediately before injection with equal volume of compatible diluent.

Compatible solutions: D_5W, 0.9% NaCl, sterile water for injection

ACTIONS

Facilitates action of gamma-aminobutyric acid (GABA, major inhibitory neurotransmitter), produces CNS depression • Results in reduction of anxiety, mild to moderate sedation, hypnotic effects, lack of recall • Minimal respiratory depressant effects at usual dose • No analgesic effects

PHARMACOKINETICS

ROUTE	ONSET	PEAK	DURATION
PO	15-45 min	2 hr	12-24 hr
IM	Rapid	60-90 min	6-8 hr
IV	Rapid	15-20 min	4 hr

DISTRIBUTION
Wide: crosses blood-brain barrier

ELIMINATION
Metabolized by liver, eliminated by kidney; half-life 12-16 hr

INDICATIONS

Management of anxiety disorders, short-term relief of anxiety symptoms • Preop to provide sedation, light anesthesia; diminish patient recall • SL route used when rapid onset of action desired; comparable to IM route *Unlabeled/investigational:* Status epilepticus; chemotherapy-related nausea, vomiting; chronic insomnia; psychogenic catatonia; acute alcohol withdrawal • Short-term use in mechanically ventilated patients to relieve anxiety, ↓ resistance to ventilation

PRECAUTIONS/CONTRAINDICATIONS

Precautions: Use in at-risk patients (e.g., older adults, debilitation, concurrent CNS depressants) or high doses may cause excessive sedation, partial airway obstruction. • IV administration may cause hypotension, respiratory depression, especially with advanced age, debilitation, limited pulmonary reserve, when administered too rapidly.

Use caution with: COPD, limited pulmonary reserve • Hepatic/renal disease, older adults, debilitation, low serum albumin; reduce dose.

L

---

italic = common side effects   **bold** = life-threatening reactions

D Pregnancy category: Risk of congenital malformations, prolonged CNS depression, withdrawal symptoms in newborn; use only if safer alternative unavailable and risk explained to woman.

Contraindications: Hypersensitivity to lorazepam • Acute alcohol intoxication with VS depression • Acute angle-closure glaucoma • Pregnancy, lactation • Not recommended in hepatic/renal failure, shock, coma, profound CNS depression

ADVERSE EFFECTS

CNS: *Drowsiness, sleepiness,* unsteady gait, dizziness, confusion, depression, delirium, visual disturbances, transient amnesia

Resp: IV—**respiratory depression, partial airway obstruction**

CV: hypo/hypertension

GI: Nausea, vomiting

Local: Pain, redness, swelling at injection site; thrombophlebitis

Misc: Tolerance; psychologic/physical dependence

TOXICITY/OVERDOSE

Symptoms (acute toxicity): Somnolence, impaired coordination, slurred speech, confusion, coma, diminished reflexes • Hypotension, respiratory depression, apnea, especially with IV administration • Respiratory depression more likely with concurrent use of CNS depressants, including alcohol

Management: After recent ingestion, implement guidelines for management of acute overdose (Appendix I). • Maintain airway/support ventilation as necessary. • Use flumazenil to reverse sedation, partially re-

verse respiratory depression.

• **Hypotension:** Elevate legs, administer IV fluids; use vasopressors (e.g., norepinephrine, dopamine) if not responsive to fluids. • Do not use barbiturates to relieve paradoxical excitation. • Forced diuresis may be helpful. • Hemodialysis is generally not useful.

INTERACTIONS

alcohol, ethyl ↑ Sedation

antacids Altered absorption

antihistamines ↑ Sedation

barbiturates ↑ Sedation

digoxin ↑ Digoxin level; toxicity; monitor digoxin levels

flumazenil ↓ Sedation

levodopa ↓ Antiparkinsonian effectiveness

opiate analgesics ↑ Sedation

probenecid ↑ Sedation

propoxyphene ↑ Sedation

rifampin ↓ Sedation

scopolamine Sedation, hallucinations, irrational behavior

theophylline ↓ Sedation

Y-SITE COMPATIBILITIES

Acyclovir, atracurium, cimetidine, diltiaxem, zidovudine

Y-SITE INCOMPATIBILITIES

Buprenorphine, ondansetron, pancuronium, piperacillin, ranitidine, vecuronium

PATIENT CARE IMPLICATIONS

• Adverse effects are more likely in first few days of therapy.

• Always use smallest effective dose. Reduce dose, administer in small increments when used with opiate analgesics.

• Avoid sudden cessation of therapy, especially in patients who have received therapy for

---

P pediatric   **G** geriatric   **V** Direct IV

several months or longer (may cause withdrawal symptoms).
• Administer with food to avoid gastric irritation.
• Large quantities should not be prescribed for patients with severe depression, suicidal tendencies, history of substance abuse.

G Older adults
• Use lower, individualized dose; closely monitor for adverse effects (e.g., impaired psychomotor, mental performance).
• Assess need for continued therapy periodically.

IV/IM
• Conditions (e.g., low lighting, patient position) during procedures may interfere with assessment of cardiopulmonary status. Use additional measures (e.g., ECG monitor, pulse oximetry, automatic BP cuff) to monitor closely.
• Drug may result in heavy sedation with partial airway obstruction/hypoventilation, especially in older adults, debilitated patients, those with limited pulmonary reserve. **G**
• Have resuscitation equipment, flumazenil immediately available.
• Monitor frequently for 3-4 hr after IV administration. Patient should remain in bed at least 8 hr, requires assistance with initial ambulation.

Vital signs/hemodynamics: Monitor VS frequently in heavily sedated patients (e.g., those also receiving opiates) or during immediate postop period. • Use continuous pulse oximetry for heavily sedated patients.

Direct IV: Monitor HR, RR, BP q2-5min during and immediately after administration. • As available, monitor ECG for dysrhythmias during injection.

Physical assessment: Assess neurologic status for excessive sedation, impaired physical coordination. Reduce dose as necessary. • Assess for hypoventilation during and after parenteral administration, especially in patients with limited pulmonary reserve, those >50 yr, when **G** other CNS depressants used.
• When used to ↓ resistance to mechanical ventilation, assess for improved ventilation: ↓ airway pressures, ↓ "bucking"

Laboratory tests: Monitor: Liver enzymes, BUN, creatinine, CBC

PATIENT/FAMILY TEACHING

Purpose of medication is to reduce anxiety and cause relaxation. • May cause drowsiness or dizziness; use caution with activity until individual effects recognized. With injection, do not get out of bed for 6-8 hr.
• Medication may decrease ability to remember procedure and events immediately after procedure. • Cigarette smoking interferes with drug effectiveness.
• Inform caregiver if you may be pregnant or are considering pregnancy.

Outpatient: Avoid concurrent use of alcohol or other drugs that cause sedation for 24-48 hr after last dose and until no longer drowsy. • Avoid driving and other activities requiring mental alertness or physical coordination for 24-48 hr and until drowsiness no longer present.
• May cause psychologic/physical dependence; consult physician before increasing dose or abruptly discontinuing.
• Take with food to minimize upset stomach.

---

italic = common side effects   **bold** = life-threatening reactions

AVAILABLE FORMS

Parenteral for IM/IV use • Tablets • Concentrated PO solution

losartan potassium
(loe-sart'an)
Cozaar

Classification: Angiotensin II antagonist, antihypertensive

USUAL DOSE

PO, adults: 50 mg, once daily; up to 100 mg/day may be used • **Volume depletion, hepatic insufficiency:** 25 mg, once daily

ADMINISTRATION

PO: Given without regard to meals

ACTION

Selectively blocks the binding of angiotensin II (AT_2) to the AT_1 receptor, thus preventing AT_2 formation. Losartan blocks potent vasoconstriction, aldosterone secretion caused by AT_2; systolic/diastolic BP reduced without changes in HR • Up to 3-6 weeks required for maximal effects • Unlike angiotensin converting enzyme (ACE) inhibitors, does not affect response to bradykinin • Little effect on serum potassium

PHARMACOKINETICS

ROUTE	ONSET	PEAK	DURATION
PO	≤1 hr	1 hr	≥24 hr

DISTRIBUTION
Highly protein bound

ELIMINATION
Metabolized in liver; eliminated in urine, feces. Losartan half-life = 2 hr; active metabolite, 6-9 hr.

INDICATIONS

Hypertension; used alone or with other agents • May be less effective in black patients

PRECAUTIONS/ CONTRAINDICATIONS

Precautions: May cause hypotension, particularly with intravascular fluid volume deficit, diuretic use; correct volume depletion, use lower dose
Use caution with: CHF, renal impairment; renin-angiotensin-aldosterone inhibition may induce oliguria, acute renal failure • Hepatic insufficiency; use lower dose, monitor closely
P • **Children:** Safe use not established
C **Pregnancy category:** (first tri-
D mester, **D** (second, third trimesters) Use after first trimester associated with fetal abnormalities; discontinue as soon as possible in pregnancy
Contraindications: Hypersensitivity to losartan

ADVERSE EFFECTS

CNS: Dizziness, insomnia
Resp: Cough, dyspnea, upper respiratory infection
CV: Hypotension
GI: Diarrhea

TOXICITY/OVERDOSE

Symptoms: Hypotension, tachycardia
Management: After recent ingestion, implement guidelines for management of acute overdose (Appendix I) • For hypotension, elevate legs, administer IV fluids; consider dopamine or other vasopressors if necessary. • Hemodialysis is not likely to be helpful.

P pediatric   **G** geriatric   **V** Direct IV

INTERACTIONS

diuretics Profound hypotension if patient volume-depleted

PATIENT CARE IMPLICATIONS

• Correct fluid volume deficit before initiating therapy. Use lower starting dose in patients at risk for volume depletion (e.g., diuretic therapy).

Vital signs/hemodynamics: Monitor BP to insure effective therapy. Monitor closely for hypotension in patients with fluid volume deficit. • Monitor urinary output, particularly in patients with CHF, renal impairment

Physical assessment: Assess skin and mucous membranes for adequate hydration.

Laboratory tests: Monitor: Sodium, potassium, BUN, creat., liver enzymes

PATIENT/FAMILY TEACHING

Purpose of medication is to control high BP. • Report dizziness, excessive thirst. • Immediately report possibility of pregnancy.

Outpatient: Take exactly as prescribed. Do not stop taking medicine even if you feel better. Medication is not a cure for high BP; other therapies, including life-style modifications, must be continued. • Consult health care professional before taking nonprescription preparations.

AVAILABLE FORMS

Tablets

---

magnesium sulfate parenteral solution

Classifications: Electrolyte replacement, anticonvulsant, antidysrhythmic

USUAL DOSE

Dose individually adjusted to clinical condition, serum magnesium levels

IM, adult: Mild magnesium deficiency: 1 g q6h • Seizure control: 1 g

Direct IV, adult: Cardiac emergencies: 1-2 g; up to 4-6 g has been used with extreme caution, continuous monitoring • Seizure control: 1 g

IV, intermit inf, adult: Severe hypomagnesemia: 5 g over 3 hr • Preeclampsia/eclampsia: Initially, 4 g (may administer same dose by slow IV injection); follow with 1-2 g/hr by cont inf. Alternative dosing regimen: follow initial IV dose by 4-5 g IM into each buttock, then 4-5 g into alternate buttocks q4h. Adjust dose to serum magnesium levels, urinary excretion. Do not exceed 30-40 g/24 hr. • Renal insufficiency: Adjust dose to serum magnesium concentration. Do not exceed 20 g/48 hr.

IV, intermit inf, children: Severe seizures: 100-200 mg/kg over 1 hr, with ½ total dose in first 15-20 min.

ADMINISTRATION

Do not administer if RR < 16/ min or knee jerk reflex absent.
IM injection, adults: Use 250 mg/ml (25%) or 500 mg/ml (50%) concentration.

M

▼ Direct IV: Use 20% (200 mg/ml) solution; if more concentrated solutions used, must be diluted to ≤20%. • Inject slowly at rate not > 150 mg/min (e.g., 1.5 ml of 10% solution over at least 1 min). More rapid injection of 1-2 g/min may be used with extreme caution, continuous monitoring in life-threatening emergencies.
• *Rapid injection may cause hypotension, heart block, cardiac/respiratory arrest.*
IV, intermit inf: Preferred route • Administer dilute solution over 30-60 min. • Large doses (e.g., ≥5 g) may be infused over several hr if patient condition permits. • Dilute solutions in 500-1,000 ml may be given as continuous infusion.

PREPARATION

Direct IV: 4%, 8%, 10%, 12.5%, 20% solutions may be given undiluted. • Dilute concentrated solutions to ≤ 20%.
IV, intermit inf: Dilute in 500-1,000 ml compatible IV solution.
IV, cont inf: Dilute in 500-1,000 ml compatible IV solution.
Compatible fluids: D_5W, 0.9% NaCl, LR, most common IV solutions

ACTIONS

Serum concentrations >2.5 mEq/L depress CNS/peripheral neuromuscular transmission, resulting in anticonvulsive, sedative effects; excess magnesium believed to ↓ acetylcholine release by motor nerve impulse.
• Serum concentrations ≥4 mEq/L depress deep-tendon reflexes; concentrations ≥10 mEq/L may cause heart block, fatal respiratory paralysis. • Slows HR at SA node, prolongs conduction time; may prolong PR interval, H (atria–His bundle) interval, antegrade AV nodal effective refractory period, SA conduction time; will protect against dysrhythmias such as PVCs, ventricular tachycardia • Produces peripheral vasodilation, resulting in flushing, sweating, hypotension when large doses used • Large doses promote relaxation of bronchial smooth muscle. CNS depressant/peripheral neuromuscular blockade effects antagonized by parenteral calcium administration

PHARMACOKINETICS

ROUTE	ONSET	PEAK	DURATION
IM	1 hr		3-4 hr
IV	Immed	Rapid	30 min

DISTRIBUTION
Wide; readily crosses placenta
ELIMINATION
Excreted by kidneys at variable rate, dependent on serum levels

INDICATIONS

Rapid electrolyte replacement in severe hypomagnesemia • Cardiac emergencies such as atypical ventricular tachycardia (torsades de pointes), refractory ventricular fibrillation • Cardiac arrest with suspected hypomagnesemia • Electrolyte replacement in acute hypomagnesemia associated with malabsorption, alcoholism, hepatic cirrhosis, acute pancreatitis, prolonged IV therapy • TPN additive to prevent magnesium deficiency
• Prevention/control of seizures in severe preeclampsia/eclampsia.
• Control of seizures associated with epilepsy, glomerulonephritis, hypothyroidism • As secondary agent in acute nephritis to

control hypertension, encephalopathy, seizures

Unlabeled/investigational:
To promote bronchodilation in acute asthma • To promote osmotic diuresis in cerebral edema • To ↓ vascular resistance, ↑ CO, improve mortality in acute MI

PRECAUTIONS/CONTRAINDICATIONS

Precautions: Carefully adjust dose to serum magnesium levels; loss of knee jerk reflex (serum level ≥4 mEq/L) signals onset of magnesium intoxication. • Rapid IV injection may cause hypotension, heart block, cardiac/respiratory arrest. • May change calcium/phosphorus balance; serious hypocalcemia possible

Use caution with: Pregnancy; administration within last 2 hr of labor may cause magnesium toxicity, including respiratory depression, in newborn. • Renal impairment: magnesium intoxication possible • Concurrent administration of cardiac glycosides

Pregnancy category: Use only if safer alternative unavailable.

Contraindications: RR <16/min • Heart block • Hypermagnesemia • Hypocalcemia • Anuria • Last 2 hr of labor

ADVERSE EFFECTS

CNS: *Sweating, flushing,* drowsiness, weakness, peripheral neuromuscular blockade
Resp: ↓ RR, **respiratory paralysis**
CV: Hypotension, ↓ SVR, bradycardia, prolonged PR interval, heart block, **cardiac arrest**

TOXICITY/OVERDOSE

Symptoms: Hypotension, heart block, cardiac arrest • CNS depression, absent deep-tendon reflexes • Respiratory paralysis/arrest

Management: Provide supportive care, including artificial ventilation. • Administer calcium gluconate to reverse respiratory depression, heart block. • **Hypotension:** Elevate legs, administer IV fluids; use dopamine if necessary. • Peritoneal dialysis/hemodialysis are effective.

INTERACTIONS

anesthetics, general ↑ CNS depression
barbiturates ↑ CNS depression
digoxin Heart block if calcium required for magnesium toxicity
NMBAs Prolonged neuromuscular blockade
opiate analgesics ↑ CNS depression

Y-SITE COMPATIBILITIES

Amikacin, ampicillin, cefamandole, cefazolin, cefoperazone, cefotaxime, cefoxitin, cephapirin, dobutamine, enalaprilat, esmolol, famotidine, gentamicin, heparin, insulin, labetalol, meperidine, morphine, nafcillin, ondansetron, oxacillin, penicillin G potassium, piperacillin, potassium chloride, tetracycline, ticarcillin, vancomycin

Y-SITE INCOMPATIBILITIES

Calcium gluceptate, ciprofloxacin, procaine, sodium bicarbonate

M

---

italic = common side effects   **bold** = life-threatening reactions

PATIENT CARE IMPLICATIONS

• Have equipment for airway management/artificial ventilation, 0.9% NaCl, calcium gluconate immediately available in case of toxicity.

• Implement seizure precautions when used to prevent/manage seizures.

Vital signs/hemodynamics: Monitor VS q15min after IV dose; monitor for hypotension, respiratory/cardiac depression.

• Measure hourly UO; must be maintained at ≥100 ml for 4 hr preceding prescribed dose.

• Check RR before each dose; do not administer if <16/min

• **Direct IV/Rapid IV inf:** Continuously monitor ECG for bradycardia, ECG changes associated with hypermagnesemia: prolonged QT interval, AV block, widened QRS complex. If ECG changes or hypotension develop, stop injection, consult physician.

Physical assessment: Assess for hypermagnesemia: flushing, hypotension, confusion, weakness, depressed deep-tendon reflexes, flaccid paralysis, respiratory depression, dyspnea.

• Assess respiratory status: rate, rhythm, character. Stop infusion/withhold next dose for respiratory depression. • Assess for knee jerk reflexes before repeat doses and q1-2h with continuous infusions (excluding low doses used in TPN). If absent, do not administer additional magnesium until return of reflexes. • Assess mental status, level of consciousness.

• **Pregnancy:** Assess timing, intensity of contractions; monitor fetal HR, reactivity. Drug may slow contractions, cause fetal depression. • Carefully assess newborn for respiratory depression, hyporeflexia, CV depression if drug given <24 hr before delivery.

Laboratory tests: Monitor: Serum magnesium levels • BUN, creat., creat. cl. • Effective in cardiac emergencies such as torsades, acute MI, even when serum magnesium level within normal limits.

PATIENT/FAMILY TEACHING

Purpose of medication is to replace magnesium. • Report weakness, flushing, sweating, difficulty moving, confusion.

AVAILABLE FORMS

Parenteral for IV/IM injection/infusion • Premixed parenteral solution for IV infusion

mannitol
(man'i-tole)
Osmitrol

Classification: Osmotic diuretic

USUAL DOSE

IV, intermit/cont inf, adults: Variable; range, 50-200 g/24hr 4 **Prevention of oliguria:** 50-100 g/24 hr; concentrated solution used initially, followed by inf of 5%-10% solution • **Extreme oliguria:** Test dose of 12.5-25 g concentrated solution (e.g., 50-100 ml 25% solution); may repeat once for inadequate response, (e.g., ≤30-50 ml/hr of urine for 2-3 hr after administration); follow successful test dose with intermit or cont inf; do not exceed 100 g/24 hr. ↑ **ICP:** 1.5-2.0 g/kg using 25% so-

lution; administer 1-1.5 hr before surgery in preop patients.
• **Edema/ascites:** 100 g using 10%-20% solution • **Diuresis of toxins:** Loading dose of 25 g followed by continuous infusion adjusted to maintain UO of 100-500 ml/hr
IV, intermit/cont inf, children: Dose for children ≤12 yr not well established; suggested dose, 0.25-1 g/kg using 15%-20% solution • Test dose in oliguria, 0.2 g/kg

ADMINISTRATION

IV: Infuse over 30-90 min.
• Give test dose over 3-5 min.
• For edema/ascites, infuse over 2-6 hr. • Inline 0.22-μm filter or filter needle required

PREPARATION

IV: Solution may crystallize at cool temperatures, especially if ≥15% concentration. Visually inspect for crystals by holding bottle up to bright light. If crystals observed, warm bottle in hot water bath (remove, shake at intervals) or autoclave; microwave warming not recommended; cool to body temperature before administration.
• May be stored in blanket or warmer to prevent crystallization • Do not administer solutions with undissolved crystals.
Compatible fluids: Avoid addition to other solutions; may cause precipitation.

ACTIONS

Greatly elevates osmotic pressure of glomerular filtrate, discourages tubular reabsorption of water/solutes, thus promoting diuresis; sufficient renal blood flow/glomerular filtration necessary for effective action • Other

desired effects; ↑ renal blood flow, ↓ renal vascular resistance, ↓ blood viscosity • Promotes excretion of some electrolytes, including sodium, potassium, chloride, calcium, others • Dilutes urine, protects kidneys by limiting exposure of nephrons to high concentrations of toxins
• With cerebral edema or ascites/edema, osmotic effect encourages fluid shifts, resulting in reduction of edema. Rebound increases in ICP may occur approx 12 hr after administration.

PHARMACOKINETICS

ROUTE	ONSET*	PEAK	DURATION
IV	30-60 min	1 hr	6-8 hr

DISTRIBUTION
Remains in extracellular compartment
ELIMINATION
Minimally metabolized, most excreted unchanged in urine; half-life 100 min; clearance impaired with CHF, cirrhosis, shock

*Diuretic effects. Reduction of CSF occurs within 15 min, lasts 3-8 hr.

INDICATIONS

Prevention/treatment of acute renal failure associated with massive hemorrhage, trauma, shock, burns, transfusion reactions, major surgery, other conditions • Reduction of greatly ↑ ICP, cerebral/spinal cord edema, particularly with evidence of herniation, pending brainstem compression • Diuresis of edema/ascites associated with nephrotic syndrome, cirrhosis, heart failure • Encourages excretion, protects kidneys from toxins such as aspirin, barbiturates, bromides, lithium, carbon monoxide, ethylene glycol, or imipramine

M

---

italic = common side effects   **bold** = life-threatening reactions

PRECAUTIONS/ CONTRAINDICATIONS

Precautions: Inadequate UO or too rapid administration of large doses may cause mannitol accumulation, excessive extracellular fluid, circulatory overload, water intoxication, CHF. • Failure to replace fluids/correct electrolytes may lead to excessive diuresis, electrolyte depletion, hypovolemia, tissue dehydration. • Mannitol-induced hyponatremia/ hyperkalemia may result in serious effects, death. • Mixing with blood may cause agglutination, erythrocyte dehydration.

Use caution with: Cerebral edema; rebound ↑ ICP possible • Oliguria/renal impairment; use test dose, establish adequate renal function before administration.

c Pregnancy category: Use only if safer alternative unavailable.

Contraindications: Hypersensitivity to mannitol • Anuria unresponsive to test dose • Severe CHF, pulmonary edema • Severe dehydration • Progressive renal insufficiency • Active intracranial bleeding (except during craniotomy)

ADVERSE EFFECTS

CNS: Headache, blurred vision, dizziness, **cerebral dehydration, seizures**
Resp: Rhinitis, **pulmonary edema**
CV: *Extracellular volume expansion,* **circulatory overload, CHF,** dehydration, hypotension, hypertension, tachycardia
GI:Thirst, dry mouth, nausea, vomiting, diarrhea

GU: *Extreme diuresis,* urinary retention
F&E: Hypo/hypernatremia, hyper/hypokalemia, acidosis, dehydration, electrolyte imbalance
Local: Edema/skin necrosis with extravasation

TOXICITY/OVERDOSE

Symptoms: Water intoxication with altered mental status, pulmonary edema, CHF • Electrolyte imbalance, hypokalemia, dysrhythmias • Dehydration, hypotension, tachycardia, seizures
Management: Slow or stop infusion. • Support respiration as needed with O_2 and/or mechanical ventilation. • **Circulatory overload:** Administer furosemide or other potent diuretic, or initiate hemodialysis. • Correct fluid/electrolyte imbalances.

INTERACTION

lithium Increased urinary excretion of lithium

Y-SITE COMPATIBILITIES

Ondansetron, piperacillin-tazobactam sodium

INCOMPATIBILITIES

Addition of KCl or NaCl to mannitol 20, 25% may result in precipitation.

PATIENT CARE IMPLICATIONS

• Replace fluids/correct electrolytes before use; avoid use in uncorrected hypovolemic shock or circulatory overload (e.g., pulmonary edema, CHF).
• Evaluate response to therapy, considering diuretic response, fluid balance, weight, electrolytes. Adjust dose accordingly.

Frequent ongoing assessment of fluid/electrolyte balance, urine pH is essential when used for forced diuresis of toxins.

• If patients with pre-renal failure become progressively more oliguric or azotemic, discontinue use.

• When used to lower ↑ ICP, administer stat, keep head of bed ≥3° and head in neutral alignment.

Vital signs/hemodynamics: Monitor BP, HR, CVP, PAP, UO q1-2h. Consult physician for ↑ or ↓ CVP, PAP, hypotension, UO <30-50 ml/hr. • Indwelling urinary catheter is recommended for accurate assessment of diuretic response. • As available, continuously monitor ECG. Note presence of dysrhythmias, ECG changes. If present, check electrolytes, correct as necessary.

• Hemodynamic monitoring recommended; monitor closely for circulatory overload or excessive diuresis, ↑ ↓ filling pressures.

• When used to lower ↑ ICP, monitor neurologic status, CSF drainage, cerebral perfusion pressure (CPP). Consult primary health care provider for inadequate response to mannitol, failure to maintain ICP <15 mmHg, CPP >60 mmHg. Rebound ↑ in ICP may occur 12 hr after administration

Physical assessment: Assess for signs/symptoms of dehydration: thirst, dry oral mucosa, poor skin turgor, fever, ↓ CVP/PCWP. •Assess for signs/symptoms of fluid overload: bibasilar crackles (rales), ↑ CVP/PCWP, dyspnea, edema. • Assess for signs/symptoms of electrolyte imbalance: dysrhythmias, confusion, dizziness, weakness, muscle cramps, headache, pares-

thesias, thirst, anorexia, vomiting. • Assess for perfusion/oxygenation deficit caused by hypovolemia: chest discomfort, decreased level of consciousness, activity intolerance, hypotension, dizziness. • Evaluate infusion site frequently to prevent extravasation, local irritation, tissue necrosis. • Weigh patient daily.

Laboratory tests: Monitor: Electrolytes, especially sodium, potassium; promptly correct imbalances. • BUN, creatinine • Serum osmolality; increases >325 m Osm/kg do not improve effectiveness • May interfere with lab tests for inorganic phosphorus, ethylene glycol.

PATIENT/FAMILY TEACHING

Purpose of medication is to eliminate excess body fluid, reduce swelling. • Remain in bed during and for several hours after therapy. Call for assistance when getting out of bed. • Immediately report breathing difficulty, palpitations, dizziness, chest pain, headache, numbness/tingling, muscle cramps, nausea, vomiting.

AVAILABLE FORMS

Solutions in various concentrations (5%, 10%, 15%, 20%, 25%) for IV use

M

---

meperidine HCl
(me-per′i-deen)
Demerol
meperidine with promethazine
Mepergan

Classifications: Opiate agonist, narcotic analgesic

Schedule II controlled substance

USUAL DOSE

Use in smallest effective dose to minimize CNS depression/tolerance. *Use caution, reduced dose in elderly or debilitated patients*

IM/SC, adults: 50-150 mg q3-4h as needed • **Preop:** 50-100 mg 30-90 min before anesthesia

IM/SC, children: 1.1-1.8 mg/kg q3-4h; single dose not to exceed 100 mg

Direct IV, adults: 10-50 mg q2-4h as needed for pain

IV, cont/PCA inf, adults: 15-35 mg/hr by slow, continuous infusion or as incremental, patient-administered boluses

PO: 50-150 mg q3-4h

ADMINISTRATION

Direct IV, adults: Inject each dose slowly over 4-5 min. • Titrate frequently for pain control without respiratory depression.
• Too rapid administration may cause apnea, hypotension.
• Have naloxone, resuscitation equipment nearby.

IV, cont inf, adults: Titrate for pain control without depressing RR, BP. • Infusion pump necessary; may be patient activated
• Have naloxone, resuscitation equipment nearby.

PREPARATION

Direct IV, adults: Dilute each dose in at least 5 ml sterile water or normal saline for injection.

IV, cont/PCA inf, adults: Dilute in D_5W or 0.9% NaCl for concentration of 1 mg/ml.
• More concentrated solutions up to 10 mg/ml may be used.

ACTIONS

Synthetic opiate agonist that acts at specific receptor sites in CNS/other tissues to inhibit pain perception, produce analgesia
• Causes respiratory, CNS depression; duration of respiratory depression < that of morphine.
• Less likely to cause intense smooth muscle spasm, constipation than morphine • Suppresses cough reflex only at analgesic doses • Active metabolite, normeperidine has mild analgesic/strong CNS stimulant effects
• Meperidine, 75 mg IM or 300 mg PO, is analgesic equivalent of morphine, 10 mg IM. • More rapid onset/shorter duration than morphine

PHARMACOKINETICS

ROUTE	ONSET	PEAK	DURATION
PO	30 min	60 min	2-4 hr
IM	10-45 min	30-50 min	2-4 hr
IV	5 min	<30 min	2 hr

DISTRIBUTION

Wide; crosses placenta

ELIMINATION

Metabolized in liver, excreted in urine; half-life 3-5 hr, prolonged with hepatic impairment • Normeperidine half-life 8-21 hr.

INDICATIONS

Relief of moderate to severe pain, associated apprehension
• Preop sedation, anesthesia supplement • Analgesia during term labor • Sometimes used in acute pulmonary edema to promote vasodilation, reduce preload, relieve anxiety

PRECAUTIONS/ CONTRAINDICATIONS

Precautions: Severe respiratory depression possible, especially with IV use • May increase SVR, ventricular

response rate, cause tachycardia • May cause hypotension, especially with rapid IV administration • Accumulation of metabolite, normeperidine, may cause toxic CNS stimulation (e.g., seizures, tremors, agitation) with high-dose/prolonged therapy, hepatic/renal dysfunction.
• Commercial preparations may contain sulfites, which can cause serious allergic reactions.

G **Use caution with:** Older adults: ↑ Incidence of adverse reactions, generally avoided; if used must use reduced dose • Hepatic/renal dysfunction, debilitation; reduce dose. • COPD • CNS depression, head injury • Seizure disorder • Hypotension, shock, tachycardia • Prostatic hypertrophy, urethral stricture • Adrenal insufficiency

P • Children

C **Pregnancy category:** Use only if safer alternative unavailable.

Contraindications: Hypersensitivity to meperidine • Undiagnosed acute abdominal conditions • Respiratory depression • Diarrhea caused by poisoning • Concurrent or recent use of MAO inhibitors

ADVERSE EFFECTS

G ↑ Incidence of all SE in older adults. Profound confusion, agitation, ↑ pain may occur.
CNS: *Sedation, confusion,* dizziness, coma, euphoria, weakness, restlessness, nervousness, **seizures**
EENT: Pupillary constriction, visual disturbances
Resp: **Respiratory depression, apnea**
CV: *Orthostatic hypotension,* **hypotension,** reflex tachycar-

dia, bradycardia, sweating, flushing
GI: Nausea, vomiting
GU: Urinary retention, oliguria
Local: Phlebitis, injection site pain
Misc: Tolerance; physical/psychologic dependence

TOXICITY/OVERDOSE
Acute toxicity/overdose:
Profound CNS depression, coma • Respiratory depression, bradycardia, hypotension • Hypothermia with cool, clammy skin • **Severe overdose:** Apnea, pulmonary edema, circulatory collapse, cardiopulmonary arrest
Chronic toxicity: Tolerance; psychologic/physical dependence • Physical dependence results in withdrawal symptoms when drug abruptly discontinued.
Management: After recent ingestion, implement guidelines for management of acute overdose (Appendix I). • **Hypoventilation:** Establish/maintain airway, administer O_2; muscular rigidity may interfere with mechanical ventilation; administration of NMBA may be necessary. • **Hypotension:** Elevate legs, administer IV fluids; use vasopressors (e.g., dopamine, norepinephrine) for circulatory collapse. • **Antidote:** Opiate antagonist, naloxone (Narcan), used to reverse respiratory depression, other symptoms

INTERACTIONS
alcohol, ethyl ↑ CNS depression
anesthetics, general ↑ CNS depression
antihistamines ↑ CNS depression; enhanced analgesia
cimetidine ↑ CNS depression

M

MAO inhibitors Severe reaction: hypertension, rigidity, excitation, coma, death
naloxone Reversal of effects; acute withdrawal in opiate-dependent patients
opiate agonist-antagonists Acute withdrawal in opiate-dependent patients
opiate analgesics ↑ CNS depression
phenothiazines ↑ ↓ Analgesia; ↑ CNS depression
sedatives, tranquilizers ↑ CNS depression; enhanced analgesia
TCAs ↑ CNS depression

COMPATIBILITIES

Amikacin, ampicillin, atenolol, cefamandole, cefazolin, cefotaxime, cefotetan, cefoxitin, ceftazidime, ceftizoxime, ceftriaxone, cefuroxime, cephalothin, cephapirin, chloramphenicol, clindamycin, dexamethasone, diphenhydramine, diltiazem, dobutamine, dopamine, doxycycline, droperidol, famotidine, fluconazole, gentamicin, heparin, insulin, labetalol, lidocaine, magnesium sulfate, metoclopramide, metoprolol, ondansetron, oxacillin, penicillin G, piperacillin, potassium chloride, propranolol, ranitidine, ticarcillin, tobramycin, vancomycin, verapamil

INCOMPATIBILITIES

Acyclovir, cefoperazone, furosemide, imipenem-cilastatin, nafcillin

PATIENT CARE IMPLICATIONS

• Administer prn doses before pain becomes severe. Regularly scheduled or PCA dosing usually more effective than prn scheduling

• Administer with peripherally acting, nonnarcotic analgesics (e.g., acetaminophen, ibuprofen) for additive analgesic effects.
• Administer with antihistamines (e.g., hydroxyzine) or phenothiazines (e.g., promethazine) to potentiate effects.
• Have naloxone, resuscitation equipment immediately available, with IV/IM/SC use.
• Long-term therapy not recommended because normeperidine accumulation, ↑ risk of toxicity
• Tolerance develops in patients receiving opiate analgesics for long-term pain control; progressively higher doses necessary.
• Gradually discontinue drug after long-term use to prevent withdrawal symptoms.
• PO: Administer with food or milk to enhance oral absorption. Administer solutions mixed in water or fruit juice to avoid transient topical anesthetic effect on mucous membranes.

Vital signs/hemodynamics: Assess BP, RR, pulse before and periodically during administration; IV injection: q5min for first 15 min, frequently thereafter; IM injection: q15-30min, thereafter according to patient condition. Consider pulse oximetry for PCA, continuous infusions, individuals at risk for hypoventilation

Physical assessment: Assess type, location, intensity of pain before and after administration. • Assess ventilation: note rate/depth of respirations, auscultate breath sounds. • Assess bowel function: bowel sounds, abdominal distention, elimination patterns. • Monitor I&O. Assess for urinary retention, bladder distention.

PATIENT/FAMILY TEACHING

Purpose of medication is to relieve pain. • Request medication before pain becomes severe.
• Change position slowly to minimize dizziness. • Change position, cough, deep breathe q2h to prevent lung problems.
• Do not perform hazardous tasks requiring mental alertness, physical coordination. Call for assistance when ambulating (initial therapy). • Drink plenty of fluids; eat high-fiber foods. Use stool softeners if necessary to minimize constipation.
Outpatient: Avoid concurrent use of alcohol or other sedatives while taking this medication.

AVAILABLE FORMS

Parenteral for IV/IM/SC use
• Tablets • PO solution • Premixed IV solution

---

metaproterenol sulfate
(met-a-proe-ter′e-nole)
Alupent, Metaprel

Classification: Beta-2-adrenergic agonist

USUAL DOSE

Metered-dose inhal, adults/children>12 yr: 2-3 puffs q3-4h
Nebulization/IPPB, adults/children >12 yr: 0.2-0.3 ml (10-15 mg) 5% solution in 2.5 ml diluent 3-4 times daily • 2.5 ml 0.4% or 0.6% solution 3-4 times daily • With acute bronchospasm, doses may be administered up to q4h.
Nebulization, children 6-12 yr: 0.1 ml (5 mg) 5% solution in 2.9 ml diluent 3-4 times daily

PO, adults/children >9 yr: 20 mg 3-4 times daily
PO, children 6-9 yr: 10 mg 3-4 times daily

ADMINISTRATION

Metered-dose inhal: Allow 2 min between each inhalation
Nebulization/IPPB: Dilute each dose of 5% solution with 0.45%-0.9% NaCl for final volume of 3 ml. • Adjust flow rate of nebulizer to deliver over 5-15 min.

ACTIONS

Stimulates beta-adrenergic receptors; predominant effects on beta-2 (bronchial, uterine, vascular smooth muscle) receptors; minimal beta-1 (cardiac) effects, although effects less selective than albuterol • Results in bronchodilation, mild vasodilation, slight ↓ in BP • Little or no effect on alpha-adrenergic receptors • Cardiac/CNS stimulatory effects more likely at higher doses

PHARMACOKINETICS

ROUTE	ONSET	PEAK	DURATION
Inhal	1-5 min	60 min	4-6 hr
PO	15 min	60 min	4-6 hr

DISTRIBUTION
Not clearly established.

ELIMINATION
Extensive first-pass metabolism; eliminated in urine

INDICATIONS

Relief of bronchospasm in asthma, chronic bronchitis, emphysema • Longer duration, less likely to cause cardiac stimulation than isoproterenol. Less cardioselective than albuterol.

M

PRECAUTIONS/ CONTRAINDICATIONS

Precautions: Tolerance may develop with prolonged use.
• Repeated or excessive use may lead to paradoxical bronchoconstriction.
Use caution with: Cardiac disorders • Hypertension • Hyperthyroidism • Diabetes mellitus • Seizure disorders • Children <6 yr: Safe use not clearly established
ⓒ **Pregnancy category:** Use only if safer alternative unavailable.
Contraindications: Hypersensitivity to metaproterenol

ADVERSE EFFECTS

CNS: *Tremors, nervousness,* insomnia, headache, dizziness
EENT: Dry, irritated nose/throat
Resp: Cough, paradoxical bronchospasm
CV: *Tachycardia, palpitations,* hypo/hypertension, dysrhythmias
GI: Nausea, vomiting
Misc: Tolerance

INTERACTIONS

aminophylline Dysrhythmias
beta-blockers ↓ Metaproterenol effectiveness
sympathomimetics CV toxicity

PATIENT CARE IMPLICATIONS

• For optimal benefits in controlling bronchospasm, schedule doses at regular intervals.
• Administer PO doses with meals.
Vital signs/hemodynamics: Monitor ECG for tachycardia, dysrhythmias. • Monitor VS for hypo/hypertension, improved RR. • Use pulse oximeter to evaluate O_2 saturation before and after administration.
Physical assessment: Assess work of breathing, ventilatory excursion, breath sounds.
• Evaluate forced expiratory volume peak flow, or other pulmonary function measurements before and after treatment.
Laboratory tests: Monitor: ABGs

PATIENT/FAMILY TEACHING

Purpose of medication is to relieve bronchospasm, improve breathing. • Report ↑ breathing difficulty, chest pain, palpitations. • Sips of water or sugarless gum may help dry mouth.
• Take oral doses with meals to decrease stomach irritation.
• Check with health care professional before taking cold or cough preparations. • Use metered-dose inhaler as demonstrated. Be certain to exhale completely before use, close lips firmly around mouthpiece, inhale deeply while activating inhaler. Hold breath for as long as possible; exhale slowly.
• Use exactly as directed. If ineffective, do not ↑ dose/frequency of use; consult health care professional.

AVAILABLE FORMS

Solution for PO inhal therapy
• Metered-dose inhaler • Standard tablets • PO solution

---

metaraminol bitartrate
(met-ah-ram'i-nole)
Aramine

Classifications: Vasopressor, sympathomimetic

USUAL DOSE

Direct IV/ET, adults: 0.5-5 mg
• May follow with IV cont inf

Direct IV/ET, children: 0.01 mg/kg as single dose • May follow with IV cont inf

IV, cont inf, adults/children: Variable according to condition; titrate to desired BP.

ADMINISTRATION

Direct IV: Administer each dose over ≥1 min. • May be given undiluted

IV, cont inf: Use slow flow rate; increase in small increments to correct hypotension.
• Titrate q10-15min; more rapid adjustment may cause excessive vasoconstriction, dysrhythmias.
• Infuse via central or other large vein; avoid hand veins. Infusion pump required.

ET instillation, adults/ children: Dilute desired dose in 10 ml sterile 0.9% NaCl for adults; use 1-2 ml for children. Provide several quick ventilations, then expel via catheter passed just beyond ETT. Follow with several quick ventilations.

PREPARATION
IV inf

DILUTION	CONCENTRATION
1 mg/25 ml (children)	4 µ/ml
50 mg/250 ml	200 µg/ml
100 mg/250 ml	400 µg/ml

More concentrated solutions, up to 1 mg/ml, may be used if necessary to limit fluid intake.

Compatible fluids: D_5W, NaCl

ACTIONS

Directly stimulates alpha-1-adrenergic and beta-1-adrenergic receptors, resulting in vasoconstriction, inotropic cardiac stimulation; indirectly stimulates CV system by stimulating release of norepinephrine from its storage sites • Prolonged use depletes norepinephrine stores, causing reduced effectiveness, refractoriness to effects. • Effects similar to but more prolonged than norepinephrine • **CV/hemodynamic:** Arterial/venous vasoconstriction, ↑ SBP, DBP, reflex bradycardia; CO usually ↑; excessive doses or prolonged use ↓ CO. Coronary artery blood flow is enhanced because ↑ systemic BP, coronary vasodilation. Inotropic effects ↑ myocardial workload, O_2 consumption; causes ventricular irritability; pulmonary vasoconstriction elevates PVR. • **Renal:** Initially ↓ renal blood flow because of renal vasoconstriction; renal blood flow may ↑ as BP restored; less likely to produce renal vasoconstriction than norepinephrine.
• May reduce circulating plasma volume because of postcapillary vasoconstriction • With hepatic cirrhosis, may ↑ excretion of water, sodium, potassium

PHARMACOKINETICS

ROUTE	ONSET	PEAK	DURATION
SC	5-20 min		20-90 min
IM	10 min		20-90 min
IV	1-2 min	10-15 min	20 min

DISTRIBUTION

Does not cross blood-brain barrier

ELIMINATION

Effects terminated by tissue uptake, urinary excretion

INDICATIONS

Hypotension associated with drug reactions, surgical complications, hemorrhage, neurogenic shock, septicemia, cardiogenic

M

---

italic = common side effects   **bold** = life-threatening reactions

shock; indicated after failure to respond to fluid administration, other specific resuscitative measures • With acute MI, drug-induced ↑ in myocardial O_2 demand may outweigh beneficial effects • Dopamine preferable if severe CHF present because of renal vasodilatory effects • Used for treatment/prevention of acute hypotension associated with spinal anesthesia

PRECAUTIONS/ CONTRAINDICATIONS

Precautions: ↑ Myocardial workload may lead to imbalance of myocardial O_2 supply/demand, resulting in ischemia, infarction. • Prolonged administration may ↓ venous return, ↓ CO. • May cause dysrhythmias, especially with hepatic cirrhosis and when myocardium sensitized to catecholamines (e.g., acute MI, hypoxia, acid-base imbalance, digoxin, anesthetics) • Adjust dose carefully to avoid hypertension, acute pulmonary edema, dysrhythmias, cardiac arrest. • Hypotension more likely to recur after metaraminol than after norepinephrine administration; may be caused by depletion of tissue stores of norepinephrine; norepinephrine administration may be necessary to replace depleted stores. • If extravasation occurs, tissue necrosis and sloughing may result. Area of extravasation should be infiltrated with phentolamine (Appendixes K and L).
Use caution with: CAD • Occlusive vascular disease • Hypertension • Hepatic cirrhosis • Thyroid disease • Diabetes; insulin requirements may ↑.
• Hypoxia, acid-base imbalances; may ↓ drug effectiveness, ↑ adverse effects
c Pregnancy category: Use only if safer alternative unavailable.
Contraindications: Hypersensitivity to metaraminol • Peripheral/mesenteric infarction • Cyclopropane, halothane anesthesia • Commercial preparations may contain sulfites, which can cause serious allergic reactions.
P Children: Safety not established

ADVERSE EFFECTS

CNS: Apprehension, dizziness, headache, tremors
CV: **Dysrhythmias, ventricular tachycardia,** palpitations, hypertension, hypotension after drug cessation
GI: Nausea
Derm: Flushing, sweating; tissue necrosis, sloughing at injection site
Misc: Resistance to effects with prolonged use

TOXICITY/OVERDOSE

Symptoms: Severe hypertension • Dysrhythmias • Convulsions, cerebral hemorrhage
Management: Discontinue infusion. • **Hypertension:** If severe or persistent, manage with nitroprusside or phentolamine. • **Dysrhythmias:** Use beta-adrenergic blocker (e.g., propranolol).

INTERACTIONS

alpha blockers ↓ Effectiveness; profound hypotension
anesthetics Dysrhythmias
atropine ↑ Pressor response; blocks reflex bradycardia
beta-blockers Excessive hypertension; bradycardia; ↓ CO
digoxin Dysrhythmias

P pediatric   **G** geriatric   **V** Direct IV

MAO inhibitors Profound hypertension
phenothiazines Blocked alpha effects; profound hypotension
sympathomimetics Dysrhythmias
TCAs Hypertension, dysrhythmias

Y-SITE COMPATIBILITIES

Amiodarone, amrinone, cephalothin, cephapirin, cimetidine, dobutamine, ephedrine, epinephrine, lidocaine, potassium chloride, sodium bicarbonate, tetracycline, verapamil

Y-SITE INCOMPATIBILITIES

Erythromycin lactobionate, methicillin, nafcillin, penicillin G potassium, phenytoin, ranitidine, thiopental sodium

PATIENT CARE IMPLICATIONS

• Correct hypovolemia before initiating therapy.
• Monitor for/correct hypoxemia, hypercapnia, acidosis before and during drug administration.
• Discontinue IV infusion very gradually to avoid recurrent hypotension. Reinstate infusion or administer other pressor agent (norepinephrine, dopamine) if SBP falls below 70-80 mm Hg.
• Prolonged use may deplete norepinephrine stores, rendering metaraminol ineffective. Vasodilation and hypotension are possible. Patients with depleted norepinephrine stores (e.g., prolonged critical illness, lengthy major surgery, profound shock) may be minimally responsive to metaraminol. Exogenous norepinephrine may be necessary.
Vital signs/hemodynamics: Monitor BP, pulse q5-15min according to stability, titration schedule. Be aware that full effects are not apparent for 15-30 min after administration or adjustment of dose. To avoid cumulative dose/possible toxicity, titrate infusion no more often than q10-15min. • Establish clear parameters for titration of IV infusion (e.g., desired BP, CO, UO). Use lowest possible dose to achieve desired effect.
• Continuously monitor ECG for dysrhythmias, ischemic changes (e.g., T wave inversion, ST depression/elevation).
• Monitor CO, PCWP, CVP, SVR as available. Immediately correct hypovolemia. • Monitor UO: consult physician if ≤5 ml/kg/hr or ≤30 ml/hr.
Physical assessment: Assess for evidence of diminished peripheral perfusion: coolness, ↓ pulse intensity, paresthesias, delayed capillary refill. • Assess for perfusion/oxygenation deficit: changes in mentation, hypotension, chest discomfort.
• Check infusion site frequently for signs of extravasation (e.g., blanching along vein pathway, coldness, hardness). If this occurs, change injection site immediately, infiltrate affected area with phentolamine (Appendixes K and L).
Laboratory tests: Monitor: Electrolytes • ABGs • Blood glucose, especially in patients with diabetes

PATIENT/FAMILY TEACHING

Purpose of medication is to improve BP, cardiac performance.
• Immediately report chest pain or discomfort, palpitations, pain at infusion site.

AVAILABLE FORMS

Concentrate for parenteral use

methyldopa, methyldopate HCL
(meth-ill-doe'pa)
Aldomet, Novo-Medopa ✦, Nu-Medopa ✦
methyldopa with chlorothiazide
Aldoclor
methyldopa with hydrochlororthiazide
Aldoril

Classifications: Antihypertensive, central adrenergic inhibitor

USUAL DOSE
PO, adults: Initially 250 mg bid or tid; gradually increase as needed at 2-day intervals. • Maximum dose, 3 g/day
P PO, children: Initially 10 mg/kg/g day bid, tid, or qid; gradually increase as needed at 2-day intervals. • Maximum dose, 65 mg/kg/day or 3 g/day, whichever less
IV, intermit inf, adults: 250-500 mg q6h • Maximum dose, 1,000 mg q6h
P IV, intermit inf, children: 5-10 mg/kg q6h • Maximum dose, 65 mg/kg/day or 3 g/day, whichever less

ADMINISTRATION
G-tube: Use oral suspension (250 mg/5 ml). Flush before and after administration.
IV: Infuse over 30-60 min. • Rate-controlling device recommended.

PREPARATION
IV: Add desired dose to 100 ml D_5W or use concentration of 100 mg/10 ml D_5W.

Compatible fluids: D_5W, 0.9% NaCl, LR, prepared combinations of these solutions

ACTIONS
Stimulates central inhibitory alpha-2-adrenergic receptors, decreases peripheral vascular resistance, lowers BP; minimal changes in HR, CO; reduction of plasma renin activity contributes to BP lowering • Slight ↑ in renal blood flow, GFR possible • May cause orthostatic hypotension • Tolerance often develops with long-term therapy

PHARMACOKINETICS

ROUTE	ONSET	PEAK	DURATION
PO	2 hr	4-6 hr	12-24 hr
IV	60 min	4-6 hr	10-16 hr

DISTRIBUTION
Weakly bound to plasma proteins
ELIMINATION
Metabolized by liver, GI tract; excreted in urine

INDICATIONS
Moderate to severe hypertension; usually reserved for patients who do not respond to other therapies. More effective if used with diuretics • Effective in managing hypertension in pregnancy • Not recommended for hypertensive crisis because of slow onset of action

PRECAUTIONS/CONTRAINDICATIONS
Precautions: Rebound hypertension, ↑ catecholamines, agitation may occur with abrupt cessation of therapy. • May cause serious complications, including hemolytic anemia, hepatic dysfunction • Commercial preparations may contain sulfites, which can cause serious allergic reactions.

P pediatric   G geriatric   V Direct IV

Use caution with: Hepatic impairment • Cerebrovascular disease • Renal impairment; lower dose • Dialysis patients; drug removal during dialysis may cause hypertension.

B Pregnancy category: Safety not clearly established

Contraindications: Hypersensitivity to methyldopa • Active liver disease • Pheochromocytoma

ADVERSE EFFECTS

CNS: *Drowsiness, sedation, weakness,* ↓ mental acuity, dizziness, psychiatric disturbances

CV: Orthostatic hypotension, **syncope,** bradycardia, **CHF, angina**

GI: Nausea, vomiting, diarrhea, dry mouth, constipation, ↑ liver enzymes, jaundice

GU: *Decreased libido, impotence,* nocturia

Hema: *Positive direct Coombs' test,* **hemolytic anemia, leukopenia, thrombocytopenia**

Derm: Rash, urticaria, eczema

Misc: *Fever, flulike symptoms;* sodium retention, weight gain, edema; SLE-like syndrome

TOXICITY/OVERDOSE

Symptoms: Hypotension, bradycardia, heart block • Deep sedation, coma • Vomiting, diarrhea

Management: After recent ingestion, implement guidelines for management of acute overdose (Appendix I). If sedation present, do not induce emesis; use gastric lavage with airway protection. • Establish/maintain airway; support breathing as needed with O_2 and/or mechanical ventilation. • **Hypotension:** Elevate legs, administer IV flu-

ids to encourage urinary excretion; if not responsive to fluids, use vasopressors (e.g., dopamine, norepinephrine). • Manage dysrhythmias according to ACLS guidelines (Appendix P). • Hemodialysis, peritoneal dialysis are effective in drug removal.

INTERACTIONS

anesthetics, general Profound hypotension

antihypertensives Hypotension

diuretics Hypotension

haloperidol Psychomotor impairment

levodopa Hypotension, psychosis

lithium Lithium toxicity

MAO inhibitors Cognitive/mental impairment

norepinephrine ↑ Pressor effects

opioid analgesics Excessive sedation

phenothiazines ↓ Methyldopa effectiveness

TCAs ↓ Methyldopa effectiveness

COMPATIBILITIES

Esmolol, meperidine, morphine

PATIENT CARE IMPLICATIONS

• Adjust dose to individual response, Older adults, renal-impaired patients usually respond to lower doses.

• Use precautions to protect sedated patients, especially when initiating therapy or increasing dose. Increase dose in evening to avoid daytime sedation.

• Use with diuretics increases effectiveness.

• Abrupt cessation of therapy may result in rebound hypertension. Withdraw gradually.

Vital signs/hemodynamics: Closely monitor BP, HR, espe-

italic = common side effects   **bold** = life-threatening reactions

cially with parenteral/initial therapy.

Physical assessment: Assess for excessive sedation, lethargy, depression. Dose adjustment may improve these symptoms.

• Assess for fluid volume overload: bibasilar crackles (rales), dyspnea, peripheral edema, neck vein distention, weight gain.

• Monitor fluid balance; weigh daily.

Laboratory tests: Monitor: CBC with differential • BUN, creatinine • Liver enzymes, bilirubin • Monitor hepatic function closely during first 6-12 wk of therapy. • If positive Coombs' test occurs, test for hemolytic anemia. If present, discontinue methyldopa.

PATIENT/FAMILY TEACHING

Purpose of medication is to lower BP. • May cause sedation, hypotension; change positions slowly. • Dry mouth relieved by frequent oral hygiene, use of sugarless gum or candy. • Report signs of anemia: weakness, shortness of breath, confusion, chest discomfort. • Urine may darken if left standing. • Medicine is not cure for high BP; other therapies, including lifestyle modifications, must be continued.

Outpatient: Take medication exactly as prescribed. Do not stop taking medicine even if you feel better. If medication abruptly discontinued, you may develop dangerously high BP, serious withdrawal symptoms.

• Avoid alcohol, sedatives, other CNS depressants. • Use caution in performing hazardous tasks requiring mental alertness or physical coordination, especially during first 1-2 wk of therapy.

• Weigh twice/wk; notify physician of weight gain, edema.

• Consult health care professional before taking cold, cough, or allergy preparations.

• Report unexplained fever, flu-like symptoms.

AVAILABLE FORMS

Tablets • PO suspension • Parenteral for IV use

methylprednisolone
(meth-ill-pred-niss'oh-lone)
Medrol
methylprednisolone acetate
Depo-Medrol, depMedalone, Depoject, Depopred, Depo-Predate, Duralone, Medralone, Methylone, Rep-Pred
methylprednisolone sodium succinate
Solu-Medrol, A-methaPred

Classifications: Adrenocortical steroid, corticosteroid, glucocorticoid, antiinflammatory agent

USUAL DOSE

Methylprednisolone: PO, adult: 5-15 mg q4h, depending on patient condition • Gradually decrease dose with cessation of therapy.

P PO, children: 0.12-1.66 mg/kg daily in 3-4 equally divided doses • Dose dependent on patient condition • Gradually decrease dose with cessation of therapy.

Methylprednisolone acetate: IM, adult: 10-80 mg once daily • Gradually decrease dose with cessation of therapy.

P pediatric   **G** geriatric   **V** Direct IV

Methylprednisolone sodium succinate: IM/IV, adult: Dose variable, adjusted to patient condition • Initially 10-250 mg; may repeat q2-6h as necessary • Shock: Initially 30 mg/kg, followed with same dose q4-6h or as slow continuous infusion over 12 hr; ≥1,000 mg q4h or sometimes used with severe shock • Do not use high-dose therapy >72 hr. • Pulse therapy: 1 g infused over 1 hr once daily for 3 consecutive days • IV route preferred; IM route contraindicated in shock, high-dose therapy. • Gradually decrease dose with cessation of therapy.

Ⓟ IM/IV, children: Dose variable, adjusted to patient condition • Initially 0.03-0.2 mg/kg q12-24h • Pulse therapy: 30 mg/kg infused over 1 hr, once daily for 6 doses • Do not use high-dose therapy >72 hr. • IV route preferred; IM route contraindicated in shock high-dose therapy. • Gradually decrease dose with cessation of therapy.

ADMINISTRATION

PO: When possible, administer with meals to minimize gastric irritation

▼ Direct IV: Inject each dose of ≤25 mg over at least 1 min • Administer single doses >250 mg over 3-15 min • May dilute or add to compatible solution for infusion • Check label carefully; USE PARENTERAL SOLUTION ONLY, suspension not for IV use

IV, intermit inf: Administer single dose over 15 min. • Administer pulse therapy doses over 1 hr. • Check label carefully; USE PARENTERAL SOLUTION ONLY, suspension not for IV use

PREPARATION

IV: Reconstitute from Mix-O-Vial by removing outer cap, turning rubber stopper ¼ turn, pressing down on stopper; diluent released into lower chamber to mix with powdered medication. Shake or twirl gently to mix solution. Withdraw from vial using sterile technique. • Initial dilution must be with solution provided by manufacturer. • May be further diluted in 0.9% NaCl or D_5W to facilitate administration.

IV, intermit inf: Add reconstituted solution to 50-250 ml compatible fluid. • 500 mg/250 ml yields concentration of 2.0 mg/ml.

Compatible fluids: D_5W, 0.9% NaCl, prepared combinations of these solutions

ACTIONS

Antiinflammatory glucocorticoid with complex action affecting almost all body systems • Stabilizes lysosomal membranes in leukocytes, prevents release of acid hydrolases; inhibits macrophage accumulation in inflamed tissues; reduces leukocyte adhesion to capillary walls; decreases capillary permeability, edema • Antagonizes histamine/kinin release • Suppresses immune response by producing lymphocytopenia, decreasing Ig/complement, reducing volume/activity of lymphatic system • Minimal mineralocorticoid activity; does not cause sodium retention • 4 times potency of hydrocortisone sodium succinate

M

PHARMACOKINETICS

ROUTE	ONSET	PEAK	DURATION
PO	<60 min	1-2 hr	Dose
IV	Rapid	30 min	dependent

DISTRIBUTION
Widely distributed throughout body tissue

ELIMINATION
Metabolized in liver, eliminated by kidneys; half-life 18-36 hr

INDICATIONS

Autoimmune conditions (e.g., SLE, rheumatic carditis, polymyositis) • Severe allergic conditions • Reduction of cerebral edema • Profound shock unresponsive to conventional therapy (controversial) • Acute life-threatening infections, along with massive antibiotics (controversial). • Inflammatory respiratory, GI, neuromuscular disorders refractory to other therapies • Acute idiopathic thrombocytopenic purpura (ITP), hemolytic anemia • To prevent rejection of transplanted organs • Not used alone in treatment of adrenocortical insufficiency because of lack of mineralocorticoid properties
Unlabeled/investigational:
Acute spinal cord injury, severe lupus nephritis, adjunct to *Pneumocystis* antiinfective therapy in AIDS patients.

PRECAUTIONS/ CONTRAINDICATIONS

Precautions: Prolonged therapy suppresses adrenal synthesis of glucocorticoids/mineralocorticoids, resulting in withdrawal symptoms with abrupt discontinuation. • May mask signs of infection, ↓ resistance to infection • May cause edema, particularly in renal impairment • May worsen systemic fungal infections; use only if hypersensitivity reaction to antifungal drug • Peptic ulceration possible in high-risk patients (e.g., history of peptic ulcer, liver/intestinal disease, nephrotic syndrome, critical illness) • Frequent articular injections may damage joint tissue. • Some preparations contain tartrazine dye (FD&C yellow no. 5), which could cause severe allergic reactions in susceptible individuals.
Use caution with: Diabetes; insulin requirements may increase. • Renal insufficiency, chronic nephritis, acute glomerulonephritis • Osteoporosis • Seizure disorder • CHF • Concurrent anticholinesterase therapy • Acute MI • Recent CVA • Phlebitis • Active tuberculosis; use only in severe cases and as adjunct to chemotherapy. • Chronic active hepatitis; may promote liver failure
C Pregnancy category: Use only if safer alternative unavailable.
Contraindications: Hypersensitivity to methylprednisolone, any corticosteroid, tartrazine (some preparations) • Systemic fungal infections • Recent administration of live viral vaccine (e.g., smallpox) • IM route with ITP

ADVERSE EFFECTS

CNS: *Euphoria, insomnia, mood swings, depression,* psychosis, headache, paresthesias, **seizures,** ↑ **ICP** (children)
CV: *Hypertension,* thrombophlebitis, **thromboembolism**
GI: *Nausea,* vomiting, *anorexia,* weight gain, **peptic ulceration, GI bleeding**
Endo: *Adrenal suppression, menstrual irregularities,* hy-

perglycemia, suppression of growth in children, "steroid-induced" diabetes mellitus

F&E: Hypokalemia, hypokalemic alkalosis, fluid retention

MS: *Muscle wasting, osteoporosis,* aseptic joint necrosis

Derm: ↓ *Wound healing, petechiae, ecchymosis, hirsutism, acne, thinning of skin,* hypo/hyperpigmentation

Misc: *Cushingoid appearance, ↑ susceptibility to infection, ↓ symptoms of infection*

TOXICITY/OVERDOSE

Symptoms: Cushingoid: Moon face, central obesity, hirsutism, acne, hypertension, osteoporosis, diabetes mellitus, hyperlipidemia, peptic ulcers, myopathy, immunosuppression, fluid/electrolyte imbalance • **Acute adrenal insufficiency:** Fever, anorexia, malaise, nausea, dizziness, fainting, dyspnea, hypoglycemia, myalgia, arthalgia: these symptoms follow rapid withdrawal of therapy

Management: After recent ingestion, implement guidelines for management of acute overdose (Appendix I). • **Hypotension:** Elevate legs, administer IV fluids; use vasopressor (e.g., dopamine, norepinephrine) or inotrope (e.g., dopamine, dobutamine) as appropriate. • **Severe fluid overload:** Administer diuretics; replace potassium as necessary • **Adrenal insufficiency:** Supplement with additional corticosteroid; taper dose gradually before withdrawal.

INTERACTIONS

antidiabetic agents, PO: insulin ↑ Antidiabetic drug requirements

barbiturates ↓ Corticoid effects

carbamazepine ↓ Corticoid effects

ketaconazole ↑ Corticoid effects

phenytoin ↓ Corticoid effects

rifampin ↓ Corticoid effects

Y-SITE COMPATIBILITIES

Amrinone, enalaprilat, famotidine, heparin, meperidine, morphine, piperacillin-tazobactam, sodium bicarbonate, ticarcillin

Y-SITE INCOMPATIBILITIES

Ciprofloxacin, diltiazem insulin, ondansetron, potassium chloride, tetracycline

PATIENT CARE IMPLICATIONS

• Administer daily in AM to coincide with physiologic peak in cortisol levels.

• Administer PO dose with meals to avoid gastric irritation.

• Dosage increases are necessary when patients subjected to severe emotional/physical stress.

• Dosage depends on condition being treated, patient response.

• Prolonged therapy suppresses hypothalamic-pituitary-adrenal axis, may lead to suppression of adrenal synthesis of glucocorticoids/mineralocorticoids. Drug dose must be tapered when discontinuing. Abrupt discontinuation may cause withdrawal symptoms: fatigue, anorexia, nausea, hypotension, hypoglycemia, depression, fever, dizziness, joint pain, malaise, fainting.

• Drug-related immunosuppression may mask signs of infection. Monitor closely; initiate antibiotic therapy as soon as infection suspected.

• Use in management of shock, particularly septic shock, is controversial; if used, therapy

M

---

italic = common side effects   **bold** = life-threatening reactions

should be initiated in early rather than late phase.

Vital signs/hemodynamics: Frequency of VS monitoring depends on patient condition rather than drug effects. Hypovolemic shock possible with adrenal crisis; monitor VS q15min or more often until condition stabilizes.

Physical assessment: Assess for adrenal insufficiency: fever, anorexia, malaise, nausea, dizziness, fainting, dyspnea, hypoglycemia, myalgia, arthralgia. Presence of these symptoms indicates insufficient dosage or too rapid withdrawal of therapy. • Assess for cushingoid symptoms: moon face, central obesity, hirsutism, acne, hypertension, osteoporosis, diabetes mellitus, hyperlipidemia, peptic ulcers, myopathy, immunosuppression, fluid/electrolyte imbalance. Presence of these symptoms indicates excessive dosage. • Assess for weight gain, peripheral edema, dyspnea, crackles (rales). Consult physician if present • Check stools, emesis for occult blood. • Monitor I&O; weigh daily. • **Cerebral edema:** Assess neurologic status before and throughout therapy. Maintain cerebral perfusion pressure of 60-80 mm Hg or other specified range.

Laboratory tests: Monitor: Electrolytes, especially sodium, potassium, calcium, • Blood glucose • CBC with differential • May cause hypokalemia, hyperglycemia.

PATIENT/FAMILY TEACHING

Purpose of medication is to reduce inflammation of affected area or body system. • Take exactly as prescribed. Do not double dose if missed. Suddenly stopping therapy may cause adrenal insufficiency: weakness, fatigue, nausea, low BP, low blood sugar. • Take with meals to minimize stomach upset. • Drug causes suppression of immune system, may mask signs of infection. Avoid individuals with contagious illnesses. Report fever, prolonged malaise, any symptom of infection immediately. • Report rapid weight gain, unusual swelling, very dark or bloody stools, vomiting of blood, sores slow to heal, significant behavior changes. • Inform physicians, dentists, other health care providers of medication regimen before treatment. • Carry Medic-Alert ID describing medication regimen.

AVAILABLE FORMS

Parenteral suspension for IM injection • Tablets • Parenteral solution for IV/IM injection

metoclopramide HCl
(met-oh-kloe'-pramide)
Clopra, Maxeran ✤,
Maxolon, Myclopramide,
Octamide, Reclomide,
Reglan

Classifications: Antiemetic, upper GI stimulant

USUAL DOSE

PO, adults: Diabetic gastric stasis: 10 mg 4 times daily, 30 min before each meal and hs for 2-8 wk until symptoms resolved • **Gastroesophageal reflux:** 10-15 mg 4 times daily, 30 min before each meal and hs

• **Hiccups:** 10-20 mg 4 times daily for up to 7 days
IV/IM, adults: 10 mg q4-6h, as needed; 20 mg sometimes used.
G Older adults/debilitation: 5-mg dose may be used
Chemotherapy-induced emesis: 1-2 mg/kg 30 min before chemotherapy; up to 2-3 additional doses administered as needed q2-3h

ADMINISTRATION

G-tube: Dilute PO concentrate with water or other liquid.
V Direct IV: Inject ≤10 mg slowly over 1-2 min, dilution not necessary. • Too-rapid injection may result in intense anxiety, restlessness followed by drowsiness. • Infuse doses >10 mg.
IV, intermit inf: Infuse over at least 15 min

PREPARATION

IV, intermit inf: Dilute single-dose in 50 ml compatible solution
Compatible fluids: 0.9% NaCl (most stable diluent), 0.45% NaCl, D_5W, LR, prepared combinations of these solutions

ACTIONS

Increases resting tone, contractility of GI smooth muscle • Accelerates gastric emptying, intestinal transit time • Increases lower esophageal sphincter pressure; relaxes pyloric sphincter • Results in coordinated gastric, pyloric, duodenal activity without increases in gastric, biliary, pancreatic secretions • Anticholinergic agents may abolish effects on motility. • Antagonizes central dopamine receptors, resulting in antiemetic/sedative ef-

fects • May produce extrapyramidal reactions

PHARMACOKINETICS

ROUTE	ONSET	PEAK	DURATION
PO	30-60 min	1-2 hr	1-2 hr
IM	10-15 min	30 min	1-2 hr
IV	1-3 min	30 min	1-2 hr

DISTRIBUTION

Concentrated in GI tract, liver, biliary system, CNS

ELIMINATION

Excreted in urine, feces; terminal-phase half-life 2.5-6 hr

INDICATIONS

Disorders of motility, including diabetic/postop gastric stasis (gastroparesis), gastroesophageal reflux • Prevent postop/chemotherapy-induced emesis • Facilitate intubation of small intestine; stimulate gastric, intestinal emptying of barium during radiologic exams
Unlabeled/investigational: Peptic ulcer, antiemetic with drugs other than neoplastic agents, vertigo, migraine, intractable hiccups; empty stomach of blood before endoscopy

PRECAUTIONS/CONTRAINDICATIONS

Precautions: Extrapyramidal reactions (e.g., dystonic reactions, motor restlessness, parkinsonian symptoms) may occur, **P** especially in children, young adults, with high-dose therapy. • Commercial preparations may contain sulfites, which can cause serious allergic reactions.
Use caution with: History of mental depression or suicidal tendencies • Parkinsonian syndrome • Renal dysfunction • CHF • Hepatic cirrhosis • Hypertension/pheochromocytoma; may induce hypertensive

M

---

italic = common side effects   **bold** = life-threatening reactions

crisis • Breast cancer; may elevate prolactin levels • Infants/children: Increased incidence of extrapyramidal reactions

B Pregnancy category: Safety not clearly established

Contraindications: Hypersensitivity to metoclopramide • Pheochromocytoma • Seizure disorder • Concurrent therapy with phenothiazines, butyrophenones, other agents associated with extrapyramidal reactions • Conditions in which stimulation of gastric motility contraindicated (e.g., obstruction, perforation, some gastric surgery)

ADVERSE EFFECTS

CNS: *Restlessness, drowsiness, fatigue, lassitude,* insomnia, headache, dizziness, anxiety, agitation, depression, suicidal ideation, delirium, extrapyramidal reactions (esp. motor restlessness), dystonia, parkinsonian symptoms

CV: Hypotension, hypertension, SVT, transient flushing of face/upper body

GI: Nausea, diarrhea, constipation

GU: Urinary frequency, incontinence

Endo: ↑ Prolactin, galactorrhea, gynecomastia, menstrual disorders, impotence, ↑ Aldosterone, fluid retention

TOXICITY/OVERDOSE

Symptoms: Drowsiness, disorientation, extrapyramidal reactions

Management: After recent ingestion, implement guidelines for management of acute overdose (Appendix I). • **Extrapyramidal reaction:** Use diazepam, benztropine (Cogentin),

and/or diphenhydramine depending on symptoms. • Hemodialysis in not likely to be helpful.

INTERACTIONS

alcohol Excessive sedation
butyrophenones (e.g., droperidol) Extrapyramidal reactions
cyclosporine ↑ Cyclosporine levels
digitalis glycosides ↓ Digoxin levels with some preparations; use Lanoxin or Lanoxicaps
phenothiazines Extrapyramidal reactions

Y-SITE COMPATIBILITIES

Acyclovir, bleomycin, cisplatin, ciprofloxacin, diltiazem, doxorubicin, droperidol, famotidine, fluconazole, heparin, meperidine, methotrexate, mitomycin, morphine, ondansetron, piperacillin-tazobactam, vinblastine, vincristine, zidovudine

Y-SITE INCOMPATIBILITIES

Furosemide

PATIENT CARE IMPLICATIONS

• IV infusion preferred over IV injection; must infuse doses >10 mg.
• Extrapyradimal reactions more likely with direct IV injection.
• When used for diabetic gastric stasis, insulin dosage and/or timing may need adjustment.

Vital signs/hemodynamics: IV/IM: Check BP, HR after administration.

Physical assessment: Assess for nausea, vomiting, abdominal distention, bowel sounds before and after administration. • Assess for extrapyramidal reactions: motor restlessness, dysphoria, anxiety, involuntary movements of limbs, facial spasms, rigidity, trembling of hands, possible upper airway obstruction. Consult physician for any reaction. Have diazepam, benzotropine (Cogentin), diphenhydramine (Benedryl) readily available.

PATIENT/FAMILY TEACHING

Purpose of medication is to reduce nausea/vomiting, improve stomach emptying. • May cause drowsiness, dizziness, mental confusion; avoid activities requiring mental alertness or physical coordination. • May enhance effects of alcohol, sedatives, some pain relievers • Immediately report involuntary movements of face, tongue, eyes, limbs.

AVAILABLE FORMS

Tablets • PO solution: 1 mg/ml • Concentrated PO solution: 10 mg/ml • Parenteral for IV/IM use

---

metoprolol succinate
(met-oh'proe-lole)
Toprol XL

metoprolol tartrate
Lopressor
metoprolol with hydrochlorothiazide
Lopressor HCT

Classifications: Class II antidysrhythmic, cardioselective beta-adrenergic blocker, antihypertensive, antianginal

USUAL DOSE

PO, adults: Hypertension: 100 mg once daily or 50 mg bid; may increase up to 400 mg/day as needed to control BP • **Chronic stable angina:** 50-200 mg bid • **Acute MI:** 50 mg 15 min after completion of IV dosing; repeat q6h for 48 hr. Use lower dose of 25-50 mg for patients unable to tolerate full IV dose. Thereafter, administer 100 mg bid.

IV, adults: Acute MI: When stable, administer initial dose of 5 mg. Repeat 5 mg dose q2min × 2 doses for total dose of 15 mg. If possible, initiate therapy within 12 hr after onset of MI symptoms.

ADMINISTRATION

PO/IV doses not interchangeable; carefully check dose, route
G-tube: Metoprolol tartrate (Lopressor) may be crushed, dissolved in water to facilitate administration. Do not crush metoprolol succinate (Toprol XL).
▼**Direct IV, adults:** Inject each dose of ≤5 mg over at least 1 min. Monitor ECG, BP as available throughout administration. Discontinue for symptomatic bradycardia, HR <45, hypotension, 2nd/3rd degree heart block
IV, intermit inf, adults: May dilute in D_5W or 0.9% NaCl for infusion

ACTIONS

Blocks sympathetic nervous system stimulation of beta-1-adrenergic receptors of myocardium • In usual doses has little effect on beta-2 receptors of vasculature, bronchial smooth muscle • Decreases HR, force of contraction, BP, myocardial O_2 consumption • ↓ O_2 consumption reduces risk of myo-

M

cardial reinfarction. • Depresses AV conduction/myocardial automaticity, particularly in SA node • Suppresses renin-angiotensin-aldosterone system • Doses >100 mg/day result in loss of cardioselectivity.

PHARMACOKINETICS

ROUTE	ONSET	PEAK	DURATION
PO	10 min	90 min-4 hr	24 hr
IV	Immed	10 min	5-8 hr

DISTRIBUTION

Wide; crosses blood-brain barrier

ELIMINATION

Eliminated mainly by liver, small amounts excreted into urine; half-life 3-4 hr, prolonged with liver impairment

INDICATIONS

Hypertension • Chronic stable angina pectoris • May reduce mortality, risk of reinfarction in acute/post-MI patients • Less risk of bronchospasm/hypoglycemia than propranolol, preferred in patients with COPD, diabetes mellitus • Less likely to produce cardiac failure in patients with catecholamine excess (e.g., pheochromocytoma, acute withdrawal of adrenergic blockers) than propranolol
Unlabeled/investigational:
IV to control/convert multifocal atrial tachycardia

PRECAUTIONS/ CONTRAINDICATIONS

Precautions: May cause symptomatic bradycardia, hypotension, CHF, particularly with pre-existing cardiac impairment • Abrupt cessation may induce angina, ventricular dysrhythmias, acute MI. • Additive impairment of cardiac contractility may occur when used with general anesthesia; drug may be withdrawn before elective sur-

gery. • May mask symptoms of hyperthyroidism, hypoglycemia

G Use caution with: Older adults; reduce dose. • Hepatic **P** impairment; reduce dose. • Children: Safety/efficacy not established

c Pregnancy category: Use only if safer alternatives unavailable

Contraindications: Hypersensitivity to metoprolol • Symptomatic bradycardia, 2nd/3rd degree heart block, HR <45 • CHF (unless resulting from tachycardia) • Cardiogenic shock

ADVERSE EFFECTS

CNS: *Fatigue, dizziness,* depression, confusion, short-term memory impairment
Resp: Dyspnea, wheezing, nasal stuffiness, sore throat
CV: *Bradycardia,* **hypotension, heart failure, angina, worsened AV heart block,** claudication, **arterial insufficiency,** peripheral edema
GI: Diarrhea, gastric pain, heartburn, constipation, ↑ liver enzymes
Endo: Blocked symptoms of hypoglycemia/hyperthyroidism
Hema: Agranulocytosis
Derm: Rash, pruritus, hair loss

TOXICITY/OVERDOSE

Symptoms: Severe bradycardia, advanced heart block • Profound hypotension • Loss of consciousness • Heart failure • Bronchospasm • Hypoglycemia
Management: After recent ingestion, implement guidelines for management of acute overdose (Appendix I). • **Bradycardia, heart block:** Administer atropine, epinephrine, isoproter-

P pediatric   **G** geriatric   **V** Direct IV

enol according to ACLS guidelines (Appendix P). • Bronchospasm: Use aminophylline, isoproterenol. • **Heart failure:** Provide inotropic support (e.g., dobutamine, dopamine), diuretics, possibly cardiac glycosides (e.g., digoxin) • **Hypotension:** Elevate legs, administer IV fluids; use vasopressors (e.g., dopamine, norepinephrine) for severe hypotension refractory to fluids, inotropic agents. • **Hypoglycemia:** Administer IV glucose.

INTERACTIONS

amiodarone Severe bradycardia; ventricular dysrhythmias

anesthetics, local (e.g., lidocaine) Hypertension, particularly if anesthetic contains epinephrine

antidiabetics (insulin, PO agents) Prolonged recovery from hypoglycemic episodes; masked hypoglycemia

barbiturates Reduced metoprolol effectiveness

calcium channel blockers Extreme bradycardia; hypotension

disopyramide ↓ CO

epinephrine, other sympathomimetics: Blocked epinephrine beta effects; unopposed alpha stimulation (hypertension, bradycardia, dysrhythmias); reduced effectiveness in anaphylaxis

isoproterenol ↓ Bronchodilatory effectiveness

lidocaine ↑ Lidocaine levels; ↓ CO

NSAIDs ↓ Hypotensive effectiveness

phenothiazines Hypotension; enhanced effects of either agent

prazosin Hypotension; especially with initial dose

quinidine Additive cardiac depression

rifampin ↑ Beta-blocker metabolism; higher doses required

theophylline ↓ Bronchodilation

COMPATIBILITIES

Meperidine, morphine

PATIENT CARE IMPLICATIONS

• Use lowest possible dose for dysrhythmia control.

• Gradually withdraw therapy to avoid rebound hypertension, angina, possible acute MI.

• Identify patients with COPD, asthma. Monitor closely; avoid high-dose therapy (>100 mg/day), which may precipitate bronchospasm.

• Observe hyperthyroid patients for symptoms of thyrotoxicosis (e.g., tachycardia, hypertension) when withdrawing therapy.

IV use in acute MI

• Begin therapy as soon as eligibility established, patient hemodynamically stable, usually within 12 hr of onset of MI symptoms.

Vital signs/hemodynamics: Monitor ECG with IV use and as available during initiation of therapy. Note development/ advancement of heart block, symptomatic bradycardia, HR <45, prolongation of PR interval, widening of QRS complex. If present, hold next dose, consult physician. • Measure CVP, PAP, CO as available. Consult physician for ↓ CO or ↑ filling pressures associated with other symptoms of heart failure.

Physical assessment: Assess for perfusion/oxygenation deficit: ↓ level of consciousness, activity intolerance, hypotension, chest discomfort, dizziness.

M

---

italic = common side effects   **bold** = life-threatening reactions

• Assess for CHF/pulmonary edema: bibasilar crackles (rales), S_3 gallop, neck vein distention, breathing difficulty, peripheral edema. • When used for angina, assess/record frequency/duration of chest pain. • When used for migraine prophylaxis, assess/record patient response. • Assess for respiratory distress in patients with history of COPD, asthma. • Assess patients with diabetes for sweating, because tachycardia/tremors associated with hypoglycemia may be blocked by therapy. • Monitor I&O; weigh daily.

Laboratory tests: Monitor: Electrolytes • Blood sugar in diabetic patients • Liver enzymes • CBC

PATIENT/FAMILY TEACHING

Purpose of medication is to control BP, reduce heart's work. • Change positions slowly to avoid dizziness, low BP. • Report breathing difficulty, palpitations, dizziness, activity intolerance, chest pain, extreme fatigue.

Outpatient: Take medication exactly as prescribed. Do not stop taking medicine even if you feel better. If medication abruptly discontinued, you may develop dangerously high BP, serious heartbeat irregularities, angina. • Check/record resting pulse each day, BP each week. Contact primary health care provider if pulse <50 or BP significantly different. • Medication is not cure for high BP; other therapies, including lifestyle modifications, must be continued. • Take with or directly after meals. • Medication may cause drowsiness. Avoid driving and other activities requiring mental alertness until individual response to drug known. • Drinking alcohol may cause extreme dizziness, drowsiness, impaired mental alertness. • You may experience increased sensitivity to cold. • Avoid excessive amounts of coffee, tea, or caffeinated soft drinks, which may counteract drug's BP-lowering effects. • Consult physician or pharmacist before taking over-the-counter preparations (e.g., aspirin, cold or sinus preparations). • Carry Medic-Alert ID identifying drug, dosage, specific indication. • Notify health care providers of therapy before any treatment. • Report severe depression, rash, unusual bleeding, fever, persistent sore throat. • Therapy blocks elevated HR/BP, so hyperthyroid/diabetic patients must be aware of other symptoms of crisis.

AVAILABLE FORMS

Tablets • Extended-release tablets • Parenteral for IV use

metronidazole/ metronidazole HCl

(me-troe-ni′da-zole)
Flagyl, Metro IV, Metryl IV, Novo-Nidazol ✦, Trikacide ✦

Classification: Miscellaneous antibiotic

USUAL DOSE

PO, adults: Trichomoniasis: 2 g as single dose or in 2 divided doses 12 hr apart; alternately, 500 mg q12h for 7 days • Antibiotic-associated pseudomembranous colitis (AAPC): 250-500 mg q6-8h

P PO, children: 15 mg/kg/24 hr in divided doses q8h

IV, adults: Loading dose of 15 mg/kg (approx 1 g) followed by maintenance dose of 7.5 mg/kg (approx 500 mg) q6h • Do not exceed 4 g/24hr. • **Severe hepatic impairment:** Reduce dose and/or frequency.

ADMINISTRATION

IV, intermit inf: Infuse each dose over 60 min. • If possible, discontinue primary solution during infusion. Do not infuse simultaneously with any other agent. • Avoid solution contact with aluminum in needles, cannulae, other sources; reddish discoloration may result. • Rotate infusion sites; use dilute solution, large vein, small catheter/needle to reduce risk of phlebitis.

PREPARATION

IV: All preparations prediluted, ready for use except Flagyl IV, which must be diluted, neutralized. If prediluted solution not available, consult pharmacist or specialized reference.
Compatible fluids: D_5W, 0.9% NaCl, LR
Stability: Reconstituted IV solution stable for at least 24 hr at room temperature; refrigeration of neutralized solutions may result in formation of crystals, which usually dissolve when warmed to room temperature; do not use crystallized solutions.

ACTIONS

Bactericidal, amebicidal, trichomonacidal antibiotic that disrupts bacterial DNA/protein synthesis • Active against many anaerobic gram-negative bacilli, including *Bacteroides fragilis* • Active against anaerobic gram-positive cocci, including *Clostridium, C. difficile, C. perfringens, Peptococcus* • Also active against *Gardnerella vaginalis* and protozoa, including *Trichomonas vaginalis, Giardia lamblia, Entamoeba histolytica* • Not active against aerobic organisms

PHARMACOKINETICS

ROUTE	ONSET	PEAK	DURATION
PO	Rapid*	1-3 hr	Approx 6-12 hr
IV	Immed	End infusion	

DISTRIBUTION

Wide; good CSF penetration; distribution similar with IV/PO routes

ELIMINATION

Metabolized in liver, eliminated in urine/feces; half-life 6-8 hr, prolonged with hepatic impairment

M

*Decreased with food.

INDICATIONS

Treatment of anaerobic bacterial infections of GI tract, reproductive structures, bones/joints, respiratory tract, CNS • Intestinal, hepatic amebic infections • Trichomoniasis • Bacterial vaginosis • Choice agent for treatment of sexually transmitted trichomoniasis • Topical gel used for acne rosacea
Unlabeled/investigational: *Clostridium difficile,* AAPC, active Crohn's disease

PRECAUTIONS/ CONTRAINDICATIONS

Precautions: Bacterial or fungal overgrowth possible • Breast/colon cancer associated with long-term use in Crohn's disease

---

italic = common side effects   **bold** = life-threatening reactions

Use caution with: Blood dyscrasias • Severe hepatic impairment; reduce dose. • CHF, corticosteroid therapy, other conditions associated with edema; contains 28 mg sodium/g • Children: Safety of IV formulation not established

Pregnancy category: Safety not clearly established

Contraindications: Hypersensitivity to metronidazole, other nitroimidazole derivatives • First trimester of pregnancy

ADVERSE EFFECTS

CNS: *Headache,* dizziness, peripheral neuropathy, including numbness, paresthesias; **seizures** (rare)

GI: *Nausea, dry mouth, metallic taste,* vomiting, diarrhea, abdominal discomfort

GU: Dark or reddish urine, dysuria, cystitis, polyuria

Hema: Leukopenia, thrombocytopenia

Local: Thrombophlebitis (IV)

Misc: Superinfection, colonization; hypersensitivity, including serum sickness with fever, joint pain

TOXICITY/OVERDOSE

Symptoms: Peripheral neuropathy, seizures

Management: After recent ingestion, implement guidelines for management of acute overdose (Appendix I). • Initiate symptomatic/supportive measures, including airway management/ventilation.

• Hemodialysis removes drug.

INTERACTIONS

alcohol, ethyl Disulfiram (Antabuse)-type reaction with flushing, headache, vomiting

antacids ↓ Absorption of PO metronidazole

anticoagulants, PO ↑ **Anticoagulation**

cholestyramine ↓ Absorption of PO metronidazole

disulfiram (Antabuse) Confusion, psychotic reaction

phenytoin ↓ Metronidazole effectiveness

Y-SITE INCOMPATIBILITIES

Simultaneous infusion with other agents not recommended

PATIENT CARE IMPLICATIONS

• Obtain specimens for culture and sensitivity before initiating antibiotic therapy. Initiate therapy before results received.

• Do not administer to patients with recent (within 2 wk) disulfiram (Antabuse) therapy.

PO: Administer with food or milk to reduce GI irritation.

• Stagger schedules if patient also taking antacids or cholestyramine.

Vital signs: Monitor VS for indicators of infection, complications.

Physical assessment: Assess for improvement in primary infection or symptoms of super/suprainfection: appearance of sputum, urine, stool, wound drainage; presence of fever, candidiasis, vaginitis. • Observe for hypersensitivity: rash, pruritus, wheezing, laryngeal edema, hypotension.

Laboratory tests: Monitor: Electrolytes • CBC with differential • Liver enzymes, bilirubin • PT with concurrent PO anticoagulant therapy

---

P pediatric   **G** geriatric   **V** Direct IV

PATIENT/FAMILY TEACHING

Purpose of drug is to limit growth of infection-causing bacteria or similar organisms. • Inform nurse/physician if pregnancy suspected. • Take all of medication exactly as prescribed. Do not stop taking medicine even if you feel better. Failure to take all of antibiotic may result in recurrence or additional infection. Do not save or share unused medicine.
• Urine may be dark or reddish brown. • Frequent oral hygiene and sugarless gum may relieve discomfort associated with dry mouth, unpleasant taste. • Trichomoniasis is sexually transmitted; all sexual contacts should be treated, even if asymptomatic. Infection may be transmitted during treatment period. Refrain from sexual intercourse or use condom to prevent infection. • Take with food or milk to reduce stomach irritation.
• Report diarrhea, blood in stool, fever, vaginal itching or discharge, furry growth on tongue, numbness or tingling of arms or legs. • May cause dizziness; use caution when performing hazardous tasks requiring mental alertness or physical coordination. • Avoid alcoholic beverages during and for at least 1 day after therapy. Failure to avoid alcohol may result in severe abdominal cramps, nausea, vomiting, headaches, flushing.
• Avoid taking antacids at same time as medication.

AVAILABLE FORMS

Capsules • Powder for PO solution • Topical gel • Parenteral for IV use

midazolam
(mye-da'zoe-lam)
Versed

Classifications: Benzodiazepine, sedative-hypnotic, general anesthetic, skeletal muscle relaxant
Schedule IV controlled substance

USUAL DOSE

Individualize dosage, increase cautiously.
IM, adults: Preop: 0.07-0.08 mg/kg or approx 5 mg for average adult; reduce dose by 30%-50% if given with opiate analgesics. • Use lower dose for Ⓖ older adults or debilitated patients. • May repeat as needed in 3-4 hr or after 1 hr in acute conditions • Do not exceed 30 mg within 8-hr period.
Direct IV, adults <60: *Administer in small increments. Excessive or rapid IV bolus doses can cause respiratory arrest.* • Conscious sedation: Initially 0.5 mg; administer additional 0.5 mg doses as necessary up to total dose of 2.5 mg over at least 2 min. Wait 2 min from last dose; if necessary, administer additional doses in 0.5-mg increments; total dose >5 mg rarely necessary. • Reduce dose by 30%-50% if narcotics or other CNS depressants also used. • Maintenance of conscious sedation: Use 25% of sedating dose; administer in 0.5 mg increments, titrate to desired effects; use only if clearly indicated.
Ⓖ **Direct IV, adults ≥60/debilitation:** *Administer in small increments. Excessive or rapid IV bolus doses can cause respiratory arrest* • Conscious se-

M

dation: Initially 0.5 mg; administer additional 0.5-mg doses as necessary up to total dose of 1.5 mg over at least 2 min. Wait 2 min from last dose; if necessary, administer additional doses in 0.5-mg increments, giving no more than 1 mg over 2 min; total dose >3.5 mg rarely necessary. • Reduce dose by 50% if narcotics or other CNS depressants also used.
• **Maintenance of conscious sedation:** Use 25% of sedating dose; administer in 0.5 mg increments, titrate to desired effects; use only if clearly indicated.

IV, cont inf, adults: 1-5 mg/hr; up to 10 mg/hr used for short periods with extreme agitation in mechanically ventilated patients

ADMINISTRATION

IM: Inject deeply into large muscle.
▼**Direct IV:** Use 1 mg/ml concentration for ease in titration. • Inject each dose in small increments over 2 min; stop injection for slurred speech, respiratory depression. • Closely monitor respiratory/CV status throughout administration: Supplemental O_2, continuous pulse oximetry, ECG monitoring recommended • *Too-rapid injection may result in severe respiratory depression/arrest; have emergency resuscitation equipment, flumazenil (antidote) immediately available.* • Avoid using small veins; may cause burning, irritation
IV, cont inf: Start with 1 mg/hr and titrate at 5–10 min intervals to control agitation without depressing respirations. Closely monitor respiratory/CV status

throughout administration. Infusion pump required.

PREPARATION

IV, cont inf: mix 20 mg/100 ml compatible solution for concentration of 0.2 mg/ml. More concentrated solutions may be used.
Compatible fluids: 0.9% NaCl; D_5W and 0.9% NaCl in dilute solution of ≤0.5 mg/ml (up to 24 hr).

ACTIONS

Short-acting benzodiazepine; facilitates action of gamma-aminobutyric acid (GABA, major inhibitory neurotransmitter), produces CNS depression • Reduces anxiety; causes mild to deep sedation, hypnotic effects, lack of recall • High doses used for induction of general anesthesia result in depression of ventilation, decreased sensitivity to respiratory stimulating effect of CO_2 for ≥15 min. • Duration/extent of respiratory depression greater in patients with COPD • IV use causes slight to moderate decrease in MAP, CO, SV, SVR. • No analgesic effects

PHARMACOKINETICS

ROUTE	ONSET	PEAK	DURATION
IM	5-15 min	20-60 min	2 hr
IV	1-5 min	≤15 min	15-60 min*

DISTRIBUTION

Highly lipophilic; widely distributed; 94%-97% protein bound; readily crosses blood-brain barrier

ELIMINATION

 Metabolized by liver, eliminated by kidneys; half-life 1-4 hr, prolonged in older adults, obesity, liver/kidney disease

*Approx; up to 6 hr with high doses.

INDICATIONS

Preop to relieve anxiety, provide sedation, diminish recall of surgery or procedure • IV used to produce sedation without loss of consciousness, control agitation, reduce recall of minor surgery, endoscopy, CV procedures • IV also used for induction/maintenance of anesthesia • 3-4 times as potent as diazepam

PRECAUTIONS/ CONTRAINDICATIONS

Precautions: *IV use associated with severe respiratory depression, including arrest, especially when used for conscious sedation.* Death, hypoxic brain damage have resulted from lack of prompt recognition. • Risk of hypoventilation, apnea ↑ in older adults, debilitated patients, those with limited pulmonary reserve, when administered too rapidly

Use caution/lower dose with: COPD • CHF • Hepatic/renal disease • Older adults • Debilitation, chronic illness • Acute uncompensated illness (e.g., fluid/electrolyte disorders) • Low serum albumin

Pregnancy category: Established risk to fetus (congenital malformations, excessive sedation); use only in life-threatening situations when potential benefits outweigh risk.

Contraindications: Hypersensitivity to midazolam • Acute angle-closure glaucoma • Shock • Coma • Respiratory depression • Acute alcohol intoxication with VS depression • Children: Safety/efficacy not established

ADVERSE EFECTS

CNS: *Retrograde amnesia, drowsiness, slurred speech,* headache, confusion, anxiety, restlessness, tonic/clonic movements, muscle tremors
EENT: Nystagmus, visual disturbances
Resp: *Severe respiratory depression, apnea*
CV: Dysrhythmias, hypotension, vasovagal response
GI: Acid taste, excessive salivation, retching
Local: Injection site swelling, burning, pain

TOXICITY/OVERDOSE

Symptoms: Respiratory depression, apnea • Hypotension • Excessive sedation, confusion, coma • Toxicity more likely with concurrent use of other CNS depressants
Management: Specific antidote: Administer flumazenil, benzodiazepine antagonist to reverse sedation, respiratory depression. Maintain airway, administer O_2, support ventilation as needed • **Hypotension:** Elevate legs, administer IV fluids; use vasopressors (e.g., dopamine, norepinephrine) if not responsive to fluids.

INTERACTIONS

alcohol, antihistamines, barbiturates, beta-blockers, cimetidine, disulfiram (Antabuse), opiate analgesics, propoxyphene, ranitidine Excessive sedation
flumazenil, theophylline ↓ Sedation

Y-SITE COMPATIBILITIES

Atracurium, famotidine, fluconazole, pancuronium, vecuronium

M

---

italic = common side effects   **bold** = life-threatening reactions

Y-SITE INCOMPATIBILITIES

Foscarnet

PATIENT CARE IMPLICATIONS

• Reactions such as agitation, involuntary movements, hyperactivity, combativeness may occur. Evaluate reactions carefully; consider inadequate/excessive dosing, too-rapid administration, cerebral hypoxia, other drugs administered, true paradoxical reaction.
• Have emergency resuscitation equipment/personnel and flumazenil immediately available.
 • Hypotension, respiratory depression are more likely in older adults, debilitation, limited pulmonary reserve, when other CNS depressants used.

IV

• ***Too-rapid administration may result in hypotension, dysrhythmias, apnea, cardiac arrest.***
• **Conscious sedation:** Administer in small increments; closely monitor respiratory/CV status throughout administration. Carefully individualize/titrate each dose. Stop injection for respiratory depression, hypotension, slurred speech.
• Monitor frequently for 3-4 hr after IV administration. Patient should remain in bed for at least 3 hr, requires assistance with initial ambulation.

Vital signs/hemodynamics:

Conditions (e.g., low lighting, patient position) during procedures may interfere with observation/assessment of cardiopulmonary status. Use additional measures (e.g., ECG monitor, pulse oximetry, automatic BP cuff) to monitor patient closely during procedures. Must use these measures with conscious sedation • Monitor VS frequently according to route of administration, patient condition. If given IV Monitor VS q2-5min during and immediately after injection.

PHYSICAL ASSESSMENT

Assess for hypoventilation/respiratory decompensation frequently during and after administration esp. in patients with history of COPD, cardiac impairment. Stop injection/infusion with slowing of respirations, which may preceed apnea. Assess neurologic status for level of sedation during and immediately after administration. Slurred speech generally indicates effective conscious sedation.

PATIENT/FAMILY TEACHING

Purpose of medication is to reduce anxiety, promote relaxation during procedures or before surgery. • Medication may decrease ability to remember procedure and events immediately after procedure. • Medication causes drowsiness. Call for assistance when getting out of bed, walking. • Inform caregiver if you may be pregnant.
• Avoid driving and other activities requiring mental alertness or physical coordination for 24 hr after administration and then only if not drowsy. • Avoid alcohol or other drugs that cause sedation for at least 24 hr after administration.

AVAILABLE FORMS

Parenteral for IV/IM use

---

milrinone lactate
(mill-re'none)
Corotrope, Primacor

Classification: Positive inotrope

USUAL DOSE

IV, adults: Initial loading dose of 50 µg/kg (4 mg for 80-kg person) given over 10 min; follow with maintenance infusion of 0.375-0.750 µg/kg/min, which is 0.59-1.13 mg/kg/24 hr. 1.13 mg/kg/24 hr is maximum recommended dose. Usually administered for 48-72 hr, but has been given for up to 5 days.
• **Renal impairment:** Used reduced dose according to creatinine clearance.

ADMINISTRATION

IV, loading inf: Administer over 10 min. May dilute to facilitate administration.
Maintenance inf: Frequent titration not usually necessary because half-life is ≥2 hr. Adjust infusion q2-4h to optimal hemodynamic response: decreased PCWP/SVR, increased CO/CI
• Must use infusion pump • See Infusion Rate table, (Appendix Q).

Inf Rate

DOSE (µg/kg/min)	80-KG PERSON (ml/hr)
0.375	8
0.500	12
0.600	16
0.750	21

*Concentration: 200 µg/ml.

PREPARATION

IV, loading inf: Dilute each 1 mg (1 ml) in 1 ml of 0.45% or 0.9% NaCl to facilitate administration.

Maintenance inf:

DILUTION	CONCENTRATION
20 mg/100 ml	200 µg/ml
40 mg/100 ml	400 µg/ml

Compatible fluids: D_5W, 0.45% NaCl, 0.9% NaCl

ACTION

Selectively inhibits cyclic adenosine monophosphate (cAMP) phosphodiesterase in cardiac, vascular tissue; increases myocardial contractility and causes vasodilation; results in increased CO. Similar to, but more potent than, amrinone. Not a digitalis glycoside or catecholamine
• Used for up to 72 hr without evidence of diminished effectiveness (tachyphylaxis) • Use for longer periods may result in tachyphylaxis; larger doses may be required to achieve the same effect. • **Hemodynamics:** Decreases PCWP, SVR, increases CO. From 25%-42% dose-related improvement in CI. May decrease BP. HR usually unchanged; may increase with higher dosages • ↑ Ventricular response may occur with atrial flutter/fibrillation.

PHARMACOKINETICS

ROUTE	ONSET	PEAK	DURATION
IV	5 min	5-15 min	2-6 hr

ELIMINATION

Renal elimination of unchanged drug, metabolites. Half-life = 2.3 hr.

INDICATIONS

• Short-term management of congestive heart failure; often used with diuretic, digoxin therapy
Unlabeled/investigational:
Used for weeks to months in patients with severe cardiomy-

M

---

italic = common side effects   **bold** = life-threatening reactions

opathy while waiting for heart transplant

PRECAUTIONS/ CONTRAINDICATIONS

Precautions: May cause ventricular tachycardia, other ectopy, particularly in patients with sensitized myocardium (severe CHF, dilated cardiomyopathy) • May cause hypotension, especially with volume depletiion or at higher dosages
Use caution with: Undigitalized atrial fibrillation/flutter; may increase ventricular response • Concurrent diuretic therapy; improved CO may promote additional diuresis; assure adequate hydration, monitor potassium; reduction in diuretic dose may be necessary • Acute MI; experience limited; extreme caution indicated because of possible increase in myocardial O₂ requirements • Children: safe use not established

Pregnancy category: Use only if safer alternative not available.

Contraindications: Hypersensitivity to milrinone • Aortic/pulmonic stenosis, IHSS; may worsen outflow obstruction

ADVERSE EFFECTS

CNS: Headache, tremor
CV: ***Hypotension, ventricular tachycardia, chest pain,*** supraventricular dysrhythmias
F&E: Hypokalemia
Hema: Thrombocytopenia

TOXICITY/OVERDOSE

Symptoms: Hypotension
Management: Reduce rate or discontinue • **Hypotension:** Elevate legs, administer IV fluids. Because of short duration, other measures not usually necessary;

if not responsive, consider dopamine, norepinephrine according to ACLS guidelines

INTERACTIONS

digoxin Potentiation of inotropic effects
disopyramide Potentiation of inotropic effects
diuretics Excessive diuresis, hypokalemia

Y-SITE COMPATIBILITIES

Digoxin, propranolol, quinidine gluconate

Y-SITE INCOMPATIBILITIES

Bumetanide, furosemide, procainamide

PATIENT CARE IMPLICATIONS

• Correct hypovolemia before initiating therapy.
• Optimize tissue oxygenation via supplemental oxygen according to patient condition.
• Establish clear criteria for titration: desired CO, PCWP, UO. Use lowest effective dose.
• Evaluate fluid volume status; monitor UO, consult physician if <0.5 ml/kg/hr (approx. 30 ml/hr). Concentrated solutions frequently necessary to limit fluid intake in patients with heart failure
• Digitalize patients with atrial fibrillation/flutter before administering milrinone; enhanced AV conduction could promote tachydysrhythmias.
Vital signs/hemodynamics: Monitor BP, HR q5-15min during initial bolus/infusion; progressively advance according to titration schedule, hemodynamic stability. • Continuously monitor ECG for dysrhythmias; have defibrillator, ACLS drugs immedi-

ately available in case of ventricular tachycardia. • Monitor filling pressures/CO frequently; significant changes in CO may occur with minimal changes in HR, BP. Immediately correct low filling pressures/hypovolemia

Physical assessment: Assess for resolution of signs/symptoms of CHF: peripheral edema, dyspnea, orthopnea, crackles, S_3 gallop, weight gain

Laboratory tests: Monitor: Electrolytes, particularly potassium • Administer supplemental potassium as necessary to maintain normal levels.

PATIENT/FAMILY TEACHING

Purpose of drug is to improve heart's blood-pumping ability. • Immediately report chest pain/discomfort, palpitations, lightheadedness • Change positions slowly to minimize dizziness, prevent injury.

AVAILABLE FORMS

Parenteral for IV injection/infusion

---

morphine sulfate
(mor'feen)
MS, MSO$_4$
preservative-free
Astramorph, Duramorph, Infumorph
extended release
MS Contin, Oramorph
rectal supp
RMS, Roxanol
oral solution
Rescudose, MSIR OMS

Classifications: Opiate agonist, narcotic analgesic

Schedule II controlled substance

USUAL DOSE

Use smallest effective dose to minimize CNS depression/tolerance. *Use caution, reduced dose in elderly/debilitated patients.*
PO, adults: 10-30 mg q4h
PO, ext, adults: 15-30 mg q8-12h
Rectal, adults: 10-20 mg q4h
IM/SC, adults: 10 mg q4h
• Range, 5-20 mg according to patient response
IM/SC, children: 0.1-0.2 mg/kg (up to 15 mg) q4h
Direct IV, adults: 2.5-15 mg q2-4h; titrate to control pain; dose individualized to patient response/tolerance. • **Pain associated with acute MI:** 2-5 mg q5-30min
Direct IV, children: 0.05-0.1 mg/kg q1-4h; titrate to control pain.
IV, cont inf, adults: Optional loading dose of ≥15 mg followed by continuous infusion of 0.8-10 mg/hr • Titrate according to analgesic effect, VS stability. • Large doses of 20-150 mg/hr may be required for patients with severe chronic pain, tolerance; very high doses, up to 440 mg/hr, occasionally used for short-term relief of severe pain in patients with established opiate tolerance.
IV, cont inf, children: Postop pain: 0.01-0.04 mg/kg/hr • Sickle cell crisis: 0.03-0.15 mg/kg/hr • Severe chronic cancer pain: 0.025-2.6 mg/kg/hr; higher end of dose range used with established tolerance • Titrate according to analgesic effect, VS stability.
Epidural/intrathecal, adults: Epidural: 5-10 mg/24 hr; initial

M

dose usually 5 mg; after 1 hr increase dose gradually by 1-2 mg, up to 10 mg total daily dose; 20-30 mg/day has been used for chronic severe pain.
• **Intrathecal:** Approx 1/10 epidural dose or 0.2-1 mg as single dose in patients without opiate tolerance; repeat doses not generally recommended

ADMINISTRATION

Check label carefully; preparations available in multiple concentrations. Verify dose before use.
G-tube: Use oral solution, verify concentration/dose. Roxanol compatible with Isocal, Vironex.
▼ Direct IV, adults: Dilute each dose in 4-5 ml sterile water; inject each dose of ≤15 mg slowly over 4-5 min. • Too-rapid IV administration may cause ↓ BP, respiratory depression, apnea. • Have naloxone, resuscitation equipment nearby.
IV, cont inf: Titrate according to pain relief, stability of VS.
• Use rate-controlling device; may be patient activated. • Have naloxone, resuscitation equipment nearby.
Epidural/intrathecal: *Caregiver must be thoroughly familiar with specific infusion device/technique to avoid life-threatening overdose.*
• Have naloxone, resuscitation equipment nearby.

PREPARATION

Direct IV: Dilute each dose in 4-5 ml sterile water.
IV inf: Usual concentration is 0.1-1 mg/ml in D_5W (e.g., 50 mg morphine in 50 ml D_5W): More concentrated solutions may be used. • Do not use discolored solutions.

Epidural/intrathecal: Use preservative-free morphine (Astramorph, Duramorph, Infumorph). Withdraw from ampule using microfilter ≤5 μm.
Compatible fluids: D_5W, 0.9% NaCl, LR

ACTIONS

Opium derivative that acts at specific receptor sites in CNS/other tissue to inhibit pain perception, produce analgesia • Reduces apprehension associated with pain • Causes sedation, CNS depression • Suppresses coughing; depresses respiratory centers in brainstem • Depression of vasomotor center and/or stimulation of histamine release causes peripheral vasodilation/ ↓ SVR, may lead to hypotension.
• GI effects result in nausea, vomiting, constipation, delayed gastric emptying. • Increases tone in biliary system, may cause spasm • Stimulates vasopressin release, may lead to oliguria

---

P pediatric   **G** geriatric   **▼** Direct IV

PHARMACOKINETICS

ROUTE	ONSET	PEAK	DURATION
PO	Var	60 min	4-5 hr
PO, ext rls	Var		8-12 hr
SC	20 min	50-90 min	4-7 hr
IM	10-30 min	30-60 min	4-7 hr
Rectal	20 min	20-60 min	4-5 hr
IV	5-8 min	20 min	4-5 hr
Epidural	6-30 min		16-24 hr
Intrathecal	Minutes		Up to 24 hr

DISTRIBUTION

Wide; variably absorbed from GI tract; readily crosses placenta; approx ⅓ bound to albumin and inactive

ELIMINATION

Metabolized in liver, CNS, kidneys, lungs, placenta; excreted in urine; half-life 1.5-2 hr

INDICATIONS

To relieve severe pain, apprehension associated with traumatic injury, malignancies, manipulation/instrumentation, other painful conditions and during immediate postop period • Preop sedation • Anesthesia supplement • Analgesia during term labor • Drug of choice for relief of pain associated with acute MI; used in left ventricular failure, pulmonary edema to decrease preload/afterload, decrease work of breathing, relieve anxiety • Continuous IV administration sustains effective blood levels/pain relief, less likely to produce excessive CNS depression associated with IV/IM bolus dosing.

PRECAUTIONS/ CONTRAINDICATIONS

Precautions: May cause severe respiratory depression, especially with rapid IV administration, epidural/intrathecal admin-istration • May cause hypotension, especially with rapid IV administration, in hypovolemia, when administered with phenothiazines/general anesthetics • Transient elevation of plasma amylase/lipase possible • Stimulates vasopressin release, may contribute to water intoxication in postop patients • Commercial preparations may contain sulfites, which can cause serious allergic reactions.
Use caution with: Hepatic/renal dysfunction; reduced dose indicated • Shock, acute MI; risk of hypotension • COPD, asthma, pulmonary disease; risk of respiratory depression
G • Older adults, debilitated patients; reduce dose indicated • CNS depression, head injury, craniotomy; may increase respiratory depression • Seizure disorder; may precipitate seizures • Untreated myxedema • Prostatic hypertrophy • Urethral stricture • Hypothyroidism • Addison's disease • Infants, children
P
C **Pregnancy category:** Use only if safer alternative unavailable.
Contraindications: Hypersensitivity to morphine • Respiratory depression, status asthmaticus • Acute alcohol intoxication with VS depression • Undiagnosed acute abdominal conditions • Biliary colic, biliary tract surgery • Acute ulcerative colitis • Diarrhea from poison-**P** ing • Premature infants, labor, delivery of premature infants • IM route contraindicated with hypothermia, shock, hypotension, impaired circulation.

ADVERSE EFFECTS

CNS: *Sedation, confusion,* dizziness, hallucinations, depres-

M

---

italic = common side effects   **bold** = life-threatening reactions

sion, coma, euphoria, dysphoria, weakness, restlessness, nervousness, **seizures**
EENT: Pupillary constriction, visual disturbances
Resp: *Respiratory depression, apnea*
CV: *Orthostasis;* hypotension; reflex tachycardia; bradycardia; sweating, flushing, warmness of face, neck, upper thorax
GI: *Constipation,* nausea, vomiting, delayed absorption of PO agents
GU: Urinary retention, oliguria
Derm: Itching, wheals, phlebitis/pain at injection site
Misc: Hypothermia, tolerance, physical/psychologic dependence

TOXICITY/OVERDOSE
Acute toxicity/overdose:
Profound CNS depression
• Respiratory depression, apnea
• Bradycardia, hypotension, circulatory collapse • Pupillary constriction • Hypothermia with cool, clammy skin • Serious, potentially fatal complications, including pneumonia, shock, pulmonary edema
Chronic toxicity: Tolerance, psychologic/physical dependence may develop. • Physical dependence results in withdrawal symptoms when drug abruptly discontinued.
Management: After recent ingestion, implement guidelines for management of acute overdose (Appendix I). • *Gastric lavage may be effective even hours after ingestion, because pylorospasm may cause much of drug to remain in stomach.* • Hypoventilation: Establish/maintain airway; administer O_2; if ventilatory efforts hindered by muscular rigidity, NMBA may be necessary • Hypotension: Elevate legs, administer IV fluids; use vasopressors (e.g., dopamine, norepinephrine) for circulatory collapse. • Antidote: Naloxone, opiate antagonist used to reverse respiratory depression, other symptoms

INTERACTIONS
alcohol, ethyl Additive CNS depression
anesthetics, general Additive CNS depression
antihistamines Additive CNS depression; enhanced analgesia
diuretics ↓ Effectiveness in patients with CHF
MAO inhibitors Additive CNS depression; hypotension
nalmefene Reversal of effects; acute withdrawal in opiate-dependent patients
naloxone Reversal of effects; acute withdrawal in opiate-dependent patients
opiate agonist-antagonists (e.g., buprenorphine, butorphanol, nalbuphine, pentazocine) Acute withdrawal in opiate-dependent patients
phenothiazines Enhanced/antagonized analgesia; additive CNS depression
sedatives Additive CNS depression
TCAs Additive CNS depression
tranquilizers Additive CNS depression, ↑ analgesia

COMPATIBILITIES
Syringe: Atropine, butorphanol, chlorpromazine, cimetidine, diphenhydramine, droperidol, fentanyl, glycopyrrolate, hydroxyzine, metoclopramide, midazolam, pentazocine, promazine, ranitidine, scopolamine

---

P pediatric   **G** geriatric   **V** Direct IV

Y-site: Amikacin, aminophylline, ampicillin, atenolol, atracurium, bumetanide, calcium chloride, cefamandole, cefazolin, cefoperazone, cefotaxime, cefotetan, cefoxitin, ceftazidime, ceftizoxime, ceftriaxone, cefuroxime, cephalothin, cephapirin, chloramphenicol, digoxin, diltiazem, dopamine, enalaprilat esmolol, famotidine, gentamicin, heparin, insulin, lidocaine, magnesium sulfate, metoclopramide, nafcillin, oxacillin, pancuronium, piperacillin, propranolol, potassium chloride, ticarcillin, vancomycin, vecuronium

INCOMPATIBILITIES

Syringe: Meperidine, pentobarbital, prochlorperazine (some preparations).
Y-site: Cefepime, furosemide

PATIENT CARE IMPLICATIONS

• Administer PRN doses before pain becomes severe. Regularly scheduled, continuous, or PCA dosing is usually more effective than PRN scheduling.
• Administer concurrently with antihistamines (e.g., hydroxyzine) or tranquilizers (e.g., prochloperazine) to potentiate effects.
• One third of morphine is protein-bound and inactive, but readily dissociates. Critically ill patients who are hypoalbuminemic, acidotic, or receiving other protein-bound medications may experience exaggerated effects. Reduce dose accordingly.
• Patients receiving morphine for pain control do not develop psychologic dependence. As tolerance develops, progressively higher doses may be necessary

to relieve pain during long-term therapy.
• Gradually discontinue drug after long-term use to prevent withdrawal symptoms.
• **PO:** Do not break or crush extended-release tablets. Administer with food or milk to enhance oral absorption. Solutions may be mixed with fruit juice immediately before administration to improve taste.
• **IM/IV/epidural/intrathecal:** Have naloxone, resuscitation equipment immediately available.
Vital signs/hemodynamics: Assess BP, pulse, and RR, before and frequently during initial administration. For IV injection: q5min for first 15 min and frequently thereafter; during epidural/intrathecal administration: q5min for first 15 min, then once daily during and for 24 hr after last dose • When used in patients with acute MI, CHF, pulmonary edema, evaluate CVP, PCWP, CO as available.
Physical assessment: Assess type, location, intensity of pain before and after administration.
• Assess ventilation; note rate/depth of respirations; auscultate breath sounds. If used as adjunct in treatment of pulmonary edema, check for resolution of crackles. • Assess bowel function: bowel sounds, abdominal distention, elimination patterns.
• Monitor I&O; assess for urinary retention, bladder distention.

PATIENT/FAMILY TEACHING

Purpose of medication is to relieve pain. • Request medication before pain becomes severe.
• Change position slowly to

M

---

minimize dizziness. • Do not perform hazardous tasks requiring mental alertness or physical coordination. Call for assistance when ambulating (initial therapy). • Change position, cough/deep breathe every 2 hr to prevent lung problems. • Drink plenty of fluids, eat high-fiber food. Request stool softeners if necessary to relieve constipation.
Outpatient: Avoid concurrent use of alcohol or other sedatives while taking this medication. • Do not break or chew extended-release tablets. Rapid release of drug could cause release of potentially toxic dose.

AVAILABLE FORMS

Parenteral injection for IV/IM/SC use • Parenteral injection, preservative free, for epidural/intrathecal/IV use • Premixed solution for IV infusion via PCA infusion device • Highly concentrated solution for IV infusion via continuous, controlled microinfusion devices • PO solution • Tablets • Extended-release tablets • Suppositories

---

nadolol
(nay-doe′lole)
Corgard
nadolol with bendroflumethiazide
Corzide

Classifications: Class II antidysrhythmic, nonselective beta-adrenergic blocker, antihypertensive, antianginal

USUAL DOSE

PO, adults: Hypertension: 40-80 mg once daily; may increase gradually as needed to control BP; do not exceed 640 mg/day. • Angina: 40 mg once daily; may increase gradually to 240 mg/day • **Cardiac dysrhythmias:** 60-160 mg once daily or 30-80 mg bid

ACTIONS

Blocks sympathetic stimulation of beta-1-adrenergic receptors of myocardium, beta-2-adrenergic receptors of vasculature/bronchial smooth muscle • Decreases HR, BP, force of contraction; reduces myocardial O_2 consumption • Depresses AV conduction/myocardial automaticity, particularly in SA node • Suppresses renin-angiotensin-aldosterone system • Blocking of beta-2 receptors causes bronchial constriction, ↑ airway resistance, ↓ efficacy of ventilation, particularly with asthma.

PHARMACOKINETICS

ROUTE	ONSET	PEAK	DURATION
PO	<1 hr	2-4 hr	24 hr

DISTRIBUTION
Wide; 30% protein bound

ELIMINATION
Not metabolized, eliminated by kidneys; half-life 10-24 hr

INDICATIONS

Control of hypertension • Chronic, stable angina pectoris *Unlabeled/investigational:* Ventricular dysrhythmias/tachycardia, migraine prophylaxis, tremors, antipsychotic-induced akathisia, situational anxiety, reduction of intraocular pressure, prevention of variceal

---

rebleeding associated with portal hypertension

PRECAUTIONS/CONTRAINDICATIONS

Precautions: May result in symptomatic bradycardia, CHF, hypotension, particularly with preexisting cardiac disease • Abrupt cessation may induce angina, ventricular dysrhythmias, acute MI.

Use caution with: Heart failure, valvular heart disease • Asthma, COPD; use lower dose, monitor for bronchospasm. • General anesthesia; may cause additive impairment of cardiac contractility; may withdraw before surgery • Diabetes, hyperthyroidism; beta-blocking effects mask symptoms • Renal/hepatic impairment; reduce dose. • Children: Safety/efficacy not established

P

C **Pregnancy category:** Use only if safer alternative unavailable.

Contraindications: Hypersensitivity to nadolol • Severe bradycardia • 2nd/3rd degree heart block • CHF (unless resulting from tachycardia) • Cardiogenic shock • Bronchial asthma, severe COPD

ADVERSE EFFECTS

CNS: *Dizziness, fatigue,* sleep disturbances, depression, confusion, hallucinations, visual disturbances
Resp: Dyspnea, wheezing, nasal stuffiness, **bronchospasm**
CV: *Bradycardia,* **hypotension, heart failure, worsened AV heart block, peripheral arterial insufficiency,** peripheral edema
GI: *Nausea,* abdominal pain, vomiting, diarrhea, constipation
GU: Diminished libido, impotence
Endo: Blocked symptoms of hypoglycemia/hyperthyroidism
Hema: Agranulocytosis, thrombocytopenic/nonthrombocytopenic purpura (rare)
Derm: Rash, pruritus, alopecia, dry skin

TOXICITY/OVERDOSE

Symptoms: Symptomatic bradycardia, HR <45, advanced heart block • Profound hypotension, dizziness, loss of consciousness • Heart failure • Bronchospasm
Management: After recent ingestion, implement guidelines for management of acute overdose (Appendix I). • **Symptomatic bradycardia, heart block:** Atropine, isoproterenol according to ACLS guidelines (Appendix P) • **Bronchospasm:** Isoproterenol, aminophylline • **Heart failure:** Inotropic agents (e.g., dobutamine, dopamine), diuretics, possibly digoxin • **Hypoglycemia:** IV glucose • **Hypotension:** Elevate legs, administer IV fluids; use vasopressors (e.g., dopamine, norepinephrine) if severe, refractory to inotropic agents. • Hemodialysis may be helpful.

INTERACTIONS

amiodarone Severe bradycardia; ventricular dysrhythmias
anesthetics, local (e.g., lidocaine) Hypertension, particularly if anesthetic contains epinephrine
antidiabetics (insulin, PO agents Prolonged recovery from hypoglycemic episodes; masked

N

---

italic = common side effects   **bold** = life-threatening reactions

hypoglycemia-associated tachycardia; hyperglycemia

calcium channel blockers Extreme bradycardia; hypotension

disopyramide ↓ CO

epinephrine, possibly other sympathomimetics Blocked epinephrine beta effects; unopposed alpha stimulation (hypertension, bradycardia, dysrhythmias); ↓ effectiveness in anaphylaxis

isoproterenol ↓ Bronchodilatory effectiveness

lidocaine Excessive lidocaine levels; negative inotropy ↓ CO

NSAIDs ↓ Hypotensive effectiveness

phenothiazines Hypotension; enhanced effects of either agent

prazosin Hypotension, especially with initial dose

quinidine Additive cardiac depression

rifampin ↑ Beta-blocker metabolism; higher doses required

theophylline ↓ Bronchodilation

PATIENT CARE IMPLICATIONS

• Use lowest possible dose for dysrhythmia control.
• Monitor closely if other antidysrhythmics or hypotensive agents used.
• Gradually withdraw therapy to avoid rebound hypertension, angina, possible acute MI.
• Tablets may be crushed, dissolved in water to facilitate administration.
• **COPD, asthma:** Monitor closely; avoid high-dose therapy, which may precipitate bronchospasm. Consider use of cardioselective beta-blocker (e.g., atenolol).
• **Hyperthyroidism, diabetes, heart disease, vascular disease:** Special precautions necessary (see Precautions)

Vital signs/hemodynamics: Monitor BP, HR, RR closely when initiating therapy, adjusting dose. Hold next dose, consult physician for hypotension, symptomatic bradycardia, tachypnea. • As available, observe ECG for heart block, symptomatic bradycardia, prolongation of PR interval, widening of QRS complex. If present, hold next dose, consult physician.
• Measure CVP, PAP, CO as available. Note signs of heart failure: ↑ CVP/PAP, ↓ CO. Consult physician for ↓ CO, ↑ filling pressures associated with other symptoms of heart failure.

Physical assessment: Assess for perfusion/oxygenation deficit: ↓ level of consciousness, activity intolerance, hypotension, chest discomfort, dizziness.
• Assess for CHF/pulmonary edema: increased RR, bibasilar crackles, frothy sputum; especially important in patients with preexisting heart disease.
• When used for migraine prophylaxis, assess/record patient response. • Assess diabetic patients for sweating, since tachycardia/tremors associated with hypoglycemia may be blocked by therapy.

Laboratory tests: Monitor: Blood glucose regularly in patients with diabetes • CBC regularly throughout therapy

PATIENT/FAMILY TEACHING

Purpose of medication is to lower BP or regulate abnormal heartbeats. • May cause drowsiness, dizziness, low BP; change positions slowly, particularly when getting out of bed. • Report breathing difficulty, palpitations, dizziness, chest pain, extreme fatigue. • You may experience increased sensitivity to cold. • Avoid excessive amounts of coffee, tea, or caffeinated soft drinks, which may counteract drug's BP-lowering effects.

Outpatient: Take medication exactly as prescribed. Do not stop taking medicine even if you feel better. If medication abruptly discontinued, you may develop dangerously high BP, serious heartbeat irregularities, angina. • Check/record resting pulse each day, BP each week. Contact caregiver if pulse <50 bpm or BP significantly different. • Medication is not cure for high BP; other therapies, including lifestyle modifications, must be continued. • Avoid driving and other activities requiring mental alertness until individual response to drug known. • Drinking alcohol may cause extreme dizziness, drowsiness, impaired mental alertness. • Consult health care professional before taking over-the-counter preparations, particularly cold or allergy preparations. • Carry Medic-Alert ID identifying drug, dosage, specific indication. • Notify health care providers of therapy before any treatment. • Therapy blocks elevated HR, BP, so with hyperthyroid disease or patients with diabetes must be aware of other symptoms of crisis.

AVAILABLE FORMS
Tablets

---

nafcillin sodium
(naf-sill'in)
Nafcil, Nallpen, Unipen

Classification: Penicillinase-resistant penicillin antibiotic

USUAL DOSE
PO, adults: 250-500 mg q4-6h • 1 g q4-6h used for more severe infections
PO, children >1 mo: 50-100 mg/kg/24 hr in equally divided doses q6h
IV/IM, adults: 500 mg-1g q4-6h • **Severe infections:** 1-2 g q4h
IV/IM, children >1 mo: 50-100 mg/kg/24 hr in equally divided doses q6-12h • **Severe infections:** 100-200 mg/kg/24 hr in equally divided doses q4-6h

ADMINISTRATION
PO: Give 1 hr before or 2 hr after meals, for best absorption.
IM: Inject deep into large muscle mass (e.g., gluteus maximus, lateral thigh).
Direct IV: Inject dilute solution slowly over 5-10 min. • Too-rapid injection causes vein irritation.
IV, intermit inf: Infuse prepared solution over 30-60 min.

PREPARATION
IM: Reconstitute each 500 mg with 1.7 ml sterile water for injection or 0.9% NaCl. Use 3.4 ml for 1-g vial, 6.8 ml for 2-g vial. Resulting concentration is 250 mg/ml.
Direct IV: Reconstitute as for IM injection. • Further dilute with 15-30 ml 0.9% NaCl.
IV, intermit inf: Reconstitute as for IM injection. • Further di-

N

---

italic = common side effects   **bold** = life-threatening reactions

lute with 50-100 ml compatible IV solution. • Concentrated solutions of 40 mg/ml may be used for fluid-restricted patients.
Compatible fluids: D$_5$W, 0.9% NaCl, LR, prepared combinations of these solutions.
Compatible dialysis solutions: Dianeal 137 1.5 or 4.25%
Stability: Reconstituted solution stable for 24 hr at room temperature

ACTIONS

Penicillinase-resistant penicillin with bactericidal activity resulting from interference with bacterial cell wall synthesis/division • Notable activity against penicillinase-producing *Staphylococcus aureus, S. epidermidis,* most other gram-positive/gram-negative aerobic cocci • Generally not active against gram-negative bacilli such as Enterobacteriaceae, *Pseudomonas* • As with other penicillinase-resistant penicillins, nafcillin ineffective against methicillin-resistant strains of *S. aureus* (MRSA).

PHARMACOKINETICS

ROUTE	ONSET	PEAK	DURATION
PO	≤30 min	30 min-2 hr	Approx 6 hr
IM	Rapid	30-60 min	
IV	Immed	End infusion	

DISTRIBUTION
Erratically absorbed from GI tract; widely distributed

ELIMINATION
Metabolized in liver, excreted in bile; half-life 30-90 min

INDICATIONS

Used only for infections caused by penicillinase-producing strains of *S. aureus/S. epidermidis,* including septicemia, osteomyelitis, pneumonia, septic arthritis, endocarditis, meningitis • Not to replace natural penicillins for treatment of streptococcal infections • Adverse renal/hepatic effects less likely than with methicillin, oxacillin

PRECAUTIONS/CONTRAINDICATIONS

Precautions: Possible bacterial or fungal overgrowth • May contribute to fluid overload, electrolyte imbalance, including hypokalemia • May impair coagulation, cause abnormal bleeding (rare)
Use caution with: Hypersensitivity to cephalosporins, other drugs; risk of allergic reaction
c **Pregnancy category:** Safety not clearly established
Contraindications: Hypersensitivity to any penicillin

ADVERSE EFFECTS

CNS: Neuromuscular irritability/ **seizures** with high-dose therapy
GI: *Nausea, vomiting, diarrhea, epigastric pain,* gastritis, ↑ AST/ALT
GU: ↑ BUN/creatinine, **interstitial nephritis** (rare)
Hema: Eosinophilia, hemolytic anemia, other blood dyscrasias, coagulation disorders
Derm: *Rash,* urticaria, pruritus
Local: *Painful injection,* thrombophlebitis IV (use)
Misc: *Hypersensitivity,* **anaphylaxis,** serum sickness; superinfection, colonization

---

P pediatric   **G** geriatric   **V** Direct IV

TOXICITY/OVERDOSE

Symptoms: Neurotoxicity, including seizures • Acute allergic reaction, including anaphylaxis
Management: Initiate symptomatic/supportive measures.
• For acute allergic reaction, see Appendix P. • Minimal removal occurs with hemodialysis or peritoneal dialysis.

INTERACTIONS

aminoglycosides (e.g., amikacin, gentamicin) Synergistic antibacterial activity
anticoagulants, PO Prolonged bleeding time
cephalosporins Unpredictable synergism or inactivation
chloramphenicol Inhibition of bactericidal activity
probenecid Higher/prolonged naficillin blood levels
rifampin Inhibition of bactericidal acitivty
tetracycline Inhibition of bactericidal activity

Y-SITE COMPATIBILITIES

Atropine, enalaprilat, esmolol, famotidine, fentanyl, fluconazole, heparin, hydromorphone, magnesium sulfate, morphine, norepinephrine, potassium chloride

Y-SITE INCOMPATIBILITIES

Aminoglycosides (e.g., amikacin, gentamicin, tobramycin), droperidol, insulin (regular), labetalol, meperidine, nalbuphine, pentazocine, succinylcholine, verapamil

PATIENT CARE IMPLICATIONS

• Obtain specimens for culture and sensitivity before initiating antibiotic therapy. Initiate therapy before results received.
• Determine previous antibiotic use, including reactions to penicillins, cephalosporins. Cross-reactivity with cephalosporin allergies may occur.
• Have epinephrine, antihistamine, resuscitation equipment readily available for use with severe allergic reaction.
• Do not discharge patient for at least 30 min after IV/IM antibiotic administration.
• High sodium content of parenteral formulation may cause fluid retention, contribute to edema, electrolyte abnormalities, dysrhythmias, heart failure, particularly with high-dose therapy in susceptible patients.
• To avoid drug incompatibility/interaction, administer at separate site; stagger schedules when aminoglycosides (e.g., amikacin, gentamicin, tobramycin), tetracycline, chloramphenicol also prescribed.
IV
• Reduce risk of thrombophlebitis by using large veins and small catheters, rotating infusion sites.
• IV route must be used for severe infections, when shock present.
Vital signs/hemodynamics: Monitor VS at beginning and throughout therapy. • Monitor I&O for imbalance; older, debilitated, seriously ill, or renal-impaired patients at greater risk for nephrotoxicity.
Physical assessment: Assess for improvement in primary infection or symptoms of super/suprainfection: appearance of sputum, urine, stool, wound drainage; presence of fever, candidiasis, vaginitis. • Observe for

N

G

---

italic = common side effects   **bold** = life-threatening reactions

symptoms of hypersensitivity: rash, pruritus, wheezing, laryngeal edema, hypotension. • Assess for unusual or occult bleeding, including ecchymosis, bleeding from gums/mucous membranes, excessive bleeding from venipuncture site/surgical incision. Note blood in urine, other body fluids. Check emesis, stools for occult blood. • Assess for fluid overload, electrolyte imbalance caused by sodium content, esp. in patients with cardiac impairment.

Laboratory tests: Monitor: Electrolytes • BUN, creatinine • Liver enzymes • CBC with differential.

May cause: Positive direct antiglobulin (Coombs') test

PATIENT/FAMILY TEACHING

Purpose of drug is to limit growth of infection-causing bacteria. • Immediately report rash, swelling, intense itching, difficulty breathing, other signs of allergic reaction. • Report diarrhea, fever, vaginal itching or discharge, furry growth on tongue. • Report unusual bruising, skin discoloration, bleeding from venipuncture, nose, mouth, urine, in stools/emesis.

Outpatient: Take medication at least 1 hr before or 2 hr after meals. Take at evenly spaced intervals over each 24-hr period. • Take all of medication exactly as prescribed. Do not stop taking medicine even if you feel better. Failure to take all of antibiotic may result in recurrence or additional infection. Do not save or share unused medicine.

AVAILABLE FORMS

Capsules • Tablets • Parenteral for IV/IM use

---

nalbuphine HCl
(nal'byoo-feen)
Nubain

Classification: Opiate agonist-antagonist, narcotic analgesic, Schedule II controlled substance

USUAL DOSE

SC/IM/Direct IV, adults: 10 mg q3-6h; up to 20 mg may be used if needed to relieve pain. Maximum total dose is 160 mg/day • **Opiate dependency:** Give test dose of 2.5 mg or approximately 25% of usual dose; if no evidence of withdrawal, carefully increase dose until effective • **Renal/hepatic insufficiency:** Reduced dose indicated

ADMINISTRATION

V Direct IV: Administer each dose of ≤10 mg over 2-3 min. Dilution not necessary

ACTION

Mixed opiate agonist-antagonist that acts at central opioid receptor sites to inhibit pain perception, produce analgesia. Abuse potential low because of mixed agonist-antagonist properties • Does not produce significant CV changes in patients with acute MI • 10 mg nalbuphine has analgesic and respiratory depressant properties similar to 10 mg morphine. Unlike morphine, at higher doses nalbuphine less likely to cause additional respiratory depression

---

PHARMACOKINETICS

ROUTE	ONSET	PEAK	DURATION
IM	<15 min	30 min	3-6 hr
IV	2-3 min	30 min	3-6 hr

ELIMINATION

Metabolized by liver, excreted in urine. Half-life 5 hr.

INDICATIONS

Relief of moderate to severe pain • Perioperative analgesia; anesthesia supplement

PRECAUTIONS/ CONTRAINDICATIONS

Precautions: May cause respiratory depression • May precipitate withdrawal in opioid-dependent patients • Commercial preparations may contain sulfites, which could cause severe hypersensitivity reactions in susceptible individuals.
Use caution with: COPD, asthma, respiratory disorders; may cause respiratory depression, use reduced dose
• Hepatic/renal insufficiency; use reduced dose • Acute MI; may contribute to nausea, vomiting, dysrhythmias • Pancreatitis, biliary tract disorders; may cause spasm of sphincter of Oddi • CNS depression, head injury, craniotomy; may cause additive respiratory depression, contribute to increased intracranial pressure • Children: safe use not established
B Pregnancy category: Safe use not established; use only if clearly indicated.
Contraindications: Hypersensitivity to nalbuphine

ADVERSE EFFECTS

CNS: *Sedation,* dizziness, headache
Resp: Depression

CV: Hypertension, hypotension, tachycardia, bradycardia
GI: Nausea, vomiting
Misc: Diaphoresis, miosis

TOXICITY/OVERDOSE

Symptoms: Sedation, dysphoria, respiratory depression
Management: Naloxone, nalmefene are specific antidotes.
• Maintain airway, support ventilation, administer IV fluids as indicated.

INTERACTIONS

alcohol, anesthetics, antihistamines, opioid analgesics, phenothiazines, sedatives, tranquilizers Additive CNS depression

SYRINGE COMPATIBILITIES

Atropine, cimetidine, diphenhydramine, droperidol, glycopyrrolate, hydroxyzine, midazolam, prochlorperazine, ranitidine

SYRINGE INCOMPATIBILITIES

Diazepam, ketorolac, pentobarbital

Y-SITE INCOMPATIBILITIES

Nafcillin, piperacillin-tazobactam

PATIENT CARE IMPLICATIONS

• Administer prn doses before pain becomes severe. Regularly scheduled, continuous, or PCA dosing is usually more effective than prn scheduling.
• Administer concurrently with antihistamines or tranquilizers to potentiate effects.
• Patients receiving nalbuphine for pain control do not develop psychologic dependence. As tolerance develops, progressively

---

italic = common side effects   **bold** = life-threatening reactions

higher doses may be necessary to relieve pain.
• Gradually discontinue drug after long-term use to prevent withdrawal symptoms.
• Have naloxone, resuscitation equipment immediately available.

Vital signs/hemodynamics: Assess BP, pulse, and PR before and frequently during initial administration. • Use continuous pulse oximetry in heavily sedated patients.

Physical assessment: Assess type, location, intensity of pain before and after administration.
• Assess ventilation: note rate/depth of respirations, auscultating breath sounds. • Assess for signs of opioid withdrawal in patients with established opioid dependency: restlessness, sweating, abdominal cramps, vomiting, hypertension, elevated temperature

PATIENT/FAMILY TEACHING

Purpose of drug is to relieve pain. • Request medication before pain becomes severe.
• Change position slowly to minimize dizziness. • Do not perform hazardous tasks requiring mental alertness or physical coordination. • Call for assistance with ambulation. • Avoid concurrent use of alcohol or other sedatives when taking this medication.

AVAILABLE FORMS

Parenteral for IV/IM/SC use

---

nalmefene HCl
(nal-mi'feen)
Revex

Classification: Opiate antagonist, antidote for opiate toxicity

USUAL DOSE

IM: Use IM route only if unable to achieve IV access; because of inability to titrate for effect, avoid repeated IM doses.

Direct IV, Opioid overdose, adults: Non–opioid-dependent patients: 0.5 mg/70 kg, which is 0.5 ml of 1 mg/ml solution (green label). If inadequate response after 2-5 min, follow with second dose of 1.0 mg/kg; total dose >1.5 mg/70 kg not likely to have additional effects. Repeat doses not usually necessary; however, if respiratory depression recurs, may administer incremental doses titrated to clinical condition.
• Opioid-dependent patients: Challenge dose of 0.1 mg/70 kg, which is 0.1 ml of 1 mg/ml solution (green label). If no evidence of withdrawal in 2 min, administer usual dose as described above

Direct IV, Postop opioid depression, adults: 0.25 µg/kg (see table) given in incremental doses q2-5min, until desired degree of opioid reversal. Do not exceed total dose of 1.0 µg/kg
• Patients at risk for cardiovascular complications: 0.1 µg/kg dilute solution given in incremental doses q2-5min, until desired degree of opioid reversal. Excessive reversal increases risk of hypertension, adverse cardiovascular effects

---

Table 1: Reversal of postop opioid depression

BODY WEIGHT (kg)	NALMEFENE DOSE (ml)*
50	0.125
60	0.150
70	0.175
80	0.200
90	0.225
100	0.250

*100 g/ml solution.

ADMINISTRATION

Two strengths are available: Green-labeled ampule contains 2 ml of 1 mg/ml solution for use with opioid overdose. Blue-labeled ampule contains 1 ml of 100 µg/ml solution for use in reversal of postop opioid depression. Verify labeling, dose before administration.

▼ **Direct IV:** Administer each dose of 1.0 mg or less over 60 seconds. Slow injection necessary to minimize hypertension, dizziness, particularly in patients with renal impairment

PREPARATION

IV: 1 mg/ml or 100 µg/ml concentrations may be given undiluted • **100 µg/ml concentration (blue label):** May use tuberculin syringe or dilute to facilitate administration. Dilution: Combine each 100 µg (1 ml) in 9 ml 0.9% NaCl or sterile water for total volume of 10 ml. Resulting concentration will be 10 µg/ml.
Compatible fluid: 0.9% NaCl

ACTION

Opiate antagonist that blocks central opioid receptors • Prevents/reverses effects of morphine, fentanyl, other opioids, including respiratory depression, sedation, hypotension • Longer duration of action than naloxone • No effect on patients who have not recently received opioids

PHARMACOKINETICS

ROUTE	ONSET	PEAK	DURATION
IV	2-5 min	5 min	2-6 hr

ELIMINATION
Metabolized by liver, excreted in urine. Half-life = 10.8 hr.

INDICATIONS

Reversal of respiratory depression, sedation, hypotension caused by natural/synthetic opioids (e.g., morphine, fentanyl, meperidine, pentazocine, others)

PRECAUTIONS/CONTRAINDICATIONS

Precautions: Use with other resuscitative measures in acute opiate overdose • Rapid opioid reversal may lead to adverse cardiovascular effects, including hypertension, hypotension, ventricular tachycardia/fibrillation, pulmonary edema, especially in patients with CV disease, use of potentially cardiotoxic drugs • May precipitate withdrawal in opioid-dependent patients • May not completely reverse respiratory depression, other effects associated with buprenorphine
Use caution with: Cardiovascular disease, presence of cardiotoxic drugs • Long-acting opioids (e.g., methadone); recurrence of respiratory depression possible; monitor closely • Children: safe use not established
B Pregnancy category: Use only if clearly indicated
Contraindications: Hypersensitivity to nalmefene

italic = common side effects   **bold** = life-threatening reactions

ADVERSE EFFECTS

CNS: Dizziness, headache
CV: Tachycardia, hypertension, vasodilation, hypotension, dysrhythmias
GI: Nausea, vomiting
Misc: Postop pain, fever

TOXICITY/OVERDOSE

Doses of up to 24 mg used without significant adverse effects

INTERACTIONS

buprenorphine Incomplete reversal of respiratory depression
flumazenil   Risk of seizures
opioids, long-acting   Possible recurrence of respiratory depression

COMPATIBILITIES

Not determined

PATIENT CARE IMPLICATIONS

• Have resuscitation equipment, O_2, ACLS drugs immediately available.
• Postop administration of nalmefene does not preclude use of subsequently administered opioid analgesics.
• If nalmefene fails to improve respiratory depression/sedation, consider other causes, including nonopioid drugs, injury, disease process.
Vital signs/hemodynamics: Assess BP, pulse, RR frequently until there is no longer a risk of recurrent respiratory depression. Effects of nalmefene outlast the duration of most opioid analgesics; recurrent respiratory depression possible with some long-acting opioids, such as methadone. • Monitor ECG continuously for dysrhythmias.

• Use continuous pulse oximetry for heavily sedated patients.
Physical assessment: Assess level of consciousness frequently until risk of excessive sedation has passed and condition stabilizes. • Assess for signs of opioid withdrawal: restlessness, sweating, abdominal cramps, vomiting, hypertension, elevated temperature. • Assess level of pain when used postop. Use smallest effective dose to reverse respiratory depression while maintaining analgesia.

PATIENT/FAMILY TEACHING

Purpose of drug is to reverse effects of morphine, other opioid drugs.

AVAILABLE FORMS

Parenteral for IV injection

---

naloxone HCl
(nal-ox'own)
Narcan

Classifications: Opiate antagonist, antidote for opiate toxicity

USUAL DOSE

Direct IV, adults: Opiate overdose: Initially 0.4-2 mg, may repeat q2-3min up to total dose of 10 mg; duration of opiate often greater than that of naloxone; additional doses or continuous IV infusion may be required. If IV unavailable IM/SC route may be used.
• Postop reversal of opiate anesthesia: 0.1-0.2 mg q2-3min; titrate to avoid complete reversal of analgesic effects.
🅟 Direct IV, children: Opiate overdose: Initially 0.01 mg/kg, may repeat q2-3min until de-

sired response; single dose of 0.1 mg/kg may be used if initial dose ineffective. Duration of opiate often greater than that of naloxone; additional doses may be required. If IV unavailable, IM/SC route may be used.

• **Postop reversal of opiate anesthesia:** 0.005-0.01 mg q2-3min; titrate to avoid complete reversal of analgesic effects.

IV, cont inf, adults: Initial loading dose of 0.4 mg IV, followed by continuous infusion of 0.4 mg/hr, titrated according to patient response • Infusion pump necessary

ADMINISTRATION

▼**Direct IV:** Inject each dose of ≤0.4 mg over 15 sec.

PREPARATION

Direct IV: May be given undiluted

IV, cont inf:

COMMON DILUTION	CONCENTRATION
2 mg/500 ml	0.004 mg/ml

Compatible fluids: D_5W, 0.9% NaCl, prepared combinations of these solutions

Stability: Stable for 24 hr

ACTIONS

Pure opiate antagonist; believed to compete for specific opiate receptor sites within CNS • Antagonizes respiratory depressant, sedative, analgesic, other effects of morphine/related opiates • Duration of action usually shorter than opiate effects, repeat doses often required. • Little or no effect on patients who have not recently received opiates • In shock states, believed to antagonize beta-endorphins, enhance action of prostaglandins/catecholamines in stabilizing circulation

PHARMACOKINETICS

ROUTE	ONSET	PEAK	DURATION
IV	1-2 min	Rapid	30-45 min

ELIMINATION

Metabolized in liver, excreted in urine; half-life 60-90 min

INDICATIONS

Reversal of respiratory depression, sedation, hypotension caused by natural/synthetic opiates (e.g., morphine, heroin, meperidine, pentazocine, others) • Diagnosis of suspected acute opiate overdose

Unlabeled/investigational:
Stabilization of circulation in endotoxic, hemorrhagic, cardiogenic, neurogenic, anaphylactic shock; high-altitude pulmonary edema; acute respiratory failure; reversal of acute alcoholic coma

PRECAUTIONS/ CONTRAINDICATIONS

Precautions: Use with other resuscitative measures in acute opiate overdose. • Duration of action of some opiates exceeds that of naloxone; repeat doses may be necessary. • May cause vomiting with potential for aspiration • Rapid opioid reversal may lead to excitement, hypertension, tachycardia. • May cause hyper/hypotension, pulmonary edema, ventricular tachycardia/fibrillation, especially in patients with CV disease or in association with potentially cardiotoxic drugs • May precipitate withdrawal in opioid-dependent patients, including neonates of opioid-dependent mothers

---

italic = common side effects   **bold** = life-threatening reactions

B Pregnancy category: Use only if clearly indicated.
Contraindications: Hypersensitivity to naloxone

ADVERSE EFFECTS

CNS: Tremors, excitement, **seizures** (rare)
Resp: Hyperventilation, pulmonary edema
CV: Hypotension, hypertension, **ventricular tachycardia/ fibrillation**
GI: Nausea, vomiting

TOXICITY/OVERDOSE

Symptoms: High doses may cause slight drowsiness. Doses ≥1 mg/kg have been used without significant adverse effects.
Management: Treat symptomatically.

INTERACTIONS

Opiate agonists, mixed opiate agonist-antagonists Acute opiate withdrawal

COMPATIBILITIES

Syringe: Heparin

INCOMPATIBILITIES

Do not mix with bisulfites, sulfites, highly alkaline solutions.

PATIENT CARE IMPLICATIONS

• Have resuscitation equipment, O_2, ACLS drugs immediately available.
• If 10 mg naloxone fails to improve respiratory depression/ sedation, consider other causes, including nonopiate drugs, injury, disease process.
Vital signs/hemodynamics: Assess BP, pulse, RR frequently until opiate effects wear off. Repeat doses of naloxone may be necessary, depending on opi-

ate dose, duration. • Monitor ECG continuously for dysrhythmias. • Use continuous pulse oximetry in heavily sedated patients.
Physical assessment: Assess level of consciousness frequently until opiate effects wear off/condition stabilizes. • Assess for signs of opioid withdrawal: restlessness, sweating, abdominal cramps, vomiting, hypertension, elevated temperature.
• Assess level of pain when used postop. Use small, frequent doses of naloxone to reverse respiratory depression while maintaining analgesia.

PATIENT/FAMILY TEACHING

Purpose of drug is to reverse effects of morphine, other opiates.

AVAILABLE FORMS

Parenteral for IV/IM/SC use

---

neomycin sulfate
(nee-oh-mye′sin)
Mycifradin, Neo-Fradin, Neo-tabs
neomycin sulfate with bacitracin zinc, polymyxin B
Mycitracin, Neosporin

Classification: Aminoglycoside antibiotic

USUAL DOSE

PO/NG, adults: Acute hepatic encephalopathy: 1-3 g q6h for 5-6 days; administered PO or via enteral feeding tube
• Preop intestinal antisepsis: 1 g qh for 4 doses, followed by 1 g q4h for 5 doses; • **Renal impairment:** Reduce dose.

P pediatric   **G** geriatric   **V** Direct IV

Rectal retention enema, adults: Acute hepatic encephalopathy: 100-200 ml 1% solution retained for 20-60 min 4 times daily

P Eyes/Ears, adults/children: Ophth ointment: Small amount into conjunctival sac of affected eye q4-24h • Ophth solution: 1-2 drops onto affected eye 2-4 times daily • Otic solution/suspension: Small amount into affected ear 3-4 times daily

ACTIONS

Bactericidal; inhibits bacterial cell protein synthesis, causing cellular death • Active against many aerobic gram-negative bacteria, some aerobic gram-positive bacteria • When administered PO or by retention enema, numbers of intestinal bacteria reduced; most of drug not absorbed • In hepatic encephalopathy, reduced numbers of intestinal bacteria result in ↓ bacterial formation of ammonia, other toxic nitrogenous substances.

PHARMACOKINETICS

Approx 3% absorbed from GI tract; impaired motility increases absorption, risk of toxicity. • Not absorbed from intact skin; readily absorbed through open wounds, burns, ulcers, peritoneum, surgical sites • Unabsorbed drug excreted unchanged in feces

INDICATIONS

As adjunct in treatment of acute hepatic encephalopathy; not indicated for chronic encephalopathy because of potential otonephrotoxicity • Preop intestinal antisepsis before colorectal surgery • Treatment of diarrhea caused by *Escherichia coli* • Superficial eye infections • Otitis externa • Prevention/treatment of superficial skin infections

PRECAUTIONS/ CONTRAINDICATIONS

Precautions: Possible bacterial or fungal overgrowth • Systemic absorption with toxicity/death possible when used for peritoneal instillation, wound irrigation, or topically with burns/large areas of denuded skin, particularly in renal impaired patients • Malabsorption syndrome possible with prolonged PO administration • Some preparations contain sulfites, which can cause serious allergic reactions in susceptible individuals.

Use caution with: Renal impairment, advanced age, preexisting hearing disorder, high-dose/prolonged therapy; oto/nephrotoxicity more likely • Preexisting neuromuscular disease, NMBAs; neurotoxicity more likely • Concurrent use of other oto/nephrotoxic agents, including other aminoglycosides • Chronic otitis media, perforated tympanic membrane; systemic absorption possible

D Pregnancy category: Risk of fetal damage, avoid pregnancy; use only if safer alternative unavailable and risks explained to woman.

Contraindications: Hypersensitivity to neomycin, other ingredients in specific formulation • Intestinal obstruction (enteral use)

ADVERSE EFFECTS

CNS: *8th cranial nerve damage, ototoxicity,* **permanent hear-**

N

ing loss (rare), **neuromuscular blockade** (systemic absorption)

GI: PO/rectal—malabsorption syndrome with diarrhea, electrolyte imbalance, impaired vitamin K absorption

GU: *Nephrotoxicity* (systemic absorption)

Misc: Hypersensitivity; superinfection, colonization

TOXICITY/OVERDOSE

Symptoms: Systemic absorption of large amounts can produce oto/nephrotoxicity. • Possible neurotoxicity with neuromuscular blockade, respiratory paralysis, seizures

Management: Discontinue drug; initiate symptomatic/supportive measures, including airway management/ventilation. • Hemodialysis or peritoneal dialysis may be helpful.

INTERACTIONS

anticoagulants, PO   Additive prolongation of PT

digoxin   ↓ Digoxin absorption; monitor serum levels

penicillin, PO   Greatly ↓ penicillin levels

PATIENT CARE IMPLICATIONS

• **Preop bowel preparation:** Usually combined with cathartics, enemas, erythromycin, low-residue diet • **Burns >20% body surface area:** Restrict topical use to once daily.

Physical assessment: Monitor for symptoms of ototoxicity: tinnitus, roaring in ears, hearing loss, dizziness, vertigo, nausea; particularly important with advanced age, preexisting hearing disorder, renal impairment, high-dose/prolonged therapy. • He-

patic encephalopathy: Monitor neurologic status; administer via enteral feeding tube or as retention enema if unable to swallow.

Laboratory tests: Monitor: Urinalysis • BUN, creatinine, serum ammonia

PATIENT/FAMILY TEACHING

Purpose of drug is to limit bacterial growth. Report rash, diarrhea, hearing difficulty, dizziness. • Topical ointment not to be used for self-treatment of infected or serious wounds except as directed by health care professional.

AVAILABLE FORMS

PO solution • Tablets • Topical cream, ointment; alone, combined with other topical antibiotics and/or antiinflammatory agents • Concentrate for GU irrigant • Ophth ointment, solution, suspension combined with other topical antibiotics and/or antiinflammatory agents • Otic solution, suspension combined with other topical antibiotics and/or antiinflammatory agents

**neostigmine bromide
neostigmine
methylsulfate**
(nee-oh-stig′meen)
Prostigmin

Classifications: Cholinergic stimulant, anticholinesterase agent

USUAL DOSE

PO, adults: Initial: 15 mg tid • Maintenance: Range, 15-375 mg/day in divided doses q2-6h; adjust dose to individual requirements

PO, children: Initial: 7.5-15 mg 3-4 times daily; adjust dose to individual requirements.

IM/SC injection, adult: Post-op urinary retention: 0.5-1 mg q3h for up to 5 doses • Myasthenia gravis: 0.5-2.5 mg IM/SC as needed; administer 0.6-1.2 mg atropine to counteract muscarinic effects associated with large doses.

Direct IV, adult: Reversal of neuromuscular blockade: 0.5-2.5 mg; repeat as necessary to restore return of voluntary respiration; total dose usually <5 mg. Administer with 0.6-1.2 mg atropine or 0.2-0.6 mg glycopyrrolate to counteract muscarinic effects. • Myasthenia gravis: 0.5 increments; carefully titrate to individual requirements. Administer with 0.6-1.2 mg atropine to counteract muscarinic effects.

PO: Poorly absorbed; administer on empty stomach to improve absorption. Administer 30 min before meals for patients experiencing chewing/swallowing difficulty.

ADMINISTRATION

Direct IV: Inject each 0.5 mg increment slowly over at least 1 min. • When used for reversal or neuromuscular blockade, peripheral nerve stimulator recommended to assess responsiveness • Dilution not necessary • Have atropine immediately available.

Compatible fluids: D₅W, 0.9% NaCl, prepared combinations of these solutions

ACTIONS

Inhibits breakdown of acetylcholine by competing for attachment to acetylcholinesterase; acetylcholine accumulates at cholinergic synapses, facilitates transmission of myoneural impulses; results in stronger, more sustained muscle contraction • Produces generalized cholinergic responses such as miosis, increased muscle tone, bronchial constriction, bradycardia, increased salivation, sweating

PHARMACOKINETICS

ROUTE	ONSET	PEAK	DURATION
PO	1-2 hr	2-4 hr	6-8 hr
IV	10-30 min	20-30 min	2-4 hr

DISTRIBUTION
Moderate doses do not cross blood-brain barrier.

ELIMINATION
Metabolized in liver/other tissue, excreted in urine; half-life 60 min

INDICATIONS

To reverse effects of nondepolarizing NMBAs (e.g., tubocurarine, pancuronium) • In myasthenia gravis to improve muscle strength and as diagnostic aid • Prevention/treatment of postop abdominal distention, urinary retention

Unlabeled/investigational:
SVT caused by tricyclic overdose in children

PRECAUTIONS/CONTRAINDICATIONS

Precautions: Severe cholinergic reaction possible • Transient cardiac dysrhythmias may occur when given with atropine to reverse NMBAs. • Respiratory depression possible with large doses • Peristaltic stimulation may disrupt recent ileorectal anastomoses.

---

italic = common side effects   **bold** = life-threatening reactions

Use caution with: Epilepsy
• Asthma • Bradycardia • Cardiac disease, dysrhythmias
• Hyperthyroidism • Peptic ulcer
• PO route with megacolon, decreased GI motility

c Pregnancy category: Use only if safer alternative unavailable.

Contraindications: Hypersensitivity to neostigmine • PO formulation with bromide sensitivity • Peritonitis • Mechanical intestinal obstruction: possibility of nonviable bowel • Mechanical urinary obstruction

ADVERSE EFFECTS

CNS: Weakness, dizziness, **seizures, paralysis**
EENT: Miosis, blurred vision, tearing
Resp: *Excessive secretions,* **bronchospasm, laryngospasm, respiratory depression, respiratory arrest**
CV: *Bradycardia,* tachycardia, AV block, hypotension, **cardiac arrest**
GI: *Nausea, vomiting, diarrhea, cramping*
GU: Urinary frequency, incontinence
Derm: *Sweating,* rash, urticaria, flushing

TOXICITY/OVERDOSE

Symptoms: Cholinergic crisis: Vomiting, diarrhea, excessive salivation/tearing, bradycardia, tachycardia, hypotension, bronchospasm, excessive bronchial secretions, weakness, fasciculation, paralysis • Death possible from respiratory paralysis, pulmonary edema, cardiac arrest
Management: After recent ingestion, implement guidelines for management of acute overdose (Appendix I). • Ensure airway, maintain adequate ventilation; ET intubation or tracheostomy usually necessary; frequent suctioning, position changes used to mobilize/clear excessive secretions. • Administer atropine, 0.6 mg IV q5-30min as needed; atropine does not reverse muscle relaxation, respiratory paralysis.

INTERACTIONS

atropine   Antagonizes muscarinic effects
corticosteroids   Inhibits neostigmine effects
opiate analgesics   Potentiates CNS sedation
pancuronium, other nondepolarizing neuromuscular blockers   Antagonizes neuromuscular blockade
succinylcholine, other depolarizing neuromuscular blockers   Prolongs neuromuscular blockade

Y-SITE COMPATIBILITIES

Heparin, potassium chloride, vitamin B complex with C

PATIENT CARE IMPLICATIONS

• PO/parenteral doses not interchangeable
• Tolerance may develop with prolonged therapy in myasthenic patients. Decreasing dosage or withdrawing therapy for several days may improve responsiveness. High-dose corticosteroid therapy has been used in critically ill patients to restore responsiveness; however, temporary worsening of condition may occur.
• Parenteral doses often administered with atropine, which can mask symptoms of toxicity.

• **IV/IM/SC:** Atropine must be immediately available to counteract severe cholinergic reactions. High doses may cause respiratory depression/paralysis; emergency resuscitation, airway management equipment must be immediately available.
• **Reversal of NMBAs:** Use peripheral nerve stimulator to monitor effectiveness.
• **Postop urinary retention:** If no response within 1 hr of administration, insert Foley catheter.
Vital signs/hemodynamics: Monitor ECG continuously during IV use or when testing for myasthenia gravis. Observe for bradycardia, tachycardia, AV block, dysrhythmias. • With parenteral use, monitor BP, RR q30-60min or more often.
Physical assessment: Closely monitor respiratory status: rate, depth of ventilation, presence of excessive secretions/bronchospasm. Measure vital capacity when testing for myasthenia gravis or increasing dose. • Assess for improved neuromuscular status: muscle strength, hand grasp, gait, ventilatory effort, chewing, swallowing. • Use peripheral nerve stimulator to monitor reversal of NMBAs. Recovery of muscle function usually occurs in following order: diaphragm, intercostals, glottis, abdominal muscles, limbs, jaws, eyelids. • In postop patients, assess for abdominal distention, presence of bowel sounds. • Monitor I&O. Assess for urinary retention/incontinence.

PATIENT/FAMILY TEACHING

Purpose of medication is to improve muscle strength. • Medicine relieves symptoms of myasthenia but is not cure. • Take all doses precisely as scheduled. Late dosing may precipitate myasthenic crisis. Early dosing may cause cholinergic crisis.
• Wear Medic-Alert ID describing myasthenia condition, medicines used. • Report breathing difficulty, palpitations, progressive weakness, muscle cramps, excessive sweating/salivation, vomiting, diarrhea.

AVAILABLE FORMS

Parenteral for IV injection
• Tablets • Sustained-release tablets, capsules

nicardipine HCl
(nye-card'i-peen)
Cardene

Classifications: Calcium channel blocker, antianginal, antihypertensive, vasodilator

USUAL DOSE

PO, adults: 20-40 mg q8h Ext rel: 30-60 mg bid • After initial dosing, dose should not be increased for 3 days to ensure steady-state plasma levels.
• **Hepatic/renal insufficiency:** Reduce dose and/or frequency
IV, cont inf, adults: Initially, 5.0 mg/hr (50 ml/hr of 0.1 mg/ml solution). As necessary, increase by 2.5 mg/hr increments q15min up to rate of 15.0 mg/hr; for rapid BP reduction may adjust rate q5min. When desired BP is reached, reduce infusion rate to 3 mg/hr (30 ml/hr). Stop infusion for hypotension, tachycardia; resume at low dose (3-5 mg/hr) when condition stabilized. • **Oral replace-**

ment therapy: For usual oral dose of 20-40 mg q8h, use IV rate of 0.5-2.2 mg/hr

ADMINISTRATION

IV, cont inf, adults: Stop infusion for hypotension, tachycardia; resume at lower dose when condition stabilized. Must use infusion pump. If administered via peripheral vein, manufacturer recommends changing infusion site q12h to avoid vein irritation

PREPARATION

DILUTION	CONCENTRATION
25 mg/250 ml	0.1 mg/ml

Compatible fluids: D_5W, 0.9% NaCl, and prepared combinations of these solutions
Incompatible fluids: LR

ACTIONS

Inhibits movement of calcium ions across myocardium, vascular smooth muscle • Dilates coronary, peripheral arteries; decreases peripheral vascular resistance • Afterload reduction reduces myocardial O_2 demand • May slightly ↑ ↓ effective refractory period (ERP) in AV node, slightly ↓ ERP in His-Purkinje system; SA node automatically usually unaffected; AV conduction time, QT interval may ↑ slightly. • CO, HR may ↑

PHARMACOKINETICS

ROUTE	ONSET	PEAK	DURATION
PO	20 min	0.5-2hr	3 hr
IV	Immed	≤15 min	2 hr

DISTRIBUTION
Wide; 95% bound to plasma protein
ELIMINATION
Metabolized in liver, eliminated by kidneys; half-life 2-4 hr

Therapeutic level: 28-50 ng/ml

INDICATIONS

Management of chronic stable angina in patients unable to tolerate nitrates or beta-adrenergic blocking agents • Management of essential hypertension • Afterload reduction in CHF • Has been used in combination with aminocaproic acid to prevent vasospasm in patients after subarachnoid hemorrhage
IV: Short-term treatment of hypertension • During surgery for cerebral aneurysm to promote vasodilation.

PRECAUTIONS/CONTRAINDICATIONS

Precautions: May cause hypotension 1-2 hr after dosing • Angina may increase when dosage initiated or increased.
Use caution with: Conduction disorders, artificial pacemakers • CHF, left ventricular failure; negative inotropic effects may worsen condition • Renal/hepatic insufficiency • Pheochromocytoma
c Pregnancy category: Use only if safer alternative unavailable.
Contraindications: Hypersensitivity to nicardipine • Advanced aortic stenosis

ADVERSE EFFECTS

CNS: *Headache, weakness,* somnolence, sleep disturbance, malaise, paresthesias, confusion, anxiety

Resp: Shortness of breath, dyspnea, wheezing

CV: *Tachycardia, peripheral edema, angina,* **heart block,** syncope, **hypotension, MI,** PVCs

GI: *Tachycardia, nausea,* abdominal discomfort, dry mouth, vomiting, constipation

GU: Polyuria, nocturia (rare)

Derm: *Flushing,* rash, dermatitis

TOXICITY/OVERDOSE

Symptoms: Profound hypotension • Palpitations, bradycardia, 2nd/3rd degree heart block, junctional rhythms • Flushing, confusion, slurred speech

Management: After recent ingestion, implement guidelines for management of acute overdose (Appendix I). • **Hypotension:** Elevate legs, administer IV fluids. Except in patients with hypertrophic cardiomyopathy, use beta-adrenergic agonists and IV calcium chloride; vasopressors (e.g., norepinephrine, dopamine) used if unresponsive to other measures. For patients with hypertrophic cardiomyopathy or IHSS, use alpha-adrenergic agents (e.g., methoxamine, phenylephrine) for hypotension. • **Symptomatic bradycardia, heart block:** Use IV atropine, calcium, epinephrine, possibly isoproterenol; consider temporary pacemaker. Manage asystole, other dysrhythmias according to ACLS guidelines (Appendix P). • Calcium may be helpful in reversing adverse hemodynamic effects but may not always reverse electrophysiologic toxicity. • Dialysis is not likely to be helpful.

INTERACTIONS

antihypertensives Profound hypotension

beta-blockers Profound hypotension; exacerbation of heart block

calcium ↓ Nicardipine effectiveness

cimetidine ↑ Nicardipine levels/toxicity

cyclosporine ↑ Cyclosporine levels; monitor closely

disopyramide ↑ negative inotropy

fentanyl Profound hypotension

vasodilators Profound hypotension

Y-SITE COMPATIBILITIES

Potassium chloride

Y-SITE INCOMPATIBILITIES

Sodium bicarbonate

PATIENT CARE IMPLICATIONS

• Older adults may experience profound hypotension. Use lowest effective dose; monitor closely.

• Nitrates, O_2 can be used to manage chest pain while initiating therapy.

IV: If possible, infuse via central vein to reduce peripheral vein irritation.

Vital signs/hemodynamics: Monitor BP 1-2 hr after initial dose and again in 8 hr. Monitor closely when increasing dosage. In acutely ill patients, continuously monitor cardiac rhythm for signs of ischemia (e.g., T wave inversions, ST segment elevation) or heart block. • **IV:** Monitor BP, HR q5-15min until stable. Stop infusion for hypo-

tension, tachycardia; resume at lower dose when stable. Use lower dose and titrate slowly in patients with cardiac, hepatic, renal impairment.
Physical assessment: Monitor for ↑ frequency, duration, severity of chest pain when drug initiated or dosage increased. • Assess for perfusion/oxygenation deficit: ↓ level of consciousness, hypotension, activity intolerance, chest discomfort. • If used after subarachnoid hemorrhage, assess neurologic status frequently.

PATIENT/FAMILY TEACHING

Purpose of medication is to control high BP or relieve angina pain. • Initiation of therapy: May cause dizziness; use caution, change positions slowly. • Report dyspnea, chest pain, palpitations, activity intolerance, breathing difficulty. • Avoid taking medication with high-fat meals, which may delay absorption. Sustained-release capsules should never be broken, chewed, or swallowed. Do not stop taking medicine without consulting primary health care provider.

AVAILABLE FORMS

Capsules, Ext. rel. capsules

---

nifedipine
(nye-fed′i-peen)
Adalat, Apo-Nifed ✦,
Procardia, Procardia XL

Classifications: Calcium channel blocker, antidysrhythmic, antianginal, antihypertensive

USUAL DOSE

PO, adult: 10-20 mg q8h; not to exceed 30 mg in a single dose or 180 mg/day • Sus rel: 30-60 mg qAM; not to exceed 120 mg/day • **Hepatic impairment:** Reduce dose by 50% • **Renal impairment:** Reduce dose and/or frequency
SL, adult:
Unlabeled/investigational:
Hypertensive crisis: 10-20 mg. **Must use fluid-filled standard capsule.** Have patient bite and then chew capsule before swallowing; may be repeated in 20-30 min. • Rapid onset, potent activity; monitor BP q5min until stable.

PREPARATION

G-tube: Contents of fluid-filled standard capsule may be aspirated with large-bore needle/syringe or extruded for administration via feeding tube. • Mix contents in small volume of water or normal saline; flush feeding tube after administration. • Do not attempt to crush or dissolve sustained-release preparations.

ACTIONS

Inhibits movement of calcium ions across myocardium, vascular smooth muscle • Coronary, systemic arteries dilated; BP reduced • Little if any effect on AV conduction/refractoriness of AV node • Afterload reduction decreases myocardial O_2 demand. • Serum calcium levels remain unchanged. • May decrease myocardial contractility; negative inotropic properties not usually evident without prior ventricular dysfunction

---

P pediatric   **G** geriatric   **V** Direct IV

PHARMACOKINETICS

ROUTE	ONSET	PEAK	DURATION
PO, std	20 min	0.5-6 hr	7-8 hr

DISTRIBUTION
Wide; 92%-98% bound to plasma proteins

ELIMINATION
Metabolized in liver, eliminated by kidneys, in feces; half-life 2-5 hr

Therapeutic level: 25-100 ng/ml

INDICATIONS

Management of variant/chronic stable angina • Control of essential hypertension • Sustained-release preparations used exclusively for control of hypertension

Unlabeled/investigational:
SL dosing used during hypertensive crisis; also used for migraine headaches, Raynaud's syndrome, cardiomyopathy, CHF, primary pulmonary hypertension

PRECAUTIONS/ CONTRAINDICATIONS

Precautions: May cause profound hypotension • ↑ Angina may occur during initiation of therapy and when dosage ↑ . • When used for angina, condition may worsen with sudden cessation of therapy.
Use caution with: Chronic heart failure, aortic stenosis, beta-blocker therapy may worsen or precipitate heart failure • Children: Safety not established
c **Pregnancy category:** Use only if possible benefits outweigh risk and safer alternatives unavailable.
Contraindications: Hypersensitivity to nifedipine • Lactation

ADVERSE EFFECTS

CNS: *Dizziness, lightheadedness, giddiness, headache,* hot sensation, balance disturbance, mood swings, nervousness
Resp: **Dyspnea, cough, sore throat,** nasal congestion, wheezing
CV: *Hypotension, peripheral edema,* **exacerbation of heart failure, angina**
GI: *Nausea,* constipation, cramps, flatulence, ↑ liver enzymes
MS: Joint stiffness, muscle cramps
Derm: Pruritus, urticaria, sweating

TOXICITY/OVERDOSE

Symptoms: Profound hypotension • Bradycardia, 2nd/3rd degree heart block, palpitations, junctional rhythms • Dizziness, drowsiness, confusion, slurred speech
Management: After recent ingestion, implement guidelines for management of acute overdose (Appendix I). • **Hypotension:** Elevate legs, administer IV fluids. Except in patients with hypertrophic cardiomyopathy, use beta-adrenergic agonists, IV calcium chloride. Vasopressors (e.g., norepinephrine, dopamine) may be used if unresponsive to other measures. For patients with hypertrophic cardiomyopathy or IHSS, use alpha-adrenergic agents (e.g., methoxamine, phenylephrine) for hypotension. • **Symptomatic bradycardia, heart block:** Use IV atropine, epinephrine, possibly isoproterenol; consider temporary pacemaker, IV calcium. Manage asystole, other dysrhythmias according to

N

---

italic = common side effects   **bold** = life-threatening reactions

ACLS guidelines (Appendix P). • Calcium may be helpful in reversing adverse hemodynamic effects but may not always reverse electrophysiologic toxicity. • Dialysis is not likely to be helpful.

INTERACTIONS

antihypertensives Profound hypotension

beta-blockers Profound hypotension; exacerbation of heart block; CHF

calcium ↓ Nifedipine effectiveness

cimetidine ↑ Nifedipine levels/toxicity

digoxin ↑ Digoxin levels; monitor closely

fentanyl Profound hypotension

phenytoin ↑ Phenytoin levels; monitor closely

ranitidine ↑ Nifedipine levels/toxicity

PATIENT CARE IMPLICATIONS

G • Older adults may experience profound hypotension. Use lowest effective dose; monitor closely.
• Nitrates, O_2 can be used to manage chest pain while initiating therapy.
• Never puncture or crush sustained-release preparations, because acute overdose with profound hypotension will result.

Vital signs/hemodynamics: During initiation of therapy and in acutely ill patients, continuously monitor cardiac rhythm for signs of ischemia/infarction (e.g., T wave inversion, ST segment depression/elevation,) or heart block. • Monitor BP 1-2 hr after initial dose and when increasing dosage. When used in hypertensive emergencies, monitor BP q5-10min until stable. • Monitor central hemodynamics, CO as available. Monitor for ↑ PCWP, ↓ CO, other indicators of left ventricular failure.

Physical assessment: Monitor for ↑ frequency, duration, severity of chest pain during initiation of therapy and when dose ↑. • Assess for perfusion/oxygenation deficit, ↓ level of consciousness, hypotension, activity intolerance, chest discomfort.
• Assess for CHF/pulmonary edema; bibasilar crackles (rales), S_3 gallop, breathing difficulty, peripheral edema.

PATIENT/FAMILY TEACHING

Purpose of medication is to control high BP or relieve angina pain. • Initiation of therapy: May cause dizziness; use caution, change positions slowly. • Report dyspnea, chest pain, palpitations, activity intolerance, other signs of heart failure. • Sustained-release tablets should never be broken, chewed, crushed. • Abrupt cessation of therapy may cause serious complications, including chest pain, profound hypertension. Do not stop taking medicine without consulting primary health care provider.

AVAILABLE FORMS

Standard capsules • Sustained-release tablets

---

nimodipine
(nye-mode'i-peen)
Nimotop

Classifications: Calcium channel blocker, vasodilator

USUAL DOSE

PO, adult: 30-60 mg q4-6h
• **Subarachnoid hemorrhage (SAH):** Initiate therapy within 96 hr of bleeding; continue for 21 consecutive days. • **Hepatic impairment:** Reduce dose by 50%

PREPARATION

G-tube: Contents of fluid-filled capsule may be aspirated with large-bore needle/syringe or extruded • Mix contents in small volume of sterile water or normal saline; flush feeding tube after administration.

ACTIONS

Inhibits movement of calcium ions across myocardium, neuronal cells, vascular smooth muscle, resulting in vasodilation • Greatest vasodilatory effect on cerebral arteries, possibly because of easier passage across blood-brain barrier, beneficial effects for patients with SAH believed to result from dilation of small cerebral resistance vessels, with resultant increase in collateral circulation and/or prevention of calcium overload in neurons • Relative selectivity for vascular vs myocardial receptors with minimal electrophysiologic/negative inotropic effects

PHARMACOKINETICS

ROUTE	ONSET	PEAK	DURATION
PO	30 min	0.5-2hr	4 hr

DISTRIBUTION

Wide; 95% bound to plasma proteins; readily crosses blood-brain barrier

ELIMINATION

Metabolized in liver, eliminated by kidneys; half-life 1-2 hr

INDICATIONS

Recent SAH to decrease severity of ischemic neurologic deficits, reduce incidence of cerebral infarction/mortality
Unlabeled/investigational:
Migraine headache, acute ischemic CVA, cerebral vasospasm associated with severe traumatic head injury

PRECAUTIONS/ CONTRAINDICATIONS

Precautions: May cause hypotension • May ↑ liver enzymes, cause hepatitis, jaundice
Use caution with: Hepatic impairment • CHF; may cause fluid retention • Children: Safety not established
C Pregnancy category: Safety not established; use only if safer alternatives unavailable.
Contraindications: Hypersensitivity to nimodipine

ADVERSE EFFECTS

CNS: Headache, dizziness, depression
Resp: Shortness of breath, dyspnea, wheezing
CV: ***Hypotension,*** peripheral edema, flushing, bradycardia
GI: Diarrhea, nausea, vomiting, ↑ liver enzymes
Derm: Rash, sweating

TOXICITY/OVERDOSE

Symptoms: Profound hypotension • Bradycardia, 2nd/3rd degree heart block, palpitations, junctional rhythms • Dizziness, drowsiness, confusion, slurred speech

Management: After recent ingestion, implement guidelines for management of acute overdose (Appendix I). • **Hypotension:** Elevate legs, administer IV fluids. Except in patients with hypertrophic cardiomyopathy, use beta-adrenergic agonists, IV calcium chloride. Vasopressors (e.g. norepinephrine, dopamine) may be used if unresponsive to other measures. In patients with hypertrophic cardiomyopathy or IHSS, use alpha-adrenergic agents (e.g., methoxamine, phenylephrine) for hypotension. • **Symptomatic bradycardia, heart block:** Use IV atropine, epinephrine, possibly isoproterenol; consider temporary pacemaker, IV calcium. Manage asystole, other dysrhythmias according to ACLS guidelines (Appendix P). • Calcium may be helpful in reversing adverse hemodynamic effects but may not always reverse electrophysiologic toxicity. • Dialysis is not likely to be helpful.

INTERACTIONS

antihypertensives Profound hypotension
beta-blockers Profound hypotension; CHF
calcium ↓ Nimodipine effectiveness
fentanyl Profound hypotension
phenytoin ↑ Phenytoin levels

PATIENT CARE IMPLICATIONS

G • Older adults may experience profound hypotension. Use low-

est effective dose; monitor closely.
• Initiate therapy within 96 hr of SAH.

Vital signs/hemodynamics: Monitor BP q30-60min during initiation of therapy and until stable. Monitor especially closely in patients with hepatic impairment. • As available, monitor ICP, maintain pressures <15 mm Hg or specified range. Consult physician for elevated ICP promptly.

Physical assessment: Evaluate effectiveness of therapy by assessing neurologic status: level of consciousness, movement, signs of ↑ ICP, changes in respiratory patterns.

PATIENT/FAMILY TEACHING

Purpose of medication is to improve blood flow through brain tissue. • Immediately report severe headache pain, sudden change in alertness. • May cause dizziness; use caution, change positions slowly.

AVAILABLE FORMS

Capsules

---

nitroglycerin
(nye-troe-gli'ser-in)
SL: Nitrostat
IV
Nitro-Bid, Nitrol,
Nitrostat, Tridil
Ointment
Nitro-Bid, Nitrol
Transdermal
Deponit, Minitran,
Nitrocine, Nitro-Dur
**Sustained-release
tablets**
Nitro-Bid, Nitrocine
Timecaps, Nitrong

Classifications: Antianginal,
vasodilator, nitrate

USUAL DOSE

Adjust dose carefully to individual response. Always use lowest effective dose.
SL, adults: Acute angina: 1 tablet (0.15-0.6 mg) dissolved under tongue at onset of anginal attack; if symptoms not relieved, may repeat q5min up to total of 3 tablets in 15 min • Angina prophylaxis: 1 tablet dissolved under tongue 5-10 min before activity associated with angina
IV, cont inf, adults: Initially, 5-10 μg/min; increase by 5-10 μg/min q5-10min until angina subsides or patient becomes hypotensive. • Some patients with low-normal PCWP may respond to very low doses (e.g., ≤5 μg). • Maxmium dose not established, although doses >200 μg/min likely to cause hypotension without increase in effectiveness • Use non-PVC administration sets. If PVC administration sets must be used, anticipate signifi-

cant absorption/higher dosage requirements, particularly when beginning infusion.
Ointment, adults: 1-2 inches (25-50 mm) q8h • Maximum dose, 5 inches (125 mm) q3-6h
Transdermal, adults: 0.2-0.4 mg/hr unit applied for 10-12 hr/day • Maximum dose, 0.8 mg/hr for 10-12 hr/day
PO, sust rel, adults: 2.5-2.6 mg 3-4 times daily; may increase slowly as needed to control symptoms • Tolerance requiring dose adjustment may develop. Up to 26 mg/day has been used.
Transmucosal (buccal), sust rel, adults: 1-3 mg between cheek and gum q4-6h while awake
Translingual aerosol spray, adults: Acute angina: 1-2 sprays (0.4-0.8 mg, respectively) under or onto tongue at onset of anginal attack; if symptoms not relieved, may repeat q5min up to total of 3 sprays (1.2 mg) in 15 min • Angina prophylaxis: 1 spray 5-10 min before activity associated with angina

ADMINISTRATION

SL: Place tablet under tongue until completely dissolved.
IV, cont inf: Titrate by 5-μg/min increments (3 ml/hr 100 μg/ml concentration) q3-5min until angina subsides or patient becomes hypotensive. Occasionally, 10-20-μg/min increments may be necessary. • Always use lowest effective dose. • Withhold further increases in dosage if BP decreases precipitously or SBP <90-100 mm Hg • Use rate-controlling device. • Absorbed by many soft plastics, IV filters; if available, use nonabsorbing, non-PVC IV tubing

italic = common side effects **bold** = life-threatening reactions

(e.g., high-density polyethylene). • If special tubing/filter not available, attempt to "saturate" administration set by running 10-15 ml solution through tubing before administering to patient. • Avoid filtering or use special nonabsorbing filter. • See Appendix Q.

Ointment: Remove previous dose. • Carefully measure onto dosing paper; apply to area of skin not covered by hair, taking care to avoid distal extremities, open or irritated skin, calluses. • Spread into thin layer with dosing paper during application. • Do not massage or rub. • Rotate sites to avoid skin irritation. • For accidental skin contact, wash affected area immediately.

Transdermal: Remove previous dose. • Apply to area of skin not covered by hair, taking care to avoid distal extremities, open/irritated skin, calluses. • Use gentle pressure, especially around edges, to apply firmly to skin. • Rotate sites to avoid skin irritation. • Do not bend, cut, or otherwise manipulate unit. • Replace units that are loose or have fallen off. • Leave unit in place for 10-12 hr, then remove for 10-12 hr. • Do not substitute one brand for another; doses may not be equivalent.

Transmucosal (buccal), sust rel: Place under upper tip or between cheek and gum until completely dissolved. • DO NOT PLACE UNDER TONGUE.

Translingual aerosol spray: Spray under or onto tongue; patient should avoid inhalation. • DO NOT SHAKE CANNISTER BEFORE SPRAYING. • Patient should not swallow immediately after spray.

PREPARATION

IV, cont inf: Dilute drug concentrate into compatible solution in GLASS or nonabsorbable container. • Use nonabsorbing, non-PVC IV tubing (e.g., high-density polyethylene), or follow manufacturer's recommendations.

DILUTION	CONCENTRATION
25 mg/250 ml	100 µg/ml
50 mg/250 ml	200 µg/ml
100 mg/250 ml	400 µg/ml

Compatible fluids: D_5W, 0.9% NaCl, prepared combinations of these solutions

ACTIONS

Relaxes vascular smooth muscle, promoting vasodilation; venous dilation greater than arteriolar dilation • Venodilation encourages peripheral pooling of blood volume, thus reducing right/left ventricular filling pressures (preload). • Arteriolar dilation decreases SVR/PVR, reduces resistance to ventricular ejection (afterload). • Myocardial O_2 consumption/workload reduced • Dilation of coronary arteries enhances myocardial perfusion. • ↓ Myocardial O_2 consumption, improved perfusion relieve ischemic chest pain. • Therapeutic doses slightly reduce SBP, DBP, mean BP without compromising coronary arterial perfusion.

PHARMACOKINETICS

ROUTE*	ONSET	PEAK	DURATION
SL	1-3 min	5-15 min	30-60 min
TO	30-60 min	30 min	2-12 hr
TD	30-60 min	CCR†	24 hr
PO	20-45 min	90 min	3-8 hr
IV	1-2 min	2-5 min	3-5 min

DISTRIBUTION

Widely distributed throughout body tissue; 60% protein bound

ELIMINATION

Metabolized in liver, eliminated in urine; half-life 1-4 min

---

*TO, Topical ointment; TD, transdermal; PO is sustained-release tablets.
†Continuous controlled release.

INDICATIONS

Relief of acute angina pectoris • Prevention of anginal attacks when administered before likely precipitating events • Relief of ischemic pain, CHF, or pulmonary edema associated with acute MI • BP reduction in severe hypertension, especially when associated with CAD, acute left ventricular failure • Control of perioperative hypertension, particularly with CV procedures

Unlabeled/investigational:

To facilitate venous cannulation in children <1 yr; with variceal bleeding to counteract cardiotoxic effects of IV pitressin, ↓ portal pressure

PRECAUTIONS/ CONTRAINDICATIONS

Precautions: Orthostatic hypotension, cerebral hypoperfusion common • >15% reduction in DBP may precipitate myocardial ischemia, angina pectoris. • Severe hypotension, bradycardia have been reported when used in first 24 hr of acute MI. • Angina associated with hypertrophic cardiomyopathy may be worsened by nitrates. • Tolerance to drug effects, cross-tolerance to other nitrates may develop with long-term repeated use; short-acting preparations less likely to cause tolerance • Gradually withdraw therapy to avoid exacerbation of angina. • **Transdermal:** May burn patient, damage paddles if not removed before cardioversion/defibrillation

Use caution with: Acute MI; may cause severe hypotension, bradycardia • Hypovolemia • Hypotension • Severe renal/hepatic impairment • **Children:** Safety/efficacy not established

Pregnancy category: Safety not established; use only if safer alternative unavailable.

Contraindications: Hypersensitivity to nitroglycerin, nitrates • ↑ ICP, inadequate cerebral perfusion • Constrictive pericarditis, pericardial tamponade • Severe hypotension • Severe anemia • **Long-acting forms:** Not indicated for use during acute MI • PO, sust rel: Do not use in patients with GI hypomotility or partial obstruction. **Transdermal/topical/sust rel PO:** Not indicated for management of acute angina pectoris

ADVERSE EFFECTS

CNS: *Headache, dizziness,* weakness, restlessness, confusion, insomnia, twitching, uncoordination
EENT: Blurred vision, diplopia
Resp: Bronchitis, pneumonia, possible dyspnea
CV: **Hypotension,** *orthostatic hypotension,* ↑ **chest pain/pressure,** *tachycardia,* paradoxical bradycardia, dysrhyth-

N

---

italic = common side effects   **bold** = life-threatening reactions

mias, syncope, rebound hypertension

GI: *Nausea,* vomiting, diarrhea, abdominal pain, bowel incontinence

GU: Urinary frequency, incontinence, dysuria, impotence

Derm: Sweating, flushing, rash, pruritus

Local: Redness/vesicles in contact area (ointments, transdermal units)

Misc: *Burning sensation in contact area* (sublingual); tolerance to this drug, cross-tolerance to other nitrates/nitrites; **methemoglobinemia** (rare)

TOXICITY/OVERDOSE

Symptoms: Hypotension, flushing, diaphoresis • Tachycardia, paradoxical bradycardia, heart block, circulatory collapse • ↑ ICP with confusion, fever • Methemoglobinemia: acidosis, cyanosis, coma, seizures; death possible

Management: After recent ingestion, implement guidelines for management of acute overdose (Appendix I). • Support breathing as needed with O_2 and/or mechanical ventilation. • **Hypotension:** Stop or slow infusion. Elevate legs, administer IV fluids; if unresponsive to fluid replacement, use vasopressors (e.g., norepinephrine, dopamine). Inotropic agents (e.g., dobutamine, dopamine) may be used to stimulate contractility. Avoid epinephrine, which is ineffective in correcting hypotension. • Bradycardia, heart block: Manage according to ACLS guidelines (Appendix P).

INTERACTIONS

alcohol Profound hypotension; CV collapse

calcium channel blockers Profound hypotension

epinephrine Unopposed beta effects (tachycardia, hypotension)

ergot alkaloids ↓ Coronary vasodilation

heparin ↓ Heparin effects; check PTT when nitroglycerin added/discontinued

hypotensive agents Profound hypotension

phenothiazines Profound hypotension

Y-SITE COMPATIBILITIES

Amiodarone, amrinone, atracurium, diltiazem, dobutamine, dopamine, famotidine, heparin, lidocaine, nitroprusside, pancuronium bromide, ranitidine, streptokinase, vecuronium

Y-SITE INCOMPATIBILITIES

Alteplase, hydralazine, phenytoin

PATIENT CARE IMPLICATIONS

• Correct hypovolemia before administration.

• Patient must be supine before administering rapid-onset formulations (e.g., SL, IV, transmucosal, buccal, aerosol).

• If headache develops, administer acetaminophen or other prescribed analgesic. Do not lower dose of nitroglycerin. Consult physician for severe or persistent headache.

• Generally, antianginal effects occur before hemodynamic effects.

• Protect patient from injury associated with falls caused by orthostatic hypotension.

• Lower dose, use extreme caution when administering to patients with ethanol intoxication.

P pediatric   **G** geriatric   **V** Direct IV

• Gradually reduce dose to avoid rebound hypertension, increased angina.

• Commercial preparations contain stabilizers to reduce explosive risk.

• See Usual Dose/Administration for specific requirements associated with various routes of administration. • **SL:** Store tablets in original container, close tightly after each use. Label bottle when opened, replace after 6 mo. • **Transdermal:** Remove for 10-12 hr each day to decrease incidence of tolerance. Use beta-blockers or calcium channel blockers as necessary during rest periods to control symptoms. Remove transdermal unit before defibrillation/cardioversion to avoid injury to patient or damage to equipment. **Vital signs/hemodynamics: IV, SL, translingual, buccal:** Monitor BP, HR q3-5min until stable. For hypotension with IV infusion, reduce rate or stop infusion; consult physician for hypotension not immediately responsive to rate adjustment. With other routes, elevate legs, administer IV fluids, hold next dose until stable. • **IV, acute MI:** Continuously monitor for ECG. Report new ST segment depression/elevation or T wave inversion, serious dysrhythmias.

• Continuous hemodynamic monitoring recommended with acute MI, severe CHF, cardiogenic shock, hemodynamic instability; note filling pressures (e.g., CVP, PCWP), SVR; titrate IV nitroglycerin to optimize CO/CI. **Physical assessment:** Assess for perfusion/oxygenation deficit: chest discomfort, breathing difficulty, ↓ level of consciousness, activity intolerance, hypotension, dizziness. • Assess for CHF/pulmonary edema: bibasilar crackles (rales), S_3 gallop, neck vein distention, peripheral edema, breathing difficulty.

• Check peripheral pulses hourly if used to enhance peripheral perfusion.

PATIENT/FAMILY TEACHING

Purpose of drug is to relieve angina pectoris and/or lower BP.

• May cause headaches; take acetaminophen or other prescribed analgesic as needed.

• May cause dizziness, low BP, especially during initiation of therapy; use caution when changing positions, walking. Alcohol, hot weather, vigorous activity, prolonged standing make these symptoms more likely.

• Lie down immediately if lightheaded or dizzy.

Outpatient: Do not skip doses even if feeling better. Do not stop taking without notifying physician. Sudden cessation may trigger angina. Consult pharmacist or physician before using other brands or formulations. • Do not consume alcohol while taking this drug. • Use SL tablets or other rapid-acting nitroglycerin to relieve symptoms of acute angina. • **SL:** Use under tongue only. Do not swallow whole. Dry mouth decreases absorption of drug. Use when seated or lying down. Immediately contact EMS, notify physician if pain unrelieved by total of 3 tablets taken at 5-min intervals. Store tablets in original container, close tightly after each use. Replace after 6 mo.

• **Transdermal:** See Administration, transdermal. Bathing and swimming do not affect

unit. Physical activity, warm body temperature may cause more rapid release of medicine.
• **PO, sust rel:** Take before meals. Do not break, crush, chew, which could result in overdose, dangerous effects.
• **Transmucosal:** Place between cheek and gums, allow tablet to dissolve over 3-5 hr. Do not chew or swallow whole. Hot liquids, manipulation of tablet with tongue increase rate of absorption. • **Translingual:** Spray under or onto tongue; avoid inhalation. DO NOT SHAKE CANNISTER BEFORE SPRAYING. Do not swallow immediately after spray.

AVAILABLE FORMS

Parenteral for IV infusion • Premixed IV infusion • SL tablets • Ointment, transdermal systems for topical use • PO tablets, capsules • Transmucosal (buccal) sustained-release tablets • Translingual aerosol spray

nitroprusside sodium
(nye-troe-pruss'ide)
Nipride, Nitropress

Classifications: Antihypertensive, vasodilator

USUAL DOSE

Adjust dose carefully to individual response. Always use lowest effective dose.
P **IV, cont inf, adults/children:** Initially 0.3 µg/kg/min (e.g., 6 ml/hr of 200 µg/ml [50 mg/250 ml] concentration for 70-kg patient); increase by small increments q2-3min until BP controlled. • Monitor daily serum thiocyanate concentrations for

infusion rates >3 µg/kg/min.
• Do not exceed rates of 10 µg/ kg/min; use this for very brief therapy (<10 min), and only if essential. • **Severe renal impairment:** 0.3 µg/kg/min; increase by small increments q2-3min until BP controlled. Maintain infusion rate <1 µg/ kg/min. Monitor serum thiocyanate concentrations.

ADMINISTRATION

IV, cont inf: Titrate by small increments every 2-3 min until BP controlled. • Use infusion pump. • See Infusion Rate Tables, Appendix Q.

PREPARATION

IV, cont inf: Reconstitute immediately before use. Dilute powder in vial with 2-3 ml D_5W or sterile water for injection without preservatives. Further dilute according to desired concentration:

DILUTION	CONCENTRATION
50 mg/250 ml	200 µg/ml
100 mg/250 ml	400 µg/ml
200 mg/250 ml	800 µg/ml

Compatible fluids: D_5W
Stability: Reconstituted solution stable for 24 hr if protected from light • Use light-resistant covering over IV bottle/bag (e.g., opaque plastic, aluminum foil) to protect solution. • Usual appearance is light brown; exposure to light causes solution to discolor, degrade. • Do not use discolored solutions.

ACTIONS

Relaxes vascular smooth muscle, promotes vasodilation • Effects more profound in hypertensive than normotensive patients • Lowers both arterial, venous BP; reduces preload, afterload • No direct effect on myocardium but may dilate coronary arteries • Effects on CO depend on BP, hydration, cardiac status; hypertensive patients have slightly ↓ CO, whereas heart failure/acute MI patients usually have slightly ↑ CO. • Myocardial O_2 demand reduced • Promotes renal vasodilation without increase in renal blood flow • Effects not inactivated by adrenergic blockers or vagotomy

PHARMACOKINETICS

ROUTE	ONSET	PEAK	DURATION
IV	Immed	1-2 min	1-10 min

DISTRIBUTION

Widely distributed

ELIMINATION

Metabolized by erythrocytes, other tissue; eliminated in urine; half-life 2 min

INDICATIONS

Rapid reduction of BP in hypertensive crises; consistently effective even in refractory hypertension; provides excellent control of BP within desired range by titration • To produce controlled hypotension during surgery to reduce blood loss • To reduce afterload, improve CO in patients with acute congestive heart failure, often in conjunction with positive inotropic agents (e.g., dopamine, dobutamine). Venodilation and preload reduction result in ↓ ventricular filling pressures and additional beneficial effects.

PRECAUTIONS/ CONTRAINDICATIONS

Precautions: Sudden, severe drop in BP possible; close monitoring of BP, HR required • Metabolized to cyanide/thiocy-anate, which may be toxic or lethal • Methemoglobinemia, impaired O_2 extraction may develop. • Controlled hypotension during surgery may affect ventilation/perfusion ratio.• **Renal impairment:** Dosages >4 µg/kg/min, prolonged therapy increase risk of toxicity.

Use caution with: Renal/hepatic impairment • Hypothyroidism • Hyponatremia • Low vitamin B_{12} level • Metabolic acidosis, drug tolerance; consider alternative therapy • Pre-existing ↑ ICP; may ↑ ICP, extreme caution indicated • Young healthy males; higher doses required

c Pregnancy category: Safe use not established

Contraindications: Hypersensitivity to nitroprusside • Compensatory hypertension (e.g., arteriovenous shunt, coarctation of aorta) • During surgery when cerebral circulation inadequate

ADVERSE EFFECTS

CNS: *Headache, dizziness,* weakness, apprehension, restlessness, hyperreflexia, twitching, **seizures, ↑ ICP, CVA**
EENT: Tinnitus, blurred vision
Resp: Nasal stuffiness, tachypnea (with acidosis)
CV: *Hypotension,* tachycardia, paradoxical bradycardia, ECG changes, palpitations, **angina, MI**
GI: Nausea, vomiting, abdominal pain
GU: Increased creatinine
Derm: Flushing, rash
Local: Injection site irritation, venous streaking
Misc: Decreased platelet aggregation, **methemoglobinemia, thiocyanate toxicity**

---

italic = common side effects   **bold** = life-threatening reactions

TOXICITY/OVERDOSE

Symptoms: Acute: Severe hypotension, tachycardia, diaphoresis, paradoxical bradycardia, ischemic ECG changes, impaired perfusion of vital organs
• **Methemoglobinemia:** More likely with dose >4 μg/kg/min or prolonged therapy (>2-3 days); results in acidosis, cyanosis, coma, seizures, death
• **Early cyanogen toxicity:** Increasing tolerance to hypotensive effects, abdominal pain, metabolic acidosis, dyspnea, confusion, venous hyperoxemia (impaired O_2 extraction resulting in bright-red venous blood)
• **Late cyanogen toxicity:** Coma, diminished pulse, absent reflexes, dilated pupils, distant heart sounds, shallow breathing, pink skin color
Management: Slow or stop infusion. • Support breathing as needed with O_2 and/or mechanical ventilation. • **Hypotension:** Elevate legs, administer IV fluids; consider other causes if not improved within minutes. • **Cyanogen toxicity:** Administer 100% O_2. Initially, amyl nitrite inhal; as soon as available, infuse 4-6 mg/kg 3% sodium nitrite solution over 2-4 min; follow with 10% or 25% sodium thiocyanate at 150-200 mg/kg (approx 50 ml 25% solution for average adult); may repeat sodium nitrite/sodium thiocyanate at half original dose in 2 hr. • Hemodialysis is ineffective for removal of cyanogen but effective for thiocyanate.

INTERACTIONS

antihypertensives, calcium channel blockers, ganglionic blockers (e.g., reserpine), general anesthetics, negative inotropic agents (e.g., diltiazem, propranolol) Additive hypotension

INCOMPATIBILITIES

Solution reacts to even very small quantities of other substances. Mix only in D_5W. Do not mix with or infuse with other drugs or solutions. If using heparinized venous access device, flush thoroughly before initiating infusion.

PATIENT CARE IMPLICATIONS

• Correct hypovolemia before administration.
• Patient must remain in bed with appropriate safety precautions throughout administration. Assist patient with initial ambulation.
• Symptoms of cyanogen toxicity (see Toxicity/Overdose) are more likely with high doses (>3-4 μg/kg/min), prolonged therapy, renal impairment, but may develop within few hours of initiating therapy.
• Convert to PO, other antihypertensive therapy as soon as possible. Gradually reduce dose to avoid rebound hypertension.
Vital signs/hemodynamics: Initially, monitor BP continuously, preferably via arterial pressure tracing. When stable, monitor BP, HR at 5–15-min intervals. For hypotension, reduce rate or stop infusion, elevate legs. Consult physician for hypotension not immediately responsive to rate adjustment.
• Continuously monitor ECG, noting tachycardia, bradycardia, ECG changes. • Hemodynamic monitoring necessary with acute MI, severe CHF, cardiogenic

---

shock, concurrent use of positive inotropic agents (e.g., dopamine); note filling pressures (e.g., CVP, PCWP), SVR; titrate agents to optimize CO/CI.
• Consider continuous pulse oximetry to evaluate O_2 saturation. Progressive clinical signs of impaired O_2 delivery without change in O_2 saturation may indicate methemoglobinemia; consult physician immediately.
Physical assessment: Assess for perfusion/oxygenation deficit; chest discomfort, shortness of breath, ↓ level of consciousness, confusion, dizziness. • Assess for CHF/pulmonary edema: bibasilar crackles (rales), S_3 gallop, neck vein distention, peripheral edema, breathing difficulty. • Monitor neurologic status for signs of ↑ ICP: ↓ level of consciousness, change in breathing patterns, widening pulse pressure, bradycardia.
Laboratory tests: Evaluate renal, hepatic, hematologic status before initiating therapy. In hypertensive crisis, samples may be drawn immediately while starting therapy. • Monitor ABGs, electrolytes; evaluate acid-base balance because metabolic acidosis is early sign of cyanogen toxicity. • Monitor thiocyanate/cyanogen levels daily with renal/hepatic impairment or prolonged/high infusion rates (>2 µg/kg/min).

PATIENT/FAMILY TEACHING

Purpose of drug is to lower BP and/or reduce cardiac workload. • May cause dizziness, low BP; do not attempt to get out of bed. • Immediately report chest discomfort, breathing difficulty, dizziness, muscle twitching.

AVAILABLE FORMS

Parenteral for IV infusion

nizatidine
(nye-zat'i-deen)
Axid

Classification: Histamine H_2 antagonist

USUAL DOSE

PO, adults: 300 mg once daily hs or 150 mg bid • **Maintenance:** 150 mg once daily hs • **Renal impairment:** Reduce dose and/or frequency according to creatinine clearance.

ACTIONS

Inhibits action of histamine on H_2 receptors of parietal cells, thus reducing gastric acid secretion • Reduces basal, nocturnal, stimulated gastric acid secretion • Decreases in volume of gastric juice result in ↓ pepsin secretion. • No antiandrogenic effects • Less likely than cimetidine, ranitidine to interact with other medications • Not an anticholinergic

PHARMACOKINETICS

ROUTE	ONSET	PEAK	DURATION
PO	≤1 hr	0.5-3 hr	4-12 hr
ELIMINATION			

Partially metabolized, excreted in urine; half-life 1-2 hr, prolonged with renal impairment

INDICATIONS

Short-term treatment of active gastric, duodenal ulcers to reduce pain, promote healing • In reduced doses to prevent ulcer recurrence • Short-term relief of gastroesophageal reflux, esophagitis • GI reflux

---

italic = common side effects   **bold** = life-threatening reactions

PRECAUTIONS/
CONTRAINDICATIONS

Use caution with: Renal dysfunction; dosage reduction indicated

c Pregnancy category: Safety not established; use only if safer alternative unavailable.

Contraindications: Hypersensitivity to nizatidine, other histamine H_2 blockers • Children: Safety/effectiveness not established

ADVERSE EFFECTS

CNS: *Headache, dizziness, drowsiness,* reversible mental confusion

GI: Nausea, ↑ bilirubin/liver enzymes

Hema: Thrombocytopenia

Derm: *Sweating,* itching, rash

Misc: Fever, hyperuricemia, **anaphylaxis** (rare)

TOXICITY/OVERDOSE

Symptoms: No data available on overdose in humans

Management: After recent ingestion, implement guidelines for management of acute overdose (Appendix I). • Initiate appropriate symptomatic/supportive measures. • Hemodialysis is not likely to be helpful.

INTERACTIONS

antacids ↓ Nizatidine absorption

ketoconazole ↓ Ketoconazole absorption

PATIENT CARE
IMPLICATIONS

• Do not administer within 1 hr of antacids.

Vital signs/hemodynamics: Monitor BP, HR for orthostatic changes in acutely ill patients.

Physical assessment: Assess for epigastric/abdominal pain. Consult physician for persistent or severe pain. • Monitor for evidence of GI bleeding: occult blood in emesis/stool, orthostatic changes.

Laboratory tests: Monitor: Liver enzymes, total bilirubin • CBC with differential • May cause: False-positive test for urobilinogen

PATIENT/FAMILY TEACHING

Purpose of medication is to reduce stomach acid. • May cause drowsiness, mental confusion; use caution, avoid activities requiring mental alertness until response to therapy established. • Smoking decreases effectiveness; smoking cessation programs/therapy recommended.

Outpatient: Take all doses as prescribed, even if feeling better. • Report black tarry stools, blood in stools/emesis, dizziness, changes in mentation to caregiver. • Avoid coffee, caffeine, alcohol, aspirin, ibuprofen, other food or drugs that may cause gastric irritation.

AVAILABLE FORMS

Capsules

norepinephrine bitartrate
(nor-ep-in-ef'rin)
Levarterenol, Levophed

Classifications: Sympathomimetic, vasopressor

USUAL DOSE

IV, cont inf, adults: Initially 0.5-2 µg/min; titrate q2-3min to maintain BP • Range, 2-12 µg/

P pediatric   **G** geriatric   **V** Direct IV

min; higher doses may be necessary. Concurrent administration of low dose dopamine (1-2 µg/kg/min) recommended in ACLS guidelines to preserve renal blood flow

P IV, cont inf, children: 1-2 µg/min; titrate q2-3min to maintain BP.

ADMINISTRATION

IV, cont inf: Titrate in small increments q2-3min to maintain desired SBP or mean BP (usually SBP ≥90 or mean ≥60).
• Always use lowest effective dose to avoid dysrhythmias, ↓ UO, organ ischemia. • Administer via central, antecubital, or other large vein. • Infusion pump is necessary. • See Appendix Q.

PREPARATION

DILUTION	CONCENTRATION
4 mg/500 ml	8 µg/ml
4 mg/250 ml	16 µg/ml
8 mg/250 ml	32 µg/ml

May add 5-10 mg phentolamine and/or 1,000 U heparin to infusion solution to protect against complications of extravasation thrombosis.

Compatible fluids: D_5W, D_5W with NaCl or LR; must be diluted in dextrose-containing solution to prevent loss of potency

ACTIONS

Potent naturally occurring catecholamine that produces peripheral venous/arterial vasoconstriction, cardiac stimulation • Cardiac stimulatory (beta-1) effects similar to epinephrine but much more potent vascular vasoconstrictive (alpha-1) effects; relatively little effect on beta-2 receptors • **CV/hemodynamics:** Alpha-1 stimulation increases SVR, SBP, DBP. Beta-1 stimulation increases HR, myocardial contractility. Rate-increasing effects usually overcome by vagal activity/reflex bradycardia occurring in response to ↑ arterial pressure. Positive inotropic effects may ↑ contractility, but ↑ SVR increases afterload, resulting in little change or ↓ CO, especially with heart failure. ↑ Myocardial O_2 demand can exacerbate myocardial ischemia, especially if coronary vasoconstriction induced by stimulation of coronary alpha receptors. Reduces circulating plasma volume, especially with prolonged use, because of postcapillary vasoconstriction, extracellular third spacing • **Pulmonary vasculature:** Produces pulmonary vasoconstriction, ↑ PAPs; may block hypoxic pulmonary vasoconstrictor responses, ↑ shunt fraction, and contribute to hypoxemia • **Other:** ↓ Renal, splanchnic, skin, skeletal muscle blood flow. Local vasoconstriction with possible hemostasis, necrosis. ↑ Glycogenolysis, ↓ insulin release; may result in mild hyperglycemia. Body temperature, O_2 consumption increased

PHARMACOKINETICS

ROUTE	ONSET	PEAK	DURATION
IV	Immed	1-2 min	1-2 min

DISTRIBUTION

Concentrates in sympathetic nervous tissue; does not cross blood-brain barrier

ELIMINATION

Rapidly metabolized in nervous tissue, excreted in urine

INDICATIONS

Short-term support of BP in low-resistance hypotension/

N

shock, including anesthesia, blood reactions, drug reactions, allergic reactions, pheochromocytomectomy, septicemia, sympathectomy, during cardiac arrest • In patients with ischemic heart disease, use only if refractory to other agents, because myocardial O_2 consumption increases, and ischemia is exacerbated. • For short-term use only until underlying abnormality corrected • Low-dose dopamine used concurrently to counteract renal vasoconstriction

PRECAUTIONS/ CONTRAINDICATIONS

Precautions: Used in hypovolemic states only as temporizing measure to maintain blood flow to vital organs until fluid volume replacement achieved • With severe vasoconstriction, norepinephrine may be ineffective, cause additional damage to vital organs because of ↓ blood flow • Drug-related ↑ in myocardial workload may lead to imbalance between myocardial O_2 supply/demand. • Hemodynamic monitoring should be initiated as soon as possible to assess changes in PCWP, SVR, CO. • May block hypoxic pulmonary vasoconstrictor responses, increase shunt fraction, contribute to hypoxemia • If extravasation occurs, tissue necrosis/sloughing may result; area should be infiltrated with phentolamine; see Appendixes K and L. • Commercial preparations may contain sulfites, which can cause serious allergic reactions.
Use caution with: Hyperthyroidism • Cardiogenic shock, acute MI, CHF, cardiomyopathy, any condition associated with severely compromised myo-

cardial function • Concurrent digitalis glycoside therapy; increased likelihood of dysrhythmias • Hypoxia, hypercapnia, acidosis; ↓ effectiveness, ↑ dysrhythmias are possible
c Pregnancy category: Reduces uterine blood flow; use only if necessary and safer alternative unavailable.
Contraindications: Mesenteric/peripheral vessel thrombosis, except as urgent life-saving measure • Significant hypovolemia • Profound hypoxia, hypercapnia • Cyclopropane, halothane anesthesia

ADVERSE EFFECTS

CNS: Headache, restlessness, tremor, weakness, dizziness, anxiety
Resp: Dyspnea, **apnea**
CV: *Increased peripheral resistance,* reflex bradycardia, hypertension, tachycardia, ↓ CO, dysrhythmias, **ventricular tachycardia/fibrillation,** chest pain, splanchnic/renal vasoconstriction
GU: Oliguria, renal failure
Endo: Hyperglycemia
Derm: Sloughing/necrosis at infusion site
Misc: Tissue hypoxia, lactic acidosis, 3rd spacing/plasma volume depletion, fever

TOXICITY/OVERDOSE

Symptoms: Severe hypertension, ↑ peripheral vascular resistance, reflex bradycardia, ↓ CO • Dysrhythmias
Management: Reduce infusion rate or discontinue until condition stabilizes. • Correct fluid/electrolyte imbalances.
• Dysrhythmias: Manage according to ACLS guidelines (Appendix P). • Short duration

of action; other treatment usually not necessary.

INTERACTIONS

amphetamines Potentiates pressor effects

anesthetics Dysrhythmias

antihistamines Potentiates pressor effects

atropine Potentiates pressor effects

beta-blockers Blocks cardiac stimulating effects; ↑ pressor effects

bretylium Dysrhythmias

digitalis glycosides Dysrhythmias

guanethidine Potentiates pressor effects

MAO inhibitors Potentiates pressor effects

phenytoin Bradycardia, hypotension; risk of seizures

phentolamine ↓ Pressor effects

sympathomimetics Dysrhythmias

TCAs Potentiates pressor effects

COMPATIBILITIES

Amiodarone, amrinone, diltiazem, famotidine, haloperidol, heparin, potassium chloride, vitamin B complex with C

INCOMPATIBILITIES

Aminophylline, amobarbital, cephalothin, lidocaine, pentobarbital, phenobarbital, sodium bicarbonate, thiopental, any highly alkaline solution

PATIENT CARE IMPLICATIONS

• Correct hypovolemia before initiating therapy; in emergencies may be administered in hypovolemic state with simultaneous fluid volume replacement.

• Infuse via central, antecubital, or other large vein. Avoid using veins in hands, ankles, legs.

• Monitor for/correct hypoxemia, hypercapnia, acidosis before and during drug administration.

• Monitor for significant dysrhythmias, hypertension, chest pain, other anginal symptoms, ECG evidence of ischemia. Consult physician for positive findings.

• May add 5-10 mg phentolamine and/or 1,000 U heparin to infusion solution to protect against thrombosis, complications of extravasation.

• Decrease dose gradually to avoid abrupt, severe hypotension; correct hypovolemia before weaning.

Vital signs/hemodynamics: Monitor BP, HR q2min initially and q5-15min thereafter according to titration schedule, stability; continuous arterial pressure monitoring preferred for BP measurements, because severe peripheral vasoconstriction can result in inaccurate auscultatory pressures. • Continuously monitor ECG for dysrhythmias, ischemic changes: T wave inversion, ST segment depression/elevation. • Establish clear parameters for titration (e.g., desired BP, CO, UO). Use lowest possible dose to achieve desired effect. • Monitor CO, PCWP, CVP, SVR frequently, immediately correct hypovolemia. Hemodynamic monitoring is necessary in patients with any condition associated with severely compromised myocardial function. • Monitor UO; consult physician if ≤5 ml/kg/hr or ≤30 ml/hr.

Physical assessment: Assess for perfusion/oxygenation deficit: changes in mentation, hypotension, chest discomfort. • Assess patient for ↓ peripheral perfusion: coolness, ↓ pulse intensity, paresthesias, delayed capillary refill. • Check infusion site frequently for signs of extravasation (e.g., blanching along vein pathway, coldness, hardness). If this occurs, change injection site immediately, infiltrate affected area with phentolamine (Appendix L).

Laboratory tests: Monitor: Electrolytes • ABGs • Blood glucose, especially in patients with diabetes

PATIENT/FAMILY TEACHING

Purpose of medication is to increase BP. • Immediately report chest pain or discomfort, palpitations, pain at infusion site.

AVAILABLE FORMS

Parenteral solution for IV infusion

---

nystatin
(nye-stat′in)
Mycostatin, Nadostine ✦,
Nilstat, Nyaderm ✦,
Nystat-Rx

Classification: Antifungal antibiotic

USUAL DOSE

PO, adults: Intestinal candidiasis: 500,000-1 million U tid
Ⓟ **PO, adults/children:** Oral candidiasis: PO suspension, 400,000-600,000 U 4 times daily or PO lozenge, 200,000-400,000 U 4-5 times daily

Ⓟ **PO, infants:** Oral candidiasis: PO suspension, 200,000 U 4 times daily
Topical: Apply cream, ointment, or powder to affected area bid-tid.
Vaginal: 100,000 U tablet inserted high into vagina 1-2 times daily

ACTIONS

Binds with structures in fungal cell membranes, resulting in loss of cellular integrity • Active against *Candida albicans,* other fungi • Poor absorption from GI tract limits usefulness. • Not active against bacteria, viruses, protozoa

INDICATIONS

Topical formulations used in treatment of *C. albicans* infections, including oral candidiasis, vulvovaginal candidiasis, diaper rash • PO formulations used in treatment of intestinal candidiasis

PRECAUTIONS/ CONTRAINDICATIONS

Precautions: Lozenges not for use in young children, obtunded patients, other conditions when risk of improper use exists
Ⓑ **Pregnancy category:** Safety not clearly established
Contraindications: Hypersensitivity to nystatin

ADVERSE EFFECTS

GI: Nausea, vomiting, diarrhea, GI distress
Local: Irritation, contact dermatitis from preservatives in some formulations

---

PATIENT CARE IMPLICATIONS

• If unresponsive to therapy after 14 days, confirm diagnosis by cultures before initiating additional therapy.
Vital signs: Monitor VS for indicators of infection, complications.
Physical assessment: Assess for improvement in primary infection. • Observe for symptoms of irritation with local application.

PATIENT/FAMILY TEACHING

Purpose of drug is to limit growth of infection-causing fungal organisms. • When used for oral candidiasis, hold suspension in mouth, "swish" before swallowing. • Good oral hygiene, including denture care, is important in resolution/prevention of oral infections. • Take all of medication exactly as prescribed. Do not stop taking medicine even if you feel better. Failure to take entire prescription may result in recurrence or additional infection. Do not save or share unused medicine. • Not necessary to interrupt or discontinue vaginal therapy during menstruation; vaginal douches not necessary, may be harmful.

AVAILABLE FORMS

Tablets for PO use • Suspension for PO use • Topical powder, ointment, cream • Vaginal tablets

---

ofloxacin
(o-flox'a-sin)
Floxin

Classification: Fluoroquinolone antibiotic

USUAL DOSE

IV, intermit inf/PO, adults: 200-400 mg q12h • IV used for ≤10 days; convert to PO therapy after 10 days. • **Renal insufficiency:** Reduce dose and/or frequency for creatinine clearance ≤50 ml/min. NOT FOR IM USE

ADMINISTRATION

IV, intermit inf: Infuse prepared solution over 60 min.
• Too-rapid infusion causes hypotension. • Use dilute solution, large vein, small catheter/needle to reduce risk of vein irritation.

PREPARATION

IV, intermit inf: Dilute each 200-mg dose in 50 ml compatible IV solution; dilute 400-mg dose in 100 ml; yields concentration of 4 mg/ml, which is maximum final concentration recommended. • Less concentrated solutions may be used.
• Premixed solution containing 4 mg/ml is available.
Compatible fluids: D_5W, 0.9% NaCl, D_5W and 0.9% NaCl, D_5W, and LR
Stability: Reconstituted solution stable for at least 24 hr at room temperature.

ACTIONS

Bactericidal antibiotic that interferes with bacterial enzyme necessary for DNA replication
• Broad spectrum of activity against many gram-positive bac-

O

teria, gram-negative aerobes • Gram-positive activity includes penicillinase-producing and non–penicillinase-producing staphylococci, most streptococci. • Gram-negative activity includes *Pseudomonas aeruginosa,* most Enterobacteriaceae; gram-negative activity generally less than ciprofloxacin. • Moderate activity against *Mycobacterium tuberculosis, Chlamydia trachomatis, Enterococcus faecalis* • Most anaerobic bacteria resistant

PHARMACOKINETICS

ROUTE	ONSET	PEAK	DURATION
PO	Rapid	30-120 min	Approx 12 hr
IV	Immed	End infusion	12 hr

DISTRIBUTION

Widely distributed; CSF levels variable

ELIMINATION

<10% metabolized, most eliminated in urine; half-life 4-8 hr, slightly longer in **G** older adults

INDICATIONS

Mild to moderate aerobic bacterial infections, particularly when multidrug-resistant organisms involved; often used for skin/bone infections, nosocomial pneumonia, urinary tract infections, prostatitis • Treatment of gonorrhea, *Chlamydia* infection • IV route no more potent than PO, generally reserved for conditions when PO route not feasible
• Not indicated for community-acquired infections (e.g., otitis media, sinusitis, pneumonia) when penicillin or cephalosporin could be used • Not used alone for intraabdominal, other infections involving anaerobic organisms

PRECAUTIONS/CONTRAINDICATIONS

Precautions: Bacterial or fungal overgrowth possible: Urinary crystal formation reported with other quinolones, particularly with high-dose therapy, alkaline urine
Use caution with: Epilepsy, CNS disorders; may precipitate seizures. • Concurrent theophylline therapy, excessive caffeine use; dysrhythmias, seizures, respiratory failure, cardiac arrest reported • Hepatic/renal impairment; reduce dose/frequency
c Pregnancy category: Risk of fetal damage unknown; use only if safer alternative unavailable.
Contraindications: Hypersensitivity to ofloxacin, other quin-**P** olones • Children <18 yr: safety not established

ADVERSE EFFECTS

CNS: Headache, dizziness, insomnia, fatigue, ↑ **ICP** (rare)
GI: *Nausea,* vomiting, diarrhea, abdominal pain, anorexia, ↑ liver enzymes
GU: Vaginitis
Derm: Rash, wheals, itching, photosensitivity, Stevens-Johnson syndrome
Local: Irritation, pain
Misc: Severe hypersensitivity, **anaphylaxis;** superinfection, colonization, joint inflammation, arthralgia

TOXICITY/OVERDOSE

Symptoms: Toxic reactions include vomiting, psychosis, CNS stimulation, seizures. • Severe allergic reactions/anaphylaxis possible
Management: After recent ingestion, implement guidelines for management of acute over-

dose (Appendix I). • Initiate symptomatic/supportive measures, including airway management/ventilation. • For acute allergic reaction, see Appendix K. • Maintain hydration to reduce risk of crystalluria. • Hemodialysis or peritoneal dialysis is not likely to be useful.

INTERACTIONS

aminophylline, theophylline, other xanthines ↑ Theophylline levels; dysrhythmias, seizures; interaction less likely than with other quinolones
antacids ↑ PO absorption
anticoagulants, PO Prolonged PT
iron/mineral supplements Impaired PO absorption; ↓ antibiotic levels
sucralfate Impaired PO absorption; ↓ antibiotic levels

PATIENT CARE IMPLICATIONS

• Obtain specimens for culture and sensitivity before initiating antibiotic therapy. Initiate therapy before results received.
• Have epinephrine, antihistamine, resuscitation equipment readily available for use with severe allergic reaction.
• If concurrent sucralfate, antacid, iron/mineral supplement therapy, stagger schedules to avoid administration within 2 hr of PO ofloxacin.
• If concurrent theophylline therapy, observe for evidence of theophylline toxicity, monitor theophylline levels, adjust dose as necessary; excessive theophylline levels especially likely in older adults. See Theophylline for symptoms of toxicity, therapeutic levels.

• Do not discharge patient for at least 30 min after parenteral antibiotic administration.
Vital signs/hemodynamics: Monitor VS for indicators of infection, complications. • Carefully monitor UO; evaluate I&O ratio. Keep patient well hydrated by PO/parenteral fluids.
Physical assessment: Assess for improvement in primary infection or additional symptoms of infection or sepsis, additional symptoms of infection or sepsis: presence of fever; appearance of sputum, urine, stool, wound drainage; candidiasis, vaginitis.
• Observe for symptoms of hypersensitivity: rash, pruritus, wheezing, laryngeal edema, hypotension.
Laboratory tests: Monitor: Electrolytes • Liver enzymes • PT, PTT • CBC with differential • Urinalysis, BUN, creatinine

PATIENT/FAMILY TEACHING

Purpose of drug is to limit growth of infection-causing bacteria. • Immediately report rash, swelling, intense itching, difficulty breathing, other signs of allergic reaction. • Report diarrhea, fever, vaginal itching or discharge, furry growth on tongue. • Drink plenty of fluids to avoid formation of crystals in urine.
Outpatient: Do not use antacids while taking this medication. • Avoid direct sunlight, wear protective clothing, because severe sunburn possible. • Take at evenly spaced intervals over each 24-hr period. • Take all of medication exactly as prescribed. Do not stop taking medicine even if you feel better. Failure to take all of antibiotic

may result in recurrence or additional infection. Do not save or share unused medicine.

AVAILABLE FORMS
Parenteral for IV use • Tablets

oxazepam
(ox-a'ze-pam)
Serax

Classifications: Benzodiazepine, sedative-hypnotic, antianxiety agent
Schedule IV controlled substance

USUAL DOSE
Individualize dosage, increase cautiously.
PO, adults: Moderate anxiety: 10-15 mg 3-4 times daily; may take larger dose (up to 30 mg) hs • Severe anxiety, acute alcohol withdrawal: 15-30 mg 3-4 times daily
G • Older adults, debilitation: Initially 10 mg tid; may increase cautiously up to 15 mg 3-4 times daily

ACTIONS
Facilitates action of gamma-aminobutyric acid (GABA, major inhibitory neurotransmitter), produces CNS depression • Reduces anxiety, causes mild to moderate sedation, promotes sleep • May result in mild lack of recall • Minimal respiratory depressant effects at usual dose • No analgesic effects

PHARMACOKINETICS

ROUTE	ONSET	PEAK	DURATION
PO	45-90 min	3 hr	6-12 hr

DISTRIBUTION
Wide; crosses blood-brain barrier
ELIMINATION
Metabolized by liver, eliminated by kidneys; half-life 8.2 hr

INDICATIONS
Management of anxiety disorders, anxiety associated with depression; short-term relief of anxiety symptoms • Management of agitation, tremulousness, other symptoms associated with acute alcohol withdrawal

PRECAUTIONS/ CONTRAINDICATIONS
Precautions: Adverse effects more likely in first few days of therapy • Rarely causes hypotension, but more likely in older adults • Serax (15 mg) contains tartrazine dye (FD&C yellow no. 5), may cause allergic response, especially in those with aspirin sensitivity.
G **Use caution with:** Older adults, debilitation, low serum albumin; reduced dose indicated • Presence of other CNS depressants (e.g., opiate analgesics, alcohol, phenothiazines); reduced P dose indicated • Children: Safety/effectiveness not well established
D **Pregnancy category:** Risk of congenital malformations, prolonged CNS depression, withdrawal symptoms in newborn; use only if safer alternative unavailable and risk explained to woman.
Contraindications: Hypersensitivity to oxazepam • Acute angle-closure glaucoma • Acute alcohol intoxication with VS de-

pression • Pregnancy, lactation • Children <6 yr

ADVERSE EFFECTS

CNS: *Drowsiness, dizziness,* headache, tremor, slurred speech, blurred vision, paradoxical excitement, especially in psychiatric patients
CV: Hypotension, edema
GI: Nausea, hepatic dysfunction (rare)
Misc: Leukopenia, tolerance, psychologic/physical dependence

TOXICITY/OVERDOSE

Symptoms (acute toxicity): Somnolence, confusion, coma, diminished reflexes • Hypotension, particularly in older adults • Respiratory depression, particularly if other CNS depressants also ingested • Toxicity more likely with concurrent ingestion of alcohol, other CNS depressants
Management: After recent ingestion, implement guidelines for management of acute overdose (Appendix J). • Maintain airway/support ventilation as necessary. • Administer IV fluids. • Flumazenil is specific antidote and reverses effects.
• Hypotension: Elevate legs, administer IV fluids; use vasopressors (e.g., norepinephrine, dopamine) as necessary. • Do not use barbiturates for paradoxical excitation. • Forced diuresis may be helpful in patients with normal kidney funciton. • Hemodialysis is not generally useful.

INTERACTIONS

alcohol, ethyl ↑ Sedation
antihistamines ↑ Sedation
barbiturates ↑ Sedation
clozapine respiratory depression, apnea
digoxin ↑ Digoxin levels; toxicity; monitor closely
flumazenil ↓ Sedation
levodopa ↓ Antiparkinsonian effectiveness
opiate analgesics ↑ Sedation
probenecid ↑ Sedation
propoxyphene ↑ Sedation

PATIENT CARE IMPLICATIONS

• Adverse effects more likely in first few days of therapy
• Administer with food to reduce gastric irritation.
• Avoid sudden cessation of therapy, especially in patients who have received therapy for several months or longer (may cause withdrawal symptoms).
• Large quantities should not be prescribed for patients with severe depression, suicidal tendencies, history of substance abuse.
Older adults: closely monitor for adverse effects (e.g., impaired psychomotor/mental performance). Assess need for continued therapy periodically.
Physical assessment: Assess neurologic status for excessive sedation, impaired physical coordination.
Laboratory tests: Monitor: Liver enzymes • CBC with differential

PATIENT/FAMILY TEACHING

Purpose of medication is to reduce anxiety, promote relaxation. • Medication may cause drowsiness or dizziness, especially during the first few days of therapy. Use caution with activity until individual effects established. • Cigarette smoking interferes with drug effectiveness. • Inform nurse or physician if you may be pregnant or are considering pregnancy.

Outpatient: Avoid concurrent use of alcohol or other drugs that cause sedation while taking this medication. • Avoid driving and other activities requiring mental alertness or physical coordination until effects of medication established. • This medication may cause psychologic/physical dependence. Consult primary health care provider before increasing dose or abruptly discontinuing. • Take with food if desired to minimize upset stomach.

AVAILABLE FORMS

Tablets, capsules

---

pancuronium bromide
(pan-kyoo-roe′nee-um)
Pavulon

Classification: Nondepolarizing neuromuscular blocking agent (NMBA)

USUAL DOSE

P Direct IV, adults/children: Initially 0.04-0.1 mg/kg; up to 0.16 mg/kg used but may cause severe tachycardia • Maintenance: 0.01-0.015 mg/kg q25-60min as needed for skeletal muscle relaxation • **Major burns:** Resistance to neuromuscular blocking effects usually occurs; ↑ doses may be necessary.

ADMINISTRATION

V Direct IV: Inject each dose over 60-90 sec. • Dilution not necessary • *Causes respiratory depression, paralysis; means for airway management/continuous artificial ventilation must be in place or provided immediately after injection.*

Compatible fluids: D$_5$W, 0.9% NaCl, prepared combinations of these solutions

ACTIONS

Causes skeletal muscle paralysis by interfering with transmission of nerve impulses at neuromuscular junction • Competes with/blocks activity of acetylcholine (neurotransmitter normally producing electrical depolarization) • First muscles affected include eyes, face, neck; followed by limbs, abdomen, chest; diaphragm affected last. Recovery usually occurs in reverse order. • Higher doses may produce ↑ HR because of direct effect on cardiac acetylcholine receptors. • No analgesic/sedative effects

PHARMACOKINETICS

ROUTE	ONSET	PEAK	DURATION
IV	2-3 min	3-6 min	≥45 min*
DISTRIBUTION			
Throughout extracellular fluid			
ELIMINATION			
Minimally metabolized, urinary/biliary excretion; half-life 2 hr			

*Additional doses ↑ duration.

INDICATIONS

Adjunct to general anesthesia to produce skeletal muscle relaxation during surgery • Facilitate ET intubation • Increase lung compliance, facilitate mechanical ventilation in critically ill patients • No effects on consciousness/pain threshold; used only after induction of general anesthesia or with appropriate analgesics/anxiolytics.

Unlabeled/investigational: Control of muscle spasms associated with seizure states when conventional therapy ineffective

PRECAUTIONS/CONTRAINDICATIONS

Precautions: *Causes respiratory paralysis; must use with artificial airway, ventilatory support, O$_2$ administration*
• Long-term use to facilitate mechanical ventilation associated with prolonged paralysis, skeletal muscle weakness
• Burn patients may develop resistance to neuromuscular blocking effects, particularly if burn exceeds 25% body surface area; ↑ doses usually necessary.
Use caution with: Renal insufficiency; delayed excretion results in prolonged neuromuscular blockade. • Liver impairment • Pulmonary impairment, respiratory depression • Advanced age • Debilitation • Myasthenia gravis; extreme caution indicated • Neonates • Electrolyte disturbances, hyperkalemia, digitalization; may cause release of intracellular potassium into plasma or potentiate drug effects
c Pregnancy category: Use only if safer alternative unavailable.
Contraindications: Hypersensitivity to pancuronium, bromides • Tachycardia, conditions in which tachycardia undesired

ADVERSE EFFECTS

CNS: Muscle weakness, **paralysis**
EENT: Excessive salivation
Resp: **Respiratory depression, prolonged apnea, bronchospasm**
CV: *Tachycardia,* hypotension
Misc: Excessive doses may trigger histamine release with erythema, wheals, itching, wheezing, bronchospasm, hypotension.

TOXICITY/OVERDOSE

Symptoms: Erythema, wheals, itching • Wheezing, bronchospasm • Hypotension, cardiac dysrhythmias
Management: Provide airway/continuous artificial ventilation
• Neostigmine or pyridostigmine with atropine q5-30min to reverse neuromuscular blockade; may worsen severe overdose
• **Hypotension:** Elevate legs, administer IV fluids; use dopamine if necessary. • Manage cardiac dysrhythmias according to ACLS guidelines (Appendix P).

INTERACTIONS

aminoglycoside antibiotics, amphotericin B, beta-blockers, calcium channel blockers, corticosteroids, diuretics (potassium wasting), lidocaine, magnesium sulfate   Prolonged neuromuscular blockade
opiate analgesics   Respiratory depression

Y-SITE COMPATIBILITIES

Aminophylline, cefazolin, cefuroxine, cimetidine, dobutamine, dopamine, epinephrine, esmolol, fentanyl, gentamicin, heparin, isoproterenol, lorazepam, midazolam, morphine, nitroglycerin, nitroprusside, ranitidine, vancomycin

Y-SITE INCOMPATIBILITIES

Diazepam

PATIENT CARE IMPLICATIONS

• Drug has no effect on consciousness/pain threshold; pa-

tient is fully awake, feels all sensations. *Use only with general anesthesia or analgesics (e.g., morphine)/anxiolytics (e.g., diazepam, midazolam).*
• *Causes respiratory depression, paralysis; use only for intubated patients with continuous mechanical ventilation.*
• Prevent corneal drying by instillation of artificial tears, eye patching.
• Cholinesterase inhibitors such as neostigmine, pyridostigmine, edrophonium used to reverse effects; multiple doses may be necessary.
• Long-term use with mechanical ventilation associated with prolonged paralysis, skeletal muscle weakness. Monitor closely; use lowest effective dose.
• Patients thought to have recovered from neuromuscular blockade may develop apnea when given certain drugs that potentiate pancuronium (see Interactions).
• Avoid administration until after succinylcholine effects subside.
Vital signs/hemodynamics: Monitor ECG continuously. Observe for tachycardia, dysrhythmias. • Monitor BP, observing for hypotension, q3-5min during initiation of therapy and frequently thereafter. • Use continuous pulse oximetry to monitor oxygenation immediately after extubation and until stable
• Monitor I&O; Foley catheter required.
Physical assessment: Closely monitor respiratory status: rate, depth, pattern of ventilation, until fully recovered. Secretions may be increased; suction as necessary. • Use peripheral

nerve stimulator to monitor effectiveness of NMBAs. Paralysis of muscle groups usually occurs in following order: eyelids, jaws, limbs, abdomen, glottis, intercostals, diaphragm. Recovery occurs in reverse order. Assess frequently for residual muscle weakness, respiratory distress until fully recovered from effects.
Laboratory tests: Monitor potassium closely, because drug may cause release of intercellular potassium into plasma; severe hyperkalemia likely to occur with electrolyte disturbances, digitalization, major trauma, burns, spinal cord injury, degenerative muscle disorders, paraplegia. • Hypermagnesemia may block release of acetylcholine, potentiate effects of NMBAs. • Hypocalcemia may increase muscle excitability, potentiate effects of NMBAs.

PATIENT/FAMILY TEACHING

Purpose of medication is to paralyze body muscles temporarily to facilitate procedures, surgery.
• When recovering from effects, it may be difficult to swallow, talk; these effects temporary.
• Drug does not affect consciousness; explain all procedures, provide information/emotional support, remind family to communicate with patient.

AVAILABLE FORMS

Parenteral for IV injection
Storage: Refrigerated storage recommended for optimal stability; stable for 6 mo at room temperature; do not store in plastic syringes.

penicillin G benzathine
(pen-i-sill'in ben'za-theen)
Bicillin, L-A

penicillin G benzathine with penicillin G procaine
Bicillin C-R

Classifications: Penicillin antibiotic, natural penicillin

USUAL DOSE
IM, adults: 1.2-2.4 million U as single dose; may be repeated at weekly intervals × 2 for syphilis >1 yr duration.
IM, children 1 mo-12 yr: Given as single IM dose • Weight <27 kg: 300,000-600,000 U. • Weight ≥27 kg: 900,000-1.2 million U

ADMINISTRATION
IM injection: Injected deep into large muscle mass (e.g., gluteus maximus, lateral thigh). • Z-track method recommended • Inject slowly; withdraw immediately for sudden, severe pain. • Use caution to avoid SC injection, injection near nerve. • Inject large doses at 2 different sites. • **Do not give IV.**

ACTIONS
Bactericidal antibiotic that interferes with bacterial cell wall synthesis/division • Formulation results in slow absorption from muscle tissue, prolonged but lower levels than those resulting from equivalent IM dose of penicillin G potassium. • Good activity against streptococci, including *S. pneumoniae,* group A beta-hemolytic streptococci, non-penicillinase-producing strains of straphylococci • Active against spirochetes, including *Treponema pallidum* (syphilis), some anaerobic bacteria • Activity against some gram-negative aerobes, some anaerobic bacteria

PHARMACOKINETICS

ROUTE	ONSET	PEAK	DURATION
IM	≤1 hr	1-4 hr	21-28 days; slow absorption from muscle tissue

DISTRIBUTION
Widely distributed; CSF levels minimal
ELIMINATION
Very slow elimination via urine; half-life 30-60 min

INDICATIONS
Wide variety of infections, including pneumococcal pneumonia, streptococcal pharyngitis, syphilis • Choice agent for treatment of early syphilis (≤1 yr duration) except when neurosyphilis suspected • Rheumatic fever prophylaxis • Follow-up to parenteral therapy with penicillin

PRECAUTIONS/CONTRAINDICATIONS
Precautions: Intravascular injection may cause microemboli, severe vascular damage, gangrene. • Injection into or near nerve may cause permanent neurologic damage, paralysis. **Use caution with:** Hypersensitivity to cephalosporins, other drugs; ↑ risk of allergic reaction • Renal insufficiency; use lower dose/frequency. **B Pregnancy category:** Safety not clearly established; use only if clearly needed.

---

italic = common side effects   **bold** = life-threatening reactions

Contraindications: Hypersensitivity to any penicillin, benzathine

ADVERSE EFFECTS

CNS: Nerve irritation and paralysis, Hoigne's syndrome (rare) —bizarre behavior, anxiety, combativeness, **seizures** immediately after IM injection
GI: *Nausea, vomiting, diarrhea*
GU: Interstitial nephritis
Hema: Eosinophilia, hemolytic anemia, other blood dyscrasias
Derm: *Rash,* wheals, itching
Local: Pain, sterile abscess, severe neurovascular damage with inadvertent vascular or nerve injection
Misc: *Hypersensitivity,* **anaphylaxis,** serum sickness, *Jarisch-Herxheimer reaction*—fever, arthralgia, tachycardia within 2-12 hr after injection in syphilis patients

TOXICITY/OVERDOSE

Symptoms: Within 2-12 hr after initiation of therapy 50%-75% of syphillis patients experience syndrome of fever, arthralgia, tachycardia; attributed to endotoxin release; usually subsides within 12-24 hr; severity of reaction ↓ by corticosteroids
Management: Discontinue drug. • Initiate symptomatic/supportive measures, including airway protection. • For acute allergic reaction, see Appendix N.

INTERACTION

Probenecid   Higher/prolonged penicillin blood levels

PATIENT CARE IMPLICATIONS

• Obtain specimens for culture and sensitivity before initiating antibiotic therapy. Initiate therapy before results received.
• CSF examination necessary in patients with suspected neurosyphilis, including most HIV-infected individuals; if positive, alternate therapy required.
• Determine previous antibiotic use, including reactions to penicillins, cephalosporins. Cross-reactivity with cephalosporin allergies may occur.
• Have epinephrine, antihistamine, resuscitation equipment readily available for use with severe allergic reaction.
• Do not discharge patient for at least 30 min after administration.
• For IM administration only. Ice packs applied locally reduce pain associated with inadvertent SC injection. Take measures to avoid inadvertent intravascular injection or injection into or near nerve, because serious neurovascular damage may result.
Vital signs: Monitor VS before and 30 min after injection.
Physical assessment: Assess for improvement in primary infection or additional symptoms of infection or sepsis: presence of fever; appearance of sputum, urine, stool, wound drainage; candidiasis, vaginitis. • Observe for symptoms of hypersensitivity; rash, pruritus, wheezing, laryngeal edema, hypotension.
Laboratory tests: Monitor: Culture results; alternate therapy indicated for penicillinase-resistant strains, CSF infections
• **May cause:** Positive direct antiglobulin (Coombs') test

P pediatric   G geriatric   V Direct IV

PATIENT/FAMILY TEACHING

Purpose of drug is to limit growth of infection-causing bacteria. • Immediately report rash, swelling, intense itching, difficulty breathing, other signs of allergic reaction. • Report diarrhea, fever, vaginal itching or discharge, furry growth on tongue, or if symptoms do not improve. • As indicated, return visits for follow-up injections are necessary to prevent infection (rheumatic fever prophylaxis) or recurrence of infection (syphilis ≥1 yr duration).

AVAILABLE FORMS

Parenteral for IM use

---

penicillin G potassium
Pfizerpen
penicillin G sodium

Classification: Penicillin antibiotic

USUAL DOSE

Ⓟ **PO, children 1 mo-12 yr:** 25,000-90,000 U/kg/24 hr in divided doses q4-8h • **Rheumatic fever prophylaxis:** 200,000 U q12h
IV/IM, adults: 10-20 million U/24 hr in divided doses q4-6h; use IV route for doses ≥10 million U. • **Serious infections:** 20-40 million U/24 hr in divided doses q4h • **Renal impairment:** Reduce dose and/or frequency.
Ⓟ **IV/IM, children 1 mo-12 yr:** 25,000-50,000 U/kg/24 hr in divided doses q6h • **Serious infections:** 100,000-400,000 U/kg/24 hr in divided doses q4-6h
PO, adults: 200,000-500,000 U q6-8h or 800,000 U q12h

• **Rheumatic fever prophylaxis:** 200,000-250,000 U q12h

ADMINISTRATION

IM injection: Inject deep into large muscle mass (e.g., gluteus maximus, lateral thigh). • Use IV route for doses ≥10 million U.
IV, intermit inf: Infuse prepared solution over 30-60 min. • Too-rapid infusion may cause dangerous hyperkalemia (penicillin G potassium only). • Use large veins, small catheters to ↓ risk of thrombophlebitis.

PREPARATION

IM: Use sterile water for injection for initial dilution. • Direct stream against side of vial, add slowly while rotating vial. • Shake vigorously to dissolve. • Use volume of diluent as recommended by manufacturer on side of vial to provide desired U/ml. • Concentrations up to 100,000 U/ml used with minimal discomfort • Vials with 10 or 20 million U for IV use only
IV, intermit inf: Reconstitute as for IM injection. • Add to compatible IV solution for slow infusion.
Compatible fluids: D_5W, 0.9% NaCl, RL, prepared combinations of these solutions • Antimicrobial activity may be lost if mixed in peritoneal dialysis fluids.
Stability: Reconstituted solution stable for 24 hr at room temperature

ACTIONS

Bactericidal antibiotic that interferes with bacterial cell wall synthesis/division • Excellent activity against gram-positive cocci, including *Streptococcus*

P

---

italic = common side effects   **bold** = life-threatening reactions

pyogenes, S. pneumoniae, some *S. viridans* • Active against some gram-negative aerobes, including strains of *Neisseria meningitidis,* non–penicillinase-producing *N. gonorrhoeae, Haemophilus influenzae* • Active against some anerobes, including strains of *Bacteroides, Clostridium* • Activity against spirochetes, including *Treponema pallidum* (syphilis), *Bacteroides burgdorferi* (Lyme's disease)

PHARMACOKINETICS

ROUTE	ONSET	PEAK	DURATION
PO	≤30 min	30-60 min	Approx 4-6 hr; dose dependent
IM	Rapid	15-30 min	
IV	Immed	End infusion	

DISTRIBUTION

Widely distributed; CSF levels higher with meningeal inflammation or probenecid administration

ELIMINATION

Primarily excreted in urine; half-life 30-60 min

INDICATIONS

Wide variety of infections, including upper/lower respiratory tract • **PO:** Mild to moderate infections, streptococcal prophylaxis, follow-up after parenteral penicillin • **Parenteral:** Serious infections such as septicemia, meningitis, pericarditis, endocarditis, severe pneumonia; with aminoglycosides for enterococcal infections; to treat syphilis, clostridial infections, Lyme disease; IV route used for non–penicillinase-producing gonococcal infections

PRECAUTIONS/ CONTRAINDICATIONS

Precautions: Bacterial or fungal overgrowth may occur. • High potassium content of penicillin G potassium may cause potentially fatal dysrhythmias; risk ↑ in renal impairment or with rapid IV administration. • High sodium content of penicillin G sodium may cause edema, electrolyte abnormalities, dysrhythmias and contribute to heart failure. • Some PO preparations contain tartrazine dye (FD&C yellow no. 5), which may cause serious allergic reactions in susceptible individuals.

Use caution with: Hypersensitivity to cephalosporins or other drugs; ↑ risk of allergic reaction • Renal insufficiency; lower dose/frequency; avoid use of penicillin G potassium.

B Pregnancy category: Safety not clearly established; use only if clearly indicated.

Contraindications: Hypersensitivity to any penicillin

ADVERSE EFFECTS

CNS: Nerve irritation/paralysis with IM injection; neurotoxicity (rare)/**seizures,** especially with high dose/renal insufficiency

GI: *Nausea, vomiting, diarrhea,* epigastric pain, oral thrush

GU: Interstitial nephritis, vaginitis

Hema: Eosinophilia, hemolytic anemia, other blood dyscrasias

Derm: *Rash,* wheals, itching

F&E: Hyperkalemia, hypernatremia

Local: IM—*pain,* sterile abscess; IV—phlebitis, thrombophlebitis

Misc: *Hypersensitivity,* **anaphylaxis,** serum sickness; superinfection, colonization; *Jarisch-Herxheimer reaction*—fever, arthralgia, tachycardia within 2-12 hr after injection in syphilis patients

TOXICITY/OVERDOSE

Symptoms: Neurotoxicity, including seizures/coma, particularly with high-dose therapy or renal insufficiency
Management: Discontinue drug. • Initiate symptomatic/supportive measures, including airway management/ventilation. • After recent ingestion, implement guidelines for management of acute overdose (Appendix I). • For acute allergic reaction, see Appendix N. • Hemodialysis is effective in drug removal; minimal removal with peritoneal dialysis.

INTERACTIONS

aminoglycosides (e.g., amikacin, gentamicin) Synergistic antibacterial activity
anticoagulants, PO Prolonged bleeding time with high-dose IV penicillin
diuretics, potassium sparing Hyperkalemia
heparin Prolonged bleeding time with high-dose IV penicillin
potassium supplements ↑ potassium levels
probenecid Higher/prolonged penicillin blood levels

Y-SITE COMPATIBILITIES
Penicillin G potassium:
Amiodarone, diltiazem, enalaprilat, esmolol, fluconazole, heparin, labetalol, lidocaine, magnesium sulfate, meperidine, morphine, potassium chloride, verapamil

Y-SITE INCOMPATIBILITIES
Penicillin G potassium/penicillin G sodium: Aminoglycosides (e.g., amikacin, gentamicin, tobramycin), aminophylline, sodium bicarbonate

PATIENT CARE IMPLICATIONS

• Obtain specimens for culture and sensitivity before initiating antibiotic therapy. Initiate therapy before results received.
• Determine previous antibiotic use, including reactions to penicillins, cephalosporins. Cross-reactivity with cephalosporin allergies may occur.
• Have epinephrine antihistamine, resuscitation equipment readily available for use with severe allergic reaction.
• Do not discharge patient for at least 30 min after parenteral antibiotic administration.
• High potassium (penicillin G potassium) content may cause electrolyte abnormalities, potentially fatal dysrhythmias.
• High sodium (penicillin G sodium) content may cause edema, electrolyte abnormalities, dysrhythmias and contribute to heart failure.
• To optimize absorption, administer PO dose at least 1 hr before or 2 hr after meals.
• IV route must be used for large doses (≥10 million U), severe infections, or when shock present.
Vital signs: Monitor VS before and 30 min after IV/IM use for possible hypersensitivity reaction. • Monitor I&O for imbalance; older, debilitated, seriously ill, renal-impaired patients at greater risk for nephrotoxicity.

---

italic = common side effects   **bold** = life-threatening reactions

Physical assessment: Assess for improvement in primary infection or additional symptoms of infection or sepsis; presence of fever, appearance of sputum, urine, stool, wound drainage; candidiasis, vaginitis; WBC.

• Observe for symptoms of hypersensitivity: rash, pruritus, wheezing, laryngeal edema, hypotension.

Laboratory tests: Monitor: Electrolytes, BUN, creatinine, CBC with differential (IV or prolonged use) particularly important in patients with renal/cardiac impairment, elderly/debilitated patients • **May cause:** Hypernatremia: monitor for edema, pulmonary crackles • Hyperkalemia: monitor for weakness, paresthesias peaked T wave • Positive direct antiglobulin (Coombs') test

PATIENT/FAMILY TEACHING

Purpose of drug is to limit growth of infection-causing bacteria. • Immediately report rash, swelling, intense itching, difficulty breathing, other signs of allergic reaction. • Report diarrhea, fever, vaginal itching or discharge, furry growth on tongue.

Outpatient: Take medication at least 1 hr before or 2 hr after meals. Take with full glass of water, not fruit juice or other beverage. Take at evenly spaced intervals over each 24-hr period. • Take all of medication exactly as prescribed. Do not stop taking medicine even if you feel better. Failure to take all of antibiotic may result in recurrence or additional infection. Do not save or share unused medicine.

AVAILABLE FORMS

Parenteral for IV/IM use • Premixed solution for IV infusion • Tablets

pentobarbital, pentobarbital sodium
(pen-toe-bar′bi-tal)
Nembutal,
Nova-Rectal ✦,
Pentogen ✦

Classification: Barbiturate, sedative/hypnotic, anticonvulsant, Schedule II controlled substance

USUAL DOSE

Dose is individualized according to specific patient/clinical response. Reduced dose indicated with advanced age, debilitation, renal/hepatic impairment

PO/PR, adults: 100 mg, hs
• **Daytime sedation:** 20 mg 3-4 times daily
IM, adults: 150-200 mg
PO/PR/IM, children: 2-6 mg/kg/day; not to exceed 100 mg/day
Direct IV, adults: Initially, 100 mg over 2 min. After at least 1 min, additional small incremental doses may be given, up to 500 mg.
Direct IV, children: 1-3 mg/kg given over ≥2 min. Do not exceed 100 mg/day.
Therapeutic coma: Patient must be mechanically ventilated. Loading dose: 3-5 mg/kg given at rate of 25-50 mg/min. Maintenance dose: 1.0-3.0 mg/kg/hr. Breakthrough seizures may necessitate additional small bolus dose and increase in maintenance rate. Infusion adjusted to maintain therapeutic pentobarbi-

tal level (2.5-4.0 mg/dl) or desired ICP (e.g., 15-20 mm Hg). Alternate dosing regimens used.

ADMINISTRATION

G-tube: Use elixir; flush tubing with 30 ml water before and after administration

▼**Direct IV:** Administer slowly at rate of 25-50 mg/min. Dilution not necessary, but preferred to facilitate accurate administration. Too-rapid injection may cause profound hypotension, laryngospasm, apnea. Take care to avoid extravasation, which could cause severe tissue necrosis; stop injection if patient experiences burning or pain. See Appendixes K, L, for management of extravasation.

PREPARATION

Direct IV: May dilute 2 ml (100 mg) with 8 ml sterile water or 0.9% NaCl for concentration of 10 mg/ml.
IV, cont inf: Dilute in convenient volume for infusion. For example, 20 ml of 50 mg/ml solution (1,000 mg) in 250 ml of compatible solution results in concentration of 4 mg/ml. Use only clear, colorless solutions.
Compatible fluids: D_5W, 0.9% NaCl, 0.45% NaCl, LR

ACTIONS

Rapid-acting barbiturate that depresses sensory cortex, decreases motor activity, alters cerebellar function. Decreases excitability of pre/postsynaptic membranes. Results in drowsiness, sedation, sleep induction, respiratory depression, anticonvulsant activity. Minimal analgesic activity • Reduces rapid eye movement (REM) stage of sleep; abrupt cessation of therapy may cause sleep disturbances • Rapid onset of action, shorter duration relative to phenobarbital

PHARMACOKINETICS

ROUTE	ONSET	PEAK	DURATION
PO/PR	15-60 min	30-60 min	1-4 hr
IM	10-25 min	30-60 min	1-4 hr
IV	Immed	<15 min	15 min

DISTRIBUTION

35%-45% protein bound

ELIMINATION

Metabolized by liver, excreted in urine. Half-life = 15-50 hr

Therapeutic level: 2.5-4.0 mg/dl

INDICATIONS

Control of status epilepticus, other acute seizure disorders • Preoperative sedation • Short-term management of insomnia ***Unlabeled/investigational:*** Coma induction in patients with increased ICP due to cerebral ischemia, trauma, other causes. Believed to reduce cerebral blood flow, thereby reducing cerebral edema/intracranial pressure • Greatest efficacy in patients ≤35 yrs and in closed head injury.

PRECAUTIONS/ CONTRAINDICATIONS

Precautions: IV administration may cause profound hypotension, laryngospasm, bronchospasm, respiratory arrest; use only in critical situation with close monitoring; extreme caution indicated in patients with CV, pulmonary disorders, or shock states • May cause status epilepticus if withdrawn too rapidly • Habit-forming; tolerance, psychological/physical dependence may develop • Nem-

P

---

italic = common side effects   **bold** = life-threatening reactions

butal 100 mg capsules contain tartrazine (FD&C yellow no. 5); allergic reactions possible
Use caution with: Status asthmaticus, other pulmonary disorders; profound respiratory depression possible • Postictal state; may add to depressive state • Severe pain; paradoxical excitation may occur • Children: paradoxical excitement, hyperactivity possible • Elders: adverse effects including paradoxical excitement, confusion, hypothermia more likely • Hepatic/renal insufficiency; reduced dose indicated
Pregnancy category: May cause birth defects, neonatal hemorrhagic disorders; do not use during pregnancy
Contraindications: Hypersensitivity to pentobarbital • Severe COPD, pulmonary disorders • Severe liver disorders • Porphyria

ADVERSE EFFECTS

CNS: *Sedation,* CNS depression, confusion, agitation, hallucinations, insomnia, nightmares
CV: Hypotension, bradycardia, syncope
Resp: Hypoventilation, apnea
GI: Nausea, vomiting, constipation, liver damage
Misc: Hypersensitivity, incl. angioedema, exfolative dermatitis

TOXICITY/OVERDOSE

Symptoms: CNS and respiratory depression, hypotension, tachycardia, hypothermia, coma, respiratory arrest, death. One-gram dose may cause toxicity in adults; death occurs with 2-10 g
Management: After recent ingestion, implement guidelines for management of acute overdose (Appendix I) • Maintain airway, support ventilation, administer IV fluids if hypotensive. Use vasopressors (e.g., dopamine) if unresponsive to fluids. • Forced diuresis and alkalinization of urine will promote elimination in patients with normal renal function. Hemodialysis may be helpful for anuric patients.

INTERACTIONS

anticoagulants, oral ↓ Anticoagulation
corticosteroids ↑ Corticosteroid metabolism
CNC depressants (alcohol, anesthetics, antihistamines, opiates, doxycycline ↓ Doxycycline effectiveness
phenothiazines, sedatives, tranquilizers) Additive CNS depression
steroidal hormones ↑ Steroidal metabolism; oral contraceptives may not be effective

COMPATIBILITIES

Syringe: Atropine, hydromorphone, scopolamine
Y-site: Acyclovir, insulin

INCOMPATIBILITIES

Syringe: Butophanol, chlorpromazine, cimetidine, diphenhydramine, droperidol, fentanyl, glycopyrrolate, meperidine, midazolam, morphine, nalbuphine, pentazocine, prochlorperazine, promethazine, ranitidine
Y-site: Atracurium, cephalosporins, isoproterenol, metaraminol, norepinephrine, penicillin G, succinylcholine, tetracycline

PATIENT CARE IMPLICATIONS

• Gradually discontinue drug to prevent withdrawal symptoms, which could include seizures.
• Large quantities should not be prescribed for patients with severe depression, suicidal tendencies, history of substance abuse.
• **IV use:** Monitor closely; have ACLS, emergency equipment immediately available. Profound respiratory depression, hypotension possible. Precautions necessary; see Administration.
• **Seizure control:** Use minimal effective dose to avoid contributing to CNS/respiratory depression immediately after seizures.
• **Therapeutic coma:** Patient must be mechanically ventilated. Obtain baseline EEG as indicated. Correct fluid volume deficit, maintain adequate hydration to prevent hypotension; hemodynamic monitoring recommended. Closely monitor/maintain fluid balance; weigh daily. Gradually taper therapy as clinical condition improves.

Vital signs/hemodynamics: Assess BP, pulse, and RR; monitor q3-5min with IV bolus or loading dose; monitor q15-60min with continuous IV use. • Use continuous pulse oximetry in heavily sedated patients. • Monitor ICP/cerebral perfusion pressure (CPP) in patients with therapeutic coma. Anticipate ICP reduction of 10 mm Hg within 10 min. Maintain ICP of 15-20 mm Hg or other predetermined range.

Physical assessment: Assess adequacy of ventilation: note rate/depth of respirations, breath sounds. • Assess neurologic status, level of consciousness; seizure activity, including precipitating factors, type, duration.
• Examine skin for irritation, eruptions that may precede potentially fatal exfoliative dermatitis; if present, consult physician immediately. • Observe for bruising, petechiae, bleeding tendencies, signs of infection, which could signal hematologic toxicity.

Laboratory tests: Monitor: CBC with differential • Electrolytes, with therapeutic coma • Therapeutic level: 2.5-4.0 mg/dl

PATIENT/FAMILY TEACHING

Purpose of drug is to provide sedation/promote sleep/prevent seizures • Change positions slowly to minimize dizziness; call for assistance with ambulation. • Report pregnancy/possibility of pregnancy.

Outpatients: Do not perform hazardous tasks requiring mental alertness or physical coordination. • Avoid concurrent use of alcohol or other sedatives when taking this medication.
• This medication may cause psychologic/physical dependence. Seizures may develop if you abruptly stop taking this medicine. Consult prescriber before increasing or abruptly discontinuing dose.

AVAILABLE FORMS

Parenteral for IV/IM use • Capsules • Elixir • Rectal suppositories

P

---

italic = common side effects   **bold** = life-threatening reactions

phenobarbital, phenobarbital sodium
(fee-noe-bar'bi-tal)
Barbita, Luminal, Solfoton

Classifications: Barbiturate, sedative/hypnotic, anticonvulsant Schedule II controlled substance

USUAL DOSE

Dose is individualized according to specific patient/clinical response. Reduced dose indicated **G** with advanced age, debilitation, renal/hepatic impairment
PO, adults: 100-320 mg, hs
• Seizure prophylaxis: 50-100 mg 3-4 times daily; maintain therapeutic level
P PO/IM, children: 1-3 mg/kg, preop
IM, adults: 100-200 mg, preop
Direct IV, adults: Use minimal effective dose • Sedation: 30-60 mg q8-12h • **Seizure prophylaxis:** 200-320 mg
• **Status epilepticus:** Loading dose of 10-20 mg/kg given at rate of 50-100 mg/min; may give additional 5 mg/kg q15-30min up to total dose of 20-30 mg/kg. Alternately, 200-600 mg may be used. Maintenance dose is 1-3 mg/kg/24 hr in divided doses q8-12hr; maintain therapeutic level
P Direct IV, children: Use minimal effective dose • **Sedation:** 1-3 mg/kg • **Seizure prophylaxis:** 3-5 mg/kg/day in divided doses q12h • **Status epilepticus:** 15-20 mg/kg given over 10-15 min; children <11 yr may need somewhat higher doses

ADMINISTRATION

G-tube: Use elixir; flush tubing with 30 ml water before and after administration
Compatible enteral formulas: Ensure, Ensure HN, Ensure Plus, Ensure Plus HN, Osmolite, Osmolite HN, Vital
IM: Inject deeply into large muscle mass to avoid tissue necrosis.
V Direct IV: Administer slowly at rate ≤60 mg/min. Dilution not necessary, but preferred to facilitate accurate administration. Too-rapid injection may cause profound hypotension, laryngospasm, apnea. Take care to avoid extravasation, which could cause severe tissue necrosis; stop injection if patient experiences burning or pain. See Appendixes K, L for management of extravasation.

PREPARATION

Direct IV: Dilution with sterile water to concentration of 5-10 mg/ml recommended. For example, dilute 130-mg/ml vial with 12 ml of sterile water for total volume of 13 ml, concentration will be 10 mg/ml. Use only clear, colorless solutions.
Compatible fluids: D_5W, 0.9% NaCl, 0.45% NaCl, LR

ACTIONS

Long-lasting barbiturate that depresses sensory cortex, decreases motor activity, alters cerebellar function • Decreases excitability of pre/postsynaptic membranes • Results in drowsiness, sedation, sleep induction, respiratory depression, anticonvulsant activity • Minimal analgesic activity • Reduces REM sleep; abrupt cessation of therapy may cause sleep disturbances, contribute to withdrawal symptoms • Slow onset, long duration relative to other barbiturates

PHARMACOKINETICS

ROUTE	ONSET	PEAK	DURATION
PO	60 min	8-12 hr	10-12 hr
IV	5 min	15-30 min	10-12 hr

DISTRIBUTION

Low lipid solubility

ELIMINATION

Metabolized by liver, excreted in urine. Half-life = 80-110 hr.

Therapeutic level: 10-25 µg/ml

INDICATIONS

Emergency management of status epilepticus, other acute seizure disorders • Long-term treatment of seizure disorders • Preoperative/daytime sedation; benzodiazepines (e.g., alprazolam [Xanax]) preferred • Short-term management of insomnia

PRECAUTIONS/ CONTRAINDICATIONS

Precautions: IV administration may cause profound hypotension, laryngospasm, respiratory arrest; use only in critical situation with close monitoring; extreme caution indicated in patients with CV, pulmonary disorders or shock states • May cause status epilepticus if withdrawn too rapidly • Habit-forming; tolerance, psychological/physical dependence may develop

Use caution with: • Status asthmaticus, other pulmonary disorders; profound respiratory depression possible • Postictal state; may add to CNS/respiratory depression • Severe pain;

paradoxical excitation may occur • Children: paradoxical excitement, hyperactivity possible • Elders: adverse effects including paradoxical excitement, confusion, hypothermia more likely • Hepatic/renal insufficiency; reduced dose indicated

Pregnancy category: May cause birth defects, neonatal hemorrhagic disorders; do not use during pregnancy

Contraindications: Hypersensitivity to pentobarbital • Severe COPD, pulmonary disorders • Severe liver dysfunction • Porphyria

ADVERSE EFFECTS

CNS: *Sedation,* CNS depression, confusion, agitation, hallucinations, insomnia, nightmares

CV: Hypotension, bradycardia, syncope

Resp: Hypoventilation, apnea

GI: Nausea, vomiting, constipation, liver damage

Misc: Hypersensitivity, incl. angioedema, exfoliative dermatitis

TOXICITY/OVERDOSE

Symptoms: CNS and respiratory depression, hypotension, tachycardia, hypothermia, coma, respiratory arrest, death • One-gram dose may cause toxicity in adults; death occurs with 2-10 g.

Management: After recent ingestion, implement guidelines for management of acute overdose (Appendix I) • Maintain airway, support ventilation, administer IV fluids if hypotensive. Use vasopressors (e.g., dopamine) if unresponsive to fluids. • Keep patient warm; use warm fluids. • Forced diuresis and urine alkalinizations will promote elimination in patients with normal renal function. Hemodialysis may be helpful for anuric patients.

INTERACTIONS

anticoagulants, oral ↓ Anticoagulation

corticosteroids ↑ Corticosteroid metabolism

CNS depressants (alcohol, anesthetics, antihistamines, opiates, phenothiazines, sedatives, tranquilizers) Additive CNS depression

doxycycline ↓ Doxycycline effectiveness

steroidal hormones ↑ Steroidal metabolism; oral contraceptives may not be effective

Y-SITE COMPATIBILITIES

Enalaprilat

INCOMPATIBILITIES

Syringe/Y-site: Atracurium, cimetidine, clindamycin, chlorpromazine, diphenhydramine, droperidol, ephedrine, hydromorphone, hydroxyzine, isoproterenol, kanamycin, norepinephrine, pancuronium, penicillin G, pentazocine, phenytoin, prochlorperazine, promethazine, ranitidine, succinylcholine, tetracycline, thiamine

PATIENT CARE IMPLICATIONS

• Gradually discontinue drug to prevent withdrawal symptoms, which could include seizures.

• Large quantities should not be prescribed for patients with severe depression, suicidal tendencies, history of substance abuse.

• **IV use:** Monitor closely; have ACLS, emergency equipment immediately available. Profound respiratory depression, hypotension possible. Precautions necessary; see Administration.

• **Seizure control:** Peak action may not occur for up to 30 min after IV administration; use minimal effective dose, monitor closely. Excessive doses will contribute to CNS/respiratory depression immediately after seizures.

Vital signs/hemodynamics: Assess BP, pulse, and RR; monitor q3-5min with IV bolus or loading dose; continue close monitoring for 30-60 min after IV dose because of slow onset of peak effects. • Use continuous pulse oximetry in heavily sedated patients.

Physical assessment: Assess adequacy of ventilation: note rate/depth of respirations, breath sounds. • Assess neurologic status, level of consciousness; seizure activity, including precipitating factors, type, duration. • Examine skin for irritation, eruptions that may precede potentially fatal exfoliative dermatitis; if present, consult physician immediately. • Observe for bruising, petechiae, bleeding tendencies, signs of infection, which could signal adverse hematologic effects.

Laboratory tests: Monitor: CBC with differential • Therapeutic level (10-25 µg/ml)

PATIENT/FAMILY TEACHING

Purpose of drug is to provide sedation/promote sleep/prevent seizures. • Change positions slowly to minimize dizziness; call for assistance with ambulation. • Report pregnancy/possibility of pregnancy.

Outpatient: Do not perform hazardous tasks requiring mental alertness or physical coordination. • Avoid concurrent use of alcohol or other sedatives when taking this medication. • This medication may cause psychologic/physical dependence. Seizures may develop if you abruptly stop taking this medicine. Consult prescriber before increasing or abruptly discontinuing dose.

AVAILABLE FORMS

Parenteral for IV/IM use • Tablets • Elixir

---

phentolamine mesylate
(fen-tole'a-meen)
Regitine

Classification: Sympatholytic, alpha-adrenergic blocker, vasodilator

USUAL DOSE

Direct IV/IM, adults: 5 mg 1-2 hr before surgical removal of pheochromocytoma; may repeat during surgery • To diagnose pheochromocytoma give 5 mg test dose; positive response is BP decline of ≥ 35 mm Hg SBP/25 mm Hg DBP.
(P) Direct IV/IM, children: 1 mg or 0.1 mg/kg 1-2 hr before surgical removal of pheochromocytoma; may repeat during surgery • 1 mg or 0.1 mg/kg test dose to diagnose pheochromocytoma; 3-mg dose used if given IM.
IV, cont inf, adults:
Unlabeled/investigational:
Initially 0.1 mg/min; titrate in increments of 0.2 mg/min q10-20 min; maximum dose, 2 mg/min.

Local infiltration, adults/
(P) children: 5-10 mg diluted in 10 ml 0.9% NaCl, infiltrated into affected area within 12 hr of alpha-adrenergic extravasation • 5 mg phentolamine may be added to each 500-ml norepinephrine infusion to prevent dermal necrosis; pressor effects of norepinephrine unaffected.

ADMINISTRATION

▼ Direct IV: Inject each 5 mg or less over 1 min
IV, cont inf, adults: Slowly titrate in increments of 0.2 mg/min q10-20min to reduce afterload, improve CO.
Local infiltration: Infiltrate dilute solution into affected area within 12 hr of alpha-adrenergic extravasation. • As available, use infiltrated IV catheter to avoid repeated injections.

PREPARATION

IV/IM: Reconstitute contents of vial with 1 ml sterile water for injection. Solution contains 5 mg phentolamine/ml. • For IV injection, may be further diluted with 5 or 10 ml 0.9% NaCl • Prepare immediately before injection.
Local infiltration, adults/
(P) children: 5-10 mg diluted in 10 ml 0.9% NaCl
IV, cont inf: Reconstitute contents of vial with 1 ml sterile water for injection; further dilute in 250-500 ml 0.9% NaCl.

COMMON DILUTIONS	CONCENTRATIONS
5 mg/500 ml	10 μg/ml
5 mg/250 ml	20 μg/ml

Compatible fluids: D_5W, 0.9% NaCl, LR, prepared combinations of these solutions;

P

0.9% NaCl recommended for dilution

ACTIONS

Blocks alpha-1- and alpha-2-adrenergic receptors; relaxes vascular smooth muscle; causes peripheral vasodilation; decreases peripheral vascular resistance; direct vasodilation contributes to reduced resistance.
• Reflexive norepinephrine release causes tachycardia, increases force of contraction, which increases CO. • PVR, PAPs usually decrease. • At lower doses BP may increase because of increased CO; at higher doses vasodilation predominates and BP decreases.
• In acute MI, beneficial effects include reduced afterload, improved left ventricular performance, increased CO. • Nonspecific effects on serotonin, histamine, acetylcholine stimulate GI smooth muscle, gastric secretions, to lesser degree respiratory/pancreatic secretions.

PHARMACOKINETICS

ROUTE	ONSET	PEAK	DURATION
IM	Rapid	20 min	30-45 min
IV	Immed	2 min	30 min

ELIMINATION
Half-life 19 min

INDICATIONS

Diagnosis of pheochromocytoma; more reliable for detection of sustained than paroxysmal hypertension • Prevention/control of hypertension immediately before or during surgical removal of pheochromocytoma • Treatment/prevention of dermal necrosis caused by infiltration of norepinephrine, other potent alpha-adrenergic agents

Unlabeled/investigational:
To reduce myocardial workload, limit infarction size during acute MI/left ventricular failure; treatment of hypertensive crises associated with catecholamine excess (e.g., reactions to MAO inhibitors, clonidine withdrawal) or sympathomimetic amines (e.g., methoxamine, phenylephrine).

PRECAUTIONS/CONTRAINDICATIONS

Precautions: Profound hypotension, shock possible • Other tests for pheochromocytoma safer, should be used when possible. • False-negative/false-positive phentolamine test results may occur.
Use caution with: Gastritis, peptic ulcer • Dysrhythmias
c **Pregnancy category:** Safety/efficacy not established; use only if clearly needed and safer alternative unavailable.
Contraindications: Hypersensitivity to phentolamine, tolazoline • CAD, angina, MI; investigational use with extreme caution in acute MI

ADVERSE EFFECTS

CNS: Weakness, dizziness, **cerebrovascular spasm/occlusion**
CV: *Profound hypotension, tachycardia, dysrhythmias,* **angina,** *flushing,* **myocardial ischemia/infarction**
Resp: Nasal stuffiness
GI: *Abdominal pain, nausea, vomiting, diarrhea, exacerbation of peptic ulcer,* metallic taste

TOXICITY/OVERDOSE

Symptoms: Hypotension, tachycardia, dysrhythmias, shock

P pediatric   **G** geriatric   **V** Direct IV

Management: Stop or slow infusion. • Support breathing as needed with O_2 and/or mechanical ventilation • **Hypotension:** Elevate legs, administer IV fluids; if unresponsive to volume expansion, use vasopressor (dopamine, norepinephrine); avoid epinephrine, which may cause further hypotension. • Manage dysrhythmias according to ACLS guidelines (Appendix P). • Avoid administration of digoxin until cardiac rhythm returns to normal.

INTERACTIONS

antihypertensives Additive hypotension

ephedrine Profound hypotension

epinephrine Profound hypotension

Y-SITE COMPATIBILITIES

Amiodarone

PATIENT CARE IMPLICATIONS

• Correct hypovolemia before administration.

• Patient must remain supine with appropriate safety precautions during and for at least 1 hr after administration. Assist patient with initial ambulation.

• Gradually reduce dose to avoid rebound hypertension.

Phentolamine test

• Withhold all sedatives, analgesics, hypotensive agents, other medications (as possible) at least 24, preferably 48-72, hr before test.

• Test not valid unless conducted during hypertensive episode.

• Use extreme caution, monitor closely; Continuous ECG monitoring, automatic BP cuff or in-

traarterial line necessary; deaths reported.

Vital signs/hemodynamics: Monitor BP, HR q5-15 min depending on patient condition, titration schedule. Phentolamine test requires systematic, very frequent monitoring; follow institutional guidelines. • Continuous monitoring of ECG, hemodynamic monitoring of left ventricular function (e.g., CO/CI, SVR, PCWP) required with continuous infusion or use in acute MI. Titrate infusion to optimize CO/CI.

Physical assessment: Assess for perfusion/oxygenation deficit: chest discomfort, shortness of breath, ↓ level of consciousness, confusion, dizziness.

• With treatment of extravasation, assess for resolution of tissue ischemia: rapid return of pink color, hyperemia. Areas of blanching require additional phentolamine infiltration.

Laboratory tests: Monitor: Electrolytes • Correct abnormalities.

PATIENT/FAMILY TEACHING

Purpose of drug is short-term lowering of BP, test for pheochromocytoma, short-term reduction of heart's workload, to improve circulation at site of medication extravasation. • May cause dizziness, hypotension; change positions slowly, do not attempt to get out of bed. • Immediately report dizziness, chest discomfort, confusion, breathing difficulty.

AVAILABLE FORMS

Parenteral for IM/IV injection

P

---

phenylephrine HCl
(fen-ill-ef'rin)
Neo-Synephrine

Classifications: Sympathomimetic, vasopressor, decongestant, ophthalmic mydriatic

USUAL DOSE
Direct IV, adults: 0.2 mg: range, 0.1-0.5 mg • May repeat q10-15min • Do not exceed 0.5 mg in single dose. • Dose variable, adjusted to patient response.
IV, cont inf, adults: Initially 100-180 µg/min • Maintenance rate, 40-60 µg/min • Titrated to SBP or mean BP • Use lowest effective dose for shortest possible time.

ADMINISTRATION
V Direct IV: Dilute, slowly inject each 0.1-0.5 mg over 1 min. • SVT: May be injected rapidly over 20-30 sec • Administer via central, antecubital, or other large vein. • Do not exceed initial dose of 0.5 mg. • Route used exclusively for hypotensive emergencies requiring strong immediate pressor effect or for SVT
IV, cont inf: Titration: Adjust q10-15min to maintain SBP >90 or mean BP >60-70 mm Hg. • Infusion pump or other rate-controlling device is necessary. • Administer via central (preferred), antecubital, or other large vein. • See Infusion Rate Table, Appendix Q.

PREPARATION
Direct IV: Dilute each 10 mg (1.0 ml) with 9 ml sterile water for injection to yield concentration of 1.0 mg/ml. May further dilute if necessary to administer in small increments.
IV, cont inf:

COMMON DILUTIONS	CONCENTRATIONS
10 mg/250 ml	40 µg/ml
20 mg/250 ml	80 µg/ml

More concentrated solutions may be used if necessary to limit fluid intake.

Compatible fluids: D_5W, 0.9% NaCl, LR

ACTIONS
Potent postsynaptic alpha-adrenergic agonist; produces arterial, slight venous vasoconstriction • Usual doses have little effect on beta receptors, although large doses may stimulate cardiac beta-1 receptors. • May trigger release of endogenous norepinephrine • **CV/hemodynamics:** Increases SBP, DBP, SVR; may trigger vagally mediated, reflex bradycardia; CO usually slightly ↓ constricts coronary, pulmonary, renal, cutaneous vascular beds; PAP ↑; may ↓ circulating volume by postcapillary vasoconstriction, loss of fluid into extracellular spaces; cardiac dysrhythmias rarely seen, even with large doses; effects similar to norepinephrine, but without significant cardiac inotropic or chronotropic (beta-1) activity, except at high doses; longer acting, less likely to produce dysrhythmias than epinephrine, ephedrine • **Other:** Constriction of renal blood vessels may result in ↓ urine formation. Topical application produces local vasoconstriction, hemostasis. Application to nasal mucosa constricts blood vessels, relieves nasal congestion.

PHARMACOKINETICS

ROUTE	ONSET	PEAK	DURATION
IV	Immed	Rapid	15-20 min

DISTRIBUTION
Throughout intravascular fluid
ELIMINATION
Metabolized in liver, intestines

INDICATIONS

Short-term augmentation of BP in low-resistance shock states or drug-induced hypotension • Control of SVT • Antidote for hypotension associated with chlorpromazine toxicity • Maintenance of BP during spinal/inhalation anesthesia • To prolong spinal anesthesia • For vasoconstriction with regional anesthesia • To correct hypotension associated with pheochromocytomectomy; carefully calculated dosage required • Topically as nasal decongestant • Ophth use as mydriatic

PRECAUTIONS/CONTRAINDICATIONS

Precautions: ↑ Myocardial workload may lead to imbalance of myocardial O₂ supply/demand, resulting in ischemia, infarction. • If extravasation occurs, tissue necrosis/sloughing may result. Area of extravasation should be infiltrated with phentolamine (Appendixes K and L).
Use caution with: General anesthesia, digoxin, acid-base imbalance; reduced effectiveness, dysrhythmias likely • Hyperthyroidism • Bradycardia, partial heart block • CV disease • Severe arteriosclerosis • Older adults • Acute pancreatic/hepatic disease

G Pregnancy category: Safety not established; use only if clearly necessary.
Contraindications: Hypersensitivity to phenylephrine • Angle-closure glaucoma • Anesthesia with halogenated hydrocarbons • Hypertension • Ventricular tachycardia • Acute MI • Commercial preparations may contain sulfites, which can cause serious allergic reactions.

ADVERSE EFFECTS

CNS: Headache, excitability, weakness, dizziness, seizures, **cerebral hemorrhage**
EENT: Ophth—*burning, stinging, lacrimation, photophobia;* nasal—*burning, stinging, mucosal drying, rebound congestion*
Resp: Distress, dyspnea
CV: **Reflex bradycardia,** tachycardia, **dysrhythmias,** hypertension, chest pain, peripheral/visceral vasoconstriction
GU: Decreased renal perfusion, reduced UO
Derm: Blanching, piloerection, pallor, sweating; sloughing/necrosis of skin at infusion site

TOXICITY/OVERDOSE

Symptoms: Hypertension, ↑ SVR • PVCs, ventricular tachycardia • Paresthesias, seizures, cerebral hemorrhage
Management: Slow or stop infusion. • **Severe/sustained hypertension:** Administer alpha-adrenergic blocker (e.g., phentolamine). • Treat dysrhythmias according to ACLS guidelines (Appendix P); resuscitate as necessary.

INTERACTIONS

alpha blockers ↓ Effectiveness; hypotension

atropine Hypertension, blocks reflex tachycardia
beta-blockers, noncardioselective Hypotension
bretylium Dysrhythmias
chloropromazine Hypotension
digoxin Dysrhythmias
epinephrine Profound hypertension
phenytoin Bradycardia, hypotension

Y-SITE COMPATIBILITIES

Amiodarone, amrinone, famotidine, zidovudine

Y-SITE INCOMPATIBILITIES

Phenytoin, strongly alkaline solutions

PATIENT CARE IMPLICATIONS

• Correct hypovolemia before initiating therapy; in emergencies, may be administered in hypovolemic state with simultaneous fluid volume replacement.
• Infuse via central, antecubital, or other large vein. Avoid using veins in hands, ankles, legs.
• For continuous infusion, use pump or other rate-controlling device.
• Monitor for/correct hypoxemia, hypercapnia, acidosis before and during drug administration.
• Monitor for significant dysrhythmias, hypertension, chest pain, other anginal symptoms, ECG evidence of ischemia. Consult physician for positive findings.
• Use lowest effective dose for shortest possible time.
• Decrease dose gradually to avoid abrupt/severe hypotension. Be certain hypovolemia corrected before weaning.

Vital signs/hemodynamics: During parenteral use, monitor BP, HR q2min initially, q5-15min thereafter according to titration schedule, stability. Continuous arterial pressure monitoring preferred for BP measurements, because severe peripheral vasoconstriction can result in inaccurate auscultatory pressures. • Continuously monitor ECG for dysrhythmias, ischemic changes: T wave inversion, ST segment depression/elevation. • Establish clear parameters for titration (e.g., desired BP, CO, UO); use lowest possible dose to achieve desired effect. • Monitor CO, PCWP, CVP, SVR frequently; immediately correct hypovolemia.
• Monitor UO; consult physician if ≤5 ml/kg/hr or ≤30 ml/hr.

Physical assessment: Assess for perfusion/oxygenation deficit: changes in mentation, hypotension, chest discomfort. • Assess for ↓ peripheral perfusion: coolness, ↓ pulse intensity, paresthesias, delayed capillary refill. • Check infusion site frequently for signs of extravasation (e.g., blanching along vein pathway, coldness, hardness). If this occurs, change injection site immediately, infiltrate affected area with 10-15 ml saline mixed with 5-10 mg phentolamine (Appendixes K and L).

Laboratory tests: Monitor: Electrolytes • ABGs

PATIENT/FAMILY TEACHING

Purpose of medication is to increase BP. • Immediately report chest pain or discomfort, palpitations, headache, dizziness, pain at infusion site. • Chronic

---

excessive use as nasal decongestant may lead to rebound congestion. • Dilation of pupils with ophthalmic use makes eyes more sensitive to light; dark glasses recommended until effects wear off.

AVAILABLE FORMS

Parenteral concentrate for IV admixture

phenytoin sodium
(fen'i-toy-in)
Dilantin, Diphenylan Sodium

Classifications: Anticonvulsant, Class IB antidysrhythmic, membrane stabilizer

USUAL DOSE

PO, adults: Loading doses; 400 mg, 300 mg, 300 mg, for total of 1000 mg; each dose given 2 hr apart. • Maintenance: 300-400 mg/day in evenly divided doses q8h (e.g., 100 mg q8h) • Extended-release capsules administered once daily when seizures well controlled with standard preparations. • Maximum dose usually 600 mg/day

PO, children: Initially 5 mg/kg/day in evenly divided doses q8h; follow with 4-8 mg/kg/day in evenly divided doses q8h.

IM, adults: 100-200 mg q4h • Erratically absorbed, only used as last resort; IV route superior for rapid control of seizures • IM dose generally increased by 50% over usual IV/PO dose

Direct IV, adults, anticonvulsant: Loading dose: 15-18 mg/kg; follow with 100-150 mg q6-8h. • Alternate dosing; 150-250

mg, initial loading dose, followed by 100-150 mg 30 min later • Do not exceed 1.5 g/24 hr.

Direct IV, adults, antidysrhythmic: 100 mg q5min until dysrhythmia controlled or severe side effects • Do not exceed total dose of 1 g.

Direct IV, children: 10-15 mg/kg in 2-3 divided doses of 5-10 mg/kg • Do not exceed 20 mg/kg/24 hr.

IV, intermit inf, adults: 10-15 mg/kg over 1-2 hr as IV loading dose • Widely used, but considered investigational

ADMINISTRATION

Two strengths of PO suspension available; check labeling/dose carefully.

G-tube: Use oral suspension; dilute with 3 parts sterile water or 0.9% NaCl to minimize drug loss due to absorption by PVC tubing. Flush with 50 ml water before and after administration. • Flush tube with at least 20 ml diluent after administration.

IM, adults: Inject deep into large muscle mass (e.g., gluteus, lateral thigh). • Avoid SC injection, which causes local tissue damage.

Direct IV: Adults: Administer each 50 mg or less slowly over at least 1 min. • **Older adults with heart disease:** Administer very slowly at rate of 50 mg over 2-3 min. • **Children:** Administer each 0.5-1.5 mg/kg slowly over at least 1 min. • Continuously monitor ECG, BP during injection; observe for marked widening of QRS complex, hypotension. • *Too-rapid administration may cause cardiac arrest.* • Solution highly alkaline, irritates veins. • Filter

P

needle or 22 µm in-line IV filter required • Flush, thoroughly clear line using 0.9% NaCl before and after injection. • Never dilute/infuse with D_5W; immediate precipitation will result.

IV, intermit inf, adults: Infuse total dose over 30-60 min; do not exceed rate of 25-50 mg/min. • Use 22-µm in-line filter. • Carefully observe solution for precipitate. • Do not infuse with or add to other solutions.

PREPARATION
IV, intermit inf, adults:

DILUTION	CONCENTRATION
100 mg/50 ml	2 mg/ml
500 mg/100 ml	5 mg/ml

Prepare solution directly before administration. Use only clear or pale-yellow solutions. Do not infuse solutions with precipitate. Do not exceed final concentration of 6.7 mg/ml.

Compatible fluids: 0.9% NaCl, 0.45% NaCl; **not compatible with dextrose-containing solutions**

ACTIONS

Promotes sodium efflux from neurons of cerebral motor cortex; reduces hyperexcitability of neurons by reducing sodium gradient, thus inhibiting spread of seizure activity • Decreases cardiac excitability by increasing threshold for electrical excitation; blocks fast sodium channels in cardiac electrical pathways; slightly decreases automaticity in SA node, ventricle, ectopic pacemakers; slightly increases conduction velocity in AV node, His-Purkinje system • No effect on effective refractory period; may decrease PR, QT intervals slightly; may widen QRS complex

PHARMACOKINETICS

ROUTE	ONSET	PEAK	DURATION
PO	30-60 min	12 hr	24 hr
PO*	30 min	1.5-3 hr	
IM	Erratic	24 hr	>24 hr
IV	Immed	1 hr	24 hr

DISTRIBUTION
Wide; 95% protein bound

ELIMINATION
Metabolized by liver, eliminated by kidneys; dose-dependent metabolism; Half-life 6-24 hr

*Prompt dissolution preparation.

Therapeutic level: 10-25 µg/ml

INDICATIONS

Suppression/prevention of tonic-clonic (grand mal) seizures, other seizure disorders • With diazepam in treatment of status epilepticus • Prevention of seizures during neurosurgery *Unlabeled/investigational:* Control of ventricular/atrial tachycardia in patients who fail to respond to cardioversion/more conventional therapy; considered choice antidysrhythmic for patients with digitalis toxicity.

PRECAUTIONS/CONTRAINDICATIONS

Precautions: Narrow range between therapeutic/toxic levels • Rapid IV administration may induce cardiac arrest; marked widening of QRS complex may precede cardiac arrest/asystole. • Severe blood dyscrasias possible • May cause lymphoma-like syndrome • Hypocalcemia, osteomalacia possible with long-term therapy • Abrupt withdrawal may precipitate status epilepticus. • Potentially fatal dermatologic conditions (e.g.,

P pediatric   **G** geriatric   **V** Direct IV

toxic epidermal necrolysis) possible

Use caution with: Hepatic disease • Renal insufficiency • SA node depression, preexisting heart block • Hypotension • CHF, acute MI, cardiomyopathy • Exercise extreme caution if IV route used in patients with cardiopulmonary disease.

▫ **Pregnancy category:** May cause birth defects; use only if clearly necessary and woman informed of risks; not recommended for discontinuation in pregnant woman with severe seizure disorders.

Contraindications: Hypersensitivity to phenytoin, other hydantoin derivatives • Sinus bradycardia, 2nd/3rd degree heart block, sinoatrial block, Stokes-Adams syndrome; unless functional ventricular pacemaker in place or readily available

ADVERSE EFFECTS

CNS: *Nystagmus, slurred speech, confusion, ataxia,* tremors, fatigue, visual disturbances, depression, headache, drowsiness, dizziness, **seizures** (rare)

CV: Hypotension, **CV collapse, new/worsened heart block, asystole,** bradycardia, **ventricular fibrillation**

GI: Nausea, vomiting, constipation, diarrhea, hepatitis, **hepatic necrosis,** swollen gums

Derm: *Various reddened rashes,* **exfoliative dermatitis,** hirsutism

Endo: Hyperglycemia

Local: "Purple-glove syndrome" —sudden purplish discoloration of extremity distal to IV site

Syst: **Blood dyscrasias,** lymph node hyperplasia, arthritis-like syndrome

TOXICITY/OVERDOSE

Symptoms: Slurred speech, nystagmus, lethargy, coma, non-reactive pupils • Hypotension, heart failure, bradycardia, heart block • Respiratory failure

Management: After recent ingestion, implement guidelines for management of acute overdose (Appendix I). • Maintain airway; support ventilation. • Hypotension: Elevate legs, administer IV fluids; use vasopressors (e.g., norepinephrine, phenylephrine) for severe hypotension. • Administer inotropic agents for heart failure (e.g., dobutamine, dopamine). • Manage symptomatic bradycardia, ventricular dysrhythmias according to ACLS guidelines (Appendix P). • Hemodialysis may be helpful.

Toxic serum level: >25 µg/ml

INTERACTIONS

Numerous serious interactions possible; pharmacist review of medications recommended

chloramphenicol ↑ Phenytoin levels; toxicity

corticosteroids ↓ Corticosteroid effectiveness

diazoxide ↓ Phenytoin levels

digitalis glycosides ↓ Digoxin levels, hypotension

disulfiram (Antabuse) **Phenytoin toxicity**

fluconazole ↑ Phenytoin levels; toxicity

furosemide ↓ Diuretic response

isoniazid **Phenytoin toxicity**

methadone Methadone withdrawal

sucralfate ↓ Phenytoin levels

sulfonamides Phenytoin toxicity

P

---

italic = common side effects   **bold** = life-threatening reactions

theophylline ↓ Theophylline
levels

INCOMPATIBILITIES

Do not mix or administer with
other agents or dextrose-containing IV solutions

PATIENT CARE
IMPLICATIONS

• Many precautions necessary
with IV/NG administration; see
Administration.
• Discontinue drug, thoroughly
evaluate patients who develop
lymph node hyperplasia, bone
marrow depression, liver enzyme elevation.
• When used for epilepsy, wean
gradually to prevent precipitation of status epilepticus.
Vital signs/hemodynamics:
IV: Continuously monitor ECG,
BP. Use lowest possible dose
for seizure/dysrhythmia control.
Note signs of toxicity, including
excessive prolongation of PR
interval/QRS complex, heart
block, bradycardia, ventricular
dysrhythmias. Stop injection,
consult physician immediately
for signs of toxicity.
Physical assessment: Assess
neurologic status, level of consciousness; seizure activity, including precipitating factors,
type, duration. Assess for perfu-
sion/oxygenation deficit: ↓ level
of consciousness, chest pain, activity intolerance, hypotension,
dizziness. • Examine skin for
reddened rashes, which may
signal onset of serious adverse
reaction. Do not administer additional medication until exam-
ined by physician.
Laboratory tests: Monitor:
Liver enzymes, bilirubin • CBC
with differential • Calcium
• Blood sugar • Plasma levels of

phenytoin; therapeutic levels:
10-25 µg/ml

PATIENT/FAMILY TEACHING

Purpose of medication is to
control seizures or manage disturbances in heart rhythm. • Report skin rash, inflammation of
skin/mucous membranes; may
signal serious skin disorder.
• Report unusual bleeding or
bruising, sore throat, fever, other
signs of infection. • Report abdominal pain, yellow tint of
skin (jaundice), dark urine, loss
of appetite, abdominal pain;
may signal liver damage. • Frequent oral hygiene will minimize gum irritation.
Outpatient: May cause drowsiness; do not perform hazardous
tasks requiring mental alertness
or physical coordination. • Patients with diabetes must monitor blood sugar closely. • Extended-release tablets should
never be broken, chewed, or
crushed.

AVAILABLE FORMS

• Prompt release capsules • Extended-release capsules • Chewable tablets • PO suspension
• Parenteral for IV/IM use

physostigmine
salicylate
(fi-zoe-stig'meen)
Antilirium

Classifications: Cholinergic
stimulant, anticholinerase agent

USUAL DOSE

IV/IM, adults: Initially 0.5-2
mg; may repeat q20min until
desired response or adverse cholinergic effects; additional dose

of 1-4 mg used q30-60min as needed for recurrence of life-threatening signs (e.g., dysrhythmias, seizures, deep coma) **IV/IM, children:** *Use for life-threatening situations only.* Initially 0.02 mg/kg; may repeat q5-10min until desired response or adverse cholinergic effects, up to maximum dose of 2 mg

ADMINISTRATION

Direct IV: Adults: Slowly inject each dose of ≤1 mg over 1-3 min. • Children: Slowly inject each dose of ≤0.5 mg over 1-3 min. • Have atropine immediately available. • Dilution not necessary • *Too-rapid injection may cause bradycardia, excessive salivation with respiratory compromise, seizures.*
Compatible fluids: Specific information not available

ACTIONS

Inhibits acetylcholinesterase, thus reducing breakdown of acetylcholine; prolongs/exaggerates acetylcholine effects • Produces generalized cholinergic responses such as pupil constriction, increased intestinal muscle tone, bronchial constriction, bradycardia, increased salivation/sweating • Very high doses produce CNS depression, respiratory paralysis, death

PHARMACOKINETICS

ROUTE	ONSET	PEAK	DURATION
IV	3-8 min	<30 min	30 min-5 hr

DISTRIBUTION
Crosses blood-brain barrier
ELIMINATION
Metabolized in liver/other tissue, excreted in urine; half-life 15-40 min

INDICATIONS

To reverse adverse CNS effects caused by anticholinergic agents (e.g., atropine, glycopyrrolate, scopolamine), other anticholinergic toxins. • To reverse severe CNS/cardiac toxicity caused by TCAs (e.g., amitriptyline, imipramine, nortriptyline), phenothiazines, antihistamines, antiparkinsonian agents, others; not helpful for dysrhythmias from other causes • Not used routinely because of potential severe adverse effects

PRECAUTIONS/ CONTRAINDICATIONS

Precautions: Severe cholinergic reaction possible (see Toxicity/Overdose) • High doses may cause bradycardia, excessive salivation with respiratory compromise, seizures • Commercial preparations contain sodium bisulfite, which may cause serious allergic reactions in susceptible individuals.
Use caution with: Epilepsy • Bradycardia • Parkinsonian syndrome
C Pregnancy category: Use only if safer alternative unavailable.
Contraindications: Hypersensitivity to physostigmine, sulfites • Asthma • Gangrene • Diabetes • CV disease • Mechanical intestinal obstruction • Mechanical urinary obstruction • Concurrent use of choline esters, depolarizing NMBAs (e.g., succinylcholine)

ADVERSE EFFECTS

CNS: *Restlessness,* weakness, dizziness, hallucinations, **seizures**

P

---

italic = common side effects   **bold** = life-threatening reactions

EENT: Miosis, blurred vision, tearing
Resp: *Excessive secretions,* **bronchospasm, respiratory depression/arrest**
CV: *Bradycardia,* hypotension
GI: *Nausea, vomiting, diarrhea, cramping, excessive salivation*
GU: Urinary frequency, incontinence
Derm: *Sweating,* rash, urticaria

TOXICITY/OVERDOSE

Symptoms: Cholinergic crisis: Vomiting, diarrhea, excessive salivation/tearing, bradycardia, tachycardia, hypotension, bronchospasm, excessive bronchial secretions, weakness, fasciculations, paralysis • Death possible from respiratory paralysis, pulmonary edema, cardiac arrest

Management: Establish airway, maintain adequate ventilation; ET intubation or tracheostomy with mechanical ventilation usually necessary. Suction frequently to mobilize/clear excessive secretions. • Administer specific antagonist, atropine 0.6 mg IV q5-30min as needed. Atropine will not reverse muscle relaxation, respiratory paralysis. Use pralidoxime chloride (Protopam chloride) to control skeletal muscle effects.
• Be prepared to manage shock, seizures as necessary

INTERACTIONS

anticholinergics Antagonized cholinergic effects
atropine Antagonizes muscarinic effects
succinylcholine, other depolarizing NMBAs Prolongs neuromuscular blockade

COMPATIBILITIES

Specific information not available

PATIENT CARE IMPLICATIONS

• Atropine must be immediately available to counteract severe cholinergic reactions: bradycardia, hypotension, bronchospasm, paralysis.
• Emergency resuscitation/airway management equipment must be immediately available.
Vital signs/hemodynamics: Monitor ECG continuously during IV use. Observe for bradycardia, AV block, dysrhythmias.
• Monitor BP, RR, HR, q15-60min according to patient condition.
Physical assessment: Monitor for symptoms of excessive cholinergic stimulation: excessive salivation, vomiting, urination, defecation. Discontinue for these symptoms. Reduce dose for nausea, excessive sweating.
• Monitor neurologic status frequently; include assessment of sensory-perceptual alterations. Use seizure precautions. Protect from self-injury. • Monitor I&O. Assess for urinary retention, incontinence.

PATIENT/FAMILY TEACHING

Purpose of medication is to control dangerous effects of certain medications or poisonings.
• Report breathing difficulty, palpitations, excessive sweating/salivation, vomiting, diarrhea.

AVAILABLE FORMS

Parenteral for IV injection

---

phytonadione
vitamin K₁
AquaMEPHYTON,
Konakion, Mephyton

Classification: Vitamin

USUAL DOSE

Dose depends on severity of prothrombin deficiency.
PO/SC/IM, adults: Hypo-prothrombinemia: 2.5-10 mg for stable patients without active bleeding; up to 25 mg has been used • May repeat PO dose in 12-48 hr; SC/IM dose may be repeated in 6-8 hr. • **Prevention of hypoprothrombine-mia during TPN:** 5-10 mg weekly
Direct IV/inf, adults: Hypo-prothrombinemia: 10-50 mg; may be repeated q4-8h based on patient response • Must use aqueous colloidal solution (AquaMEPHYTON); do not use aqueous dispersion (Konakion). • Because of risk of serious hy-persensitivity reaction, IV route used only when other routes not feasible

ADMINISTRATION

▼ Direct IV/intermit inf, adults: Administer VERY SLOWLY at rate no >1 mg/min • Dilute with at least 10 ml preservative-free dextrose or 0.9% NaCl to facilitate administration. • May be given by IV infusion; some sources recommend protecting infusion solutions from light.

ACTIONS

Vitamin required for hepatic synthesis of clotting factors II (prothrombin), VII, IX, X • Prevents/reduces bleeding from hy-poprothrombinemia • Reverses anticoagulant effects of couma-rin derivatives (e.g., warfarin)

PHARMACOKINETICS

ROUTE	ONSET	DURATION
PO	6-12 hr	
SC/IM/IV	1-2 hr	Bleeding control 3-8 hr; normal PT 12-14 hr

DISTRIBUTION
Concentrated in liver; crosses placenta

INDICATIONS

Treatment of hypoprothrombine-mia associated with PO antico-agulant overdose, salicylates, broad-spectrum antibiotics, nutritional deficiencies, includ-ing prolonged TPN, malabsorp-tion syndromes • May partially correct bleeding problems asso-ciated with liver disease.

PRECAUTIONS/
CONTRAINDICATIONS

Precautions: PT should be used to monitor effectiveness. • SC/IM route may be contrain-dicated with hypoprothrombine-mia because of risk of hemor-rhage at injection site • In liver disease, does not completely correct hypoprothrombinemia • Repeated large doses may de-press liver function, aggravate bleeding tendencies. • Does not antagonize heparin
Use caution with: Premature infants, neonates; risk of hyper-bilirubinemia, hemolytic ane-mia, brain damage, death
Contraindications: Hypersen-sitivity to phytonadione • Re-peated large doses in patients with liver disease

P

ADVERSE EFFECTS

Derm: Pain, swelling/tenderness at injection site; erythematous, indurated, pruritic plaques after repeated injection

Misc: IV injection may result in hypersensitivity reactions manifested by cramping pain, seizures, cardiac irregularities, chest pain, facial flushing, dizziness, ↓ level of consciousness, bronchospasm, dyspnea, **hypotension, shock, cardiac/respiratory arrest, death.**

TOXICITY/OVERDOSE

Symptoms: Excessive amounts given for PO anticoagulant overdose may result in near-normal PTs with return to condition that necessitated anticoagulant therapy. • Repeated large doses may depress liver function, aggravate bleeding tendencies. • Severe hypersensitivity-like reactions possible

Management: Heparin may be used to maintain anticoagulation after overdose with vitamin K₁. See Appendix N for management of acute hypersensitivity reactions.

INTERACTIONS

anticoagulants, PO Antagonistic effects
aspirin Antagonistic effects
cephalosporins, some (e.g., cefoperazone, cefamanadole, cefotetan) Antagonistic effects
cholestyramine ↓ Oral absorption
colesiptol ↓ Oral absorption
NSAIDs Antagonistic effects
sucralfate ↓ Oral absorption

Y-SITE COMPATIBILITIES

Ampicillin, epinephrine, famotidine, heparin, hydrocortisone sodium succinate, potassium chloride, vitamin B complex with C

Y-SITE INCOMPATIBILITIES

Dobutamine, phenytoin

PATIENT CARE IMPLICATIONS

• Use lowest effective dose, especially with PO anticoagulant overdose when overaggressive therapy may restore thromboembolic problems.

• Because of risk of serious hypersensitivity reaction, use IV route only in emergency situations when other routes not feasible. Have epinephrine, antihistamine, resuscitation equipment immediately available during IV administration; must use AquaMEPHYTON; do not use aqueous dispersion (Konakion).

• Avoid IM/SC injections, invasive procedures until risk of bleeding passed.

Vital signs/hemodynamics: Monitor BP, HR frequently according to severity of bleeding.
• Monitor UO for decreases or I&O imbalance.

Physical assessment: Assess for continued/recurrent bleeding until PT returns to normal or patient's baseline. • Test stools, emesis for occult blood. • Assess for hypersensitivity reaction.

Laboratory tests: Monitor: PT; in actively bleeding patients, obtain before initiating therapy and q4-8h until stable.
• Use PT, clinical condition to monitor effectiveness, need for additional doses.

PATIENT/FAMILY TEACHING

This medication is given to replace vitamin K₁, which is necessary for blood clotting. • Immediately report unusual bleeding, bruising. • Change position slowly to avoid dizziness, fainting (IV use). • Avoid activities that may result in bleeding (shaving, brushing teeth, ambulation) until risk of bleeding passed. • Long-term therapy: (1) inform physicians, dentists of vitamin K_1 therapy before treatment, surgery; (2) do not take over-the-counter medications without consulting caregiver; (3) foods high in vitamin K include green leafy vegetables, meat, dairy products; vitamin K preserved during cooking; do not drastically alter diet while taking vitamin K.

AVAILABLE FORMS

Aqueous colloidal solution (AquaMEPHYTON) for parenteral use • Aqueous dispersion FOR IM USE ONLY (Konakion) • Tablets • Drug photosensitive, protect from light.

---

piperacillin sodium
(pi-per′a-sill-in)
Pipracil

Classifications: Penicillin antibiotic, extended-spectrum penicillin

USUAL DOSE

IV/IM, adults: 2-4 g q4-8h; higher dosage used for severe infections • Maximum dose, 24 g/24 hr • **Severe renal impairment:** Reduce dose and/or frequency.

ADMINISTRATION

IM: Inject deep into large muscle mass (e.g., gluteus maximus, lateral thigh) • Slow injection/reconstitution with 0.5% or 1% lidocaine HCl reduces injection

site pain. • Do not administer more than 2 g at single site.
▼**Direct IV:** Slowly inject over 3-5 min. Intermit inf preferred since pain, thrombophlebitis, other local reactions more frequent with direct injection.
IV, intermit inf: Infuse prepared solution over 30 min. Use large vein, small catheter, rotate infusion sites to ↓ risk of thrombophlebitis.

PREPARATION

IM: Reconstitute each g with 2 ml sterile or bacteriostatic water for injection or sterile or bacteriostatic 0.9% NaCl. • May reconstitute with 2 ml 0.5% or 1% lidocaine HCl to reduce pain. • Shake vigorously to dissolve.

IV: Reconstitute each g with 5 ml sterile water; bacteriostatic water or sterile or bacteriostatic 0.9% NaCl may be used.
• Shake vigorously to dissolve.
• For intermit inf, add to 50 ml compatible IV fluid.
Compatible fluids: D_5W, 0.9% NaCl, LR
Stability: Reconstituted solution stable for 24 hr at room temperature

ACTIONS

Semisynthetic, extended-spectrum penicillin with bactericidal action; interferes with bacterial cell wall synthesis/division; more active against gram-negative bacilli than other penicillins • Active against most gram-positive, gram-negative aerobic cocci (except penicillinase-producing strains), some gram-positive bacilli, many gram-negative bacilli, including *Proteus vulgaris, P. mirabilis, Morganella morganii, Escherichia*

P

coli, Enterobacter, Citrobacter, Klebsiella • Also active against *Enterococcus faecalis, Bacteroides fragilis* • Most active penicillin against *Pseudomonas aeruginosa*

PHARMACOKINETICS

ROUTE	ONSET	PEAK	DURATION*
IM	Rapid	30 min-2 hr	6-8 hr
IV	Immed	End infusion	

DISTRIBUTION

Widely distributed; CSF levels higher with meningeal inflammation

ELIMINATION

Primarily excreted in urine; half-life 30-80 min, longer with higher dose range

*Approx; dose dependent.

INDICATIONS

Serious intraabdominal, urinary tract, gynecologic, respiratory tract, skin, bone/joint infections; septicemia • Primary use in gram-negative aerobic infections, mixed aerobic-anaerobic bacterial infections • Used empirically in febrile granulocytopenic patients, often with aminoglycoside or 3rd generation cephalosporin • Synergism with aminoglycosides frequently used to therapeutic advantage in *P. aeruginosa* infections • Not to replace natural penicillins (e.g., penicillin G) or aminopenicillins (e.g., ampicillin) for treatment of streptococcal infections

PRECAUTIONS/ CONTRAINDICATIONS

Precautions: Bacterial or fungal overgrowth may occur; indwelling lines, catheters ↑ risk. • Sodium content may contribute to electrolyte imbalance, edema, heart failure. • May impair coagulation, cause abnormal bleeding (rare)

Use caution with: Hypersensitivity to cephalosporins, other drugs; risk of allergic reaction • Severe renal insufficiency; use **P** lower dose/frequency. • Children <12 yr: Safety not clearly established

B **Pregnancy category:** Use only if clearly necessary. **Contraindications:** Hypersensitivity to any penicillin

ADVERSE EFFECTS

CNS: Headache, neuromuscular irritability/**seizures,** especially with high dose/renal insufficiency

GI: *Diarrhea,* nausea, vomiting, unpleasant taste, elevated liver enzymes

GU: Increased BUN/creatinine

Hema: Eosinophilia, hemolytic anemia, other blood dyscrasias, coagulation disorders

Derm: *Rash,* wheals, itching

Local: *Injection site pain,* thrombophlebitis (IV use)

Misc: *Hypersensitivity,* **anaphylaxis,** serum sickness; *superinfection, colonization*

TOXICITY/OVERDOSE

Symptoms: Neurotoxicity, including seizures. • Acute allergic reaction, including anaphylaxis

Management: Discontinue drug. • Initiate symptomatic/ supportive measures. • For acute allergic reaction, see Appendix N. • Hemodialysis is effective in drug removal; minimal removal with peritoneal dialysis.

INTERACTIONS

aminoglycosides (e.g., amikacin, gentamicin) Synergistic antibacterial activity

anticoagulants, PO Prolonged bleeding time

cephalosporins Unpredictable synergism/antagonism

probenecid Higher/prolonged piperacillin blood levels

vecuronium bromide Prolonged neuromuscular blockade

Y-SITE COMPATIBILITIES

Acyclovir, ciprofloxacin, diltiazem, enalaprilat, esmolol, famotidine, hydromorphone IL-2, labetalol, magnesium sulfate, meperidine, morphine, potassium chloride, ranitidine, verapamil, zidovudine

Y-SITE INCOMPATIBILITIES

Aminoglycosides (e.g., amikacin, gentamicin, tobramycin), fluconazole, ondansetron

PATIENT CARE IMPLICATIONS

• Obtain specimens for culture and sensitivity before initiating antibiotic therapy. Initiate therapy before results received.

• Determine previous antibiotic use, including reactions to penicillins, cephalosporins. Cross-reactivity with cephalosporin allergies may occur.

• Have epinephrine, antihistamine, resuscitation equipment readily available for use with severe allergic reaction.

• Do not discharge patient for at least 30 min after antibiotic administration.

• High sodium content may cause edema, electrolyte abnormalities, dysrhythmias and contribute to heart failure, particularly with high-dose therapy in susceptible patients.

• To avoid drug incompatibility/interaction, administer at separate site; stagger schedules when aminoglycosides (e.g., amikacin, gentamicin, tobramy-

cin), tetracycline, chloramphenicol also prescribed.

• Reduce risk of suprainfection by limiting use of indwelling lines, catheters.

• IV route must be used for severe infections or when shock present.

Vital signs: Monitor VS at beginning and throughout therapy.

Physical assessment: Assess for improvement in primary infection or symptoms of infection or sepsis: presence of fever; appearance of sputum, urine, stool, wound drainage; candidiasis, vaginitis; WBC. • Observe for symptoms of hypersensitivity: rash, pruritus, wheezing, laryngeal edema, hypotension.

• Assess for unusual or occult bleeding, including ecchymosis, bleeding from gums/mucous membranes, excessive bleeding from venipuncture site or surgical incision. Note blood in urine, other body fluids. Check emesis, stools for occult blood.

Laboratory tests: Monitor: Electrolytes, BUN, creatinine, liver enzymes, CBC with differential; particularly with renal/cardiac impairment, elderly/debilitated patients • Consult physician for significant changes, subtherapeutic levels. • May cause: Positive direct antiglobulin (Coombs') test

PATIENT/FAMILY TEACHING

Purpose of drug is to limit growth of infection-causing bacteria. • Immediately report rash, swelling, intense itching, difficulty breathing, other signs of allergic reaction. • Report diarrhea, fever, vaginal itching or discharge, furry growth on tongue.

P

G

AVAILABLE FORMS
Parenteral for IV/IM use

plasma protein fraction, PPF
Plasmanate, Plasma-Plex, Plasmatein, Protenate

Classifications: Blood derivative, plasma volume expander

USUAL DOSE
IV inf, adults: Dose variable according to clinical condition; range, 250-1500 ml/24 hr • **Shock:** Initially 250-500 ml at 5-8 ml/min • **Hypoproteinemia:** 1,000-1,500 ml/24 hr; larger doses may be necessary. • Do not exceed infusion rate of 5-8 ml/min. • Adjust dose, rate to clinical response. • Do not exceed adult dose of 250 g/48 hr (5,000 ml).
P IV inf, children: Dose variable according to clinical condition; range, 6.6-33ml/kg/24 hr. Rate of 5-10 ml/min used for shock states; slower rates used for other indications

ADMINISTRATION
IV inf: Rate of infusion variable according to clinical condition, fluid loss, VS, central hemodynamics, presence of venous/pulmonary congestion, plasma oncotic pressure, Hct • Range, 5-10 ml/min in hypovolemic states; slower rates used in non-hypovolemic states • Rates >10 ml/min should be avoided; too-rapid infusion may cause hypotension • Use administration set provided by manufacturer. • Administer through ≥20-gauge needle or catheter. • Do not administer near any site of infection

or trauma. • Blood type/Rh matching not required

PREPARATION
Solution should be transparent, nearly colorless to slightly brown. Do not use if solution appears turbid or contains a deposit. • Infuse within 4 hr of opening.

ACTIONS
Sterile solution of plasma proteins, albumin, globulin prepared from pooled donors • Maintains/restores plasma volume; slightly increases concentration of plasma protein; causes fluid to shift from interstitial spaces into circulation • Osmotic equivalent to equal amount of plasma • Contains 130-160 mEq sodium/L • Processing removes risk of hepatitis, HIV transmission. • Does not contain major antibodies, may be given without matching of blood type or Rh factor • Does not contain cellular elements; no risk of sensitization with repeated infusions • Does not affect blood clotting

PHARMACOKINETICS

ROUTE	ONSET	PEAK	DURATION
IV	Rapid	End infusion	Several hours; longer in volume-depleted states

DISTRIBUTION
Intravascular, except with impaired capillary permeability
ELIMINATION
Variable depending on clinical state

INDICATIONS
Plasma volume expansion/maintenance of CO in hypovolemic shock or serious hypovolemia from burns, hemorrhage,

trauma, surgery, other conditions resulting in fluid volume deficit • Also used in hypoproteinemia, but 25% albumin preferred, because large amount of albumin can be administered in relatively small volume.
Unlabeled/investigational: To bind antibodies during exchange transfusions in myasthenia gravis

PRECAUTIONS/CONTRAINDICATIONS

Precautions: Rapid infusion may cause circulatory overload. • CVP, PAPs, other central hemodynamics helpful in optimizing therapy for acutely ill patients • Restoration of volume in patients with surgery, trauma, other bleeding may increase hemorrhage. • Use with whole blood or packed cells in bleeding/anemic patients.
Use caution with: Hepatic/renal failure because of added protein, fluid, sodium load
c **Pregnancy category:** Safety not established, use only if clearly necessary.
Contraindications: Hypersensitivity to PPF • Severe anemia • Cardiac failure • Increased intravascular volume • Patients on cardiopulmonary bypass

ADVERSE EFFECTS

CV: **Circulatory overload;** elevated CVP, PCWP; hypotension, especially with rapid or intraarterial administration
Resp: Dyspnea, **pulmonary edema**
Misc: Allergic response with chills, fever, nausea, vomiting, wheals, VS instability

TOXICITY/OVERDOSE

Symptoms: Circulatory overload; ↑ CVP/PCWP • Dyspnea, pulmonary edema
Management: Stop infusion; consult physician. • Use diuretics cautiously if necessary.

Y-SITE COMPATIBILITIES

Most IV infusion fluids, plasma, whole blood

Y-SITE INCOMPATIBILITIES

Alcohol, norepinephrine

PATIENT CARE IMPLICATIONS

• Not a replacement for transfusion therapy; for actively bleeding/anemia patients, use as adjunct to whole blood or packed cells.
• Many precautions necessary during administration; see Administration.
Vital signs/hemodynamics: Monitor VS frequently during initial administration, observing for hypotension/acute allergic reactions; thereafter, monitor q1-2h, depending on indication, rate of administration; frequent monitoring necessary with acute hypovolemia, rapid administration. • Monitor CVP, PCWP, CO as available. Administer at rate/dosage to restore intravascular fluid volume/avoid overload. Stop or slow infusion; consult physician of CVP >6 mm Hg or PCWP >12 mm Hg or other established range. • Monitor UO; evaluate fluid balance.
Physical assessment: Assess for circulatory overload: crackles (rales), S_3 gallop, dyspnea, jugular venous distention • Restoration of volume in patients with surgery, trauma, other

P

---

italic = common side effects   **bold** = life-threatening reactions

bleeding increases intravascular pressure, may result in renewed/increased bleeding. Assess for indicators of bleeding. • Assess for allergic reactions such as chills, fever, hypotension, nausea, vomiting, urticaria. Slow or stop infusion; consult physician. If additional PPF is indicated, use solution from different lot. **Laboratory tests:** Monitor: Hgb/Hct • Serum albumin, protein • Electrolytes, especially sodium • May cause: Hypernatremia: monitor for edema, pulmonary crackles

PATIENT/FAMILY TEACHING

Purpose of solution is to provide necessary blood proteins. • Immediately report chills, fever, nausea, vomiting, urticaria.

AVAILABLE FORMS

5% solution
Storage: Some solutions require refrigerated storage at 2°-10° C (35°-49° F) (check manufacturer's labeling). Do not freeze.

---

pneumococcal vaccine, polyvalent
(nu-mo-kok'al)
Pneumovax 23,
Pnu-Imune

Classification: Vaccine

USUAL DOSE
P SC/IM, adults/children >2 yr: 0.5 ml

ADMINISTRATION
P SC/IM, adults/children >2 yr: • SC: Route used for individuals with bleeding disorders • IM: Inject into deltoid or lateral midthigh. DO NOT ADMINISTER IV/INTRADERMALLY.

ACTIONS

Polyvalent vaccine containing antigenic capsular polysaccharides derived from 23 types of *Streptococcus pneumoniae* • Promotes active immunity by stimulating production of serum antibodies to antigens present in vaccine • Protective antibodies against pneumococcal infection develop within 2-3 wk • Antibody response rates lower in immunosuppressed patients

PHARMACOKINETICS

ROUTE	ONSET	DURATION
SC IM	≥2-fold increase in antibodies within 2-3 wk	Protective antibody levels present for at least 5 yr

INDICATIONS

To promote active immunity to pneumococcal pneumonia and **P** bacteremia in adults/children >2 yr at ↑ risk of morbidity/mortality from pneumococcal infections • At-risk individuals include adults with chronic disease (e.g., CV/pulmonary/renal disease, diabetes mellitus, alcoholism, hepatic cirrhosis, CSF **G** leaks); older adults (>65 yr); immunocompromised adults/ **P** children (e.g., anatomic asplenia, splenic dysfunction, sickle cell disease, Hodgkin's disease, lymphoma, multiple myeloma, chronic renal failure, immunosuppression therapy); **P** adults/children >2 yr with HIV infection.

P pediatric	**G** geriatric	**V** Direct IV

PRECAUTIONS/ CONTRAINDICATIONS

Precautions: May cause serious allergic reaction, including anaphylaxis • ↑ Risk of reactions if administered within 3 yr of previous vaccination • Hemodialysis or immunosuppressed patients require higher doses; response to immunization may not be satisfactory.

Use caution with: Thrombocytopenia, hemophilia, other bleeding disorder; IM injection may cause bleeding. • Febrile or severely ill patients; defer immunization, because febrile or adverse reaction may pose significant risk.

C **Pregnancy category:** Safety not established for use in pregnancy or lactation

Contraindications: Hypersensitivity to pneumococcal polyvalent vaccine, other vaccine components (e.g., phenol, thimerosal) • Children >2 yr

ADVERSE EFFECTS

CNS: Rarely—paresthesias, acute radiculoneuropathy, Guillain-Barré syndrome

Local: *Injection site soreness, swelling, erythema, induration;* rash

Misc: *Fever,* mild myalgia, arthralgia, **anaphylaxis** (rare)

INTERACTIONS

chemotherapy (cancer), corticosteroids, immunosuppressives Diminished immune response; ↑ dose of vaccine required

PATIENT CARE IMPLICATIONS

• Determine previous vaccination history, reactions; ↑ risk of adverse reactions with repeat vaccination.

• Have epinephrine, antihistamine, resuscitation equipment immediately available at time of injection.

• Do not mix in same syringe or administer in same site as other vaccines.

Vital signs/hemodynamics: Monitor BP, HR, RR, temperature before and 30 min after injection.

Physical assessment: Assess for allergic-type or anaphylactic reactions: chills, fever, sweating, rash, itching, laryngeal edema, wheezing. • Observe outpatients for 30 min after injection.

PATIENT/FAMILY TEACHING

Vaccination provides long-term protection from organisms that cause pneumococcal pneumonia, other infections. • Low-grade fever/pain; tenderness, redness, muscle stiffness at injection site may occur. • Immediately report allergic-type reaction: chills, fever, sweating, itching, difficulty breathing. • Routine booster doses not recommended at this time; consider revaccination after 3-5 yr for children with nephrotic syndrome, asplenia, or sickle cell anemia who will be ≤10 yr at revaccination.

AVAILABLE FORMS

Parenteral solution for IM/SC use

Storage: Refrigerate at 2°-8° C (35°-46° F). Do not freeze.

P

potassium chloride
Cena-K, K-Lease, K-lor,
K-lyte, K-Norm, K-Tab,
Kalium Durules ✦,
Kay Ceil, Klor-Con,
Micro-K, Slow-K

Classification: Electrolyte replacement

USUAL DOSE
PO, adults: Prevention of hypokalemia: 20 mEq/24 hr 2-4 times daily • **Treatment of hypokalemia:** 40-100 mEq/24 hr 2-4 times daily • Do not exceed 150 mEq/24 hr.
Ⓟ PO, children: 2-3 mEq/kg/24 hr 2-4 times daily • Do not exceed 3 mEq/kg/24 hr.
IV inf, adults: 20-60 mEq/24 hr, depending on plasma levels • Up to 400 mEq/24 hr used with extreme caution/close monitoring in severe hypokalemia
Ⓟ IV inf, children: 2-3 mEq/kg/24 hr, depending on plasma levels • Do not exceed 3 mEq/kg/24 hr.

ADMINISTRATION
PO: Administer with/after meals and with 6-8 oz water/juice to reduce GI irritation.
IV inf: MUST BE DILUTED BEFORE ADMINISTRATION • Administer ≤20 mEq over at least 60 min. • With severe hypokalemia (<2.5 mEq/L serum), give up to 40 mEq/hr using extreme caution. • Monitor ECG continuously with administration of ≥10 mEq/hr. • Use large vein; small needle/catheter; Ⓟ avoid scalp veins in children. • AVOID INFUSION OF CONCENTRATED SOLUTIONS VIA CENTRAL OR JUGULAR CATHETERS. • Dose may be split, infused simultaneously via two veins when necessary to administer large dose. • Stop or slow infusion for burning, discomfort. • Use extreme care to avoid extravasation. • Do not administer IM/SC. • **Rapid infusion/high doses may cause hypotension, heart block, cardiac arrest.**

PREPARATION
IV inf: Generally, dilute to concentration of ≤40 mEq/L. In extreme emergencies, more concentrated solutions may be given via large vein with relatively high flow, but central/jugular infusion should be avoided. • Thoroughly shake prepared solution to avoid layering of potassium. • Do not add to IV bottle in hanging position. • With severe hypokalemia, prepare in nondextrose solutions, because dextrose might decrease serum potassium level.
Compatible fluids: D_5W, 0.9% NaCl, LR, most common IV solutions

ACTIONS
Necessary for nerve impulse transmission, effective contraction of cardiac, skeletal, smooth muscles • Helps maintain osmotic pressure, ion balance • Essential for acid-base balance, normal renal function, gastric secretions, carbohydrate/protein metabolism, enzyme reactions • Change of 0.1 U in plasma pH produces inverse change of 0.6 mEq/L in plasma potassium concentration.

PHARMACOKINETICS

ROUTE	ONSET	PEAK
PO	<30 min	30 min
PO, ext rel	30-60 min	1-2 hr
IV	Immed	Rapid

DISTRIBUTION

Dextrose, insulin, O_2 facilitate movement of potassium into cells

ELIMINATION

Excreted mainly by kidneys; ↑ with surgery/tissue injury

INDICATIONS

Prevention/treatment of hypokalemia associated with GI losses, hyperadrenalism, malnutrition, negative nitrogen balance, metabolic alkalosis, metabolic/diabetic acidosis, excessive urinary loss, surgery, other conditions • Prevention of potassium depletion associated with thiazide diuretics, furosemide, ethacrynic acid, corticosteroids, amphotericin B, other drugs • Treatment of dysrhythmias associated with cardiac glycoside toxicity • To elevate potassium levels to upper limits of normal, prevent tachydysrhythmias after cardiac surgery.

PRECAUTIONS/ CONTRAINDICATIONS

Precautions: Avoid infusion of concentrated solutions via central or jugular catheters, because fatal cardiotoxicity may result. • Carefully adjust dose to serum potassium levels. • Rapid injection may cause hypotension, dysrhythmias, heart block, cardiac arrest. • Intestinal/gastric ulceration has occurred with extended-release preparations. • Some commercial preparations contain tartrazine dye (FD&C yellow no. 5), which may cause serious allergic reactions. • Elixir may contain alcohol.

Use caution with: Renal impairment • Cardiac disease • Concurrent use of cardiac glycosides

A Pregnancy category: Minimal risk to fetus

Contraindications: Severe renal impairment, oliguria, anuria, azotemia • Untreated Addison's disease • Acute dehydration • Heat cramps • Extensive tissue breakdown (e.g., acute trauma/burn injury) • Concurrent use of potassium-sparing diuretics • Solid PO preparations with GI hypomotility (e.g., diabetic gastroparesis, anticholinergic therapy) • Hyperkalemia

ADVERSE EFFECTS

CNS: Confusion

CV: Peaked T waves, prolonged PR interval, widened QRS complex, ST depression, bradycardia, **ventricular dysrhythmias, heart block, cardiac arrest**

GI: Nausea, vomiting, gastric irritation, diarrhea, small bowel ulceration

Local: *Burning/pain at injection site,* phlebitis

Hyperkalemia: Fatigue, irritability, weakness, paresthesias

TOXICITY/OVERDOSE

Symptoms: ECG changes, bradycardia, ventricular dysrhythmias/fibrillation, cardiac arrest • Weakness, paresthesias, muscle paralysis, respiratory distress, death

Management: After recent ingestion, implement guidelines for management of acute overdose (Appendix I). • Monitor ECG continuously. • For severe hyperkalemia (>8 mEq/L), ad-

P

italic = common side effects   **bold** = life-threatening reactions

minister 300-500 ml/hr IV dextrose, 10%-20%, with 5-10 U regular insulin for each 20 g dextrose. Correct acidosis with sodium bicarbonate. • For absence of P waves or wide QRS complex, administer calcium gluconate or chloride (not interchangeable, calcium chloride 3 × potency of calcium gluconate). Do not use calcium for digitalized patients. • These measures cause intracellular shift of potassium, may be initiated simultaneously. • Administer sodium polystyrene sulfonate (kayexalate) PO or by retention enema to bind/remove potassium from body. • Hemodialysis or peritoneal dialysis may be useful. • *Use caution with digitalized patients, because too rapid removal of potassium may cause digitalis toxicity.*
• For extravasation, inject area with 1% procaine and hyaluronidase (Wydase) using 25–27-gauge needle (Appendixes K and L). Apply warm moist compresses.

INTERACTIONS

angiotensin-converting enzyme inhibitors Serious hyperkalemia
diuretics, potassium sparing (e.g., amiloride, spirinolactone, triamterene) Profound hyperkalemia; avoid concurrent use

Y-SITE COMPATIBILITIES

Aminophylline, amiodarone, ampicillin, amrinone, atropine, calcium gluconate, cephalothin, cephapirin, chlorpromazine, ciprofloxacin, dexamethasone, digoxin, diltiazem, dobutamine, dopamine, droperidol, enalaprilat, epinephrine, esmolol, famotidine, fentanyl, furosemide, insulin, isoproterenol, labetalol, lidocaine, magnesium sulfate, meperidine, morphine, norepinephrine, penicillin G potassium, pentazocine, piperacillintazobactam, procainamide, propranolol, sodium bicarbonate, zidovudine

Y-SITE INCOMPATIBILITIES

Diazepam, methylprednisolone sodium succinate, phenytoin

PATIENT CARE IMPLICATIONS

• Postop or stressed patients with normal renal function excrete up to 80-90 mEq potassium daily. Gastric/intestinal secretions contain large amounts of potassium (e.g., up to 60 mEq/L in diarrheal fluid), account for major losses in certain patients.
• Available in many forms, including extended-release capsules, various tablets/powders (sugar free, effervescent, extended release), for PO solution, and parenteral solutions.
• Do not crush or break extended-release preparations.
• Many precautions necessary with IV use; see Administration
• IV infusions up to 40 mEq/hr may be given in extreme situations such as severe hypokalemia with life-threatening cardiac dysrhythmias, diabetic ketoacidosis, diuretic phase of acute renal failure.
Vital signs/hemodynamics:
IV inf: Continuously monitor ECG for peaked T waves, prolonged PR interval, widened QRS complex, ST depression, bradycardia, ventricular dysrhythmias, heart block. If present, stop potassium infusion,

---

P pediatric   **G** geriatric   **V** Direct IV

consult physician. • Assess BP frequently with IV administration of large doses or within short periods (e.g., ≤1 hr).
Physical assessment: Assess for hyperkalemia: irritability, confusion, diarrhea, weakness, paresthesias, Slow or stop infusion; check serum levels. • Monitor I&O. Slow or stop infusion; consult physician for ↓ UO.
Laboratory tests: Monitor: Serum potassium levels • Digoxin levels with concurrent cardiac glycoside therapy • ABGs, acid-base status in critically ill patients • Change of 0.1 U in plasma pH will result in inverse change of 0.6 mEq/L in plasma potassium.

PATIENT/FAMILY TEACHING

Purpose of medication is to replace potassium; often used with other medications such as diuretics, digoxin. • Report weakness, fatigue, tingling of extremities, confusion, vomiting, diarrhea, bloody or dark stools, vomiting of blood.
Outpatient: It is especially important to take this medication exactly as prescribed. Do not skip or double doses. Take missed dose as soon as remembered. • Do not crush, break, chew, or dissolve extended-release preparations. Be sure to thoroughly dissolve powder, tablets before drinking. GI irritation may be caused by improper use. • Take with/after meals and with 6-8 oz water/juice to reduce GI irritation. • Follow dietary recommendations as prescribed. • Avoid salt substitutes or "lite" salt unless specifically prescribed by physician. • Follow-up exams, laboratory tests

are important in monitoring potassium levels, response to therapy.

AVAILABLE FORMS

Parenteral for IV injection • Extended-release tablets/capsules • PO solution • Powder for PO solution • Extended-release powder for PO suspension

prazosin HCl
(pra′zoe-sin)
Minipress
prazosin HCl with polythiazide
Minizide

Classifications: Vasodilator, antihypertensive, peripheral antiadrenergic agent

USUAL DOSE

PO, adults: Initially 1 mg bid-tid • Increase as needed to control BP. • Range, 6-15 mg daily in divided doses • Maximum dose, 40 mg/day • Renal impairment: use reduced dose

ACTIONS

Dilates arteriovenous vasculature, reducing peripheral vascular resistance/BP • Selectively inhibits alpha-1-adrenergic receptors • Most profound effects on DBP • HR, CO unchanged in supine patients • With CHF, results in ↓ right atrial pressure, ↓ pulmonary/systemic venous pressures and ↑ CO; HR unchanged or slightly ↓ • May ↑ CO, ↓ regurgitant volume in aortic/mitral insufficiency.

P

PHARMACOKINETICS

ROUTE	ONSET	PEAK	DURATION
PO	1 hr	1-3 hr	≤24 hour

DISTRIBUTION

Widely distributed; 92%-97% protein bound

ELIMINATION

Eliminated in urine, bile; half-life 2-3 hr

INDICATIONS

Moderate to severe hypertension in patients who have not adequately responded to diuretics, beta-adrenergic blockers, ACE inhibitors • Generally used in combination with diuretic
Unlabeled/investigational:
Along with cardiac glycosides/diuretics in management of CHF • To ↓ urinary obstruction in benign prostatic hypertrophy

PRECAUTIONS/ CONTRAINDICATIONS

Precautions: Initial dose may cause profound hypotension.
Use caution with: Renal impairment; reduce dose. • Concurrent use of other antihypertensives/diuretics, surgery, anesthesia • Narcolepsy; may worsen condition
c Pregnancy category: Safety not established; use only if safer alternatives unavailable.
Contraindications: Hypersensitivity to prazosin, other quinazolines • Children: Safety/efficacy not established

ADVERSE EFFECTS

CNS: *Headache, dizziness, fatigue, drowsiness,* paresthesias, nervousness
EENT: Blurred vision, tinnitus
Resp: Nasal congestion, dyspnea, epistaxis

CV: *Palpitations, orthostatic hypotension,* **hypotension, syncope,** tachycardia, edema
GI: *Nausea,* vomiting, dry mouth, abdominal pain, diarrhea, constipation, ↑ liver enzymes
GU: Urinary frequency, incontinence, priapism, impotence
Derm: Itching, rash
Misc: Fever, arthralgia

TOXICITY/OVERDOSE

Symptoms: Hypotension
• Drowsiness, depressed reflexes
Management: After recent ingestion, implement guidelines for management of acute overdose (Appendix I). • Support respiration as needed with O_2 and/or mechanical ventilation.
• **Hypotension:** Elevate legs, administer fluids; use vasopressors (e.g., dopamine, norepinephrine) as necessary. • Monitor renal, electrolyte, acid-base status closely. • Hemodialysis is not likely to be useful.

INTERACTIONS

beta blockers Profound hypotension
calcium channel blockers Profound hypotension
diuretics Additive hypotensive effects
indomethacin, other highly, protein-bound agents ↓ Hypotensive effects
nitroglycerin Profound hypotension

PATIENT CARE IMPLICATIONS

• Protect patient from injury associated with orthostatic hypotension, especially when initiating therapy.

• Initially and when dosage increased, administer hs to reduce dizziness.
• Effectiveness ↑ when used in combination with diuretic therapy.
• Vomiting, diarrhea, excessive perspiration, dehydration could cause excessive ↓ BP.

Vital signs/hemodynamics: Monitor BP, HR q1-2h when initiating therapy or increasing dose. • Hemodynamic monitoring useful in establishing optimal dose in patients with severe CHF receiving combination therapy.

Physical assessment: Assess for perfusion/oxygenation deficit: chest discomfort, ↓ level of consciousness, activity intolerance, hypotension, dizziness.
• Assess for fluid volume overload: bibasilar crackles (rales), dyspnea, peripheral edema, neck vein distention, weight gain.
• Monitor fluid balance, weigh daily.

PATIENT/FAMILY TEACHING

Purpose of drug is to lower BP and/or relieve symptoms of heart failure. • May cause excessive lowering of BP, dizziness, especially during initiation of therapy. Use caution when changing positions, walking. Alcohol, hot weather, vigorous activity, vomiting, diarrhea, dehydration, prolonged standing make these symptoms more likely. • Lie down immediately if lightheaded or dizzy. • Immediately report chest discomfort, shortness of breath, confusion, activity intolerance, lightheadedness, dizziness. • Medication is not cure for high BP; Other therapies, including life-style modifications, must be continued.

Outpatient: Take medication exactly as prescribed. Do not stop taking medicine even if you feel better. If medication abruptly discontinued, you may develop dangerously high BP.
• Avoid driving and other activities requiring mental alertness until individual response to drug known. • If dose increased, take first larger dose at bedtime.
• Weigh twice/wk; notify primary health care provider of weight gain, edema. • Consult physician or pharmacist before taking cough, cold, or allergy preparations.

AVAILABLE FORMS

Capsules • Capsules with poly-thiazide

prednisone
(pred′ni-sone)
Cortan, Deltasone, Meticorten, Orasone, Panasol, Prednicen-M, Sterapred

Classifications: Adrenocortical steroid, corticosteroid, glucocorticoid, antiinflammatory agent

USUAL DOSE

PO, adults: Initially, 5-60 mg daily in 2-4 divided doses, depending on patient condition. Dose gradually decreased
PO, children: Initially 0.14-2.0 mg/kg daily in 2-4 divided doses; maintenance dose depends on patient condition
• Dose gradually decreased.

---

italic = common side effects   **bold** = life-threatening reactions

ADMINISTRATION

PO: When possible, administer with meals to minimize gastric irritation.

ACTIONS

Antiinflammatory glucocorticoid with complex action affecting almost all body systems • Stabilizes lysosomal membranes in leukocytes, inhibits macrophage accumulation in inflamed tissues; reduces leukocyte adhesion to capillary walls; decreases capillary permeability, edema • Antagonizes histamine/kinin release • Suppresses immune response by producing lymphocytopenia, decreasing Ig/complement, reducing volume/activity of lymphatic system • Mineralocorticoid activity promotes sodium retention.

PHARMACOKINETICS

ROUTE	ONSET	PEAK	DURATION
PO	<60 min	1-2 hr	Dose dependent

DISTRIBUTION

Widely distributed throughout body tissue

ELIMINATION

Metabolized in liver, eliminated by kidneys; biologic half-life 18-36 hr

INDICATIONS

Inflammatory, allergic, hematologic, neoplastic, autoimmune disorders to reduce inflammation, promote immunosuppression • Replacement therapy in adrenal insufficiency • Alternate-day dosing possible in management of chronic, stable conditions.

PRECAUTIONS/ CONTRAINDICATIONS

Precautions: Prolonged therapy suppresses adrenal synthesis of glucocorticoids/mineralocorti-coids, resulting in withdrawal symptoms with abrupt discontinuation. • May mask signs of infection, ↓ resistance to infection • May cause edema, particularly in renal impairment • Peptic ulceration possible in high-risk patients (e.g., history of peptic ulcer, liver/intestinal disease, nephrotic syndrome, critical illness)

Use caution with: Diabetes; insulin requirements may ↑ . • Renal disorders • Osteoporosis • Seizure disorder • CHF • Chronic active hepatitis; may promote liver failure • Glaucoma • AIDS

C Pregnancy category: Use only if safer alternative unavailable.

Contraindications: Hypersensitivity to prednisone, any corticosteroid • Psychosis • Amebiasis • Systemic fungal infections • Tuberculosis • Recent administration of live viral vaccine (e.g., smallpox)

ADVERSE EFFECTS

CNS: *Mood swings, depression,* aggravation of psychiatric disorder, headache

CV: *Hypertension,* tachycardia, thrombophlebitis, **thromboembolism**

GI: *Nausea,* vomiting, *anorexia,* weight gain, **peptic ulceration, GI bleeding**

Endo: *Adrenal suppression, menstrual irregularities,* hyperglycemia, suppression of growth in children, "steroid-induced" diabetes mellitus

F&E: Hypokalemia, hypokalemic alkalosis, fluid retention

MS: *Muscle wasting, osteoporosis,* aseptic joint necrosis

Derm: *Diminished wound healing, petechiae, ecchymosis,*

hirsutism, acne, thinning of skin, hypo/hyperpigmentation
Misc: *Cushingoid appearance,* ↑ *susceptibility to infection,* ↓ *symptoms of infection*

TOXICITY/OVERDOSE

Symptoms: Cushingoid: Moon face, central obesity, hirsutism, acne, hypertension, osteoporosis, diabetes mellitus, hyperlipidemia, peptic ulcers, myopathy, immunosuppression, fluid/electrolyte imbalance
• Acute adrenal insufficiency: Fever, anorexia, malaise, nausea, dizziness, fainting, dyspnea, hypoglycemia, myalgia, arthralgia; follows rapid withdrawal of therapy
Management: After recent ingestion, implement guidelines for management of acute overdose (Appendix I). • For severe fluid overload, administer diuretics; replace potassium as necessary. • For symptoms of adrenal insufficiency, supplement with additional corticosteroid; taper dose gradually before withdrawal.

INTERACTIONS

amphotericin B Hypokalemia
antidiabetics (PO agents, insulin) ↑ Antidiabetic drug requirements
carbamazepine ↓ Corticoid effects
diuretics Hypokalemia
ketoconazole Enhanced corticoid effects
phenytoin ↓ Corticoid effects
rifampin ↓ Corticoid effects

PATIENT CARE IMPLICATIONS

• Administer daily dose in AM to coincide with physiologic peak in cortisol levels.

• Administer PO dose with meals to avoid gastric irritation.
• Dosage should be gradually tapered to avoid adrenal insufficiency
• Dosage increases are necessary when patients subjected to severe emotional/physical stress.
• Dosage depends on condition being treated, patient response.
• Prolonged therapy suppresses hypothalamic-pituitary-adrenal axis, may lead to suppression of adrenal synthesis of glucocorticoids/mineralocorticoids. Abrupt discontinuation may cause withdrawal symptoms: fatigue, anorexia, nausea, hypotension, hypoglycemia, depression, fever, dizziness, joint pain, malaise, fainting.
• Drug-related immunosuppression may mask signs of infection. Monitor closely, initiate antibiotic therapy as soon as infection suspected.
Vital signs: Frequency of VS monitoring depends on patient condition rather than drug effects.
Physical assessment: Assess for adrenal insufficiency or cushingoid symptoms (see Toxicity/overdose). Symptoms of adrenal insufficiency indicate insufficient dosage or too-rapid withdrawal of therapy. Cushingoid symptoms indicate excessive dosage. Assess for weight gain, peripheral edema, dyspnea, crackles (rales). • Check stools, emesis for occult blood. • Monitor I&O, weigh daily.
Laboratory tests: Monitor: Electrolytes, especially sodium, potassium, calcium • Blood glucose • CBC with differential
• Plasma cortisol (normal, 138-635 nmol/L at 8 AM)

P

---

italic = common side effects   **bold** = life-threatening reactions

PATIENT/FAMILY TEACHING

Purpose of medication is to reduce inflammation of affected area or body system. • Take exactly as prescribed. Do not double dose if missed. Suddenly stopping therapy may cause adrenal insufficiency: weakness, fatigue, nausea, low BP, low blood sugar. • Take with meals to minimize stomach upset. • Drug causes suppression of immune system, may mask signs of infection. Avoid individuals with contagious illnesses. Report fever, prolonged malaise, any symptom of infection immediately. • Report rapid weight gain, unusual swelling, very dark or bloody stools, vomiting of blood, sores slow to heal, significant behavior changes. • Inform physicians, dentists, other health care providers of medication regimen before treatment. • Carry Medic-Alert ID describing medication regimen.

AVAILABLE FORMS

Tablets • PO solution/syrup (1 mg/ml) • PO solution concentrate (5 mg/ml)

---

procainamide HCl
(proe-kane'-a-mide)
Procan SR, Procaimide SR, Promine, Pronestyl, Rhythmin

Classifications: Class IA antidysrhythmic, membrane stabilizer

USUAL DOSE

Always use lowest effective dose. • Discontinue for widened QRS complex, hypotension, aggravation of dysrhythmias.

PO, adults: Loading dose: 1,000 mg initially, followed by 375-750 mg q2-3h until dysrhythmia controlled. Do not use ext. rel. tabs for loading dose • Maintenance, standard preparation: 500-1,000 mg q4-6h • Maintenance, sustained-release preparation: 500-1,000 mg q6h

ⓅPO, children: 10 mg/kg q4-6h

Direct IV, adults: 50-100 mg q5min until dysrhythmia suppressed; do not exceed total dose of 1,000 mg. • Follow successful therapy with IV cont inf.

ⓅDirect IV, children: Loading dose: 3-6 mg/kg up to 100 mg; may repeat in 10-30 min, but do not exceed maximum dose of 30 mg/kg/24 hr. • Follow successful therapy with IV cont inf.

IV, cont inf, adults: 1-4 mg/min (15-60 ml/hr of 1 g/250 ml solution); use follows control of dysrhythmia with bolus dose

ⓅIV, cont inf, children: 0.02-0.08 mg/kg/min; use follows control of dysrhythmia with bolus dose

ADMINISTRATION

Ⅴ Direct IV: Administer slowly at rate no >20 mg/min until dysrhythmia controlled. • May be diluted to facilitate administration • Too-rapid administration may trigger serious hypotension, heart block. • Stop injection for hypotension, >50% widening of QRS complex, or when total of 1,000 mg given.

IV, cont inf: Must use infusion pump • Administer at rate of 1-4 mg/min (15-60 ml/hr of 4 mg/ml concentration) until dysrhythmias controlled with PO medication.

PREPARATION

DILUTION	CONCENTRATION
1,000 mg/250 ml	4 mg/ml
2,000 mg/250 ml	8 mg/ml

More concentrated solutions may be used if necessary to limit fluid intake.

Compatible fluids: D₅W (conflicting data), 0.9% NaCl, prepared combinations of these solutions

ACTIONS

Decrease cardiac excitability by increasing threshold for electrical excitation • Blocks fast sodium channels to suppress automaticity in His-Purkinje system, as well as ectopic atrial/ectopic ventricular pacemakers • PR, QT intervals may be prolonged. • Conduction velocity ↓ in atrium, bundle of His, ventricle. • Action potential duration ↑ • Contractility may be ↓ in damaged heart. • Anticholinergic effects cause vasodilation, may ↓ BP.

PHARMACOKINETICS

ROUTE	ONSET	PEAK	DURATION
IV	Immed	15 min	3-4 hr

DISTRIBUTION
Rapid, wide; ↓ with heart failure

ELIMINATION
Activated/metabolized by liver, excreted in urine; half-life 2.5-4.7 hr

Therapeutic level: 4-10 µg/ml

INDICATIONS

Suppression/prevention of symptomatic atrial/ventricular dysrhythmias • Used to control SVTs, atrial fibrillation only after failure of cardiac glycosides • For ventricular dysrhythmias, procainamide used only if lidocaine ineffective

PRECAUTIONS/CONTRAINDICATIONS

Precautions: May precipitate/worsen AV heart block • Effectiveness ↓ with hypoxia, electrolyte imbalance, acid-base disturbances
Use caution with: Hepatic/renal impairment, heart failure; reduced dose necessary • Preexisting 2nd/3rd degree heart block, bundle branch block, digitalis intoxication • Acute MI • Bone marrow suppression
C Pregnancy category: Safety not established; use only if safer alternative unavailable.
Contraindications: Hypersensitivity to procainamide, procaine • Tartrazine or aspirin hypersensitivity (Pronestyl Filmlok tablets containing FD&C yellow no. 5 [tartrazine]) • Torsade de pointes • 2nd/3rd degree heart block, unless functional ventricular pacemaker in place or readily available • Commercial parenteral preparations may contain sulfites, which can cause serious allergic reactions.

ADVERSE EFFECTS

CNS: Dizziness, headache, confusion, depression
Resp: Dyspnea, asthma, respiratory depression
CV: *Prolongation of PR/QT intervals, QRS complex;* **hypotension, bradycardia, heart block, torsades de pointes**
GI: Anorexia, bitter taste, nausea, vomiting, diarrhea, abdominal pain
Hema: Bone marrow depression, *neutropenia,* thrombocytopenia
Derm: Wheals
Syst: Fever, SLE-like syndrome

---

italic = common side effects   **bold** = life-threatening reactions

TOXICITY/OVERDOSE

Symptoms: Severe hypotension • Bradycardia, heart block, wide QRS complex, tachycardia, possible ventricular fibrillation • Lethargy, confusion, nausea, vomiting

Management: After recent ingestion, implement guidelines for management of acute overdose (Appendix I). • Slow or stop infusion. • **Hypotension:** Elevate legs, administer IV fluids; use vasopressors (e.g., dopamine, norepinephrine) as necessary if inadequate response to fluids. • Manage symptomatic bradycardia, ventricular dysrhythmias according to ACLS guidelines (Appendix P). Hemodialysis may be helpful.

Toxic serum level: >16 µg/ml

INTERACTIONS

antihypertensives Profound hypotension

beta-blockers Hypotension, bradycardia, toxicity

bretylium Additive cardiac depression

cimetidine ↑ Procainamide levels; toxicity

lidocaine Additive cardiac depression

NMBAs Prolonged neuromuscular blockade

phenytoin ↑ Procainamide metabolism; excessive cardiac depression

quinidine Heart block, ventricular dysrhythmias

Y-SITE COMPATIBILITIES

Amiodarone, famotidine, heparin, potassium chloride, ranitidine, vitamin B complex with C

Y-SITE INCOMPATIBILITIES

Milrinone, phenytoin

PATIENT CARE IMPLICATIONS

• Correct hypoxemia, hypokalemia, other fluid/electrolyte imbalance; O_2 therapy usually indicated.

• Continuous infusion indicated only if bolus dose suppresses ventricular dysrhythmias.

• If positive ANA titer develops or SLE symptoms occur, consult physician, consider discontinuation of drug.

Vital signs/hemodynamics: Continuously monitor ECG during loading/parenteral therapy. Use lowest possible dose for dysrhythmia control. Monitor for toxicity: widening of QRS complex, prolongation of QT interval, bradycardia, heart block, ↑ ventricular dysrhythmias. If present, consult physician immediately. • Monitor BP q5min during IV loading; stop or slow injection for hypotension. Thereafter, monitor q15-60min according to titration schedule, stability. • As available, measure CO, PCWP q1-4h. Monitor for excessive myocardial depression: decreased CO or increased PCWP, especially with history of CHF, acute MI, shock, liver disease.

Physical assessment: Assess for perfusion/oxygenation deficit: ↓ level of consciousness, chest pain, activity intolerance, hypotension, dizziness.

Laboratory tests: Monitor: ABGs • Electrolytes • Plasma levels of procainamide and its metabolite, *N*-acetylprocainamide (NAPA) in patients with constant infusion of ≥3 mg/min for ≥24 hr and in patients receiving PO therapy • Procainamide therapeutic level: 4-8 μg/ml

PATIENT/FAMILY TEACHING

Purpose of medication is to regulate beating of heart. • Immediately report chest pain, dizziness, breathing difficulty. • Sustained-release tablets should never be broken, chewed, or crushed. • Dosage intervals should be evenly spaced.

AVAILABLE FORMS

Parenteral for IV/IM use • Standard capsules, tablets • Sustained-release tablets

---

prochlorperazine, prochlorperazine edisylate, prochlorperazine maleate
(proe-klor-per′a-zeen) ✦
Compazine, Stemetil ✦

Classifications: Antiemetic, antipsychotic, tranquilizer, phenothiazine

USUAL DOSE

PO/rectal, adults: 5-10 mg 3-4 times daily; increase gradually as necessary. • Sustained release: 15 mg q AM or 10 mg q12h. Up to 100-150 mg/day used for severe psychiatric disturbances.

PO/rectal, children (>2 yr or 20 lb): According to body weight as follows:

WEIGHT (lb)	DOSE (mg)/ FREQUENCY	MAX DOSE (mg/day)
20-29	2.5 qd-bid	7.5
30-39	2.5 bid-tid	10
40-85	2.5 tid/5 bid	15

IM, adults: 5-10 mg q3-4h as needed; do not exceed 40 mg within 24-hr period. Up to 10-20 mg q2-4h used for severe psychiatric disturbances. • Convert to PO therapy as soon as possible.

IM, children: 0.06 mg/lb • Only one dose usually necessary

Direct IV/Intermit inf, adults: 5-10 mg; may repeat once if needed • Do not exceed single dose >10 mg.

Older adults, debilitation: Use ¼-⅓ usual dose

ADMINISTRATION

Direct IV: Patient should be supine. • Inject dilute solution slowly at rate of 1-5 mg/min. • Stop injection for hypotension, dysrhythmias, ECG changes.

IV, intermit inf: Patient should be supine. • Infuse over 15-20 min; do not exceed rate of 1 mg/min. • Stop infusion for hypotension, dysrhythmias, ECG changes.

PREPARATION

Avoid skin contact with solution for injection, which may cause contact dermatitis.
Direct IV: Dilute each 5 mg (1 ml) with 9 ml 0.9% NaCl for injection for concentration of 0.5 mg/ml.

IV, intermit inf: Dilute in ≥50 ml compatible IV solution
Compatible fluids: D₅W, 0.9% NaCl, LR

ACTIONS

Dopamine receptor antagonist; depresses parts of CNS that control wakefulness, basal metabolism, temperature regulation, vasomotor tone, emesis, hormonal balance • Decreases

P

---

italic = common side effects   **bold** = life-threatening reactions

anxiety/tension, relaxes muscles, sedates • Relative to other phenothiazines, has strong antiemetic, weak anticholinergic, moderate sedative, strong extrapyramidal (e.g., dystonia, motor restlessness, parkinsonism) effects • Weak peripheral alpha-adrenergic blocking activity may cause mild hypotension.
• Potentiates CNS, respiratory depressant, analgesic effects of opioid analgesics, sedatives, hypnotics, anesthetics

PHARMACOKINETICS

ROUTE	ONSET	PEAK	DURATION
PO	30-40 min	1-2 hr	3-4 hr
PO, sus rls	30-40 min		10-12 hr
IM	10-20 min	Var	3-4 hr
IV	>10 min	Rapid	3-4 hr

DISTRIBUTION

Wide; highly protein bound; readily crosses blood-brain barrier

ELIMINATION

Metabolized by liver, excreted in urine/feces; half-life 10-20 hr

INDICATIONS

Prevention/control of nausea/vomiting caused by postop status, toxins, radiation, drugs, chemotherapy, disease • Not generally effective for prevention of vertigo, motion sickness • Preop to decrease tension/anxiety, enhance anesthetic induction, potentiate anesthetic agents, ↓ postop vomiting • To ↓ hallucinations, autonomic hyperactivity, anxiety/tension other symptoms in schizophrenia, other psychiatric disorders • As adjunct in treatment of acute alcohol withdrawal (efficacy not clearly established)
Unlabeled/investigational:
IV route for severe vascular/tension headaches

PRECAUTIONS/ CONTRAINDICATIONS

Precautions: Risk of serious adverse CNS effects, including irreversible extrapyramidal reactions; initiate long-term therapy only if need clearly established • Lowers seizure threshold; may precipitate seizures • Antiemetic effects may impede diagnosis of disorders with vomiting as prominent feature (e.g., intestinal obstruction, Reye's syndrome)
Use caution with: CNS depressants, severe CV disease, hepatic/renal disease, seizure **G** disorder, older adults, debilitation, acute alcohol withdrawal, glaucoma, prostatic hypertrophy, exposure to organophosphate insecticides, exposure to temperature extremes, thermoregulatory failure, hypocalcemia; reduced dose indicated • COPD, asthma, acute respiratory infections, limited ventilatory reserve; CNS depressant effects may depress ventilatory drive. • Obtunded patients or when vomiting, aspiration likely; suppresses cough reflex
c **Pregnancy category:** Safety not established; use only if safer alternative unavailable.
Contraindications: Hypersensitivity to prochlorperazine, other phenothiazines • Hypersensitivity to tartrazine dye (FD&C yellow no. 5); avoid tablets. • Severe CNS depression • Coma • Bone marrow depression • Severe hypertension • Hypotension • Reye's syndrome • Children <2 yr or 20 **P** lb • Pediatric surgery • First trimester of pregnancy • Commercial parenteral preparations may contain sulfites, which can

---

cause serious allergic-type reactions.

ADVERSE EFFECTS

CNS: *Drowsiness,* anxiety, euphoria, paradoxical excitation, depression, weakness, headache, cerebral edema, **seizures,** *extrapyramidal reactions*—dystonia (neck and back muscle rigidity, carpopedal spasm, difficulty swallowing or talking); motor restlessness; parkinsonian signs/ symptoms; tardive dyskinesia (rhythmic involuntary movements of tongue, face, mouth, jaw, extremities); **neuroleptic malignant syndrome**—hyperthermia, hypertonicity, ↓ level of consciousness, autonomic instability

Resp: Bronchospasm, dyspnea

CV: Hypotension, *orthostatic hypotension,* tachycardia, syncope, dizziness, Q and T wave ECG changes, **circulatory collapse, sudden death**

GI: *Constipation, dry mouth,* **adynamic ileus,** hepatitis

GU: Urinary retention, pink or brownish discoloration of urine

Hema: Blood dyscrasias

Derm: *Photosensitivity,* rashes, changes in pigmentation, contact dermatitis (parenteral formulation or syrup)

Syst: Thermoregulatory failure with hypo/hyperthermia

Misc: Allergic/hypersensitivity reactions, **sudden death**

TOXICITY/OVERDOSE

Symptoms: CNS depression, coma • Hypotension, dysrhythmias, especially with IV administration • Extrapyramidal symptoms, seizures, hypo/ hyperthermia, agitation, autonomic reactions • Toxicity more likely with concurrent use of other CNS depressants

Management: After recent ingestion of large amounts, consider early gastric lavage with airway protection; *induction of vomiting not recommended, because dystonic reaction of head or neck could result in aspiration of vomitus.* • Use saline cathartics to evacuate extended-release capsules. • Maintain airway/support ventilation; administer IV fluids. • Observe closely for dystonia, extrapyramidal reactions, which could lead to airway difficulties. • **Hypotension:** Elevate legs, administer IV fluids; if necessary use norepinephrine or phenylephrine; avoid epinephrines, because phenothiazines may block alpha (pressor) effects, resulting in predominant beta effects, profound hypotension. • For acute dystonic reactions/ extrapyramidal symptoms, use diphenhydramine, anticholinergic antiparkinsonian agents. • Control seizures with diazepam or pentobarbital. • Dialysis not likely to be helpful.

INTERACTIONS

alcohol, ethyl Excessive sedation

amphetamines Mutual inhibition of therapeutic effects

antacids Impaired absorption; administer 1 hr before or 2 hr after prochlorperazine

anticholinergics Inhibition of antipsychotic effects

antihistamines ↑ Sedation

barbiturates Additive/antagonized effects

beta-blockers Hypotension

epinephrine Blocked alpha effects; profound hypotension

P

opiate analgesics ↑ Sedation, hypotension

COMPATIBILITIES

Syringe: Atropine, butorphanol, chlorpromazine, diphenhydramine, droperidol, fentanyl, glycopyrrolate, hydroxyzine, meperidine, metoclopromide, morphine, nalbuphine, pentazocine

Y-site: Fluconazole, heparin, ondansetron, potassium chloride

INCOMPATIBILITIES

Syringe: Hydromorphone, ketorolac, midazolam, pentobarbital

Y-site: Piperacillin-tazobactam

PATIENT CARE IMPLICATIONS

P G • Children/ older adults more likely to develop extrapyramidal effects, paradoxical excitation, other adverse reactions. Use lowest effective dose; monitor frequently.

• **Avoid skin contact with syrup, PO concentrate, solution for injection, which may cause contact dermatitis.**

• Drowsiness, orthostatic hypotension possible, especially during first week of therapy; use safety precautions. When possible, administer hs.

• Large quantities should not be prescribed for patients with severe depression, suicidal tendencies, history of substance abuse.

• Reserve parenteral therapy to urgent/emergency situations or when PO route unacceptable (e.g., vomiting, NPO status). Convert to PO therapy as soon as possible.

IV use

• Adverse CV effects (e.g., hypotension, tachycardia, dizziness, syncope) more likely.

• Monitor frequently. Patient should remain in bed at least 1 hr, requires assistance with initial ambulation.

• Have resuscitation equipment immediately available.

Vital signs/hemodynamics: Monitor VS frequently in heavily sedated patients (e.g., receiving opiates) or during immediate postop period. • Continuous pulse oximetry recommended for heavily sedated patients

IV: Monitor HR, BP during and frequently after administration.

• As available, monitor ECG for ↑ QT interval, ST depression, AV conduction disturbances, dysrhythmias during and immediately after injection.

Physical asssessment: Assess neurologic status for excessive sedation, dizziness, impaired physical coordination; dose reduction may be necessary. • Assess for respiratory distress in patients with history of COPD, cardiac impairment.

Laboratory tests: • Monitor: Liver enzymes • BUN, creatinine • CBC

PATIENT/FAMILY TEACHING

Purpose of medication is to reduce anxiety, promote relaxation, prevent nausea/vomiting.

• Medication may cause dizziness, drowsiness. Call for assistance when getting out of bed, walking. Change positions slowly. Reactions are less likely after first week of therapy.

• Urine may turn pink or reddish brown. • Inform caregiver if you may be pregnant or are considering pregnancy.

Outpatient: Avoid driving and other activities requiring mental alertness or physical coordination. • May contribute to devel-

---

P pediatric   **G** geriatric   **V** Direct IV

opment of heatstroke; avoid hot weather, seek air conditioning. • Avoid using alcohol or other drugs that cause sedation while taking this medication. • Take antacids 1 hr before or 2 hr after drug. • Do not break or chew extended-release capsules. • If syrup or oral concentrate used, avoid skin contact.

Long-term therapy: Report (1) sore throat, mouth, or gums, other signs of infection that could signal dangerous lowering of WBC, (2) yellowing of skin or whites of eyes, (3) tremors or muscle twitching, (4) problems with eyesight. • Avoid prolonged exposure to sunlight; use sunscreen. • May cause withdrawal symptoms; consult primary health care provider before changing dose or abruptly discontinuing.

AVAILABLE FORMS

Parenteral solution • Tablets, syrup • Ext rel. capsules • Suppositories

promethazine
(proe-meth′a-zeen)
Anergan, Histanil ✤,
K-Phen, Phenameth,
Phenazine, Phencen,
Phenergan, Phenoject,
Prometh, Prorex, V-Gan
**promethazine with
meperidine**
Mepergan
**promethazine with
phenylephrine HCl**
Phenergan VC, Pherazine
VC

Classifications: Antiemetic, antihistamine, sedative, phenothiazine

USUAL DOSE

PO/rectal, adults: 12.5-25 mg q4-6h or 25-50 mg q8-12h

PO/rectal, children >2 yr: 0.25-0.5 mg/kg q4-6h • Two strengths of syrup available, 6.25 mg/5 ml and 25 mg/5 ml; VERIFY STRENGTH/DOSAGE BEFORE ADMINISTERING.

Direct IV/IM, adults: 12.5-25 mg q4-6h; up to 50 mg IM sometimes used

IM, children: 0.25-0.5 mg/kg q4-6h; up to 1.1 mg sometimes used

Older adults, debilitation: Use ¼-⅓ usual dose

ADMINISTRATION

Direct IV: Patient should be supine. • Inject dilute solution slowly at rate of 12.5 mg/min; must be diluted to concentration of ≤25 mg/ml. • Extravasation or intraarterial injection may cause necrosis; when possible, inject through tubing of free-

P

flowing IV line • If injection painful, immediately stop, evaluate IV patency. • Too-rapid injection causes hypotension.

PREPARATION

Direct IV: Dilute each ml (25 or 50 mg) with 9 ml 0.9% NaCl; dilute solution has 2.5 or 5 mg/ml, depending on concentration used
Compatible fluids: D_5W, 0.9% NaCl, LR

ACTIONS

Dopamine receptor antagonist with potent antihistaminic (H_1 receptor–blocking), sedative effects • Antiemetic, antimotion sickness, anticholinergic, local anesthetic effects • Slight antitussive activity • In usual doses has no significant effect of CV system • Potentiates CNS, respiratory depressant, analgesic effects of opioid analgesics, sedatives, hypnotics, anesthetics

PHARMACOKINETICS

ROUTE	ONSET	PEAK	DURATION*
PO	20 min	1-2 hr	4-6 hr
IM	20 min	Var	2-6 hr
IV	3-5 min	Rapid	2-4 hr

DISTRIBUTION

Wide; 93% protein bound

ELIMINATION

Metabolized by liver, excreted in urine/feces

*Duration of sedative effects; antihistaminic effects may persist ≥12 hr.

INDICATIONS

Prevention/control of nausea/vomiting caused by postop status, toxins, radiation, drugs, chemotherapy, disease, motion sickness • With opioid analgesics, for sedation and as adjunct in pain management • Preop, to decrease tension/anxiety, enhance anesthetic induction, potentiate anesthetic agents, reduce postop vomiting • During labor/delivery, for antiemetic, sedative effects • Relief of rhinorrhea/sneezing associated with common cold or allergies; control of minor allergic reactions to blood transfusion

PRECAUTIONS/ CONTRAINDICATIONS

Precautions: Risk of serious adverse CNS effects, including irreversible tardive dyskinesia, potentially fatal neuroleptic malignant syndrome; initiate long-term therapy only if need clearly established. • Lowers seizure threshold; may precipitate seizures • Antiemetic effects may impede diagnosis of disorders with vomiting as prominent feature (e.g., intestinal obstruction, Reye's syndrome). • Risk of CNS stimulant effects ↑ in children • Extravasation or intraarterial injection may cause necrosis, gangrene of affected extremity. • Commercial parenteral preparations may contain sulfites, which can cause serious allergic reactions.

Use caution with: CNS depressants, severe CV disease, hepatic/renal disease, seizure disorder, older adults, debilitation, acute alcohol withdrawal, glaucoma, prostatic hypertrophy, exposure to organophosphate insecticides, exposure to temperature extremes, thermoregulatory failure, hypocalcemia; reduced dose indicated • COPD, asthma, acute respiratory infections, limited ventilatory reserve; CNS depressant effects may depress ventilatory drive. • Obtunded

P pediatric   **G** geriatric   **V** Direct IV

patients or when vomiting, aspiration likely; suppresses cough reflex

c Pregnancy category: Safety not established; use only if safer alternative unavailable.

Contraindications: Hypersensitivity to promethazine, other phenothiazines • Severe CNS depression • Coma • Bone marrow depression • Severe hypertension • Hypotension • Reye's syndrome • Acutely ill or dehydrated children because of increased risk of extrapyramidal effects • Children with undiagnosed vomiting • Premature or term infants

ADVERSE EFFECTS

CNS: *Drowsiness,* dizziness, confusion, disorientation, incoordination, restlessness, anxiety, euphoria, paradoxical excitation, **seizures,** catatonia, hysteria; high-dose therapy—extrapyramidal reactions, including dystonia, motor restlessness, parkinsonian signs/symptoms, tardive dyskinesia, **neuroleptic malignant syndrome** (rare)

Resp: Irregular respiration

CV: Tachycardia, bradycardia, dizziness, ↑ ↓ BP

GI: *Nausea, vomiting, constipation,* dry mouth, hepatitis

GU: Urinary retention, pink or brownish discoloration of urine

Derm: Photosensitivity, rashes

Hema: Blood dyscrasias

Local: Venous thrombosis at injection site, gangrene after extravasation or intraarterial injection

TOXICITY/OVERDOSE

Symptoms: Somnolence, CNS depression, respiratory depression, coma • Hypotension (IV) • Atropine-like effects, including dry mouth, fixed/dilated pupils, flushing, GI symptoms • Extrapyramidal symptoms, seizures, agitation, autonomic reactions also possible • Toxicity more likely with concurrent use of other CNS depressants

Management: After recent ingestion of large amounts, consider early gastric lavage with airway protection. • Centrally acting emetics not likely to be useful • Maintain airway/support ventilation; administer IV fluids. • **Hypotension:** Elevate legs, administer IV fluids; use norepinephrine or phenylephrine as necessary if unresponsive to volume replacement; avoid epinephrine because phenothiazines may block alpha (pressor) effects, causing hypotension.

• For extrapyramidal symptoms, use diphenhydramine, anticholinergic antiparkinsonian agents.

• Control seizures with diazepam or pentobarbital. • Dialysis not likely to be helpful

INTERACTIONS

alcohol, ethyl ↑ Sedation

amphetamines Mutual inhibition of therapeutic effects

antacids Impaired absorption; administer 1 hr before or 2 hr after promethazine

anticholinergics Inhibition of antipsychotic effects

antihistamines ↑ Sedation

barbiturates Additive/antagonized effects

beta-blockers Hypotension

epinephrine Blocked alpha effects; profound hypotension

opiate analgesics ↑ Sedation, hypotension

TCAs Additive CNS depression

---

italic = common side effects   **bold** = life-threatening reactions

COMPATIBILITIES

Syringe: Atropine, butorphanol, droperidol, fentanyl, glycopyrrolate, hydromorphone, meperidine, metoclopromide, midazolam, morphine, pentazocine
Y-site: Ciprofloxacin, fluconazole, ondansetron, potassium chloride

INCOMPATIBILITIES

Syringe: Heparin, ketorolac, nalbuphine, pentobarbital, thiopental
Y-site: Cefoperazone, heparin, piperacillin-tazobactam

PATIENT CARE IMPLICATIONS

P **G** • Children/older adults more likely to develop extrapyramidal reactions, paradoxical excitation, other adverse reactions; use lowest effective dose; monitor frequently.
• *Avoid skin contact with syrup, solution for injection, which may cause contact dermatitis.*
• Drowsiness, orthostatic hypotension possible, especially during first week of therapy. Monitor ambulation; use safety precautions
• Large quantities should not be prescribed for patients with severe depression, suicidal tendencies, history of substance abuse.
• Reserve parenteral therapy for urgent/emergency situations or when PO route unacceptable (e.g., vomiting, NPO status). Convert to PO therapy as soon as possible.
IV
• Adverse CV effects (e.g., hypotension, tachycardia, dizziness, syncope) more likely.

• Monitor frequently. Patient should remain in bed at least 1 hr, requires assistance with initial ambulation.
• Have resuscitation equipment immediately available.
Vital signs/hemodynamics: Monitor VS frequently with IV use, heavily sedated patients (e.g., receiving opiates), or during immediate postop period.
• Continuous pulse oximetry recommended for heavily sedated patients
Physical assessment: Assess neurologic status for excessive sedation, dizziness, impaired physical coordination; reduced dose my be necessary. • Assess for respiratory distress in patients with history of COPD, cardiac impairment.
Laboratory tests: Monitor: Liver enzymes • BUN, creatinine • CBC

PATIENT/FAMILY TEACHING

Purpose of medication is to reduce anxiety, promote relaxation, prevent nausea/vomiting.
• Medication may cause dizziness, drowsiness; call for assistance when getting out of bed, walking. Change positions slowly. Reactions are less likely after first week of therapy.
• Urine may turn pink or reddish brown. • Inform caregiver if you may be pregnant or are considering pregnancy.
Outpatient: Avoid driving and other activities requiring mental alertness or physical coordination. • May contribute to development of heatstroke; avoid hot weather, seek air conditioning.
• Avoid using alcohol or other drugs that cause sedation while taking this medication. • Take antacids 1 hr before or 2 hr af-

ter drug. • If syrup or oral concentrate used, avoid skin contact.

Long-term therapy: Report (1) sore throat, mouth, or gums, other signs of infection that could signal dangerous lowering of WBC, (2) yellowing of skin or whites of eyes, (3) tremors or muscle twitching, (4) problems with eyesight. • Avoid prolonged exposure to sunlight; use sunscreen. • May cause withdrawal symptoms with long-term therapy; consult primary health care provider before changing dose or abruptly discontinuing.

Children: Adult supervision is necessary when riding bike or participating in other activities requiring mental alertness or physical coordination. • Report hyperactivity or excessive stimulation.

AVAILABLE FORMS

Parenteral solution • Tablets, syrup, concentrated syrup • Suppositories

---

propafenone
(proe-pa-fen′one)
Rythmol

Classification: Class IC antidysrhythmic, membrane stabilizer

USUAL DOSE

PO: Initially, 150 mg q8h • Increase dosage slowly to reduce possibility of life-threatening dysrhythmias. • Do not exceed 900 mg/24 hr. • Reduce dose for significant widening of QRS, 2nd/3rd degree heartblock

ACTIONS

Decreases cardiac excitability by increasing threshold level for electrical excitation • Decreases automaticity, triggered activity • Blocks fast sodium channels, prolongs AV conduction time, increases effective refractory period • Little or no effect on sinus node recovery time; increases refractory period of accessory conduction pathways in both directions; may prolong PR interval, QRS complex • May ↓ heart rate via slight beta-adrenergic blocking effects • Negative inotropic effects may ↓ CO. • Local anesthetic effect, similar to procaine

PHARMACOKINETICS

ROUTE	ONSET	PEAK	DURATION
PO	30 min	3.5 hr	8-10 hr

DISTRIBUTION
Wide
ELIMINATION
Metabolized in liver, excreted in urine; genetically determined, rate variable; half-life 2-10 hr (fast metabolizers) or 10-32 hr (slow metabolizers)

Therapeutic level: 0.06-1 µg/ml

INDICATIONS

Suppression/prevention of sustained symptomatic ventricular dysrhythmias • Not recommended for nonsustained ventricular dysrhythmias, even if symptomatic

PRECAUTIONS/CONTRAINDICATIONS

Precautions: Initiate therapy, increase dosages in hospital. • May worsen heart failure, cardiac dysrhythmias • May exacerbate ventricular tachycardia or cause torsades de pointes • May

P

worsen AV heart block, precipitate development of new 1st heart block, prolong QRS complex • May increase pacing/sensing thresholds in patients with artificial cardiac pacemakers • Electrolyte imbalance, acid-base disturbances, hypoxia interfere with drug action, increase likelihood of adverse reactions. • Adverse reactions dose related

Use caution with: Underlying heart failure • History of MI • COPD • Renal impairment; reduced dose indicated • Hepatic impairment; reduce dose by 20%-30%

c Pregnancy category: Safety not established; use only if safer alternative unavailable.

Contraindications: Hypersensitivity to propafenone • Nonsustained ventricular dysrhythmias • 2nd/3rd degree heart block unless functional ventricular pacemaker in place or readily available • Sick sinus syndrome, bradycardia • Severe COPD • Severe hypotension • Uncontrolled CHF

ADVERSE EFFECTS

CNS: *Dizziness, fatigue,* headache, blurred vision, drowsiness, loss of balance, sleep disturbance, anxiety, weakness, confusion

Resp: *Dyspnea*

CV: **New/worsened heart block, CHF,** chest pain, palpitations, bundle branch block, **hypotension, new/worsened dysrhythmias**

GI: *Nausea, vomiting, constipation, taste alteration,* abdominal discomfort, dry mouth, diarrhea

Hema: Bone marrow depression, leukopenia, anemia, thrombocytopenia

Syst: Positive ANA titer, arthritis-like or lupuslike syndrome

TOXICITY/OVERDOSE

Symptoms: Hypotension • Severe AV heart block, bundle branch block, bradycardia, ventricular tachycardia, torsades de pointes • Lethargy, somnolence, seizures • Vomiting • Heart failure, respiratory failure

Management: After recent ingestion, implement guidelines for management of acute overdose (Appendix I). • Administer inotropic agents for heart failure (e.g., dobutamine, dopamine). • Maintain airway/support ventilation. • Hypotension: Elevate legs, administer IV fluids; use vasopressors (e.g., norepinephrine, phenylephrine) for severe hypotension. • Manage symptomatic bradycardia, ventricular dysrhythmias according to ACLS guidelines (Appendix P).

INTERACTIONS

anticoagulants, PO Prolonged bleeding time

beta-blockers Hypotension, bradycardia, toxicity

bretylium ↑ Cardiac depression

cimetidine ↑ Propafenone levels; toxicity

digitalis glycosides ↑ Digoxin levels; monitor closely

quinidine ↑ Cardiac depression; toxicity

PATIENT CARE IMPLICATIONS

• **May cause serious or fatal dysrhythmias; use reserved for sustained symptomatic ventricular dysrhythmias.**

 P pediatric   **G** geriatric   **V** Direct IV

• Correct hypoxemia, hypercapnia, other fluid/electrolyte imbalance before initiating therapy.

Vital signs/hemodynamics: Continuously monitor ECG during initial therapy. Use lowest effective dose for dysrhythmia control. Note signs of toxicity, including prolongation of PR interval/QRS complex, 2nd, 3rd degree AV heart block, ventricular dysrhythmias. Immediately consult physician. • Monitor BP frequently during initiation of therapy and when dosage increased. • Monitor patients with artificial pacemakers for failure to sense or capture.

Physical assessment: Assess for perfusion/oxygenation deficit; ↓ level of consciousness, chest pain, activity intolerance, hypotension, dizziness. • Assess for heart failure; bibasilar crackles (rales), dyspnea, peripheral edema, neck vein distention, S_3 gallop. • Assess for anemia: pallor, activity intolerance; thrombocytopenia—bruising, prolonged/occult bleeding; leukopenia—fever, sore throat, infection. • Assess for signs of liver dysfunction: jaundice, abdominal tenderness.

Laboratory tests: Monitor: Electrolytes, ABGs; immediately correct abnormalities.
• CBC for possible bone marrow suppression • BUN, creatinine • Liver enzymes, bilirubin • ANA titers • Plasma levels of propafenone: therapeutic levels, 0.06-1.0 µg/ml • Consider discontinuation of therapy if patient develops positive ANA titers with arthritis-like symptoms, ↑ liver enzymes, ↑ creatinine

PATIENT/FAMILY TEACHING

Purpose of medication is to control abnormal heartbeats.
• Take with food or milk to reduce stomach upset. • Report chest discomfort, activity intolerance, dizziness, breathing difficulty, swelling of extremities, rapid weight gain, yellow discoloration of skin or whites of eyes, joint tenderness, fever, sore throat, infection, easy bruising, blood in urine/stool.

AVAILABLE FORMS

Tablets

propofol
(proe-po'foel)
Diprivan

Classifications: General anesthetic, sedative-hypnotic

USUAL DOSE

Sedation of intubated patients: IV cont inf, adults: Initially 5 µg/kg/min (0.3 mg/kg/hr) for at least 5 min • Adjust by increments of 5-10 µg/kg/min (0.3-0.6 mg/kg/hr) q5-10min as needed to provide continuous sedation, prevent resistance to mechanical ventilation. • Usual range, 5-50 µg/kg/min • Maximum dose, 200 µg/kg/min

Anesthesia: Direct IV/cont inf, adults <55/American Society of Anesthesiologists (ASA) I/II: Induction, 2-2.5 mg/kg or approx 40 mg q10sec until induction • Maintenance infusion, generally 0.1-0.2 mg/kg/min • Intermittent bolus, 25-50 mg as needed • Direct IV/cont inf, adults >65/debilitation/hypovolemia/ASA

P

G

III/IV: Induction 1-1.5 mg/kg or approx 20 mg q10sec until induction • Maintenance infusion, generally 0.5-0.1 mg/kg/min • Intermittent bolus, 25-50 mg as needed

ADMINISTRATION

V Direct IV/cont inf: *Airway management/emergency resuscitation equipment must be immediately available.* • For maintenance of anesthesia/sedation, cont inf preferred to intermit bolus inj to avoid under/oversedation • Use large vein of forearm, antecubital fossa, injection of 1 mg 1% lidocaine to ↓ pain associated with injection. • Closely monitor respiratory/CV status • Use lowest effective dose; adjust rate q5-10min to provide desired level of sedation. • Too-rapid administration may cause severe cardiopulmonary complications. • Infusion pump necessary with cont inf • DO NOT FILTER. • Special handling required; see Preparation.

PREPARATION

IV: Minimally water soluble; available as premixed lipid emulsion in concentration of 10 mg/ml • Dilution not recommended; if necessary, use D_5W only, do not dilute to concentration <2 mg/ml • Shake well before withdrawing from ampule/vial. • Do not use if evidence of separation of lipid emulsion.
Special handling technique: Strict asepsis necessary • Wash hands/fingernails with antimicrobial soap. • Disinfect neck of ampule/stopper of vial with 70% isopropyl alcohol. • Use sterile gauze to protect fingers (ampule). • Withdraw contents with sterile syringe; connect to sterile infusion set. • Administer promptly. • Discard tubing, any unused portion at end of procedure or after 12 hr, whichever sooner.
Compatible fluids: Compatible when administered into running IV solution of D_5W, LR, 0.9% NaCl, 0.45% NaCl, prepared combinations of these solutions

ACTIONS

Dose/rate dependent; lower doses provide conscious/unconscious sedation; higher doses used for general anesthesia produce rapid hypnosis with minimal excitation, usually within 40 sec. • Rapid onset, short duration facilitate accurate titration, rapid emergence from sedation (approx 8-10 min). • When used for sedation of ventilated patients, propofol easier to control, results in faster weaning/more rapid emergence from sedation when compared with midazolam • Causes slight to moderate ↓ in DBP, MAP, SVR; may ↓ CO, particularly if concurrent opioid analgesia, mechanical ventilation or with advanced age, debilitation, preexisting CV disorders • No analgesic/amnesic effects

PHARMACOKINETICS

ROUTE	ONSET	PEAK	DURATION
IV	<40 sec	1-3 min	8-10 min

DISTRIBUTION

Extensive redistribution to other tissues; high metabolic clearance

ELIMINATION

Rapidly metabolized by liver/other tissues, eliminated by kidneys; half-life 100 min

INDICATIONS

Sedation for critically ill, intubated adults to promote comfort, prevent resistance to mechanical ventilation • Induction/ maintenance of anesthesia during inpatient/outpatient surgery • Maintenance of conscious sedation during diagnostic procedures (e.g., colonoscopy)

PRECAUTIONS/ CONTRAINDICATIONS

Precautions: Apnea occurs with bolus dosing, may last >60 sec. • When used for sedation, initiate as continuous infusion, adjust no more often than every 5 min. • Contains no preservatives; strict aseptic technique necessary to prevent microbial contamination • Not recommended for patients with ↑ ICP/impaired cerebral perfusion, because reductions in MAP may ↓ cerebral perfusion • Not recommended for obstetric use • Not an analgesic; must be used with analgesics or local anesthetics as indicated
Use caution with: Disorders of lipid metabolism (e.g., diabetic hyperlipemia, pancreatitis) • Epilepsy; may cause seizures during recovery phase
Use caution/lower dose
G **with:** Older adults • Debilitation • CV disorders • Severe respiratory disorders • Dehydration, hypovolemia
B **Pregnancy category:** Use only if clearly necessary.
Contraindications: Hypersensitivity to propofol, soybean oil, glycerol, eggs • Any contraindication to general anesthesia/
P sedation • Children: Safety/efficacy not established

ADVERSE EFFECTS

All side effects dose related, more likely during loading or supplemental bolus injection
CNS: Headache, fever, dizziness, jerking, shivering, tremors, confusion, paresthesias
Resp: ***Severe respiratory depression, apnea,*** cough, dyspnea, wheezing
CV: ***Profound bradycardia,*** *hypotension,* hypertension, tachycardia, PVC, PAC, ST segment depression
GI: *Nausea, vomiting,* cramping
GU: Green urine
Local: Pain/burning with injection
Syst: Fever

TOXICITY/OVERDOSE

Symptoms: Specific information not available
Management: Maintain airway, administer O$_2$, support ventilation as needed. • **Hypotension:** Elevate legs, administer IV fluids; use vasopressors (e.g., dopamine, norepinephrine) if unresponsive to fluids. • Use atropine for symptomatic bradycardia; manage other dysrhythmias according to ACLS guidelines (Appendix P).

INTERACTIONS

alcohol, anesthetics, barbiturates, benzodiazepines, opiate analgesics ↑ CNS depression

INCOMPATIBILITIES

Do not mix/infuse with other agents

PATIENT CARE IMPLICATIONS

• To be administered only by qualified personnel with specialized training in continuous seda-

---

italic = common side effects   **bold** = life-threatening reactions

tion/anesthesia; must have emergency resuscitation equipment/personnel immediately available
• Correct hypovolemia before initiating therapy.
• Hypotension, bradycardia, other adverse reactions more **G** likely in older adults, debilitation, preexisting CV disease, limited pulmonary reserve, use of other CNS depressants, bolus administration
• Reactions such as agitation, involuntary movements, hyperactivity, combativeness may occur. Evaluate reactions carefully; consider inadequate or excessive dosing, too-rapid administration, cerebral hypoxia, other drugs administered, true paradoxical reaction.
• Administer in small increments, closely monitor cardiopulmonary status throughout. Carefully individualize/titrate each dose.
• No analgesic/amnesic properties; administer analgesic and/or local anesthetic as indicated. Use with midazolam to reduce recall of painful procedures.
• Monitor frequently for 3-4 hr after use. Patient should remain in bed for at least 3 hr, requires assistance with initial ambulation.
• Many specific implications during administration; see Administration/Preparation.
• Rapid metabolism, little accumulation. Rapid emergence from sedation expected, even when used for relatively long periods. Weaning not necessary.
Vital signs/hemodynamics: Continuously monitor ECG for dysrhythmias. • Monitor VS frequently according to patient condition; continuous monitoring during induction/bolus

dosing necessary; direct arterial pressure monitoring recommended. • Continuous pulse oximetry recommended until patient fully alert. • Closely monitor CVP, PAP, PCWP, CO/CI, particularly during initiation of therapy in mechanically ventilated patients. Decreases in MAP, CO accentuated with positive-pressure ventilation.
• Conditions such as low lighting, patient position during procedures may interfere with observation/assessment of cardiopulmonary status. Use additional measures (e.g., ECG monitor, pulse oximetry, automatic BP cuff) to monitor patient closely during procedures.
Physical assessment: Assess neurologic status for level of sedation regularly throughout use. Titrate carefully, use lowest effective dose to provide desired level of sedation. • Assess respiratory status frequently until fully awake: rate, rhythm, character, depth of excursion.

PATIENT/FAMILY TEACHING

Purpose of medication is to provide heavy sedation or unconsciousness during procedures or before surgery. • Remain in bed for at least 3 hr after use. Call for assistance when getting out of bed for first time. • Avoid driving and other activities requiring mental alertness or physical coordination for 24 hr after use and then only if not drowsy. • Avoid use of alcohol or other drugs that cause sedation for at least 24 hr after use.

AVAILABLE FORMS

Parenteral for IV use only

P pediatric   **G** geriatric   **V** Direct IV

propranolol HCl
(proe-pran'oh-lole)
Betachron, Inderal
**propranolol HCl with
hydrochlorothiazide**
Inderide

Classifications: Class II antidysrhythmic, nonselective beta-
adrenergic blocker, antihypertensive, antianginal

USUAL DOSE

PO, IV doses not interchangeable, verify dose, route.
PO, adults: 10-60 mg 2-4
times daily • **Hypertension:**
not to exceed 640 mg/day
• **Post-MI:** not to exceed 240
mg/day
PO, sus rel, adults: 80-160
mg daily
Ⓟ **PO suspension, children:**
• Hypertension: 0.5-1.0 mg/kg
bid • Dysrhythmias: 1-2 mg/kg
bid
**Direct IV/intermit inf,
adults:** 0.5-3 mg in 0.5–1-mg
increments; if initial dose ineffective after 2 min, may repeat
once • Stop injection/infusion as
soon as rhythm converted; always use lowest effective dose.
• Do not administer additional
dose by any route for 4 hr. • **IV
route for acute life-threatening
dysrhythmias only**

ADMINISTRATION

G-tube: Use solution; flush before and after administration
**Compatible feeding formu-
las:** Isocal, Sustacal, Sustacal
HC
Ⅴ **Direct IV/intermit inf:** Injection: Inject slowly at rate not
>1 mg/min. • Infusion: Infuse 1
mg over 10-15 min. • Monitor

ECG, BP throughout administration; discontinue as soon as
rhythm is converted. • Immediately stop injection for symptomatic bradycardia, HR <45, hypotension, 2nd/3rd degree heart
block.

PREPARATION

Direct IV: Each 1 mg may be
diluted in 10 ml sterile water,
D_5W, or 0.9% NaCl for ease in
administration; concentration is
0.1 mg/ml.
IV, intermit inf: Entire dose
may be diluted in 50 ml compatible solution.
Compatible fluids: D_5W,
0.9% NaCl, LR

ACTIONS

Blocks sympathetic nervous
system stimulation of beta-1-
adrenergic receptors of myocardium, beta-2-adrenergic receptors of vasculature/bronchial
smooth muscle • Decreases HR,
BP, force of contraction, CO,
myocardial O_2 consumption
• Reduces angina, risk of myocardial reinfarction • Depresses
AV conduction, myocardial automaticity, especially in SA
node • May cause bronchial
constriction, ↑ airway resistance, ↓ efficacy of ventilation,
particularly in asthma
• Suppresses renin-angiotensin-
aldosterone system • Reduces
hepatic blood flow • May inhibit cerebral vasodilation • Reduces anxiety

P

---

italic = common side effects   **bold** = life-threatening reactions

PHARMACOKINETICS

ROUTE	ONSET	PEAK	DURATION
PO, std	<30 min	60-90 min	8-12 hr
PO, ext rel	>1 hr	6 hr	12-24 hr
IV	Immed	1 min	5 hr

DISTRIBUTION

Wide; 90% protein bound; crosses blood-brain barrier

ELIMINATION

Metabolized by liver, eliminated by kidneys; half-life 3.4-6 hr

INDICATIONS

Control of hypertension • Suppression of rapid-rate cardiac dysrhythmias, including supraventricular/ventricular tachycardia, tachycardias associated with hyperthyroid crises, pheochromocytoma • Reduction of mortality after MI • Management of chronic stable angina, particularly in patients with IHSS • Migraine prophylaxis
Unlabeled/investigational:
Acute anxiety states, prevention of recurrent GI bleeding associated with portal hypertension

PRECAUTIONS/ CONTRAINDICATIONS

Precautions: May result in symptomatic bradycardia, CHF, hypotension, particularly with preexisting cardiac disease, digoxin toxicity, WPW syndrome • Abrupt cessation may induce angina, ventricular dysrhythmias, acute MI, and/or thyrotoxicosis-like symptoms in hypertensive patients • Withdrawal of high-dose, long-term therapy may cause profound CNS disturbances. • May alter lipid profile, increase total cholesterol, triglycerides
Use caution with: Cardiac impairment, valvular heart disease • Asthma, COPD; use lower dose, monitor for bronchospasm. • General anesthesia; may cause additive impairment of cardiac contractility • Hyperthyroidism; beta-blocking effects may mask symptoms. • Diabetes; may mask symptoms of hypoglycemia or cause acute hyperglycemia

c Pregnancy category: Safety not established; use only if safer alternative unavailable.
Contraindications: Hypersensitivity to propranolol • Severe bradycardia, 2nd/3rd degree heart block • Raynaud's phenomenon • Malignant hypertension • CHF (unless resulting from tachycardia) • Cardiogenic shock not associated wtih acute MI • Bronchial asthma, severe COPD • Myasthenia gravis;
P may worsen condition • Children: Safe use not established

ADVERSE EFFECTS

CNS: *Dizziness, fatigue,* lightheadedness, sleepiness, headache, visual disturbances, depression, lethargy, confusion
Resp: Dyspnea, coughing, wheezing, nasal stuffiness, **bronchospasm, laryngoscope**
CV: *Bradycardia,* **hypotension, worsened heart block, CHF, angina, increased peripheral arterial insufficiency,** Raynaud's phenomenon, **CVA** (rare)
GI: *Nausea,* gastric pain, vomiting, flatulence, abdominal cramping, diarrhea, constipation, elevated liver enzymes, **renal/mesenteric arterial thrombosis** (rare)
GU: Increased BUN/creatinine, diminished libido
Endo: Hyperglycemia

Derm: Rash, itching, dry/scaly skin, thickened nails, dermatitis

Hema: *Eosinophilia,* other blood dyscrasias

Syst: Joint pain, altered lipid profile

TOXICITY/OVERDOSE

Symptoms: Severe bradycardia, advanced heart block • Profound hypotension, loss of consciousness • Heart failure • Bronchospasm, respiratory distress • Seizures

Management: After recent ingestion, implement guidelines for management of acute overdose (Appendix I). • **Symptomatic bradycardia:** Atropine, isoproterenol, according to ACLS guidelines (Appendix P); epinephrine may be ineffective (see Interactions). • **Bronchospasm:** Aminophylline, isoproterenol • **Heart failure:** Inotropic support (e.g., dobutamine, dopamine), diuretics, possibly digoxin • **Hypotension:** Elevate legs, administer IV fluids; use vasopressors (e.g., norepinephrine, dopamine) for severe hypotension refractory to inotropic agents, fluids. • Implement seizure precautions; administer diazepam, lorazepam, phenytoin as needed. • Hemodialysis generally ineffective

INTERACTIONS

amiodarone Severe bradycardia; ventricular dysrhythmias

antidiabetic agents Masked hypoglycemia-associated tachycardia; hyperglycemia

barbiturates ↓ Beta-blocker levels/effectiveness

bronchodilators ↓ Bronchodilation

calcium channel blockers Extreme bradycardia; hypotension

disopyramide ↑ Negative inotropy; ↓ CO

epinephrine, possibly other sympathomimetics Predominant alpha effects: hypertension, bradycardia, dysrhythmias; ↓ effectiveness in anaphylaxis

isoproterenol ↓ Bronchodilatory effectiveness

lidocaine Lidocaine toxicity; ↓ CO

phenothiazines Hypotension

prazosin Hypotension, especially with initial dose

quinidine Additive cardiac depression

rifampin ↑ Beta-blocker metabolism

Y-SITE COMPATIBILITIES

Altepase, amrinone, heparin, meperidine, milrinone, morphine, potassium chloride, verapamil, vitamin B complex with C

Y-SITE INCOMPATIBILITIES

Diazoxide

P

PATIENT CARE IMPLICATIONS

• Use lowest effective dose for dysrhythmia control.

• Monitor closely for adverse effects if other antidysrhythmic, hypotensive agents used.

• Administer with or directly after meals; food improves bioavailability.

• Gradually withdraw therapy to avoid rebound hypertension, angina, possible acute MI.

• Standard tablets may be crushed, dissolved in water to facilitate administration. Do not crush, break, or chew sust rel tablets.

---

italic = common side effects   **bold** = life-threatening reactions

• Consider dosage reduction or use cardioselective beta-blocker (e.g., atenolol) in patients with asthma, COPD.

Vital signs/hemodynamics: Monitor BP, HR, RR closely when initiating therapy, adjusting dose. Withhold next dose; consult physician of symptomatic bradycardia, HR <45, hypotension, breathing difficulty.
• As available, monitor ECG for development/advancement of heart block, prolongation of PR interval, widening of QRS complex. • Measure CVP, PAP, CO, as available. Consult physician of ↓ CO or ↑ filling pressures associated with other symptoms of heart failure.

IV:
• Continuously monitor ECG; carefully observe for dysrhythmia control, adverse effects (see Administration).
• Monitor HR, BP q2-5min during and immediately after administration.

Physical assessment: Assess for perfusion/oxygenation deficit; ↓ level of consciousness, activity intolerance, hypotension, chest discomfort, dizziness.
• Assess for CHF/pulmonary edema: breathing difficulty, bibasilar crackles (rales), S_3 gallop, neck vein distention, frothy sputum; especially important with preexisting heart disease.
• Assess for respiratory distress, wheezing in patients with asthma, COPD, cardiac impairment. • When used for migraine prophylaxis, assess/record patient response. • Assess diabetic patients for sweating, since tachycardia/tremors associated with hypoglycemia may be blocked by therapy.

Laboratory tests: Monitor: Electrolytes • CBC • Cholesterol, triglycerides • BUN, creatinine • Liver enzymes, bilirubin • Blood sugar; especially with diabetes

PATIENT/FAMILY TEACHING

Purpose of medication is to lower BP or regulate abnormal heartbeats. • May cause drowsiness, dizziness, low BP; change positions slowly, particularly when getting out of bed. • Report breathing difficulty, palpitations, dizziness, chest pain, extreme fatigue, severe depression, rash, unusual bleeding, fever, persistent sore throat. • You may experience increased sensitivity to cold. • Avoid excessive amounts of coffee, tea, caffeinated soft drinks, which may counteract drug's BP-lowering effects.

Outpatient: Take medication exactly as prescribed. Do not stop taking medicine even if you feel better. If medication abruptly discontinued, you may develop dangerously high BP, serious heartbeat irregularities, angina. • Check/record resting pulse each day, BP each week. Contact caregiver if pulse <50 bpm or BP significantly different. • Medication is not cure for high BP; other therapies, including life-style modifications, must be continued. • May cause drowsiness, dizziness; avoid driving and other activities requiring mental alertness until individual response to drug known. Alcohol worsens these effects. • Take with or directly after meals. • Do not crush, break, or chew sust rel tablets. • Consult caregiver or pharmacist before taking over-the-counter preparations. • Carry Medic-Alert ID identifying drug, dosage, specific indication. • Notify physicians, dentists of therapy before treatment. • Therapy blocks ↑ HR/BP, so hyperthyroid/diabetic patients must be aware of other symptoms of crisis.

AVAILABLE FORMS

Tablets • Sustained-release capsules • PO solution • Concentrated PO solution • Parenteral for IV injection

protamine sulfate
(proe′ta-meen)

Classification: Heparin antidote

USUAL DOSE

Direct IV, adults: Depends on heparin dose, route, time of administration • **IV heparin:** If <30 min after heparin, 1-1.5 mg protamine/100 U heparin; if 30-60 min after heparin, 0.5-0.75 mg/100 U; if ≥2 hr, 0.25-0.375 mg/100 U • **IV heparin cont. inf:** 25-50 mg after infusion discontinued • **Deep SC heparin:** 1-1.5 mg/100 U heparin or loading dose of 25-50 mg, followed by cont inf over 8-16 hr • Dose adjusted as needed according to coagulation studies

ADMINISTRATION

▼ Direct IV, adults: Inject ≤20 mg very slowly over 1-3 min. • Do not exceed 50 mg in any 10-min period. • Too-rapid administration may cause hypotension, bradycardia. • Sometimes given by cont inf; infusion pump required.

PREPARATION

Reconstitute by adding 5 ml sterile or bacteriostatic water for injection to 50-mg vial. • Shake vigorously until all particulate matter dissolved. • Solution contains 10 mg/ml. • May be further diluted with D_5W or 0.9% NaCl. • Use reconstituted solution immediately.

ACTIONS

Binds with heparin to form inactive complex without anticoagulant activity • Generally 1 mg protamine neutralizes 90-115 U heparin

PHARMACOKINETICS

ROUTE	ONSET	PEAK	DURATION
IV	Rapid	5 min	2 hr

DISTRIBUTION
Not clearly established

ELIMINATION
Heparin-protamine complex may be partially metabolized, thus freeing heparin.

INDICATIONS

Severe heparin overdose or hemorrhage related to heparin therapy • Not indicated for minor bleeding during heparin therapy
Unlabeled/investigational: To neutralize heparin administered during extracorporeal circulation, hemodialysis

PRECAUTIONS/ CONTRAINDICATIONS

Precautions: Must monitor APTT or ACT during therapy • Heparin rebound may occur up to 18 hr after heparin administration. • Potential for hypersensitivity ↑ in patients with sensitivity to fish, previous use of protamine-containing insulin or protamine therapy, males with infertility or vasectomies; consider pretreatment with corticosteroid, antihistamine.

P • Children: Safe use not established

C Pregnancy category: Use only if safer alternative unavailable.

Contraindications: Hypersensitivity to protamine

ADVERSE EFFECTS

CV: **Hypotension, bradycardia,** hypertension, transient flushing

Resp: Dyspnea, pulmonary hypertension, pulmonary edema

GI: Nausea, vomiting

MS: Back pain

Misc: Hypersensitivity, **anaphylaxis**

TOXICITY/OVERDOSE

Symptoms: Possibility of hemorrhage because of slight anticoagulant effects of protamine
• Hypotension, bradycardia

Management: Monitor coagulation studies; treat side effects symptomatically. • Administer blood, blood products, vasopressors (e.g., dopamine) for hypotension. • Administer atropine, epinephrine for bradycardia according to ACLS guidelines (Appendix P).

Y-SITE INCOMPATIBILITIES

Cephalosporin/penicillin antibiotics

PATIENT CARE IMPLICATIONS

• Assess for history of fish allergy, vasectomy, male infertility, protamine-containing insulin therapy, previous protamine therapy. Use caution and administer premedication as pre-scribed to prevent hypersensitivity reactions in these patients.
• Have epinephrine, antihistamine, resuscitation equipment immediately available during administration.
• Avoid IM/SC injections, invasive procedure until risk of bleeding passed.

Vital signs/hemodynamics: Monitor BP, HR frequently according to severity of bleeding.

Physical assessment: Assess for continued/recurrent bleeding at least 24 hr after therapy for heparin overdose. • Test stools, emesis for occult blood. • Assess for heparin rebound: return of anticoagulation/bleeding that may occur up to 18 hr after protamine administration. • Assess for hypersensitivity reaction, including wheals, itching, edema, coughing, wheezing, hypotension.

Laboratory tests: APTT or ACT necessary to monitor effectiveness; obtain coagulation tests 5-15 min after initiating therapy; tests may be repeated q2-8h up to 24 hr to check for heparin rebound.

PATIENT/FAMILY TEACHING

Purpose of medication is to neutralize effects of heparin.
• May cause dizziness, low BP; do not get out of bed without assistance. • Avoid activities that may result in bleeding (shaving, brushing teeth, ambulation) until risk of bleeding passed. • Report vomiting of blood, blood in stool, urine.

AVAILABLE FORMS

Parenteral for IV use
Storage: Store refrigerated at 2°-8° C (35.6°-46.4° F).

quinapril HCl
(kwin'a-pril)
Accupril

Classifications: Angiotensin-converting enzyme (ACE) inhibitor, antihypertensive

USUAL DOSE
PO, adults: Initially 10 mg once daily or 5 mg bid; increase to 20-80 mg once daily or 10-40 mg bid as needed to control BP. • If concurrent diuretic therapy, use initial dose of 5 mg once daily.

G PO, older adults/renal impairment: Initially 2.5-5 mg once daily; gradually increase as needed to control BP. • Observe closely for symptomatic hypotension.

ACTIONS
Long-acting ACE inhibitor that prevents conversion of angiotensin I to angiotensin II, a potent vasoconstrictor • BP reduced directly by ↓ vascular tone, indirectly by reduction in aldosterone secretion and therefore ↓ sodium/water retention • Reduces SBP/DBP, with minimal effect on HR or contractility. May improve CO in patients with heart failure, but effects of long-term use not well established. • Requires conversion in liver to be activated

PHARMACOKINETICS

ROUTE	ONSET	PEAK	DURATION
PO	1 hr	2-4 hr	24 hr

DISTRIBUTION
Wide; 96% protein bound

ELIMINATION
Eliminated in urine, feces; half-life 2 hr, prolonged with renal insufficiency

INDICATIONS
Mild to severe hypertension; may be used in conjunction with other hypotensive agents, diuretics • Symptomatic CHF alone or with digoxin, diuretics. Improves CO, exercise tolerance; relieves dyspnea, fatigue

PRECAUTIONS/ CONTRAINDICATIONS
Precautions: Initial dose may cause profound hypotension, severe allergic reaction. • May cause agranulocytosis, thrombocytopenia

Use caution with: Renal impairment; reduce dose, monitor renal function. • Concurrent diuretic use, hypovolemia, hyponatremia, surgery, anesthesia; risk of severe hypotension • CAD, cerebrovascular disease, CHF, aortic stenosis; hypotensive episodes may worsen condition. • Hepatic failure; effectiveness diminished

D Pregnancy category: Use only if necessary and woman informed of potential hazards to fetus.

Contraindications: Hypersensitivity to quinapril, other ACE **P** inhibitors • Children: Safety/efficacy not established

ADVERSE EFFECTS
CNS: *Headache, dizziness, fatigue,* paresthesias, confusion, nervousness

Resp: *Cough,* dyspnea, **angioedema/stridor** (allergic reaction)

CV: *Transient/orthostatic hypotension,* **profound hypotension,** tachycardia, palpitations

GI: *Nausea, vomiting,* abdominal pain

GU: ↓ **Renal function,** oliguria

F&E: Hyponatremia, hyperkalemia, muscle cramps

Misc: Photosensitivity, full range of allergic reactions, **anaphylaxis**

TOXICITY/OVERDOSE

Symptoms: Hypotension • ↓ Level of consciousness • MI or CVA from profound hypotension in high-risk patients

Management: After recent ingestion, implement guidelines for management of acute overdose (Appendix I). • Support respiration as needed with O_2 and/or mechanical ventilation. • Hypotension usually responsive to intravascular volume expansion with 0.9% NaCl or LR • Hemodialysis generally ineffective

INTERACTIONS

alcohol   Hypotension

antacids   ↓ Quinapril absorption

calcium channel blockers   Profound hypotension

digitalis glycosides   ↑ Digoxin levels; toxicity

diuretics   Additive hypotensive effects

diuretics, potassium sparing   Hyperkalemia

NSAIDs   ↓ Quinapril effectiveness

phenothiazines   Hypotension

potassium supplements   Hyperkalemia

sympathetic blockers   Profound hypotension

PATIENT CARE IMPLICATIONS

• Correct hypovolemia before administration.

• Evaluate renal function before initiating therapy.

• Protect patients from injury associated with orthostatic hypotension, especially when initiating therapy.

• Vomiting, diarrhea, excessive perspiration, dehydration could cause serious hypotension.

• Tablets may be crushed, dissolved in water to facilitate administration.

Vital signs/hemodynamics: Monitor BP, HR q1-2h until stable when initiating therapy, and with following uses: hypertensive crisis, acute CHF; use of additional hypotensive agents/diuretics. • Use IV 0.9% NaCl for transient hypotensive episodes during initial therapy. • As available, continuously monitor ECG for PVCs, ST segment elevation/depression, especially when initiating therapy in patients with CHF, CAD.

Physical assessment: Assess for perfusion/oxygenation deficit: chest discomfort, ↓ level of consciousness, activity intolerance, hypotension, dizziness. • Assess neurologic status q2-4h after initiation of therapy until BP controlled. • Monitor fluid balance, weigh daily.

Laboratory tests: Monitor: Electrolytes • BUN, creatinine • Bilirubin, liver enzymes • CBC with differential • Hyperkalemia, hyponatremia possible; renal impairment, CHF, diabetes mellitus, potassium-sparing diuretics, potassium supplements, salt substitutes increase risk of hyperkalemia.

PATIENT/FAMILY TEACHING

Purpose of drug is to lower BP and/or relieve symptoms of heart failure. • May cause orthostatic hypotension, dizziness, especially during initiation of therapy; use caution when changing positions, walking. Alcohol, hot weather, vigorous activity, vomiting, diarrhea, dehydration, prolonged standing make these symptoms more likely. • Lie down immediately if lightheaded or dizzy. • Medication is not cure for high BP; other therapies, including lifestyle modifications, must be continued. • Immediately report rash; swelling of extremities; fever, sore throat, infection; chest pain; swelling of face, lips, tongue, throat; difficulty breathing. • May interfere with taste perception, cause persistent coughing; report these effects if bothersome. • Notify prescriber if you may be pregnant or are planning pregnancy.

Outpatient: Take medication exactly as prescribed. Do not stop taking medicine even if you feel better. If medication abruptly discontinued, you may develop dangerously high BP. • Avoid driving and other activities requiring mental alertness until individual response to drug known. • Avoid salt substitutes or other foods high in potassium unless physician specifies otherwise. • Weigh twice/wk; notify physician of weight gain, edema. • Consult physician or pharmacist before taking cough, cold, or allergy preparations.

AVAILABLE FORMS

Tablets

quinidine sulfate
(kwin'i-deen)
Cin-Quin, Quinidex
Extentabs, Quinora

quinidine polygalacturonate
Cardioquin

quinidine gluconate
Duraquin, Quinaglute, Dura-Tabs, Quinalan, Quinatime

Classifications: Class IA anti-dysrhythmic, membrane stabilizer, antimalarial

USUAL DOSE

PO, initial therapy, adults: Use quinidine sulfate for initial dysrhythmia control. • Test dose, 50-200 mg • **SVT:** 400-600 mg q2-3h until controlled • **Atrial fibrillation:** 200-300 mg q3-4h until controlled; digitalize first to reduce incidence of tachycardia. • **Other dysrhythmias:** 200-300 mg q6-8h until controlled

PO, maintenance therapy, adults: Quinidine sulfate: 200-400 mg q6-8h • Quinidine sulfate, extended release: 300-600 mg q8-12h • Quinidine polygalacturonate: 275 mg q8-12h • Quinidine gluconate: 324-660 mg q8-12h

IV, intermit inf, initial therapy, adults: 16 mg/min (1 ml of 400 mg/25 ml solution) until dysrhythmia controlled; usually ≤300 mg. Up to 750 mg may be necessary. Stop injection for >25% widening of QRS, absent P wave, hypotension, HR ↓ to 120, or severe adverse effects.

Q

ADMINISTRATION

IV: Administer at rate of 16 mg/min (1 ml/min) with continuous ECG, BP monitoring. • Too-rapid administration may cause hypotension, heart block. • Use infusion pump or other rate-controlling device. • For hypotension >25% widening of QRS complex, immediately discontinue, consult physician.

PREPARATION

DILUTION	CONCENTRATION
800 mg/50 ml	16 mg/ml
400 mg/25 ml	16 mg/ml

Compatible fluids: D_5W, 0.9% NaCl, LR, prepared combinations of these solutions
Stability: Stable for 24 hr at room temperature when diluted with D_5W; use only clear, colorless solution.

ACTIONS

Decreases cardiac excitability by increasing threshold for electrical excitation • Prolongs effective refractory period (ERP), action potential duration • Anticholinergic properties shorten ERP, AV conduction time, may interfere with suppression of ectopic supraventricular pacemakers. • Blocks fast sodium channels, suppresses automaticity in His-Purkinje system, prevents reentry • Negative inotropic effects may reduce cardiac contractility. • Alpha-adrenergic blockade reduces peripheral resistance, BP.

PHARMACOKINETICS

ROUTE	ONSET	PEAK	DURATION
PO	30 min	1-2 hr	6-12 hr
IM	<30 min	4 hr	
IV	Immed	Rapid	4-6 hr

DISTRIBUTION
Wide; does not cross blood-brain barrier
ELIMINATION
Metabolized by liver; excreted by kidneys; urine acidity increases excretion; half-life 6-8 hr

Therapeutic level: 2-6 µg/ml

INDICATIONS

Control/prevention of atrial/ventricular dysrhythmias, including supraventricular, ventricular tachycardias; atrial fibrillation/flutter; atrial, ventricular premature contractions
• Patients with atrial fibrillation/flutter should be digitalized before receiving quinidine to prevent 1:1 conduction and possible rapid tachycardia. Combination therapy with lidocaine, propranolol may ↑ effectiveness of quinidine. • Alternative to quinine dihydrochloride in treatment of malaria

PRECAUTIONS/CONTRAINDICATIONS

Precautions: IV use may cause severe hypotension, heart block. • Reduction in degree of AV nodal block may result in 1:1 conduction and rapid ventricular rate in nondigitalized patients managed with quinidine for atrial fibrillation/flutter (quinidine effect). • Severe prolongation of QT interval, QRS complex may precipitate torsades de pointes, ventricular tachycardia/fibrillation. • May worsen/precipitate heart block, especially in patients with preexisting conduction defects • Hyper-

sensitivity reactions may go unnoticed in patients with fever, asthma, muscle weakness, because these symptoms similar to those of hypersensitivity.
• Commercial parenteral preparations contain sulfites, which can cause serious allergic reactions.

Use caution with: Renal/hepatic insufficiency; reduce dosage. • Preexisting cardiac disease; may precipitate heart failure

c **Pregnancy category:** Safety not established; use only if safer alternative unavailable.

Contraindications: Quinidine hypersensitivity • Digitalis intoxication • History of torsades de pointes • Myasthenia gravis • 2nd/3rd degree heart block unless functional ventricular pacemaker in place or readily available

ADVERSE EFFECTS

CNS: Headache, dizziness, confusion, ataxia, lethargy, jerking/twitching, **seizures**
Resp: **Respiratory distress/arrest,** acute asthma
CV: *Hypotension, prolongation of PR/QRS/QT,* new/worsened atrial/ventricular dysrhythmias, ↑ ventricular rate in atrial fibrillation/flutter, new/worsened heart block, bradycardia, **asystole** (rare)
GI: *Diarrhea, nausea,* vomiting, bitter taste, abdominal discomfort, hepatitis (rare)
Derm: Rash, flushing, pruritus, dermatitis
Syst: SLE-like syndrome, hypersensitivity

TOXICITY/OVERDOSE

Symptoms: Visual disturbances, dizziness, tinnitus • Vomiting, diarrhea, abdominal pain • Lethargy, coma, seizures • Respiratory arrest • Hypotension, SVT, ventricular tachycardia, torsades de pointes, ventricular fibrillation, bradycardia, heart block, asystole

Management: After recent ingestion, implement guidelines for management of acute overdose (Appendix I). • Maintain airway/support ventilation as necessary. • **Hypotension:** Elevate legs, administer IV fluids; use pressors (e.g., dopamine, norepinephrine, phenylephrine) as necessary. • **Symptomatic bradycardia, ventricular dysrhythmias:** Manage according to ACLS guidelines (Appendix P). Treat torsades de pointes with defibrillation, magnesium sulfate, isoproterenol infusion. • Hemodialysis may be effective.

Toxic serum level: >8 μg/ml

INTERACTIONS

acetazolamide ↑ Quinidine levels
amiodarone ↑ Quinidine levels; toxicity
antacids ↑ Quinidine levels
barbiturates ↓ Quinidine levels
cholinergic drugs Blocked cholinergic effects
cimetidine ↑ Quinidine levels
digitalis glycosides Digitalis toxicity
nifedipine ↓ Quinidine levels
NMBAs ↑ Neuromuscular blockade
phenytoin ↓ Quinidine levels
procainamide ↑ Effects of both drugs; toxicity possible
sodium bicarbonate ↑ Quinidine levels
TCAs ↑ Antidepressant levels
verapamil Profound hypotension; avoid concurrent use

Q

---

italic = common side effects   **bold** = life-threatening reactions

COMPATIBILITIES

Bretylium, cimetidine, milrinone, verapamil

INCOMPATIBILITIES

Amiodarone, furosemide, heparin

PATIENT CARE IMPLICATIONS

• Monitor for/correct hypoxemia, hypercapnia, other fluid/electrolyte imbalance before initiating therapy.
• Carefully observe for dysrhythmia control during loading so that lowest possible dose given (see Administration).
• If positive ANA titer develops or SLE symptoms occur (e.g., unexplained fever, joint pain, muscle aches), consult physician, consider discontinuing drug.

Vital signs/hemodynamics: Continuously monitor BP, ECG during loading/parenteral therapy. Monitor for new/worsened dysrhythmias (heart block, ventricular dysrhythmias); observe for prolongation of PR/QT intervals, QRS complex. For hypotension or >25% widening of QRS complex, immediately discontinue, notify physician.
• Check apical pulse, BP immediately before administering maintenance dose; withhold next dose if significant bradycardia, hypotension present.

Physical assessment: Assess for perfusion/oxygenation deficit: ↓ level of consciousness, chest pain, activity intolerance, hypotension, dizziness. • Assess for excessive diarrhea, which could cause dangerous fluid/electrolyte imbalance.

Laboratory tests: Monitor: Electrolytes • ABGs • Liver enzymes, bilirubin • ANA titers • Plasma levels of quinidine; therapeutic level, 2-6 µg/ml

PATIENT/FAMILY TEACHING

Purpose of medication is to control abnormal heartbeats.
• Never break, crush, or chew sustained-release tablets. • Take with food to reduce stomach upset. • Report dizziness, breathing difficulty, excessive diarrhea, rash, fever, joint tenderness.

AVAILABLE FORMS

Parenteral for IV/IM injection • Tablets, capsules • Extended-release tablets

ramipril
(ram-i'-prel)
Altace

Classifications: Angiotensin-converting enzyme (ACE) inhibitor, antihypertensive

USUAL DOSE

PO, adults: Initially 1.25-2.5 mg once daily; titrate at intervals ≥2 wks according to BP. Up to 20 mg once daily or 10 mg bid may be used; use initial dose of 1.25 mg once daily in patients with concurrent diuretic therapy

G PO, older adults/renal impairment: 1.25 mg once daily; gradually increase at intervals ≥2 wks according to BP • Observe closely for symptomatic hypotension.

P pediatric   **G** geriatric   **V** Direct IV

ACTIONS

Long-acting ACE inhibitor that prevents conversion of angiotensin I to angiotensin II, a potent vasoconstrictor • BP reduced directly by decreased vascular tone, indirectly by reduction in aldosterone secretion and therefore decreased sodium/water retention • Reduces SBP, DBP; little or no effect on HR, contractility (in absence of heart failure) • Requires conversion in liver to be activated

PHARMACOKINETICS

ROUTE	ONSET	PEAK	DURATION
PO	1-2 hr	1-4 hr	24 hr

DISTRIBUTION

Wide; 73% protein bound

ELIMINATION

Eliminated in urine, feces; terminal half-life 50 hr, prolonged with renal insufficiency

INDICATIONS

Mild to severe hypertension • May be used in conjunction with other hypotensive agents, diuretics
Unlabeled/investigational:
With cardiac glycosides and diuretics to improve cardiac function, relieve symptoms, improve exercise tolerance in CHF patients.

PRECAUTIONS/CONTRAINDICATIONS

Precautions: Initial dose may cause profound hypotension, severe allergic reaction. • Other ACE inhibitors cause agranulocytosis; risk not well established with ramipril.
Use caution with: Renal impairment; reduce dose, monitor renal function. • Concurrent diuretic use, hypovolemia, hyponatremia, surgery/anesthesia; risk of severe hypotension • CAD, cerebrovascular disease, CHF, aortic stenosis; hypotensive episodes may precipitate MI, CVA, oliguria, or worsen heart failure. • Hepatic failure; reduce dose, monitor closely.
D Pregnancy category: Use only if necessary and woman informed of potential harm to fetus.
Contraindications: Hypersensitivity to ramipril, other ACE **P** inhibitors • Children: Safety/efficacy not established

ADVERSE EFFECTS

CNS: *Headache, dizziness, fatigue,* depression
Resp: *Cough,* dyspnea, **angioedema/stridor** (allergic reaction)
CV: *Hypotension,* palpitations, vasodilation
GI: *Nausea, vomiting,* altered taste, abdominal pain
GU: **Decreased renal function,** oliguria, proteinuria
Hema: Anemia, eosinophilia, neutropenia (rare)
Derm: Pruritus, rash, diaphoresis
Misc: Muscle cramps, arthralgia, hyponatremia, hyperkalemia (rare), photosensitivity, **allergic reaction, anaphylaxis**

TOXICITY/OVERDOSE

Symptoms: Hypotension • ↓ Level of consciousness • MI, CVA caused by severe hypotension in high-risk patients
Management: After recent ingestion, implement guidelines for management of acute overdose (Appendix I). • Support respiration as needed with O_2 and/or mechanical ventilation. • For hypotension, elevate legs, administer IV fluids (e.g., 0.9%

R

NaCl, LR) • Hemodialysis generally ineffective

INTERACTIONS

alcohol Hypotension
antacids ↓ Ramipril absorption
antihypertensives Profound hypotension
calcium channel blockers Profound hypotension
digitalis glycosides ↑ Digoxin levels; toxicity
diuretics Hypotension
diuretics, potassium sparing Hyperkalemia
NSAIDs ↓ Ramipril effectiveness
phenothiazines Hypotension
potassium supplements Hyperkalemia
sympathetic blockers Profound hypotension

PATIENT CARE IMPLICATIONS

• Correct hypovolemia before administration.
• Evaluate renal function before initiating therapy.
• Protect patients from injury associated with orthostatic hypotension, especially when initiating therapy.
• Vomiting, diarrhea, excessive perspiration, dehydration could cause serious hypotension.
Vital signs/hemodynamics: Monitor BP, HR q1-2h until stable, with following uses: initial therapy, hypertensive crisis, acute CHF, use of additional hypotensive agents/diuretics.
• Use IV 0.9% NaCl for transient hypotensive episodes during initial therapy. • As available, continuously monitor ECG for PVCs, T-wave inversion, ST segment elevation especially in patients with CHF, CAD.
Physical assessment: Assess for perfusion/oxygenation deficit: chest discomfort, ↓ level of consciousness, activity intolerance, hypotension, dizziness.
• Assess neurologic status q2-4h after initiation of therapy until BP controlled. • Monitor fluid balance; weigh daily.
Laboratory tests: Monitor: Electrolytes • BUN, creatinine • Bilirubin, liver enzymes • CBC with differential • **May cause:** Hyperkalemia, hyponatremia. Renal impairment, CHF, diabetes mellitus, potassium-sparing diuretics, potassium supplements, salt substitutes ↑ risk of electrolyte imbalance

PATIENT/FAMILY TEACHING

Purpose of drug is to lower BP and/or relieve symptoms of heart failure. • May cause orthostatic hypotension, dizziness, especially during initial therapy; use caution when changing positions, walking. Alcohol, hot weather, vigorous activity, vomiting, diarrhea, dehydration, prolonged standing make these symptoms more likely. • Lie down immediately if lightheaded or dizzy. • Medication is not cure for high BP; other therapies, including life-style modifications, must be continued. • Promptly report rash; swelling of extremities; fever, sore throat, infection; chest pain; swelling of face, lips, tongue, throat; difficulty breathing. • May cause persistent coughing; notify prescriber if these effects bothersome.
• Report pregnancy or plans to become pregnant.
Outpatient: Take medication exactly as prescribed. Do not stop taking medicine even if you feel better. If medication abruptly discontinued, you may

develop dangerously high BP.
• Avoid driving and other activities requiring mental alertness until individual response to drug known. • Avoid salt substitutes or other foods high in potassium unless prescriber specifies otherwise. • Weigh twice/wk; report weight gain, edema.
• Consult health care professional before taking cough, cold, or allergy preparations.

AVAILABLE FORMS

Capsules

ranitidine
(ra-nye'te-deen)
Nu-Ranit ♣, Zantac

Classification: Histamine H₂ antagonist

USUAL DOSE

PO, adults: Initially 150 mg bid or 300 mg once daily, usually hs; more frequent doses may be needed for pathologic hypersecretory conditions.
• Maintenance, 150 mg once daily, usually hs • **Renal impairment:** 150 mg q24h; schedule a dose immediately after dialysis.
IV/IM, adults: 50 mg q6-8h
• Do not exceed 400 mg/day.
• **Renal impairment:** 50 mg q18-24h; schedule a dose immediately after dialysis.
IV, cont inf, adults: 6.25 mg/hr (e.g., 150 mg/250 ml D₅W at 11 ml/hr) • **Hypersecretory conditions:** Start at 1 mg/kg/hr; increase upward in 0.5 mg/kg/hr increments q4h as needed according to gastric acidity, patient condition; up to 2.5 mg/kg/hr has been used.

ADMINISTRATION

▼**Direct IV:** Inject dilute solution slowly over at least 5 min.
• Too-rapid injection causes bradycardia, dysrhythmias, dyspnea.
IV, intermit inf: Infuse pre-mixed/prepared solution over 15-20 min.
IV, cont inf: Administer at prescribed rate, usually 11 ml/hr of 0.6 mg/ml concentration which is 6.25 mg/hr • **Hypersecretory conditions:** Start at 1 mg/kg/hr; increase upward in 0.5 mg/kg/hr increments q4h as needed according to gastric acidity, patient condition. • Use infusion pump, monitor closely

PREPARATION

Direct IV: Dilute in 20 ml sterile water or 0.9% NaCl.
IV, intermit inf: 50 mg in 100 ml compatible solution
IV, cont inf:

COMMON DILUTIONS	CONCENTRATION
50 mg/100 ml	0.5 mg/ml
150 mg/250 ml	0.6 mg/ml
250 mg/250 ml	1 mg/ml

Do not exceed concentration of 2.5 mg/ml.

Compatible fluids: D₅W, 0.9% NaCl, TPN
Stability: Stable at room temperature for 48 hr

ACTIONS

Inhibits action of histamine on H₂ receptors of parietal cells, thus reducing gastric acid secretion • Reduces basal, nocturnal, stimulated gastric acid secretion • 5-12 times potency of cimetidine in controlling gastric acid hypersecretion • Small transient increases in prolactin levels after large IV bolus injections;

R

italic = common side effects   **bold** = life-threatening reactions

may inhibit vasopressin release; little if any other hormonal effects • Not anticholinergic

PHARMACOKINETICS

ROUTE	ONSET	PEAK	DURATION
PO	<2 hr	2-3 hr	12 hr
IM	Rapid	15 min	8 hr
IV	Immed	Rapid	6-8 hr

DISTRIBUTION

Wide; 10%-19% protein bound

ELIMINATION

Excreted in urine, feces; half-life 1.7-3.2 hr, increases with age, up to 6 hr in older **G** adults

INDICATIONS

Short-term treatment of active, benign gastric/duodenal ulcers to reduce pain/other symptoms, promote healing • To reduce ulcer recurrence • To reduce acid secretion, promote ulcer healing in hypersecretory conditions (e.g., Zollinger-Ellison syndrome, postop hypersecretion, short-gut syndrome) • Relief of gastroesophageal reflux that fails to respond to conventional therapy alone • Treatment of erosive gastritis
Unlabeled/investigational:
Prevention of stress ulcer; control of upper GI bleeding associated with conditions such as gastric/duodenal ulcer, hemorrhagic gastritis; prevention of mucosal damage associated with NSAID therapy; perioperatively to prevent aspiration, pneumonia

PRECAUTIONS/ CONTRAINDICATIONS

Precautions: Rapid IV injection may cause bradycardia, dysrhythmias, dyspnea, especially in cardiac patients, others predisposed to dysrhythmias • May cause reversible mental

G confusion, especially with debilitation, advanced age, renal impairment • May cause ↑ total bilirubin, AST, ALT, other liver enzymes
Use caution with: Hepatic dysfunction; may be hepatotoxic • Renal dysfunction; reduced dose indicated
B **Pregnancy category:** Safety not clearly established
Contraindications: Hypersensitivity to rantidine, other hista- **P** mine H_2 antagonists • Children: Safety not established

ADVERSE EFFECTS

CNS: *Headache, malaise,* dizziness, sleepiness, insomnia, blurred vision, reversible mental confusion
CV: Bradycardia, tachycardia, PVCs (IV)
GI: Constipation, nausea, vomiting, abdominal pain
Hema: Rarely the following— leukopenia, agranulocytosis, thrombocytopenia
Derm: Urticaria/macropapular/ pruritic rash
Local: Transient burning/itching (IV)
Misc: **Anaphlaxis** (rare)

TOXICITY/OVERDOSE

Symptoms: Similar to adverse effects
Management: After recent ingestion, implement guidelines for management of acute overdose (Appendix I). • Manage dysrhythmias according to ACLS guidelines. • Dialysis may aid in elimination.

P pediatric   **G** geriatric   **V** Direct IV

INTERACTIONS

antacids ↓ Ranitidine absorption

anticoagulants, PO   Prolonged PT; risk of bleeding

benzodiazepines ↑ Benzodiazepine levels

beta blockers ↑ Beta-blocker levels

calcium channel blockers ↑ Calcium channel–blocking effects

ketoconazole ↓ Ketoconazole levels

opiate analgesics ↑ Opiate effects; monitor closely

procainamide ↑ Procainamide effects/toxicity

theophylline ↑ Theophylline effects/toxicity

COMPATIBILITIES

Acyclovir, aminophylline, atracurium, bretylium, ceftaxidime, ciprofloxin, diltiazem, dobutamine, dopamine, enalaprilat, esmolol, heparin, labetalol, meperidine, morphine, nitroglycerin, ondansetron, pancuronium, piperacillin sodium, procainamide, vecuronium, zidovudine

INCOMPATIBILITIES

Amphotericin B, hetastarch, metaraminol

PATIENT CARE IMPLICATIONS

• Do not administer within 1 hr of antacids. Stagger dosage schedules if also taking diazepam, other benzodiazepines.

• Administer IV doses as intermittent infusion when possible.

Vital signs/hemodynamics: Monitor BP, HR for orthostatic changes in acutely ill patients. Observe for bradycardia, dysrhythmias during direct IV administration, high-dose therapy

Physical assessment: Assess for epigastric, abdominal pain. Consult physician if pain persistent/severe • Monitor for GI bleeding: occult blood in emesis/stool, orthostatic changes • Monitor gastric pH, gastric output in acutely ill patients. **G** • Assess older adults, severely ill patients for mental confusion.

Laboratory tests: Monitor: Liver enzymes (e.g., ALT, AST, alkaline phosphatase), total bilirubin • CBC with differential • BUN, creatinine

PATIENT/FAMILY TEACHING

Purpose of medication is to reduce stomach acid. • May cause drowsiness, dizziness, mental confusion; use caution and avoid activities requiring mental alertness until response to therapy established. • Report vomiting of blood, bloody or black tarry stools, dizziness, confusion. • Smoking decreases effectiveness of ranitidine, increases gastric acidity. Smoking cessation programs/therapy recommended.

Outpatient: Take all doses as prescribed, even if feeling better. • Do not take antacids, diazepam, similar medications within 1 hr of ranitidine. • Avoid coffee, caffeine, alcohol, aspirin, ibuprofen, other food or drugs that may cause gastric irritation. • Inform all health care providers of ranitidine therapy to avoid possible drug interactions

AVAILABLE FORMS

Tablets, capsules, granules • Syrup • Parenteral for IV/IM use

rocuronium bromide
(roe-kyoo-roe-nee'um)
Zemuron

Classification: Nondepolarizing
neuromuscular blocking agent

USUAL DOSE

Each dose individualized according to patient response

(P) Direct IV, adults/children:
Endotracheal intubation:
0.45-1.2 mg/kg enables intubation within 2 min in most cases.
Dose-related muscle relaxation
usually lasts 15-60 min.
• **Maintenance:** 0.1-0.2 mg/kg
for adults; 0.1-0.15 mg/kg for
older adults; 0.075-0.125 mg/kg
(P) for children. Dose-related muscle relaxation usually lasts 10-
30 min. Longer dosing intervals
may be necessary with renal/
hepatic insufficiency.

(P) IV, cont inf, adults/children:
0.01-0.012 µg/kg/min, adjust to
individual requirements. Initiate
infusion after administering initial bolus dose.

ADMINISTRATION

▼ Direct IV: Inject each dose over
15 sec; dilution not necessary.
*Causes immediate respiratory
paralysis; means for continuous
artificial ventilation must be in
place or provided immediately
after injection.* Use nerve stimulator to monitor neuromuscular
blockade. Avoid additional doses
until there is a certain response
to T_1 (first twitch).

IV, cont inf: Infusion pump
necessary. Titrate for minimal
dose required to maintain 90%
(using nerve stimulator) or desired neuromuscular blockade.
Check for a certain response to
T_1 (first twitch). If no response,

discontinue infusion until response returns.

PREPARATION

DILUTION	CONCENTRATION
50 mg/100 ml	0.5 mg/ml
100 mg/100 ml	1 mg/ml

Compatible fluids: D_5W,
0.9% NaCl, LR

ACTIONS

Causes skeletal muscle paralysis
by interfering with transmission
of nerve impulses at neuromuscular junction. • Competes with/
blocks activity of acetylcholine
(neurotransmitter normally producing electrical depolarization)
• Eye, face, neck muscles affected first; followed by limbs,
abdomen, chest, diaphragm
• Recovery occurs in reverse order. • May trigger histamine release; likelihood increased if
recommended dose exceeded
• No analgesic/sedative effects
• Dose-related rapid to intermediate onset of effects; intermediate duration relative to other
NMBAs

PHARMACOKINETICS

ROUTE	ONSET	PEAK	DURATION
IV	<1 min	1-3 min	20-90 min, depending on dose. Greatest time to recovery in elders

DISTRIBUTION
Throughout extracellular fluid; 30% pro-
tein bound
ELIMINATION
Primarily hepatic

INDICATIONS

With general anesthesia to produce skeletal muscle relaxation
during surgery • To facilitate
routine ET intubation • To provide skeletal muscle relaxation,

---

(P) pediatric   **(G)** geriatric   **▼** Direct IV

increase lung compliance during mechanical ventilation • No effects on consciousness/pain threshold • Used only after induction of general anesthesia or with analgesics/anxiolytic

PRECAUTIONS/ CONTRAINDICATIONS

Precautions: *Causes respiratory paralysis; must use with artificial airway, ventilatory support* • Peripheral nerve stimulator recommended during use • Long-term use in ICU patients not well established; tolerance, prolonged paralysis, skeletal muscle weakness are possible. Ventilator weaning may be delayed.

Use caution with: Hepatic insufficiency; excretion may be delayed • Myasthenia gravis, severe electrolyte/acid-base disturbances; drug effects may be prolonged

B **Pregnancy category:** Animal studies have not demonstrated adverse fetal effects; use only if benefit exceeds risk.

Contraindications: Hypersensitivity to rocuronium

ADVERSE EFFECTS

CNS: *Muscle weakness, paralysis,* prolonged blockade
Resp: Bronchospasm, wheezing, rhonchi
CV: Hypotension, hypertension, dysrhythmias, tachycardia
Derm: Rash, itching, injection site edema

TOXICITY/OVERDOSE

Symptoms: Overdosage has not been reported; expect prolonged neuromuscular blockade.
Management: Provide continuous artificial ventilation. • Reverse effects with anticholinesterase agent such as neostig-

mine, edrophonium, in conjunction with anticholinergic such as atropine, glycopyrrolate. • Hypotension: Elevate legs; administer IV fluids; use dopamine, other pressors if necessary • For management of acute allergic reaction, see Appendix N.

INTERACTIONS

aminoglycosides (amikacin, gentamicin), amphotericin B, beta-blockers, calcium channel blockers, corticosteroids, diuretics, inhalation anesthetics, lidocaine, magnesium, procainamide, quinidine Potentiate/prolong neuromuscular blockade

digoxin ↑ Risk of dysrhythmias
opiate analgesics Respiratory depression
succinylcholine Avoid rocuronium until patient recovered from succinylcholine

Y-SITE COMPATIBILITIES
Not determined

Y-SITE INCOMPATIBILITIES
Alkaline solutions, barbiturates

PATIENT CARE IMPLICATIONS

• Has no effect on consciousness/pain threshold; patient is fully awake and feels all sensations. *Use only with general anesthesia or analgesics (e.g., morphine) and anxiolytics (e.g., midazolam).*
• Causes respiratory paralysis, apnea; *use only for patients under direct observation and continuous mechanical ventilation.*
• Prevent corneal drying by instillation of artificial tears, eye patching.
• Cholinesterase inhibitors such as neostigmine, edrophonium

R

used to reverse effects; multiple doses may be necessary.
• Long-term use may cause prolonged paralysis, skeletal muscle weakness; use lowest effective dose.
• Patients thought to have recovered from neuromuscular blockade may develop apnea when given certain drugs that potentiate NMBAs (see Interactions).

Vital signs/hemodynamics: Monitor ECG continuously. Observe for bradycardia (unlike some other NMBAs, will not counter bradycardia caused by anesthetics or vagal stimulation), tachycardia. • Monitor BP, observing for hypotension, q3-5min during initiation of therapy and frequently thereafter.
• Use continuous pulse oximetry to monitor oxygenation during and immediately after neuromuscular blockade.

Physical assessment: Closely monitor respiratory status: rate, depth, pattern of ventilation, until fully recovered. Secretions may be increased; suction as necessary. • Paralysis of muscle groups usually occurs in the following order: Eye, face, neck muscles affected first; followed by limbs, abdomen, chest, diaphragm. Recovery occurs in reverse order. Assess frequently for residual muscle weakness, respiratory distress until fully recovered from effects. • Use peripheral nerve stimulator to monitor effectiveness of NMBAs. *Avoid additional doses of NMBAs until there is a certain response to T_1 (first twitch). If no response, discontinue infusion until response returns.* • Monitor I&O; Foley catheter required.

Laboratory tests: Monitor: Potassium; drug action potentiated by hypokalemia. Magnesium; drug action potentiated by hypermagnesemia. Calcium; drug action potentiated by hypocalcemia. Acid-base status; imbalance alters drug action. ABGs; to evaluate adequacy of ventilation.

PATIENT/FAMILY TEACHING

Purpose of medication is to paralyze body muscles temporarily to facilitate procedures, surgery.
• When recovering from effects, it may be difficult to swallow, talk; these effects are temporary. • Drug does not affect consciousness: explain all procedures.

AVAILABLE FORMS

Parenteral for IV injection
Storage: Intact vials stable for 30 days at room temp; refrigerate if stored for longer periods.

---

sodium bicarbonate, baking soda
Carbicarb ✤, Neut, Soda Mint

Classifications: Electrolyte replacement, alkalinizing agent

USUAL DOSE
PO, adults: Urinary alkalinization: 1-2 g q4h; up to 16 g/24 hr may be necessary • Acidosis/chronic renal failure: 4-6 g/24 hr in 4-5 divided doses
🅟 **PO, children:** 84-840 mg/kg/24 hr in divided doses
Direct IV, adults: Indicated only during adult cardiac arrest • Initially 1 mEq/kg; subsequent

doses, usually 0.5 mEq/kg, depending on severity of acidosis.
IV inf, adults: 2-5 mEq/kg given over 4-8 hr depending on severity of acidosis, fluid status, clinical response • Generally, initial dose should not exceed >50% of calculated deficit to avoid overcorrection.
ⓅIV/intraosseous inf, children: 0.5-1 mEq/kg, depending on severity of acidosis, fluid status, clinial response • **Cardiac arrest:** Initially 0.5-1 mEq/kg; subsequent doses, usually 0.5 mEq/kg, depending on severity of acidosis.

ADMINISTRATION

Verify patency of catheter/needle before administration; inadvertent subcutaneous injection may cause tissue necrosis.
PO: Instruct patient to thoroughly chew tablets. • Administer with full glass of water. • Effervescent tablets must be completely dissolved.
▼Direct IV, adults: Inject undiluted single dose over 1-3 min.
IV inf: Flush IV line before and after administration. • Infuse over 4-8 hr; do not exceed rate of 50 mEq/hr. • Decrease rate Ⓟ for children. • For neonates, Ⓟ children <2 yr, do not exceed rate of 8 mEq/kg/24 hr. • Too-rapid administration may cause alkalosis, hypokalemia, hypocalcemia, dysrhythmias.

PREPARATION

IV: Use of premixed solution or dilution with compatible IV solution preferred • May be given undiluted in severe emergencies
Compatible fluids: D₅W, 0.9% NaCl, 0.45% NaCl, combinations of these solutions

ACTIONS

Main component of major buffering system of body, the bicarbonate/carbonic acid buffer • Extremely effective in buffering fixed acids, bases; efficiently buffers pH, reverses acidosis • Encourages redistribution of potassium ions from extracellular to intracellular fluid • Increases urinary pH in patients with normal renal function; alkaline urine encourages excretion of certain organic acids (e.g., phenobarbital, salicylates). • Orally neutralizes gastric acid; each gram neutralizes about 12 mEq acid.

PHARMACOKINETICS

ROUTE	ONSET	PEAK	DURATION
PO	Rapid	30 min	1-3 hr
IV	Immed	Rapid	Var

DISTRIBUTION
Widely distributed throughout extracellular fluid
ELIMINATION
Renally reabsorbed or eliminated, depending on body's needs

INDICATIONS

Metabolic acidosis (blood pH <7.10) associated with severe renal disease, ketoacidosis, shock, other conditions • Hyperkalemia; to promote intracellular potassium shift • Hyponatremia: Administer with 5% sodium chloride, usually 1 part sodium bicarbonate to 3 parts sodium chloride. • Cardiac arrest with preexisting hyperkalemia/metabolic acidosis, prolonged cardiac arrest; routine use in cardiac arrest not recommended; not indicated for mild to moderate metabolic acidosis during cardiac arrest; effective ventilation/volume replacement necessary • Acute toxicity from barbiturates, salicylates, other agents to alkalinize urine, encourage renal excretion of toxin • Buffering solution to raise pH of IV fluids, medications • Orally as antacid

PRECAUTIONS/ CONTRAINDICATIONS

Precautions: Temporary therapy in metabolic acidosis; underlying disorder must be corrected. • Rapid or excessive administration may cause alkalosis, hypokalemia, hypocalcemia, dysrhythmias. • IV use may cause fluid/electrolyte disturbances, fluid overload, pulmonary edema. • Avoid overcorrection, metabolic alkalosis by carefully adjusting dose to laboratory results. • Extravasation may cause cellulitis, necrosis, ulceration, sloughing.

Use caution with: Renal impairment • CHF, corticosteroid therapy, other sodium-retaining or edematous conditions • Hypertension • Cirrhosis • Toxemia • Diabetic ketoacidosis; too-rapid correction of acidosis causes hypokalemia; acidosis generally only partially corrected to pH of 7.2 • Neonates/

P children <2 yr; too-rapid injection (>10 ml/min), excessive dose causes hypernatremia, ↓ CSF pressure, possible intracranial hemorrhage.

c Pregnancy category: Use only if safer alternative unavailable.

Contraindications: Metabolic/ respiratory alkalosis • Hypocalcemia; alkalosis may induce tetany. • Excessive, uncorrected chloride loss • Acute ingestion of strong acids (PO formulation) • PO use as antacid: Sodium restriction, renal failure

ADVERSE EFFECTS

CNS: Headache, confusion, tremors, *twitching, hypereflexia,* **tetany, seizures**

GI: Flatulence, belching, distention, acid rebound

GU: Calculi

F&E: Fluid retention, weight gain, edema, hypokalemia, hypocalcemia, metabolic alkalosis

Local: *Burning/pain at injection site*

TOXICITY/OVERDOSE

Symptoms: Ventricular dysrhythmias, cardiac arrest • Tremors, tetany, carpopedal spasm, seizures • Hypokalemia, hypocalcemia

Management: After recent ingestion, implement guidelines for management of acute overdose (Appendix I). • **Severe metabolic alkalosis:** Administer calcium gluconate and/or ammonium chloride. Correct hypokalemia. • For extravasation, infiltrate area with lidocaine or hyaluronidase using 25–27-gauge needle. Elevate extremity, apply warm moist compresses (Appendixes K and L).

INTERACTIONS

amphetamines Prolonged amphetamine effects

iron ↓ Iron absorption (PO)

lithium ↓ Lithium levels

quinidine ↑ Quinidine levels

Y-SITE COMPATIBILITIES

Acyclovir, famotidine, insulin, morphine, piperacillin-tazobactam, potassium chloride

---

P pediatric   **G** geriatric   **V** Direct IV

INCOMPATIBILITIES
Alcohol/dextrose solution, amrinone, calcium chloride, calcium gluconate, cefotaxime, ciprofloxacin, diltiazem, dobutamine, dopamine, epinephrine, isoproterenol, magnesium sulfate, norepinephrine, ondansetron, ticarcillin, verapamil

PATIENT CARE IMPLICATIONS
• All doses must be individually adjusted to severity of acidosis, laboratory values, patient's age, weight, clinical condition.
• Correct hypokalemia, hypocalcemia before or during use.
• Use in metabolic acidosis is for temporary stabilization; underlying condition must be corrected as soon as possible.
• Many precautions necessary with IV use (see Administration).
• PO use may cause premature dissolution of enteric-coated tablets.
• Do not administer with milk, because milk alkali syndrome (confusion, headache, nausea, vomiting, urinary calculi, hypercalcemia) may result.
Vital signs/hemodynamics: PO: VS according to patient condition • IV: Continuously monitor ECG for dysrhythmias, hypokalemic changes: ventricular dysrhythmias, U wave, flattened T wave. Monitor for fluid overload: ↑ PAP, PCWP, CVP, MAP. Slow or stop infusion, consult physician for fluid overload.
Physical assessment: Assess respiratory status: rate, rhythm, depth, lung sounds. • Evaluate fluid balance: I/O ratio, daily weights, edema. • Consult physician for evidence of fluid overload: hypertension, edema, dyspnea, crackles (rales), frothy sputum. • Assess for alkalosis: irritability, confusion, hyperreflexia, slow respirations, cyanosis, muscle twitching, tetany, seizures. Consult physician if alkalosis suspected.
Laboratory tests: Monitor: Electrolytes, especially sodium, potassium, calcium, chloride, bicarbonate • ABGs, especially pH, CO_2, bicarbonate, base deficit • BUN, creatinine • Urine pH when used for renal alkalinization • **May cause:** ↑ Urinary urobilinogen • False-positive urinary protein, blood lactate

PATIENT/FAMILY TEACHING
Purpose of medication is to correct excess acid in body or neutralize stomach acids (PO).
• Report breathing difficulty, swelling of hands/feet, chest pain, diarrhea, dark tarry stools, numbness, tingling, twitching.
• Thoroughly chew/dissolve tablets, drink with at least 8 oz water. • Do not take with milk.
• Do not use as antacid if on sodium restriction. • Weigh 2-3 times/wk; report weight gain.

AVAILABLE FORMS
Parenteral for IV use • Tablets • PO granules

S

sodium chloride, 3% & 5% hypertonic solution

Classification: Electrolyte replacement

---

italic = common side effects   **bold** = life-threatening reactions

USUAL DOSE

IV, intermit inf, adults: 100 ml 3% or 5% solution; after first dose, check electrolytes, evaluate need for further therapy; repeat as necessary to resolve neurologic symptoms or until serum sodium 130 mEq/L. • Do not administer >100 ml/hr.

ADMINISTRATION

IV, intermit: Infuse ⅓-½ estimated requirement over 6-8 hr; rate individualized according to patient's needs. • Solution hypertonic; use large vein, verify placement, check frequently to avoid infiltration. • Do not exceed 100 ml/hr.

PREPARATION

Available as premixed 3% or 5% solution • Do not dilute; only indicated for sodium/chloride replacement without large amount of fluid.
Compatible fluids: D_5W, LR, combinations of these solutions

ACTIONS

Sodium is major cation of extracellular fluid, helps control water distribution, fluid/electrolyte/acid-base balance, osmotic pressure. • Osmoreceptors located in the hypothalamus control serum sodium concentrations • Body fluid lost with ↓ sodium content, retained with ↑ sodium. • Sodium is readily absorbed in renal tubules, frequently exchanged for hydrogen/potassium ions. • Chloride is major anion of extracellular fluid, helps maintain acid-base balance.

PHARMACOKINETICS

ROUTE	ONSET	PEAK	DURATION
IV	Immed	Rapid	Var

DISTRIBUTION
Widely distributed throughout extracellular fluid

ELIMINATION
Renally reabsorbed or eliminated; depending on body's needs

INDICATIONS

To replace lost sodium/chloride in body, maintain electrolyte balance under conditions when sodium/chloride deficit severe and/or administration of large amounts of fluid undesired (e.g., SIADH, severe GI losses, excessive administration of hypotonic solutions, addisonian crisis, edematous states) • Sodium content of 500 ml 5% NaCl approx that of 3 L 0.9% NaCl

PRECAUTIONS/ CONTRAINDICATIONS

Precautions: Adjust therapy to electrolyte concentrations, fluid balance, clinical condition. • Rapid/excessive administration causes rapid intravascular osmotic shift, possible pulmonary edema. • Too-rapid administration may cause RBC hemolysis. • May cause hypokalemia **Use caution with:** Postop or **G** comatose patients • Older adults • Renal impairment • CHF, other sodium-retaining/edematous conditions • Hypertension • Corticosteroid therapy • Cirrhosis • Toxemia • Any patient prone to metabolic, acid-base fluid/electrolyte disorders **C Pregnancy category:** Use only if safer alternative unavailable.
Contraindications: Increased, normal, slightly decreased serum sodium concentrations

---

P pediatric   **G** geriatric   **V** Direct IV

ADVERSE EFFECTS

CNS: Disorientation, weakness, **coma**

CV: **Pulmonary edema,** CHF

F&E: Fluid retention, weight gain, edema, hypokalemia, hypernatremia

Local: *Burning/pain at injection site*

TOXICITY/OVERDOSE

Symptoms: Hypernatremia: intense thirst, fever, flushed skin, restlessness, agitation, coma • Peripheral/pulmonary edema • Hypertension, increased PAP, PCWP, CVP

Management: Immediately discontinue infusion, consult physician. • Diuretics, hemodialysis may be helpful. • Monitor closely, treat symptomatically.

INTERACTIONS

antihypertensives ↓ Antihypertensive effectiveness

lithium ↓ Lithium levels

Y-SITE COMPATIBILITIES

Ciprofloxacin

Y-SITE INCOMPATIBILITIES

Mannitol

PATIENT CARE IMPLICATIONS

• All doses must be individually adjusted to laboratory values, acid-base balance, fluid status, estimated sodium deficit, clinical condition.

• Many precautions necessary with IV use (See Administration).

Vital signs/hemodynamics: Monitor VS according to patient's clinical condition. Monitor for fluid overload resulting from rapid osmotic shift into vascular space; ↑ PAP, PCWP, CVP, MAP. Slow or stop infusion; consult physician for fluid overload.

Physical assessment: Assess respiratory status: rate, rhythm, depth, lung sounds. • Evaluate fluid balance: I/O ratio, daily weights, edema. • Monitor for fluid overload: hypertension, edema, dyspnea, crackles (rales), frothy sputum. • Assess for hypernatremia: intense thirst, fever, flushed skin, restlessness, agitation, coma. • Consult physician for fluid overload, hypernatremia.

Laboratory tests: Monitor: Electrolytes, especially sodium, potassium, chloride, bicarbonate • Serum osmolarity • ABGs, especially pH, CO_2 pressure, bicarbonate, base deficit • BUN, creatinine

PATIENT/FAMILY TEACHING

Purpose of medication is to restore normal balance of sodium/chloride in body. • Report breathing difficulty, swelling of hands/feet, intense thirst, restlessness.

AVAILABLE FORMS

Parenteral for IV use

S

sodium polystyrene sulfate
Kayexalate, SPS Suspension

Classification: Cation exchange resin

USUAL DOSE

Dose individualized according to serum potassium, patient condition

---

italic = common side effects   **bold** = life-threatening reactions

PO, adults: 15 g 1-4 times daily

Rectal, adults: Initially, 120-180 ml commercially prepared suspension q1-2h as retention enema; alternately, 30-50 g powder mixed in 100 ml appropriate solution; when stabilized, administer same dose q4-6h.
• Up to 100 g may be used.

P PO/rectal, children: 1g/kg q6h
• Individualized; 1 g resin binds approx 1 mEq potassium.

ADMINISTRATION

Use commercial suspension or freshly prepared solution. Do not use if >24 hr old.

PO: Do not administer with potassium-containing food such as orange/other citrus juice, bananas

Rectal: Administer initial cleansing enema. • Warm prepared solution to body temperature, do not overheat. • Use soft, large (e.g., 28 French for adults) rubber tube. Lubricate tip; insert approx 20 cm into rectum (adults) with tip well into sigmoid colon. Tape in place. • Stir, gently agitate suspension; administer by gravity drainage. • Flush tube with 50-100 ml of fluid, clamp, leave in place. • Elevation of hips or knee-chest position helps with retention. • Retain for at least 30-60 min. • After maximal retention, irrigate colon with 1-2 L nonsaline irrigating solution to remove resin thoroughly.
• Sealed dialysis bag or Y connector with tubing may facilitate enema administration, drainage.

PREPARATION

PO: Mix powder in 20-100 ml water, syrup (e.g., 70% sorbi-

tol), other fluid. • May be mixed in food

Rectal: Mix powder in 100-200 ml water, other solution (e.g., 25% sorbitol, 1% methylcellulose, 10% dextrose). • Mix to thick suspension; avoid paste, which ↓ exchange surface, limits effectiveness.

ACTIONS

Releases sodium in exchange for other cations of higher molecular weight, such as potassium, calcium, magnesium
• Exchange occurs primarily in large intestine. • Exchange of other cations, including iron, organic cations, lipids, steroids, proteins, may occur.

PHARMACOKINETICS

ROUTE	ONSET	PEAK	DURATION
PO	2-12 hr	Var	Until eliminated
Rectal	<1 hr	1-2 hr	

DISTRIBUTION
Not absorbed

ELIMINATION
Eliminated in feces

INDICATIONS

Mild to moderate hyperkalemia
• Severe hyperkalemia, in conjunction with other measures such as glucose/insulin infusion, sodium bicarbonate, calcium, furosemide • Single dose of 50 g lowers serum potassium by approx 0.5-1 mEq.

PRECAUTIONS/CONTRAINDICATIONS

Precautions: Slow onset of action; rapid-acting therapy must be initiated in severe hypokalemia. • Exchange of sodium for potassium may cause fluid retention, edema. • Fatal intestinal necrosis has been associated with exchange resin enemas in azotemic patients; sorbitol, omission of final cleansing enema have been implicated; use of non–sorbitol-based enemas, thorough final cleansing enema recommended.

G Use caution with: Older adults • Renal impairment • CHF, other sodium-retaining/edematous conditions • Hypertension • Digitalized patients

c Pregnancy category: Use only if safer alternative unavailable.

Contraindications: Hypersensitivity to any ingredient in specific preparation • Ileus

ADVERSE EFFECTS

GI: Constipation, nausea, vomiting, diarrhea (sorbitol), fecal impaction, gastric irritation

F&E: Hypernatremia, fluid retention, weight gain, edema, hypokalemia, hypocalcemia, hypomagnesemia

INTERACTIONS

antacids ↓ Effectiveness; systemic alkalosis

digoxin Hypokalemia, digoxin toxicity

PATIENT CARE IMPLICATIONS

• Because of slow onset of action, should not be used as sole therapy in severe hyperkalemia with ECG changes; rapid-acting therapy with calcium, bicarbonate, glucose plus insulin, and/or diuretics must be initiated first.

• Many implications with rectal use; see Administration

Vital signs/hemodynamics: Monitor VS according to patient's clinical condition. • Continuously monitor ECG. Observe for hyperkalemic (peaked

T waves, ST depression, prolonged QT interval, widened QRS complex, loss of P waves) or hypokalemic (flattened T wave, presence of U wave, ventricular dysrhythmias) changes. Onset of hyperkalemic changes suggests potassium >7-8 mEq/L, indicates immediate need for rapid-acting therapy (e.g., calcium, bicarbonate, glucose plus insulin). For hypokalemic changes, drain/expel enema, check serum potassium, consult physician. • As available, monitor for fluid overload resulting from hypernatremia; ↑ PCWP/CVP, ↑ MAP. Consult physician for fluid overload.

Physical assessment: Evaluate fluid balance: I/O ratio, daily weights, edema. • Assess for evidence of fluid overload: hypertension, edema, dyspnea, crackles (rales), frothy sputum. • Assess for hypernatremia: intense thirst, fever, flushed skin, restlessness, agitation, coma. • Assess abdomen; note frequency, character of stools. Usually administered with laxative such as sorbitol to prevent constipation. Additional advantage of sorbitol is action as osmotic cathartic, which aids in potassium removal. • With concurrent cardiac glycoside therapy, assess for symptoms of digitalis toxicity: nausea, vomiting, blurred/yellow vision, dysrhythmias.

Laboratory tests: Monitor: Electrolyes, especially sodium, potassium, calcium, magnesium • BUN, creatinine • Check serum potassium 1-2 hr after initial dose; adjust subsequent doses to electrolyte concentrations, clinical condition. Ther-

S

apy usually stopped when potassium reaches 5 mEq/L.

PATIENT/FAMILY TEACHING

Purpose of medication is to reduce potassium to normal levels. • Report diarrhea or constipation; 1 or 2 soft stools/day desired. • Report breathing difficulty, swelling of hands/feet, intense thirst, restlessness. • Shake well before use. Do not mix with citrus, prune, tomato juice, other high-potassium foods.

AVAILABLE FORMS

Powder for PO/rectal suspension • Premixed PO/rectal suspension

---

sotalol HCl
(soe-ta'lole)
Beta-Cardone ♣,
Betapace Sotacor ♣,
Sotalex ♣

Classifications: Classes II/III antidysrhythmic, nonselective beta-adrenergic blocker

USUAL DOSE

PO, adults: Initially 80 mg q12h; gradually increase at 2–3-day intervals until dysrhythmia controlled. Up to 240-320 mg/24 hr given in divided doses may be used; 480-640 mg/24 hr sometimes necessary for refractory dysrhythmias. • Initiate therapy in hospital setting with continuous cardiac monitoring. • Reduce dose, frequency for renal impairment.

ACTIONS

Blocks sympathetic stimulation of beta-adrenergic receptors (Class II effect), prolongs duration of cardiac action potential (Class III effect) • Beta-blocking effects seen at doses as low as 25 mg; Class III effects usually occur at doses ≥160 mg/24 hr. • Noncardioselective beta blockade slows AV conduction, reduces HR; in hypertensive patients, SBP/DBP decreased. • Activity against life-threatening ventricular dysrhythmias caused primarily by Class III effects, including prolonged atrial/ventricular action potentials, prolonged effective refractory period of atria, ventricle, AV accessory pathways in both anterograde/retrograde directions

PHARMACOKINETICS

ROUTE	ONSET	PEAK	DURATION
PO	<1 hr	2.5-4 hr	Steady-state levels achieved in 2-3 days

DISTRIBUTION

Throughout plasma, not protein bound; does not cross blood-brain barrier

ELIMINATION

Not metabolized, renal elimination; half-life 12 hr, ↑ with renal impairment

INDICATIONS

Documented life-threatening ventricular dysrhythmias such as sustained VT • Not indicated for non–life-threatening dysrhythmias such as symptomatic PVCs, nonsustained VT, because use may cause serious dysrhythmias (e.g., torsades de pointes, new VT/VF)

PRECAUTIONS/ CONTRAINDICATIONS

Precautions: Prodysrhythmic effects, serious dysrhythmias such as torsades de pointes (polymorphic VT with shifting ventricular axis) or new VT/VF may develop. Risk of torsades de pointes ↑ with history of sustained VT/VF, CHF, prolonged QT interval, ↓ HR, hypokalemia, hypomagnesemia. Most serious dysrhythmias occur within 7 days of initiating therapy or increasing dosage. • Diarrhea, vomiting, diuretic therapy may adversely affect electrolyte balance, contribute to severe dysrhythmias. • Abrupt withdrawal of therapy may precipitate myocardial ischemia. **Use caution with:** QT_c interval >500 msec; consider reduced dose, cessation of therapy. • Acute MI, CHF, cardiomegaly; may depress myocardial contractility, precipitate severe failure; dysrhythmias more likely • COPD; avoid if possible, if not use minimal dose, monitor for bronchospasm. • General anesthesia; may cause additive impairment of cardiac contractility; may withdraw before surgery • Diabetes, hyperthyroidism; beta-blocking effects mask symptoms. • Sick sinus syndrome; use extreme caution, may cause sinus arrest. • Renal impairment; reduced dose indicated

P • Children: Safety/efficacy not established

B Pregnancy category: Use only if safer alternative unavailable

Contraindications: Hypersensitivity to sotalol • QT_c interval >550 msec • Uncorrected hypokalemia/hypomagnesemia • Severe bradycardia • 2nd/3rd degree heart block, unless artificial ventricular pacemaker • Cardiogenic shock • Uncontrolled CHF • Bronchial asthma, severe COPD

ADVERSE EFFECTS

Serious adverse effects dose related

CNS: *Fatigue, weakness, dizziness,* headache

Resp: *Dyspnea,* bronchospasm

CV: *Bradycardia, chest pain, hypotension, palpitations,* **torsades de pointes, VT/VF, edema, heart failure**

GI: Nausea, vomiting, diarrhea

Endo: Blocked symptoms of hypoglycemia/hyperthyroidism

TOXICITY/OVERDOSE

Symptoms: Fatal ventricular dysrhythmias, including torsades de pointes • Symptomatic bradycardia, HR <45, advanced heart block • Profound hypotension, loss of consciousness • Heart failure • Bronchospasm **Management:** After recent ingestion, implement guidelines for management of acute overdose (Appendix I). • Correct electrolyte imbalance, especially hypokalemia, hypomagnesemia. • **Symptomatic bracycardia, heart block:** Atropine, beta-adrenergic agonist (e.g., epinephrine, dopamine), transvenous pacemaker • **Torsades de pointes:** Cardioversion, transvenous pacing, epinephrine, magnesium sulfate • **Bronchospasm:** Aminophylline, aerosol beta-2-receptor stimulant (e.g., isoetharine) • **Hypotension:** Elevate legs, administer IV fluids; use vasopressor (e.g., dopamine, epinephrine) if severe and refractory to inotropic agents; avoid isoproterenol, norepinephrine. • **Heart failure:** Inotropic agents (e.g., dobutamine, dopamine), diuretics • Hemodialysis may be helpful.

S

---

italic = common side effects   **bold** = life-threatening reactions

INTERACTIONS

amiodarone Severe bradycardia; ventricular dysrhythmias

antidiabetics (insulin, PO agents) Prolonged recovery from hypoglycemic episodes; masked hypoglycemia-associated tachycardia; hyperglycemia

astemizole, terfenadine Additive prolongation of QT interval

calcium channel blockers Extreme bradycardia; hypotension

digoxin Ventricular dysrhythmias

disopyramide Additive negative inotropy; ↓ CO; dysrhythmias

diuretics, nonpotassium-sparing Excessive prolongation of QT interval

isoproterenol ↓ Bronchodilatory effectiveness

phenothiazines Additive prolongation of QT interval

quinidine Additive cardiac depression

theophylline ↓ Bronchodilation

TCAs Additive prolongation of QT interval

PATIENT CARE IMPLICATIONS

• Use lowest possible dose for dysrhythmia control.

• Monitor closely if other antidysrhythmics, hypotensive agents used.

• Gradually withdraw therapy to avoid rebound hypertension, angina, possible acute MI.

• Correct hypokalemia, hypomagnesemia before initiating therapy.

• **COPD:** Monitor closely; avoid high-dose therapy, which may precipitate bronchospasm.

Vital signs/hemodynamics: Monitor BP, HR, RR closely when initiating therapy/adjusting dose. Hold next dose, consult physician for hypotension, symptomatic bradycardia, dyspnea. • When initiating therapy/increasing dose, monitor ECG for ↑ QT interval, new/increased ventricular dysrhythmias, profound bradycardia, heart block. If present, hold next dose, consult physician. • Measure PAWP, PAP, CVP, CO/CI as available. Consult physician for ↓ CO/CI, ↑ filling pressures, other symptoms of heart failure.

Physical assessment: Assess for perfusion/oxygenation deficit: ↓ level of consciousness, activity intolerance, hypotension, chest discomfort, dizziness.

• Assess for CHF/pulmonary edema: increased RR, bibasilar crackles, frothy sputum; especially important in patients with preexisting heart disease, recent MI. • Monitor for dyspnea, wheezing, bronchospasm in patients with history of COPD.

• Assess patients with diabetes for sweating, because tachycardia/tremors associated with hypoglycemia may be blocked by therapy.

Laboratory tests: Monitor: Electrolytes, especially potassium, magnesium • Blood glucose • Digoxin level in patients with cardiac glycoside therapy • Monitor fluid, electrolyte/acid-base status closely; correct promptly.

PATIENT/FAMILY TEACHING

Purpose of medication is to prevent serious, irregular beating of heart. • May cause drowsiness, dizziness, low BP; Change positions slowly, particularly when getting out of bed. • Report breathing difficulty, palpitations, dizziness, chest pain, extreme fatigue.

P pediatric   **G** geriatric   **V** Direct IV

Outpatient: Take medication exactly as prescribed. Do not stop taking medicine even if you feel better. If medication abruptly discontinued, you may develop dangerously high BP, serious heartbeat irregularities, angina. Check/record resting pulse each day, BP each week. Contact caregiver if pulse is < 50 bpm or BP significantly different. • Report severe or prolonged diarrhea, vomiting.
• Avoid driving and other activities requiring mental alertness until individual response to drug known. • Drinking alcohol may cause extreme dizziness, drowsiness, impaired mental alertness.
• Consult health care professional before taking over-the-counter preparations, particularly cold or allergy preparations. • Carry Medic-Alert ID card identifying drug, dosage, specific indication.
• Notify physicians and dentists of therapy before any treatment.
• Therapy blocks elevated HR/BP, so hyperthyroid/diabetic patients must be aware of other symptoms of crisis.

AVAILABLE FORMS
Tablets

spironolactone
(speer'on-oh-lak'tone)
Alatone, Aldactone, Novo-Spirotone ✦

spironolactone with hydrochlorothiazide
Alazide, Aldactazide, Spirozide

Classifications: Potassium-sparing diuretic, antihypertensive

USUAL DOSE
PO, adults: 25-200 mg qAM with breakfast or 25-100 mg bid with meals
PO, children: 3.3 mg/kg qAM with breakfast or divided and bid with meals.

ADMINISTRATION
Administer with food to maximize absorption.

ACTIONS
Inhibits sodium/water reabsorption by binding to aldosterone receptors of distal renal tubule, preventing sodium transport • Effects: ↑ excretion of sodium, chloride, water; ↓ excretion of potassium, phosphate, ammonium, acids • Diuresis induced only in presence of aldosterone, increases as aldosterone levels increase • GFR, renal blood flow unchanged, despite increased clearance of free water • Reduces BP in hypertensive patients, augments action of other anithypertensives • When combined with non–potassium-sparing diuretics, diuresis increases, whereas potassium excretion caused by other agent decreases.

S

PHARMACOKINETICS

ROUTE	ONSET*	PEAK*	DURATION
PO	24-48 hr	48-72 hr	28-72 hr

DISTRIBUTION

90% bound to plasma proteins; crosses placenta

ELIMINATION

Metabolized by liver, eliminated in urine/feces; half-life of active metabolite 13-24 hr

*Diuretic effect.

INDICATIONS

To reduce edema associated with excessive aldosterone secretion, CHF, liver cirrhosis, nephrotic syndrome, steroid use • Unlike loop/thiazide diuretics, conserves potassium • Often used in combination with other diuretics • Used, usually with other agents, to reduce BP in hypertensive patients • Prophylaxis/treatment of hypokalemia *Unlabeled/investigational:* Treatment of hirsuitism; adjunct in treatment of myasthenia gravis

PRECAUTIONS/ CONTRAINDICATIONS

Precautions: May induce or worsen hyponatremia, particularly if used with other diuretics • Risk of hyperkalemia in renal impairment or when potassium supplements used; avoid potassium supplements unless used with other diuretic, corticosteroid. • Reduces vascular responsiveness to norepinephrine; use caution with general anesthesia. • Has been associated with tumor formation in animal studies **Use caution with:** Renal impairment; may cause hyperkalemia • Cirrhosis, hepatic failure; reversible hypercholoremic metabolic acidosis/hyperkalemia possible

D Pregnancy category: Use in pregnancy only if potential benefits justify risk.

Contraindications: Hypersensitivity to spironolactone • Rapidly deteriorating renal status; anuria; hyperkalemia

ADVERSE EFFECTS

CNS: Lethargy, drowsiness, confusion, headache
Resp: Acidosis/compensatory hyperventilation
CV: hypotension, **dysrhythmias**/ECG changes from hyponatremia/hyperkalemia, intravascular fluid volume deficit
GI: Abdominal pain/cramping, diarrhea
GU: ↑ BUN/creatinine, oliguria
Endo: Gynecomastia
F&E: ↑ Potassium, ↓ sodium, dehydration
Derm: Rash, urticaria, macropapular/reddened skin eruptions
Misc: Drug fever, agranulocytosis, possible association with breast cancer

TOXICITY/OVERDOSE

Symptoms: Hypotension • Hyperkalemia, hyponatremia • Nausea, vomiting, abdominal cramping • Deteriorating renal function • Hyperchloremic acidosis in cirrhotic patients
Management: After recent ingestion, implement guidelines for management of acute overdose (Appendix I). • Support respiration as needed with O_2 and/or mechanical ventilation. • Administer IV fluids, replace electrolytes based on laboratory results of serum levels. Closely monitor sodium/potassium balance. Treat hyperkalemia imme-

diately with IV $D_{50}W$ or $D_{10}W$,
regular insulin (0.25-0.5) U/g
glucose). Additional measures
for hyperkalemia include IV
calcium, bicarbonate if acidotic,
and cation exchange resin.
• **Hypotension:** Elevate legs,
administer IV fluids; if unresponsive to fluid replacement,
use vasopressors (e.g., dopamine, norepinephrine). • Hemodialysis may be moderately effective.

INTERACTIONS

angiotensin-converting enzyme
    inhibitors Hyperkalemia
aspirin ↓ Diuresis
beta-blockers Hypotension
calcium channel blockers Hypo-
    tension
digitalis glycosides ↑ Digoxin
    levels, toxicity
diuretics ↑ Diuresis
diuretics, potassium-sparing
    Hyperkalemia
hypotensive agents Synergistic
    effects; hypotension
indomethacin Hyperkalemia
norepinephrine, other pressors
    ↓ Vascular responsiveness
potassium supplements Hyper-
    kalemia

PATIENT CARE IMPLICATIONS

• Avoid use in severely ill patients at risk for developing
respiratory/metabolic acidosis,
which may result in sudden increases in serum potassium. If
use unavoidable, check electrolytes, acid-base balance frequently.
• Evaluate response to therapy
considering diuretic response,
fluid balance, weight, electrolytes. Adjust dose accordingly.
• Avoid combination formulas
with potential for profound hy-

potension when initiating therapy.
• If progressive oliguria or azotemia develops, discontinue
drug.
Vital signs/hemodynamics:
Monitor BP, HR, UO. Consult
physician of hypotension, oliguria. • As available, continuously monitor ECG. Note presence of PVCs, dysrhythmias,
hyperkalemic ECG changes;
peaked T waves, prolongation
of PR interval, ST depression,
widened QRS complex. If present, check potassium level, correct as necessary. Digitalized
patients must be carefully monitored.
Physical assessment: Assess
extremities, face, sacrum for improvement in edema. • Assess
for signs/symptoms of electrolyte imbalance, including dysrhythmias, confusion, dizziness,
weakness, muscle cramps, fatigue, faintness, headache, paresthesias, thirst, anorexia, vomiting. • Assess for perfusion/
oxygenation deficit caused by
hypovolemia: chest discomfort,
↓ level of consciousness, activity intolerance, hypotension,
dizziness. • Weigh patient daily.
Laboratory tests: Monitor:
Electrolytes, especially sodium,
potassium • BUN, creatinine
• Bilirubin, liver enzymes •
CBC with differential • May interfere with laboratory tests for
plasma, urinary steroids • **May
cause:** falsely elevated serum
digoxin level when radioimmu-
noassay procedure used

PATIENT/FAMILY TEACHING

Purpose of drug is to eliminate
excess body fluid, lower BP.
• May cause dizziness, especially when starting therapy; use

S

caution when changing positions, walking. • Report signs/symptoms of heart failure: breathing difficulty, palpitations, dizziness, activity intolerance, chest pain. • Report signs/symptoms of electrolyte imbalance: confusion, weakness, dizziness, fatigue, faintness, headache, paresthesias, muscle cramps, persistent thirst, anorexia, nausea, vomiting.

Outpatient: Take medication in AM. Never double doses. • Continue taking medications as prescribed even if feeling better. Drug controls but does not cure condition. • Take with food or milk. • Avoid excessive ingestion of high-potassium foods, including salt substitues. • Avoid alcohol, which could cause dizziness, fainting. • Do not take aspirin or other nonprescription drugs without consulting physician or pharmacist. • Weigh twice/wk; notify physician of weight gain, edema

AVAILABLE FORMS
Tablets

streptokinase
(strep-toe-kye′nase)
Kabikinase, Streptase

Classification: Thrombolytic

USUAL DOSE
IV, intermit inf: Coronary artery thrombolysis: 1.5 million IU; other dosing regimens used; administer as soon as possible after onset of MI symptoms.
• Acute pulmonary embolism, deep-vein thrombosis, arterial embolism/thrombosis: Loading dose, 250,000 IU

over 30 min; followed by 100,000 IU/hr for 24-72 hr; other dosing regimens used
• **Occluded arteriovenous cannulae:** 250,000 IU in 2 ml diluent

Intracoronary inf: Coronary artery thrombolysis: 20,000 IU bolus in small volume of diluent (e.g., 3-20 ml); follow bolus with maintenance infusion of 2,000 IU/min for 60 min; other dosing regimens used; administer as soon as possible after onset of MI symptoms.

ADMINISTRATION
Must use volumetric infusion pump/syringe infusion pump; reconstituted solution alters droplet size, inaccuracies result if other infusion devices used. Use ≥0.8-μm filter; DO NOT USE STANDARD IN-LINE FILTER. After infusion complete, flush line with 25-30 ml saline.

Coronary artery thrombolysis: 1.5 million IU given over 1 hr; 750,000 IU may be administered over first 10 min.

Intracoronary inf, adults: Coronary artery thrombolysis: Administer bolus in small volume of diluent via specialized technique over 15 sec-2 min. Follow with maintenance infusion of 2,000 IU/min for 60 min. Must use volumetric infusion pump/syringe infusion pump; reconstituted solution alters droplet size, inaccuracies result if other infusion devices used. Use ≥0.8-μm filter. After infusion complete, flush line with 25-30 ml saline.

Acute pulmonary embolism, deep-vein thrombosis, arterial embolism/thrombosis: Administer loading dose of

250,000 IU over 30 min. Follow by continuous infusion of 100,000 IU/hr (or other prescribed dose) for 24-72 hr.
Injection, occluded A-V cannulae: Occluded arteriovenous cannulae: Very slowly, gently inject single dose into each occluded limb of cannula; may use volumetric infusion pump/syringe infusion pump. Use ≥0.8-μm filter. Clamp for 2 hr, then carefully aspirate contents. Flush with 0.9% NaCl; reconnect.

PREPARATION

Reconstitute each vial with 5 ml 0.9% NaCl (preferred) or D_5W. Add slowly, direct stream of diluent to sides of vial. Roll and tilt gently to dissolve. Shaking will cause foaming. • Further dilute reconstituted solutions in 0.9% NaCl or D_5W to total volume of 45-500 ml. Gently invert or swirl bag to mix thoroughly. • Visually inspect solution; discard those with large amounts of particulate matter, excessive foaming. • Use within 8 hr.

ACTIONS

Promotes thrombolysis (clot dissolution) by producing activator complex that converts plasminogen into the proteolytic enzyme plasmin • Plasmin degrades fibrin clots, fibrinogen, other clotting factors, thus dissolving clots, improving blood flow through previously occluded arteries, usually within 1-2 hr. • Prompt reperfusion of myocardial tissue promotes improved ventricular function. • Decreases in circulating clotting factors may result in bleeding complications. • Indirect effects include reduced PVR/BP with corresponding afterload reduction. • Repeated administration triggers antibodies that reduce drug effectiveness, may result in serious allergic reactions.

PARMACOKINETICS

ROUTE	ONSET	PEAK	DURATION
IV	Rapid	1-2 hr	To 12 hr

DISTRIBUTION
Does not cross placenta, but antibodies do

ELIMINATION
Rapidly cleared by antibodies, RE system; half-life biphasic with initial 18 min, subsequent 83 min

INDICATIONS

Acute MI: Restores coronary perfusion, limits infarct size, improves ventricular function, ↓ incidence of CHF/other complications; initiate therapy as soon as possible, preferably within 6 hr of symptom onset. Concomitant therapy with anticoagulants (e.g., heparin, warfarin), platelet-aggregation inhibitors (e.g., aspirin, dipyridamole) reduces reocclusion.
Acute pulmonary emboli: Dissolves emboli, restores pulmonary blood flow in acute massive pulmonary emboli; initiate therapy as soon as possible, preferably within 7 days; improves hemodynamic stability, reduces pulmonary hypertension; may reverse right ventricular dysfunction.
Other uses: Lysis of acute, extensive deep-vein thrombosis; lysis of acute arterial thrombosis/embolism; to clear occluded arteriovenous cannulae

PRECAUTIONS/ CONTRAINDICATIONS

Precautions: Bleeding, bruising, hematomas may occur, es-

S

pecially at vascular access sites, after invasive procedures, with IM injections. • Cerebral, other serious or fatal spontaneous bleeding is possible. • Atrial/ventricular dysrhythmias may occur during coronary reperfusion. • May trigger serious allergic reactions; patients with recent (5 days-6 mo) streptococcal infection of treatment with streptokinase/anistreplase possess ↑ antibodies, may fail to respond to therapy, are at greater risk for hypersensitivity reactions.

G **Use caution with:** Older adults: history of cerebrovascular disease, severe or uncontrolled hypertension

c **Pregnancy category:** Safety not established; use only if safer alternative unavailable

Minor relative contraindications: Recent (within 10 days) minor trauma, including CPR • History of cerebrovascular disease • Pregnancy • Likelihood of left-sided heart thrombus (e.g., atrial fibrillation, severe left ventricular dyskinesia) • Acute pericarditis • Subacute bacterial endocarditis • Hemostatic defects, including those associated with liver/renal dysfunction; anticoagulant therapy • Hemorrhagic ophthalmic conditions • Age >75 yr • Septic

G thrombophlebitis, occluded AV cannula at seriously infected site • Any condition in which serious bleeding likely or would be difficult to control

Major relative contraindications: Recent (within 10 days) major surgery, serious trauma, obstetric delivery, organ biopsy, puncture of noncompressible vessels • GI/GU bleeding within 10 days • Hypertension (SBP >180, DBP >110 mm Hg)

Absolute contraindications: Hypersensitivity to anistreplase, streptokinase • Active internal bleeding • Intracranial neoplasm, arteriovenous malformation/aneurysm • Recent (within 2 mo) CVA, intracranial/intraspinal surgery/trauma • Bleeding diathesis • Severe, uncon-

P trolled hypertension • Children: Safety not established

ADVERSE EFFECTS

CNS: **Cerebral hemorrhage**

Resp: Hemoptysis, noncardiogenic pulmonary edema

CV: *Reperfusion dysrhythmias,* including accelerated idioventricular rhythm, PVCs, **ventricular tachycardia/fibrillation,** PACs, atrial fibrillation, junctional rhythm, sinus bradycardia; hypotension

GI: *Nausea/vomiting,* bleeding

GU: Hematuria

EENT: Gingival bleeding, epistaxis

Hema: *Puncture site/soft tissue bleeding, bruising, ecchymosis/hematoma,* thrombocytopenia

Misc: Full range of hypersensitivity reactions, including anaphylaxis; fever

TOXICITY/OVERDOSE

Symptoms: Bleeding, bruising, hematomas; spontaneous bleeding from cerebral, retroperitoneal, GU, GI, soft tissue sources • Dose-dependent depletion of clotting proteins, production of fibrin degradation products

Management: Stop infusion. • Initiate local measures such as manual compression followed by pressure dressings. • Administer plasma volume expanders (avoid dextran), packed RBCs, fresh-frozen plasma, cryoprecipitate, as indicated by blood loss/clotting studies. • Antifibrinolytics (e.g., aminocaproic acid) may be used in cases of life-threatening bleeding (e.g., intracranial hemorrhage). • For management of acute allergic reactions, see Appendix N

INTERACTIONS

aminocaproic acid ↓ therapeutic effects

anticoagulants (e.g., heparin, warfarin) ↑ Bleeding risk

antiplatelet agents (abciximab, ↓ aspirin dipyridamole, NSAIDS, ticlopidine) ↑ Bleeding risk

cefamandol, cefoperazone, cefotetan Cephalosporin may ↓ prothrombin levels; ↑ bleeding risk

streptokinase (within 5 days-6 mo) Failed thrombolytic therapy; ↑ risk of hypersensitivity reactions

INCOMPATIBILITIES

Do not mix, dilute, or infuse with other agents.

PATIENT CARE IMPLICATIONS
Before starting therapy
• Obtain baseline 12-lead ECG.
• Review history for contraindications.
• Have emergency resuscitation equipment, including epinephrine, lidocaine, atropine, immediately available.
• Apply pressure dressings to unsuccessful venipuncture attempts.
• Start 2 or more 18-gauge or larger catheters for laboratory samples, additional medications, fluids, emergency use.

• See many precautions under Administration.
During/immediately after therapy
• Avoid unnecessary venipuncture, invasive procedures, IM injections.
• If venipuncture necessary, hold manual pressure over site for 20 min or until bleeding stops, then apply pressure dressing. Inspect frequently for bleeding.
• If arterial puncture necessary, avoid femoral site; hold manual pressure over puncture site for 30 min or until bleeding stops. Apply pressure dressing; inspect frequently for bleeding.
• Avoid arterial/venous invasive procedures in areas inaccessible to manual compression (e.g., internal jugular, subclavian).
• Transient dysrhythmias, reduced chest pain, reduction of ST segment elevation suggest successful thrombolysis/coronary reperfusion.
• Consult physician for significant dysrhythmias, unusual or excessive bleeding, change in neurologic status, unrelieved or recurrent chest pain, allergic reactions.
Vital signs/hemodynamics:
Initially, monitor BP, HR at 5–15-min intervals; when stable, progress to 30–60-min intervals during and for several hr after infusion. Hypotension may result from reperfusion dysrhythmias, hemorrhage, impaired myocardial contractility, ↓ PVR; carefully evaluate each case.
• Immediately consult physician for severe or uncontrolled hypertension (SBP >180, DBP >110 mm Hg). Prepare to initiate hypotensive therapy. • Con-

S

---

italic = common side effects   **bold** = life-threatening reactions

tinuously monitor ECG for dysrhythmias, changes in ST segment elevation. Anticipate reperfusion dysrhythmias; if symptomatic, manage according to ACLS guidelines (Appendix P).

Physical assessment: Assess/document chest pain intensity, character, location, radiation, duration. Note any associated symptoms. • Monitor all vascular access sites; assess for bleeding at 15-min intervals during and immediately after infusion, then q4h for 24 hr. If bleeding occurs, apply pressure, continue to monitor closely. Infusion may need to be discontinued if bleeding becomes excessive. • Assess peripheral pulses for diminished intensity, especially those distal to arterial puncture or other invasive procedures. • Assess neurologic procedures. • Assess neurologic status before, during, and immediately after infusion. Immediately consult physician for changes. • Assess for retroperitoneal bleeding (e.g., low back pain, flank ecchymosis). • Note blood in urine, other body fluids. Check emesis, stools for occult blood.

Laboratory tests: Monitor: CPK, CBC, PT, PTT, thrombin time (TT), fibrinogen before and after therapy • TT frequency during therapy • Cardiac enzymes for coronary thrombolysis • In patients with pulmonary embolism, deep-vein thrombosis, arterial thrombosis/embolism, failure of TT to increase after 4 hr therapy suggests ineffectiveness from streptokinase resistance. Notify physician, who may discontinue infusion. • May cause: Unrelia-

ble results with coagulation studies; notify lab of thrombolytic therapy

PATIENT/FAMILY TEACHING

Purpose of drug is to dissolve clots blocking blood flow to heart muscle. • Frequent monitoring is necessary because of many side effects. • Immediately report chest pain or discomfort, unusual bleeding (e.g., from venipunctures, nose, mouth, urine), breathing difficulty, itching. • Remain on bed rest throughout therapy. • Avoid potential trauma from shaving, toothbrushing, excessive activity for 24 hr after therapy.

AVAILABLE FORMS

Parenteral for IV injection/infusion

succinylcholine chloride
(suk-sin-ill-koe'leen)
Anectine, Sucostrin, Sux-Cert ✤, Quelicin

Classification: Depolarizing neuromuscular blocking agent

USUAL DOSE

Each dose individualized according to patient response
Direct IV, adults: Initial dose: 0.6 mg/kg (approx. 40 mg); range is 0.3-1.1 mg/kg. Maximum dose, 150 mg. Dose-related muscle relaxation usually lasts 4-6 min. Prophylactic atropine may be given to prevent bradycardia. **Maintenance:** 0.04-0.07 mg/kg q5-10min. **Test dose:** 0.1 mg may be given to test for sensitivity, predict recovery time.

Direct IV, children: Initial dose: 1-2 mg/kg; 1-mg/kg dose used for older children, adolescents. Dose-related muscle relaxation usually lasts 4-6 min. Prophylactic atropine may be given to prevent bradycardia. **Maintenance:** 0.3-1 mg/kg q5-10min.

ADMINISTRATION

Direct IV: Inject each dose over 15-30 sec; dilution not necessary. *Causes immediate respiratory paralysis; means for continuous artificial ventilation must be in place or provided immediately after injection.* In patients with repeat doses, sustained neuromuscular blockade, use nerve stimulator to monitor degree of blockade. Avoid additional doses until there is a certain response to T_1 (first twitch). **Compatible fluids:** D_5W, 0.9% NaCl

ACTIONS

Very short-acting skeletal muscle relaxant that causes paralysis by interfering with transmission of nerve impulses at neuromuscular junction • Causes depolarization (evidenced by fasciculations); then blocks activity of acetylcholine (neurotransmitter normally producing electrical depolarization) by occupying cholinergic receptor site • Face, neck muscles affected first; followed by chest, diaphragm, other skeletal muscles. • May trigger histamine release; likelihood increased if recommended dose exceeded • No analgesic/sedative effects

PHARMACOKINETICS

ROUTE	ONSET	PEAK	DURATION
IV	30-60 sec	3-4 min	5-10 min, depending on dose

ELIMINATION

Metabolized by plasma enzymes; excreted in urine

INDICATIONS

To facilitate routine ET intubation • With general anesthesia to produce skeletal muscle relaxation during surgery • No effects on consciousness/pain threshold; used only after induction of general anesthesia or with analgesics/anxiolytics

PRECAUTIONS/ CONTRAINDICATIONS

Precautions: *Causes respiratory paralysis; must use with artificial airway, ventilatory support* • Increased risk of hyperkalemia, dysrhythmias, cardiac arrest with digoxin toxicity, acid-base/electrolyte abnormalities, major burns, multiple trauma, upper motor neuron injury, abdominal infection, subarachnoid hemorrhage, central/peripheral nervous system degeneration • Neuromuscular blockade prolonged with hypokalemia, hypocalcemia • May increase intragastric pressure; result in vomiting, aspiration • May cause potentially fatal malignant hyperthermia • Symptomatic bradycardia may occur; more likely after second dose • Sustained use may result in tachyphylaxis, prolonged respiratory depression, apnea. • Do not attempt reversal with anticholinesterase agent unless multiple doses given and patient remains in Phase II block after

S

---

italic = common side effects   **bold** = life-threatening reactions

≥20 min (see specialized literature).

Use caution with: Fractures, muscle spasm; initial fasciculations may result in additional injury • Patients with decreased plasma cholinesterase (e.g., genetic disorder, pregnancy, malignancy, hepatic/renal disorders, infection, burns, heart failure); neuromuscular blockade prolonged; use reduced dose
P • Children: bradycardia, hyperkalemia more likely

C Pregnancy category: Use only if clearly needed

Contraindications: Hypersensitivity to succinylcholine • History of malignant hyperthermia, skeletal muscle myopathy • Post acute phase of burn, major trauma, upper motor neuron injury; severe hyperkalemia may cause cardiac arrest; risk of hyperkalemia peaks 7-10 days after injury • Children except for emergency intubation

ADVERSE EFFECTS

CNS: *Muscle weakness, paralysis,* prolonged blockade
Resp: ***Depression, apnea***
CV: Hypotension, hypertension, bradycardia, tachycardia, dysrhythmias, **cardiac arrest**
MS: *Fasciculation,* postop muscle pain, rhabdomyolysis
Misc: Hyperkalemia, increased intraocular pressure, excessive salivation, **malignant hyperthermia, anaphylaxis**

TOXICITY/OVERDOSE

Symptoms: Apnea, prolonged neuromuscular blockade
Management: Maintain airway, provide continuous artificial ventilation • Hypotension: Elevate legs; administer IV fluids; use dopamine, other pressors if necessary. • For management of acute allergic reactions see Appendix N.

INTERACTIONS

aminoglycosides (amikacin, gentamicin), amphotericin B, beta-blockers, calcium channel blockers, corticosteroids, diuretics, inhalation anesthetics, lidocaine, magnesium, procainamide, quinidine, terbutaline Potentiate/prolong neuromuscular blockade
cholinesterase inhibitors (e.g., neostigmine, edrophonium) Prolonged depolarizing neuromuscular blockade
digoxin ↑ Risk of dysrhythmias
opiate analgesics Respiratory depression

Y-SITE COMPATIBILITIES

Heparin, potassium

Y-SITE INCOMPATIBILITIES

Alkaline solutions, barbiturates

PATIENT CARE IMPLICATIONS

• Has no effect on consciousness/pain threshold; patient is fully awake and feels all sensations. *Use only with general anesthesia or analgesics (e.g., morphine) and anxiolytics (e.g., midazolam).*
• Causes respiratory paralysis, apnea; *use only for patients under direct observation and continuous mechanical ventilation.*
• Prophylactic atropine may be given to prevent bradycardia.
• Do not use cholinesterase inhibitors such as neostigmine, edrophonium to reverse effects unless multiple doses of succinylcholine have been given, and patient remains in deep neuromuscular blockade (Phase II)

≥20 min after the last succinyl-choline dose.

• Not recommended for sustained use because of tachyphylaxis, prolonged effects, delayed recovery.

• Patients thought to have recovered from neuromuscular blockade may develop apnea when given certain drugs that potentiate NMBAs (see Interactions).

Vital signs/hemodynamics: Monitor ECG continuously. Observe for bradycardia, tachycardia, dysrhythmias. • Monitor BP frequently, observing for hypotension, instability. • Use continuous pulse oximetry to monitor oxygenation throughout neuromuscular blockade and until fully recovered. • Monitor temperature closely to detect malignant hyperthermia; monitor continuously if multiple doses used.

Physical assessment: Closely monitor respiratory status; rate, depth, pattern of ventilation, until fully recovered. Secretions may be increased; suction as necessary. • Paralysis of muscle groups usually occurs in the following order: Face, neck, chest, diaphragm, other skeletal muscles. Recovery occurs in reverse order. Assess frequently for residual muscle weakness, respiratory distress until fully recovered from effects. • Use peripheral nerve stimulator to monitor effectiveness of NMBAs. *Avoid additional doses of NMBAs until there is a certain response to T_1 (first twitch).* • Monitor for onset of malignant hyperthermia: spasm of jaw muscles, generalized rigidity, profound hyperthermia,

acidosis. If any of these are present, withhold further dose, consult physician immediately.

• Monitor I&O; Foley catheter required.

Laboratory tests: Monitor: Potassium; drug may cause hyperkalemia in some patients (see Precautions). Magnesium; drug action potentiated by hypermagnesemia. Calcium; drug action potentiated by hypocalcemia. Acid-base status; imbalance alters drug action. ABGs; to evaluate adequacy of ventilation.

PATIENT/FAMILY TEACHING

Purpose of medication is to paralyze body muscles temporarily to facilitate procedures, surgery.

• When recovering from effects, it may be difficult to swallow, talk; these effects temporary.

• Drug does not affect consciousness: explain all procedures.

AVAILABLE FORMS

Parenteral for IV injection
Storage: Refrigerate vials. Anectine Flo-Pack does not require refrigeration.

---

sucralfate
(sue-kral'fate)
basic aluminum sucrose sulfate
Carafate, Sulcrate ✢

S

Classifications: Antiulcer agent

USUAL DOSE

PO, adults: 1 g 4 times daily 1 hr before each meal and hs for up to 8 wks. Maintenance, 1 g bid, 1 hr before meal or hs

---

ADMINISTRATION

PO: Administer on empty stomach 1 hr before meal or at bedtime.

G-tube: Use commercially prepared suspension. If unavailable, prepare suspension by placing tablet in 15-30 ml water until it disintegrates, usually within 2-3 min. • Suspension may be prepared directly in catheter-tipped syringe for ease in administration via gastric tube (place syringe tip up while tablet disintegrates).

• Mix only in water; other liquids may reduce effectiveness.

ACTIONS

Reacts with hydrochloric acid to form thick protective substance that binds to ulcers/gastric erosions, also coats gastric/duodenal mucosa • Protects from ulceration, aids in healing by forming barrier to irritating gastric/intestinal secretions • Does not significantly alter gastric pH

PHARMACOKINETICS

ROUTE	ONSET	PEAK	DURATION
PO	30 min	NE	To 6 hr

DISTRIBUTION
Minimally absorbed; 95% remains in GI tract

ELIMINATION
>90% excreted unchanged in feces

INDICATIONS

Short-term treatment of duodenal ulcer; in reduced doses for prevention of recurrence. Antacids may be used for pain relief, but should not be given within 1 hr of sucralfate.
Unlabeled/investigational:
Prevention of stress ulcers/GI bleeding in critically ill patients, may offer some advantage over antacids/histamine H_2 antagonists, since ↑ gastric pH implicated in nosocomial infections in these patients; treatment of gastric ulcer; protection from aspirin/NSAID-induced erosions; reflux esophagitis.

PRECAUTIONS/ CONTRAINDICATIONS

Precautions: Small amounts of aluminum absorbed; use caution in impaired renal function.

P • Children: Safety/effectiveness not established

B **Pregnancy category:** Safety not established

Contraindications: None reported.

ADVERSE EFFECTS

CNS: Headache, dizziness, sleepiness
GI: Constipation, diarrhea, nausea, vomiting, gastric discomfort, indigestion, dry mouth, "full" sensation
Derm: Rash, pruritus

TOXICITY/OVERDOSE

Risks of toxicity minimal with normal renal function.

INTERACTIONS

antacids, aluminum-containing Aluminum toxicity
anticoagulants, PO ↓ Anticoagulation
cimetidine, PO ↓ Absorption
ciprofloxacin, PO ↓ Absorption
digoxin, PO ↓ Absorption; decreased digoxin levels
phenytoin, PO ↓ Absorption; ↓ phenytoin levels
ranitidine, PO ↓ Absorption
tetracyline, PO ↓ Absorption
theophylline, PO ↓ Absorption; ↓ theophylline levels

PATIENT CARE IMPLICATIONS

Administer 30 min before meals on empty stomach. • Do not administer antacids within 1 hr, other PO drugs within 2 hr of sucralfate.
Vital signs/hemodynamics: Monitor BP, HR for orthostatic changes in acutely ill patients.
Physical assessment: Assess for epigastric/abdominal pain. Consult physician for persistent or severe pain. • Monitor for GI bleeding; frank or occult blood in emesis, gastric drainage, stool. • Monitor for constipation.

PATIENT/FAMILY TEACHING

Purpose of medication is to protect lining of stomach from irritating secretions. • Take 30 min before meals on empty stomach. • Do not take antacids within 1 hr of sucralfate. • Do not take other oral medications within 2 hr of sulcralfate. • For ease in swallowing, break tablet in half or allow to disintegrate in 15-30 ml water. Do not mix with other liquids; effectiveness may be reduced. • Increased fluid intake, high-bulk diet, exercise help prevent constipation. • Take all doses as prescribed, even if feeling better. • Report vomiting of blood, dark or bloody stools, dizziness. • Avoid coffee, caffeine, alcohol, aspirin, ibuprofen, other food or drugs that may cause gastric irritation. • Inform all health care providers of sucralfate therapy.

AVAILABLE FORMS

Tablets

---

sumatriptan succinate
(summa-trip'tan)
Imigran, Imitrex

Classification: Seritonin antagonist, antimigraine agent

USUAL DOSE

SC, adults: 6 mg • Do not exceed two 6-mg doses in 24 hr. • DO NOT ADMINISTER IV.

ACTIONS

Selective agonist for vascular receptor subtype (5-HT$_1$) present on cranial arteries; selectively constricts inflamed, dilated cranial blood vessels • Inhibits release of inflammatory mediators from trigeminal nerve terminals • Relieves headache, nausea, vomiting, other symptoms (e.g., photophobia, sound sensitivity) associated with migraines • Causes small transient increases in SBP, DBP

PHARMACOKINETICS

ROUTE	ONSET	PEAK	DURATION
SC	Rapid	12 min	2-4 hr

DISTRIBUTION
14%-21% protein bound
ELIMINATION
Excreted in urine; half-life 115 min

INDICATIONS

Acute treatment of migraines with or without aura • Not indicated for hemiplegic/basilar migraine • Safety/effectiveness for cluster headache not established

PRECAUTIONS/ CONTRAINDICATIONS

Precautions: May cause transient mild ↑ BP • May cause coronary vasospasm, myocardial ischemia • Serious dysrhythmias (e.g., ventricular tachycardia/

S

---

fibrillation), ischemic ECG changes, angina pectoris, acute MI have been rarely associated with use. • Not for IV administration, which could cause coronary vasospasm

Use caution with: Patients in whom unrecognized CAD may be likely (e.g., postmenopausal women, males >40, presence of coronary risk factors: hypertension, high cholesterol, obesity, diabetes, smoking, strong family history) • Renal/hepatic impairment

C Pregnancy category: Use only if safer alternatives unavailable.

Contraindications: Hypersensitivity to sumatriptan • Ischemic heart disease (angina pectoris, history of MI, silent ischemia, Prinzmetal's angina) • Uncontrolled hypertension • Use of ergotamine preparations within 24 hr • Children: Safety/efficacy not established

ADVERSE EFFECTS

CNS: *Warmth, burning, paresthesias,* numbness, atypical sensations, fatigue, *dizziness,* drowsiness
CV: Flushing, chest pressure/tightness/pain, ↑ BP, **dysrhythmias**
MS: Neck pain/stiffness, weakness, muscle pain/cramps
Local: *Injection site pain/redness*
Misc: Full range of hypersensitivity reactions, including anaphylaxis

TOXICITY/OVERDOSE

Symptoms: Coronary vasospasm has occurred with IV administration. • Limited data available; animal studies suggest

tremors, seizures, cyanosis, paralysis may occur.

Management: Manage symptomatically • Monitor for at least 10 hr. • Effectiveness of hemodialysis unknown

INTERACTION

ergotamine Additive, prolonged vasospasm

PATIENT CARE IMPLICATIONS

• May cause coronary vasospasm; administer first dose in controlled setting (physician's office, emergency department) for patients in whom unrecognized CAD may be likely (e.g., postmenopausal women, males >40, presence of coronary risk factors: hypertension, high cholesterol, obesity, diabetes, smoking, strong family history).

Vital signs/hemodynamics: Monitor BP, HR, RR 15-20 min after injection. • Continuously monitor ECG in patients who develop chest pain, other symptoms of coronary vasospasm.

Physical assessment: Assess for relief of headache, other symptoms 20-30 min after injection. If no relief after 1 hr, additional injection may be required. • Monitor for symptoms of coronary vasospasm: chest, jaw, neck, or arm pain, pressure, tightness. Consult physician; obtain 12-lead ECG.

PATIENT/FAMILY TEACHING

Purpose of medication is to relieve migraine symptoms; does not prevent/reduce number of migraines. • May cause drowsiness, dizziness; Change positions slowly, particularly when getting out of bed. • Report chest, jaw, neck, or arm pain, pressure, tightness, irregular heartbeats, difficulty breathing. **Outpatient:** Use injection only to treat actual migraine attack. Use as soon as you experience symptoms. • Second injection may be used if symptoms recur, but do not use more than 2 injections in 24 hr. • You may experience redness/pain at injection site. • Read and save "Patient Information" leaflet provided with medication.

AVAILABLE FORMS

Parenteral for SC injection

---

temazepam
(te-maz'e-pam)
Restoril

Classifcations: Benzodiazepine, sedative hypnotic
Schedule IV controlled substance

USUAL DOSE

Individualize dosage, increase cautiously.
PO, adults: 15-30 mg hs
G **PO, older adults:** 7.5-15 mg hs

ACTIONS

Facilitates action of gamma-aminobutyric acid (GABA, major inhibitory neurotransmitter), produces CNS depression • Results in mild sedation, hypnotic effects • Especially effective in reducing early morning awakening, which often affects older adults • Few morning residual or "hangover" effects • No respiratory depressant effects at usual dose • No analgesic effects

PHARMACOKINETICS

ROUTE	ONSET	PEAK	DURATION
PO	20-40 min	2-3 hr	6-12 hr

DISTRIBUTION

Wide; 96% protein bound; crosses blood-brain barrier

ELIMINATION

Metabolized by liver, eliminated by kidneys; half-life 10 hr

INDICATIONS

Short-term relief of insomnia, including difficulty falling asleep, nocturnal awakenings, early morning awakenings

PRECAUTIONS/ CONTRAINDICATIONS

Precautions: Adverse effects more likely in first few days of therapy • Adverse effects more likely in older adults
G **Use caution with:** Older adults, debilitation, low serum albumin; reduced dose indicated • Presence of other CNS depressants (e.g., opiate analgesics, alcohol, phenothiazines); reduced dose indicated
X **Pregnancy category:** *Risk of congenital malformations, prolonged CNS depression, withdrawal symptoms in newborn; do not use.*
Contraindications: Hypersensitivity to temazepam • Myasthenia gravis • Severe pulmonary disease • Acute angle-closure glaucoma • Acute alcohol intoxication with VS depression • Pregnancy, lactation
P • Children: Safety/effectiveness not established

ADVERSE EFFECTS

NOTE: Most likely during initial therapy
CNS: *Drowsiness, headache, dizziness, lethargy,* confusion, euphoria, amnesia, tremor

T

---

italic = common side effects   **bold** = life-threatening reactions

(rare), paradoxical excitement (rare)

Resp: Respiratory depression

CV: Palpitations (rare)

GI: Nausea, diarrhea, abdominal discomfort

Misc: Tolerance, psychologic/ physical dependence

TOXICITY/OVERDOSE

Symptoms (acute toxicity): Somnolence, impaired coordination, confusion, coma, diminished reflexes • Hypotension **G** particularly in older adults • Respiratory depression, particularly if other CNS depressants also ingested • Toxicity more likely with concurrent ingestion of alcohol, other CNS depressants

Management: After recent ingestion, implement guidelines for management of acute overdose (Appendix I). • Maintain airway/support ventilation as necessary. • Administer IV fluids. • Use flumazenil to reverse temazepam effects. • **Hypotension:** Elevate legs, administer IV fluids; use vasopressors (e.g., norepinephrine, dopamine) as necessary. • Do not use barbiturates for paradoxical excitation. • Forced diuresis may be helpful in patients with normal kidney function. • Hemodialysis is not generally useful.

INTERACTIONS

alcohol, ethyl ↑ Sedation

antacids Altered absorption

antihistamines ↑ Sedation

barbiturates ↑ Sedation

digoxin ↑ Digoxin levels; toxicity; monitor closely

flumazenil ↓ Sedation

levodopa ↓ Antiparkinsonian effectiveness

opiate analgesics ↑ Sedation

probenecid ↑ Sedation

propoxyphene ↑ Sedation

theophylline ↓ Sedation

PATIENT CARE IMPLICATIONS

• Adverse effects more likely in first few days of therapy

• Use appropriate safety precautions according to patient response. Assistance with ambula- **G** tion may be required, especially with older adults.

• Individualize dosage, increase cautiously. Use smallest effective dose.

• Administer with food to reduce gastric irritation.

• Avoid sudden cessation of therapy, especially in patients who have received prolonged therapy or 30-mg dosage. Taper doses to avoid withdrawal.

• Large quantities should not be prescribed for patients with severe depression, suicidal tendencies, history of substance abuse.

G • Older adults: Individualize dose; closely monitor for adverse effects (e.g., impaired psychomotor/mental performance)

• Assess need for continued therapy periodically.

Physical assessment: Assess neurologic status for excessive sedation, impaired physical coordination.

Laboratory tests: Monitor: Liver enzymes • CBC with differential regularly

PATIENT/FAMILY TEACHING

Purpose of medication is to reduce anxiety, promote relaxation. • Medication may cause drowsiness, dizziness, especially during first few days of therapy. Use caution with activity until individual effects established. • Cigarette smoking interferes

with drug effectiveness. • Report possible pregnancy.
Outpatient: Avoid concurrent use of alcohol or other drugs that cause sedation while taking this medication. • Avoid driving and other activities requiring alertness or physical coordination until effects of medication established. • This medication may cause psychologic/physical dependence. Consult prescriber before increasing dose or abruptly discontinuing. • Take with food if desired to minimize upset stomach.

AVAILABLE FORMS

Capsules

terbutaline sulfate
(ter-byoo'te-leen)
Brethine, Bricanyl

Classification: Beta-adrenergic agonist

USUAL DOSE

Metered-dose inhal: 1-2 puffs q4-6h
PO, adults: 5 mg tid • Maximum dose, 15 mg/day
Ⓟ **PO, children 12-15 yr:** 2.5 mg tid • Maximum dose, 7.5 mg/day
SC, adults: 0.25 mg; if ineffective, may administer 1 additional 0.25 mg dose in 15-30 min • Maximum dose, 0.5 mg within any 4-hr period

ADMINISTRATION

PO: Give with meals to ↓ stomach irritation.

ACTIONS

Stimulates beta-adrenergic receptors in bronchial, uterine, vascular and cardiac smooth muscle tissue • Results in bronchodilation, mild vasodilation, slight ↓ in BP; may cause reflex tachycardia, especially at higher doses • Little or no effect on alpha-adrenergic receptors

PHARMACOKINETICS

ROUTE	ONSET	PEAK	DURATION
Inhal	5-30 min	1-2 hr	3-4 hr
PO	30 min	2-3 hr	4-8 hr
SC	15 min	30-60 min	2-4 hr

ELIMINATION

Partially metabolized in liver; excreted in urine, feces

INDICATIONS

Relief of bronchospasm in asthma, chronic bronchitis, emphysema • Slower onset, longer duration, greater efficacy than metaproterenol

PRECAUTIONS/ CONTRAINDICATIONS

Precautions: Tolerance may develop with prolonged use. • Repeated/excessive drug use may lead to paradoxical bronchoconstriction.
Use caution with: Cardiac disorders • Hypertension • Hyperthyroidism • Diabetes mellitus • Children <12 yr
Ⓑ **Pregnancy category:** Safe use not clearly established
Contraindications: Hypersensitivity to terbutaline

ADVERSE EFFECTS

CNS: *Tremors, nervousness,* insomnia, headache, dizziness, restlessness, anxiety, **seizures** (rare)
EENT: Dry/irritated nose/throat
Resp: Dyspnea, paradoxical bronchospasm

---

italic = common side effects   **bold** = life-threatening reactions

CV: *Tachycardia,* palpitations, hypo/hypertension, dysrhythmias

GI: Nausea, vomiting

Misc: Tolerance

TOXICITY/OVERDOSE

Symptoms: Angina, hypotension, tachycardia, dysrhythmias • Hypokalemia, hyperglycemia followed by hypoglycemia
Management: After recent ingestion, implement guidelines for management of acute overdose (Appendix I). • Manage dysrhythmias according to ACLS guidelines (Appendix P).

INTERACTIONS

aminophylline Cardiotoxicity
beta-blockers ↓ Terbutaline effectiveness
cyclic antidepressants Dysrhythmias
MAO inhibitors Dysrhythmias
sympathomimetics Cardiotoxicity

PATIENT CARE IMPLICATIONS

• For optimal benefits in controlling bronchospasm, schedule doses at regular intervals.
Vital signs/hemodynamics: Monitor ECG for tachycardia, dysrhythmias. • Monitor VS for hypo/hypertension, improved RR. • Use pulse oximeter to evaluate O_2 saturation before and after administration.
Physical assessment: Assess work of breathing, ventilatory excursion, breath sounds.
• Evaluate forced expiratory volume, other pulmonary function measurements before and after treatment.
Laboratory tests: Monitor: ABGs • Potassium, particularly in patients susceptible to hypokalemia (e.g., diuretic/digoxin therapy)

PATIENT/FAMILY TEACHING

Purpose of medication is to relieve bronchospasm, improve breathing. • Report ↑ breathing difficulty, chest pain, palpitations. • Sips of water or sugarless gum may help dry mouth.
• Take oral doses with meals to decrease stomach irritation.
• Check with physician or pharmacist before taking cold or cough preparations. • Use metered-dose inhaler as demonstrated. Be certain to exhale completely before use, close lips firmly around mouthpiece, inhale deeply while activating inhaler. Hold breath for as long as possible, exhale slowly.
• Use exactly as directed. If ineffective, do not increase dose or frequency of use; consult prescriber.

AVAILABLE FORMS

Solution for parenteral use • Metered-dose inhaler • Tablets

tetanus immune globulin
Hyper-Tet, TIG

Classifications: Serum, immune globulin

USUAL DOSE

IM, postexposure prophylaxis, adults/children: 250 U as single dose as soon as possible after injury • Additional doses may be given q4wk if tetanus threat persists. • **Severe wounds, delay in initiating prophylaxis:** 500 U as soon as possible after injury

IM, active tetanus infection,
ⓟ adults/children: 3,000-6,000
U • Part of dose may be infiltrated around wound.

ADMINISTRATION

ⓟ IM: Adults/older children: Administer into deltoid. • Infants/
ⓟ children <3 yr • Administer
into anterolateral thigh. • Do not
administer concurrently with tetanus toxoid • May be administered concurrently with tetanus
toxoid ADSORBED, but use
separate site. • DO NOT AD-
MINISTER SC, IV, INTRA-
DERMALLY. • Solution is col-
orless/transparent or slightly
opalescent; do not use cloudy/
discolored solutions.

ACTIONS

Sterile solution of antibody-
containing globulins prepared
from plasma of adults hyperim-
munized with tetanus toxoid
• Contains antibodies to toxin
produced by organism causing
tetanus, *Clostridium tetani*
• Provides passive immunity by
neutralizing bacterial endotoxin

PHARMACOKINETICS

ROUTE	PEAK	DURATION
IM	2 days	32 days
ELIMINATION		
Half-life 28 days		

INDICATIONS

Provides temporary passive immunity to tetanus after injury in
individuals incompletely immu-
nized or when immunization
status unknown • Used with tetanus toxoid adsorbed (provides
active immunization) for
tetanus-prone wounds: contaminated wounds, puncture wounds,
avulsions, wounds from mis-

siles, crush injuries, frostbite,
burns • Not necessary for clean,
minor wounds or when ≥3
doses of tetanus toxoid or tetanus toxoid adsorbed have been
received • Used in conjunction
with other therapies in treatment
of active tetanus

PRECAUTIONS/
CONTRAINDICATIONS

Precautions: Bleeding may occur after IM injection in patients
with bleeding disorders. Inadvertent IV administration may
cause serious allergic reaction.
Use caution with: Previous
hypersensitivity to immune
globulin
c Pregnancy category: Use
only when clearly needed and
safer alternative unavailable.
Contraindications: Hypersensitivity to tetanus immune globulin, thimerosal

ADVERSE EFFECTS

Derm: Urticaria
Local: Injection site pain, redness, tenderness
Misc: Low-grade fever, sensitization (rarely, with repeated
injections), **anaphylaxis** (rare)

INTERACTIONS

live vaccines (measles, mumps,
rubella, polio) within previous
3 mo Less effective immune
response
tetanus toxoid, tetanus toxoid
adsorbed in same syringe or
at same site ↓ Effectiveness
of both medications

PATIENT CARE
IMPLICATIONS

• Administer as soon as possible after injury.
• Have epinephrine, antihistamine, resuscitation equipment

T

immediately available at time of injection.

• Thorough wound cleansing, including removal of devitalized tissue/foreign material is essential for tetanus prevention.

Vital signs/hemodynamics: Monitor BP, HR, RR, temperature before and 30 min after injection.

Physical assessment: Assess for allergic reaction: chills, fever, sweating, rash, itching, laryngeal edema, wheezing. Observe outpatients 30 min after injection.

PATIENT/FAMILY TEACHING

Tetanus immune globulin provides rapid temporary protection from tetanus. For long-term protection, vaccination with tetanus toxoid or tetanus toxoid adsorbed is necessary. • Low-grade fever/pain, tenderness, redness, muscle stiffness at injection site may occur. • Immediately report chills, fever, sweating, itching, breathing difficulty.

AVAILABLE FORMS

Vials, prefilled syringes
Storage: Store refrigerated at 2°-8° C (35°-46° F); do not freeze.

---

tetanus and diphtheria toxoids, adsorbed, adults, Td

diphtheria and tetanus toxoids, adsorbed, children, Dt

Classification: Toxoid

USUAL DOSE

P **IM, Td, adults/children >7 yr:** 0.5 ml • Primary immunization: 2nd dose 1-2 mo after initial dose; 3rd dose 6-12 mo after 2nd. • Administer emergency booster dose to injured individuals with incomplete immunization, last tetanus dose >10 yr ago, or tetanus prone wounds/last tetanus dose >5 yr ago. • Schedule routine booster dose q10yr.

P **IM, Dt, children <6yr:** 0.5 ml IM in series of 4 doses with 1st 3 q4-8wk (usually 2, 4, 6 mo), 4th dose 6-12 mo after 3rd.

ADMINISTRATION

P **IM, adults/older children:**
P Administer into deltoid. • Infants/children <3 yr: Administer into anterolateral thigh.

• May be administered concurrently with tetanus immune globulin, but use separate site.

• DO NOT ADMINISTER SC, IV, INTRADERMALLY • Solution is colorless/transparent or slightly opalescent; do not use cloudy/discolored solutions.

ACTIONS

Tetanus toxoid produces active immunity by stimulating production of serum antitoxin, which neutralizes endotoxin produced by *Clostridium tetani,* causative agent of tetanus.

• Diphtheria toxoid produces active immunity by stimulating production of serum antitoxin, which neutralizes toxin produced by *Corynebacterium diphtheriae,* causative agent of diphtheria. • With complete immunization series, protective levels last for at least 10 yr.

INDICATIONS

Td used to provide active immunity against tetanus/diphtheria in adults/children ≥ 7 yr
• Dt used in younger children when pertussis vaccine contraindicated or given separately
• Prior tetanus immunization provides protection at time of injury, eliminates need for passive immunization in most cases. • Tetanus/diphtheria toxoid recommended for incomplete immunization (<3 doses tetanus toxoid), if last tetanus dose >10 yr ago or if last tetanus dose >5 yr ago and wound tetanus prone: contaminated wounds, puncture wounds, avulsions, wounds from missiles, crush injuries, frostbite, burns
• Many adults have inadequate levels of diphtheria antitoxin; therefore, diphtheria toxoid usually administered with tetanus immunization.

PRECAUTIONS/ CONTRAINDICATIONS

Precautions: Arthus-type hypersensitivity (itching/edema, similar to giant "hive" at injection site) reactions may occur, especially in adults >25 yr who have received frequent doses of tetanus toxoid. • Immunosuppressed patients or those with recent Ig injections may not have optimal response to immunization. • Inadvertent IV administration may result in serious allergic reaction.
Use caution with: Infants with history of CNS damage/ seizures; postpone primary immunization until 2 yr old
• Thrombocytopenia, bleeding disorder: bleeding may occur after IM injection

c Pregnancy category: Safe use not established; use only if safer alternative unavailable.
Contraindications: Hypersensitivity to tetanus toxoid, diphtheria toxoid, thimerosal • Defer routine immunization during polio outbreaks or with active infection/fever.

ADVERSE EFFECTS

CNS: *Fretfulness, drowsiness,* malaise, fatigue, seizures, encephalopathy, neuropathies including Guillain-Barré syndrome
CV: Tachycardia, dizziness, hypotension
GI: Anorexia, nausea, vomiting
Derm: Urticaria, pruritus, rash, flushing
Local: *Tenderness, erythema, induration;* rarely, Arthus-type hypersensitivity (erythema, boggy edema, itching)
Misc: Fever, chills, arthralgias, **anaphylaxis** (rare)

INTERACTIONS

chemotherapy, corticosteroids, immunosuppressives ↓ Immune response to Td, Dt
tetanus immune globulin in same syringe or at same site ↓ Effectiveness of both agents

PATIENT CARE IMPLICATIONS

• Determine previous vaccination history, reactions.
• Have epinephrine, antihistamine, resuscitation equipment immediately available at time of injection.
• Avoid unnecessary/frequent (e.g., annual) booster doses; Arthus-type local hypersensitivity reactions may occur.
• Thorough wound cleansing, including removal of devitalized

T

---

italic = common side effects   **bold** = life-threatening reactions

tissue/foreign material, essential for tetanus prevention

Vital signs/hemodynamics: Monitor BP, HR, RR, temperature before and 30 min after injection.

Physical assessment: Assess for allergic or anaphylactic reactions such as chills, fever, sweating, rash, itching, laryngeal edema, wheezing. Observe outpatients for 30 min after injection.

PATIENT/FAMILY TEACHING

Td or Dt vaccination provides long-term protection from tetanus, diphtheria; full series of injections with booster doses necessary for complete protection. • Low-grade fever/pain, tenderness, redness, muscle stiffness at injection site may occur. • Immediately report allergic reaction such as chills, fever, sweating, itching, difficulty breathing.

AVAILABLE FORMS

Storage: Vials, syringes. Store all preparations refrigerated at 2°-8° C (35°-46° F); do not freeze.

---

theophylline
(thee-off'-i-lin)
Bronkodyl, Elixophyllin,
Pulmophylline ✤,
Quibrin ✤,
Respbid, Slo-bid,
Slo-Phyllin, Theo-Dur

Classifications: Bronchodilator, xanthine derivative

USUAL DOSE

Dose individually adjusted to patient response, pulmonary function, serum levels; excessive dosage results in serious toxicity; dosage calculations based on lean body weight.

P PO, adults/children: Oral loading dose of 5mg/kg. Use immediate-release product (e.g., Slo-phyllin). Maintenance dose as follows. Adjust to serum levels.

	MAINTENANCE DOSE
P 1-9 yr	4 mg/kg q6h
P 9-16 yr, smoking adults	3 mg/kg q6h
Nonsmoking adults	3 mg/kg q8h
G Older adults, cor pulmonale	2 mg/kg q8h
CHF, hepatic failure	1-2 mg/kg q12h

ACTIONS

Relaxes smooth muscles with potent action on respiratory smooth muscle • **Respiratory:** Relieves bronchospasm; flow rates, vital capacity increased; dilates pulmonary arterioles, ↓ pulmonary hypertension, ↓ alveolar CO_2 tension, ↑ pulmonary blood flow; unlike sympathomimetic bronchodilators, tolerance rarely develops. • **CNS:** Stimulates vagal, vasomotor, vomiting centers; constricts cerebral vasculature, ↓ cerebral blood flow; ↑ in CO_2 levels may stimulate respiratory center, increase rate/depth of ventilation. • **CV:** Direct arteriolar/venous dilation decreases peripheral vascular resistance, venous pressures. Vasodilation usually offset by ↑ CO; only slight ↑ BP seen at moderate doses; higher doses cause vagal stimulation with tachycardia, dysrhythmias, hypotension. • **Renal:** Mild diuresis from increased CO/slight renal arteriolar dilation.

PHARMACOKINETICS

ROUTE	ONSET	PEAK	DURATION
PO, std	30 min	1-2 hr	
PO, ext rel	4-5 hr		

DISTRIBUTION

Wide

ELIMINATION

Metabolized in liver, renal elimination; half-life 7-9 hr, increased in children/smokers, decreased with CHF/COPD/advanced age

Therapeutic levels: 10-20 µg/ml

INDICATIONS

Reversible bronchospasm associated with chronic asthma, chronic bronchitis, emphysema • To counteract bronchospasm associated with propranolol

PRECAUTIONS/ CONTRAINDICATIONS

Precautions: Simultaneous administration by more than one route or with other xanthines increases risk of toxicity, should be avoided. • Some commercial preparations contain sulfites, which may cause serious allergic reactions.

Use caution with: Smokers (cigarettes, marijuana)/ young children; Larger or more frequent doses may be necessary. • Children: Adverse CNS effects more common • Sustained high fever, active influenza, older adults, heart failure, COPD, renal/hepatic impairment; monitor serum levels closely, use reduced dose. • Peptic ulcer • Hyperthyroidism • Glaucoma • Diabetes mellitus • Severe hypoxemia • Hypertension • CV disease • Seizure disorders

c Pregnancy category: Use only if safer alternative unavailable.

Contraindications: Hypersensitivity to theophyllines, caffeine, theobromine • Uncontrolled seizure disorder

ADVERSE EFFECTS

CNS: *Headache, irritability, restlessness,* nervousness, insomnia, dizziness, hyperexcitability, **seizures**

Resp: Tachypnea

CV: *Palpitations, sinus tachycardia,* flushing, **dysrhythmias, hypotension, circulatory failure**

GI: *Nausea, vomiting, anorexia,* epigastric pain

GU: ↑ Urinary frequency

Misc: Dehydration, SIADH

TOXICITY/OVERDOSE

Symptoms: Anorexia, nausea, vomiting, extreme thirst • Headache, irritability, agitation, maniacal behavior, delirium, muscle twitching, seizures • Tachycardia, palpitations, dysrhythmias, diaphoresis, hypotension, ventricular fibrillation, cardiac standstill

Management: After recent ingestion, implement guidelines for management of acute overdose (Appendix I). • Charcoal may be administered q4h until theophylline level <20 µg/ml. • **Seizures:** Establish airway; administer oxygen, IV diazepam. • **Hypotension:** Elevate legs, administer IV fluids; use dopamine for severe hypotension. • **Extreme tachycardia:** Administer propranolol. • Consider charcoal hemoperfusion for levels >40 µg/ml.

Toxic levels: >20 µg/ml

INTERACTIONS

barbiturates ↓ Theophylline levels

T

---

italic = common side effects   **bold** = life-threatening reactions

benzodiazepines ↓ Sedative effects

beta-blockers ↓ Bronchodilation

cabamazepine ↓ Theophylline levels

calcium channel blockers ↑ Theophylline levels

cimetidine ↑ Theophylline levels

ciprofloxacin, other quinolones ↑ Theophylline levels

digoxin Cardiotoxicity

erythromycin ↑ Theophylline levels

halothane anesthesia Dysrhythmias

lithium ↑ Lithium excretion

phenytoin ↓ Theophylline and/or phenytoin levels

propranolol ↑ Theophylline levels

rifampin ↓ Theophylline levels

sympathomimetics Dysrhythmias

PATIENT CARE IMPLICATIONS

• Toxic effects occur rapidly. If present, discontinue, consult physician

• To reduce stomach irritation, administer after meals, with full glass of liquid, or with antacids. For faster absorption with PO loading, administer with full glass of water 30-60 min before or 2 hr after meals.

• Extended-release preparations (e.q., Theo-Dur) helpful in patients with continuous asthma symptoms or rapid theophylline **P** elimination (e.g., children, young smokers)

• Do not crush or chew extended-release preparations.

• Many drug interactions possible; pharmacist review of drug profile recommended

Vital signs/hemodynamics: As available, monitor ECG for tachycardia, dysrhythmias esp. if history of cardiac disorders

• Monitor VS for hypo/hypertension, improved RR. • Use pulse oximeter to evaluate O_2 saturation according to clinical condition.

Physical assessment: Assess work of breathing, ventilatory excursion, breath sounds.

• Evaluate forced expiratory volume, other pulmonary function measurements. • Monitor I&O. Diuresis may lead to dehydration in susceptible individuals (e.g., older adults, young children).

Laboratory tests: Monitor: ABGs • Theophylline levels; therapeutic range, 10-20 μg/ml

PATIENT/FAMILY TEACHING

Purpose of medication is to relieve bronchospasm, improve breathing. • Report increased breathing difficulty, symptoms of toxicity: chest pain, palpitations, nausea, vomiting, twitching, convulsions. • Dizziness possible; avoid driving and hazardous activities until individual effects established.

• Take oral doses with meals to decrease stomach irritation.

• Avoid excessive intake of caffeine (e.g., coffee, tea, carbonated beverages). • Check with physician or pharmacist before taking cold or cough preparations. • Notify physician or prescriber of change in smoking habits; dosage adjustment may be necessary.

AVAILABLE FORMS

Premixed solution for parenteral use • Standard tablets, capsules • Extended-release tablets, capsules • PO solution

---

P pediatric   **G** geriatric   **V** Direct IV

thiamine HCl
Betalin S, Betaxin ✸,
Bewon ✸, Biamine,
Vitamin B₁

Classification: Vitamin, water soluble

USUAL DOSE
℗ **PO, adults/children:** Thiamine deficiency: 5-50 mg/24 hr 1-2 times daily
IV/IM, adults: Critical illness: 10-100 mg 1-3 times daily • Use IV route for emergencies (e.g., Wernicke's encephalopathy, beriberi with high-output heart failure)
℗ **IV/IM, children:** Critical illness: 10-25 mg 1-3 times daily

ADMINISTRATION
IV: In emergencies, may inject each dose of ≤100 mg over 5 min. • If not an emergency, dilute in compatible solution and administer as infusion over 15-30 min. Do not exceed rate of 20 mg/min
IM: Use Z-track method to minimize pain.

PREPARATION
IV, intermit inf: Dilute in 50-100 ml or other convenient volume of compatible solution
Compatible fluids: D₅W, 0.9% NaCl, RL, prepared combinations of these solutions

ACTIONS
Required for metabolic processes; forms coenzyme important in carbohydrate metabolism • Advanced deficiency results in beriberi with possible CV symptoms (↓ SVR, high-output heart failure) or nervous system deterioration (paresthesias, ↓ reflexes, Wernicke's encephalopathy) • Severe deficiency results in accumulation of pyruvic acid and possible lactic acidosis.

PHARMACOKINETICS

ROUTE	ONSET	PEAK	DURATION
IV/IM	Rapid	Rapid	Stored; excreted or used as needed

DISTRIBUTION
Throughout body tissue.
PO: Readily absorbed; absorption ↓ in alcoholism, cirrhosis, malabsorption
ELIMINATION
Metabolized in liver, excreted in urine.

INDICATIONS
Prevention/treatment of thiamine deficiency • Deficiency develops after 2-3 wk of inadequate intake; results in beriberi, Wernicke's encephalopathy, peripheral neuritis; typically occurs with malabsorption, alcoholism, cirrhosis, prolonged vomiting, severe anorexia. Thiamine requirements ↑ with pregnancy, ↑ carbohydrate intake, hyperthyroidism, infection, hepatic disease • Beriberi with high-output failure; use IV route. CV symptoms usually reversible. • Wernicke's encephalopathy; use IV route. Nervous system damage may be irreversible. • Acute ethylene glycol poisoning

PRECAUTIONS/ CONTRAINDICATIONS
Precautions: Serious adverse effects, including severe hypersensitivity, vascular collapse, death have occurred, usually after repeated IV administration. • Intradermal skin testing recommended by manufacturer for

T

patients with suspected sensitivity before parenteral administration (consult labeling for specific testing procedure)

A Pregnancy category

Contraindications: Hypersensitivity to thiamine

ADVERSE EFFECTS

Hypersensitivity, adverse reactions rare, but more likely with IV administration
CNS: Weakness, restlessness
Resp: Respiratory distress, cyanosis, **pulmonary edema**
CV: Vasodilation, hypotension, **CV collapse**
GI: Nausea, diarrhea, **hemorrhage**
Local: IM injection site pain, induration
Syst: Hypersensitivity reactions, including **anaphylaxis**

TOXICITY/OVERDOSE

Symptoms: Toxicity unusual, even with high-dose parenteral therapy (e.g., 100-500 mg)
Management: See Appendix N for management of acute allergic reaction.

INTERACTIONS

NMBAs Potentiates neuromuscular blockade

Y-SITE COMPATIBILITIES

Famotidine

Y-SITE INCOMPATIBILITIES

Alkaline solutions, barbiturates, erythromycin, kanamycin, sodium bicarbonate, streptomycin, sulfites

PATIENT CARE IMPLICATIONS

• Acute symptoms of neuritis, ataxia, edema, heart failure usually respond within hours of IV administration. Confusion, psychosis are slower to respond; no response may occur if nerve damage present.
• In known or suspected thiamine deficiency, administer thiamine before or simultaneously with glucose. Glucose may cause additional depletion of thiamine stores and precipitate/worsen heart failure.
Vital signs/hemodynamics: Monitor according to patient condition. • In patients with high-output heart failure, expect ↓ SVR; ↑ PAP, PCWP, CO, CI; ↓ arterial O_2 saturation, arteriovenous O_2 difference. Hemodynamic alterations usually improve after 2-3 days of therapy.
Physical assessment: Assess for thiamine deficiency/improvement of symptoms; mild deficiency characterized by numbness, tingling, weakness; severe deficiency characterized by high-output heart failure, tachycardia, palpitations, dependent edema, arteriovenous shunting.
• Assess for pulmonary edema with high-output heart failure: bibasilar crackles (rales), distended neck veins, S_3 gallop, breathing difficulty, frothy sputum. • Assess neurologic status in patients with Wernicke's encephalopathy: level of consciousness, orientation, mental alterations, ataxia, peripheral neuropathy.
Laboratory tests: Thiamine deficiency diagnosed by ↓ erythrocyte transketolase and/or ↑ pyruvic acid concentrations in blood

---

PATIENT/FAMILY TEACHING

Purpose of medication is to replace vitamin B_1. • Report breathing difficulty, palpitations.

AVAILABLE FORMS

Parenteral for IV/IM injection • Tablets

---

thrombin
(throm'bin)
Thrombinar,
Thrombogen,
Thrombostat

Classification: Hemostatic agent

USUAL DOSE
Topical, powder/solution:
Dose depends on severity of bleeding, response to therapy. • Thrombin solution of 1,000 U/ml clots 5 ml blood in <1 sec or liter of blood in <1 min.

ADMINISTRATION
Topical, powder/solution:
Solution: Spray or flood surface using sterile syringe, small-gauge needle/catheter. • Powder: Open vial, break dried thrombin into powder using sterile instrument such as scalpel. Sponge (do not wipe) blood from area, apply powder. After application, avoid sponging or other disturbance of clot. • Absorbable gelatin sponge: Immerse strips of sponge in reconstituted solution, knead with fingers (wearing sterile gloves) to remove air/facilitate saturation. Apply saturated sponge to bleeding area, hold in place for 10-15 sec with small gauze sponge.

PREPARATION

Reconstitute by adding sterile water for injection or 0.9% NaCl. • Generally, concentration of 100 U/ml used • Concentrations as high as 1,000-2,000 U/ml may be used for profuse bleeding. • Use within 3 hr of reconstitution, or store under refrigeration or preferably freeze for use within 48 hr. • Discard partially used vials.

ACTIONS

Converts fibrinogen to fibrin to cause clotting of whole blood, plasma • Will not clot blood in absence of fibrinogen • Derived from bovine sources

PHARMACOKINETICS

ROUTE	ONSET	PEAK/DURATION
Topical	Immed	Within min
DISTRIBUTION		
Local		
ELIMINATION		
Clot resolution as tissue heals		

INDICATIONS

Aids in hemostasis with bleeding from capillaries, small venules • When used alone will not control arterial bleeding • Used with absorbable gelatin sponge for hemostasis in surgery • May be used to shorten duration of bleeding from puncture sites in heparinized patients
Unlabeled/investigational:
PO administration in upper GI bleeding; questionable effectiveness because thrombin inactivated at Ph <5

PRECAUTIONS/
CONTRAINDICATIONS
Precautions: Do not use alone to control arterial bleeding. • Do not use to moisten microfibrillar

T

---

collagen hemostat; may impair efficacy • Is antigenic, may cause hypersensitivity or allergic reactions • *Intravascular clotting, death may result from injection or other entry into large blood vessels.*

c **Pregnancy category:** Safe use not established; use only if safer alternative unavailable.

Contraindications: Hypersensitivity to thrombin, bovine

P products Children: Safety/efficacy not established.

ADVERSE EFFECTS

Resp: Dyspnea, pulmonary hypertension, pulmonary edema
CV: **Hypotension, bradycardia,** hypertension, transient flushing
GI: Nausea, vomiting
MS: Back pain
Misc: Febrile reactions, allergic reaction

TOXICITY/OVERDOSE

Treat symptomatically. • For management of acute allergic reaction, see Appendix N.

PATIENT CARE IMPLICATIONS

• Assess for history of bovine allergy.
• Have epinephrine, resuscitation equipment immediately available during administration.
• See many implications with Administration.
Vital signs/hemodynamics: Monitor BP, HR frequently according to severity of bleeding.
Physical assessment: Assess for continued/recurrent bleeding during and immediately after therapy. • Assess for hypersensitivity reaction, including fever, urticaria, edema, coughing, wheezing, hypotension.

Laboratory tests: Monitor: Hct/Hgb • Coagulation factors

PATIENT/FAMILY TEACHING

Purpose of drug is to promote clot formation and slow bleeding. • Immediately report recurrent bleeding. • Do not disturb formed clot.

AVAILABLE FORMS

Topical powder
Storage: Store refrigerated at 2°-8° C(35°-46° F).

---

ticarcillin disodium
(tye-kar-sill'in)
Ticar

Classifications: Penicillin antibiotic, extended-spectrum penicillin

USUAL DOSE

P **IV/IM, adults/children >40 kg:** 1-3 g q4-6h; up to 24 g/24 hr used for severe infections • **Severe renal impairment:** Reduce dose and/or frequency.
P **IV/IM, children 1 mo-40 kg:** 50-100 mg/kg/24 hr in equally divided doses q6-8h • **Serious infections:** 200-300 mg/kg/24 hr in equally divided doses q4-6h

ADMINISTRATION

IM: Inject deep into large muscle mass (e.g., gluteus maximus, lateral thigh) • Do not administer more than 2 g at single site.
V **Direct IV:** Slowly inject over 3-5 min. • Infusion preferred, since pain, thrombophlebitis, local reactions more frequent with injection
IV, intermit inf: Infuse prepared solution over 30 min-2 hr.

P pediatric   **G** geriatric   **V** Direct IV

PREPARATION

IM: Reconstitute with 2 ml sterile water for injection, 0.9% NaCl, or 1% lidocaine HCl.
Direct IV: Reconstitute with 4 ml sterile water for injection, for each g ticarcillin; will yield concentration of 200 mg/ml. • Dilute with compatible IV solution to final concentration of at least 50 mg/ml. In fluid-restricted patients, may use concentration of 100 mg/ml; slow injection via large vein recommended for this concentration.
IV, intermit inf: Reconstitute with ≥10 ml of 0.9% NaCl or D$_5$W for each g ticarcillin to yield concentration of 100 mg/ml; may be further diluted with compatible fluid. • Final concentration should be 10-100 mg/ml. Dilute concentrations minimize peripheral vein irritation.
Compatible fluids: D$_5$W, 0.9% NaCl, LR, 1.5% and 4.25% peritoneal dialysis fluid
Stability: Reconstituted solution stable for 24 hr at room temperature

ACTIONS

Semisynthetic extended-spectrum penicillin with bactericidal action; interferes with bacterial cell wall synthesis/division • More active against gram-negative bacilli than other penicillins • Active against most gram-positive, gram-negative aerobic cocci (except penicillinase-producing strains), some gram-positive bacilli, many gram-negative bacilli, including *Proteus vulgaris, P. mirabilis, Morganella morganii, Escherichia coli, Enterobacter* species, *Pseudomonas aeruginosa* • Less active than piperacillin against *Enterococcus faecalis, P. aeruginosa,* and *Bacteroides fragilis*

PHARMACOKINETICS

ROUTE	ONSET	PEAK	DURATION
IM	Rapid	30-75 min	Approx 6-8 hr
IV	Immed	End infusion	

DISTRIBUTION
Widely distributed
ELIMINATION
Primarily excreted in urine; half-life 30-80 min

INDICATIONS

Serious intraabdominal, urinary tract, gynecologic, respiratory tract, skin, bone/joint infections; septicemia • Primary use in gram-negative aerobic infections, mixed aerobic-anaerobic bacterial infections • Used empirically in febrile granulocytopenic patients, often with aminoglycoside or 3rd generation cephalosporin • Synergism with aminoglycosides frequently used to therapeutic advantage in *P. aeruginosa* infections • Not to replace natural penicillins (e.g., penicillin G) or aminopenicillins (e.g., ampicillin) for treatment of streptococcal infections

PRECAUTIONS/ CONTRAINDICATIONS

Precautions: Bacterial or fungal overgrowth may occur; indwelling lines/catheters ↑ risk. • May contribute to fluid overload, electrolyte imbalance, including hypernatremia, hypokalemia • May impair coagulation, cause abnormal bleeding
Use caution with: Hypersensitivity to cephalosporins, other drugs; risk of allergic reaction

T

- Severe renal insufficiency; lower dose/frequency
B Pregnancy category: Safety not clearly established
Contraindications: Hypersensitivity to ticarcillin, any penicillin

ADVERSE EFFECTS

CNS: Headache, neuromuscular irritability/**seizures,** especially high dose/renal insufficiency
GI: Nausea, vomiting, *diarrhea,* unpleasant taste, ↑ AST/ALT
GU: Hypokalemia, hypernatremia, ↑ BUN/creatinine
Hema: Eosinophilia, hemolytic anemia, other blood dyscrasias, coagulation disorders
Derm: *Rash,* urticaria, pruritus
Local: *Pain* with IM injection, *pain*/and thrombophlebitis with IV use
Misc: *Hypersensitivity,* **anaphylaxis,** serum sickness; *superinfection, colonization*

TOXICITY/OVERDOSE

Symptoms: Neurotoxicity, including seizures, particularly with high-dose therapy, renal insufficiency • Acute allergic reaction, including anaphylaxis
Management: Discontinue drug. Initiate symptomatic/supportive measures. For acute allergic reaction, see Appendix N. Hemodialysis effective in drug removal

INTERACTIONS

aminoglycosides (e.g., amikacin, gentamicin) Synergistic antibacterial activity
anticoagulants, PO Prolonged bleeding time
cephalosporins Unpredictable synergism/antagonism
chloramphenicol Inhibition of bactericidal activity

clavulanic acid Synergistic bactericidal activity
probenecid Higher/prolonged ticarcillin blood levels
tetracycline Inhibition of bactericidal activity

Y-SITE COMPATIBILITIES

Acyclovir, diltiazem, famotidine, hydromorphone, insulin (regular), magnesium sulfate, meperidine, morphine, ondansetron, verapamil

Y-SITE INCOMPATIBILITIES

Aminoglycosides (e.g., amikacin, gentamicin, tobramycin), fluconazole

PATIENT CARE IMPLICATIONS

- Obtain specimens for culture and sensitivity before initiating antibiotic therapy. Initiate therapy before results received.
- Determine previous antibiotic use, including reactions to penicillins, cephalosporins. Cross-reactivity with cephalosporin allergies may occur; higher incidence of reactions reported with cystic fibrosis patients.
- Have epinephrine, antihistamine, resuscitation equipment readily available for use with severe allergic reaction.
- Do not discharge patient for at least 30 min after antibiotic administration.
- High sodium content may cause edema, electrolyte abnormalities, dysrhythmias and contribute to heart failure.
- To avoid drug incompatibility/interaction, administer at separate site; stagger schedules when aminoglycosides (e.g., amikacin, gentamicin, tobramycin), tetracycline, chloramphenicol also prescribed.

• Reduce risk of suprainfection by limiting use of indwelling lines/catheters.
• Reduce risk of thrombophlebitis by using large veins, small catheters/needles, and rotating IV infusion sites.
• IV route must be used for severe infections or when shock present.
Vital signs/hemodynamics: Monitor VS at beginning and throughout therapy. • Monitor I&O for imbalance.
Physical assessment: Assess for improvement in primary infection or symptoms of super/suprainfection: appearance of sputum, urine, stool, wound drainage; presence of fever, candidiasis, vaginitis. • Observe for symptoms of hypersensitivity: rash, pruritus, wheezing, laryngeal edema, hypotension. • Assess for unusual or occult bleeding, including ecchymosis, bleeding from gums, mucous membranes, excessive bleeding from venipuncture site/surgical incision. Note blood in urine, other body fluids. Check emesis, stools for occult blood.
Laboratory tests: Monitor: CBC with differential; electrolytes, BUN, creatinine, liver enzymes, PT, PTT, particularly important in patients with renal/cardiac impairment, elderly/debilitated patients • Concurrent aminoglycoside therapy; Closely monitor aminoglycoside levels, because aminoglycosides sometimes inactivated by ticarcillin • May cause: Positive direct antiglobulin (Coombs') test

PATIENT/FAMILY TEACHING
Purpose of drug is to limit growth of infection-causing bacteria. • Immediately report rash, swelling, intense itching, difficulty breathing, other signs of allergic reaction. • Report diarrhea, fever, vaginal itching or discharge, furry growth on tongue. • Report unusual bruising, skin discoloration, bleeding from venipunctures, nose, mouth, urine, in stools/emesis.

AVAILABLE FORMS
Parenteral for IV/IM use

ticarcillin disodium/clavulanate potassium
(tye-kar-sill'in)
Timentin

Classifications: Penicillin antibiotic, extended-spectrum penicillin

USUAL DOSE
IV, adults > 60 kg: 3.1 g q4-6h • Severe renal impairment: Reduce dose and/or frequency.

ADMINISTRATION
IV, intermit inf: Infuse prepared solution over 30 min.

PREPARATION
IV, intermit inf: Reconstitute with 13 ml sterile water or 0.9% NaCl for injection; will yield concentration of 200 mg ticarcillin/ml. • Further dilute with 50-100 ml compatible IV solution.
Compatible fluids: D_5W, 0.9% NaCl, LR
Stability: Reconstituted solution stable for 24 hr at room temperature.

ACTIONS

Semisynthetic, extended-spectrum penicillin with bactericidal action; interferes with bacterial cell wall synthesis/division • More active against gram-negative bacilli than other penicillins • Clavulanic acid inhibits bacterial enzymes (beta-lactamases) responsible for inactivating ticarcillin, extends spectrum of activity to include many strains of bacteria resistant to ticarcillin alone. • Active against most gram-positive, gram-negative aerobic cocci, some gram-positive bacilli, many gram-negative bacilli, including *Proteus vulgaris, P. mirabilis, Morganella morganii, Escherichia coli, Enterobacter, Pseudomonas aeruginosa* • More active than ticarcillin disodium alone against *Staphylococcus aureus, Haemophilus influenzae, Moraxella catarrhalis,* Enterobacteriaceae • Less active than piperacillin against *Enterococcus species, P. aeruginosa, Bacteroides fragilis*

PHARMACOKINETICS

ROUTE	ONSET	PEAK	DURATION
IV	Immed	End infusion	Approx 6-8 hr

DISTRIBUTION
Widely distributed

ELIMINATION
Primarily excreted in urine; half-life 30-80 min

INDICATIONS

Infections caused by beta-lactamase–producing organisms when extended-spectrum penicillin alone not likely to be effective • Serious intraabdominal, urinary tract, gynecologic, respiratory tract infections; septicemia • Synergism with aminoglycosides used to therapeutic advantage in *P. aeruginosa* infections, febrile granulocytopenic patients • Not to replace natural penicillins (e.g., penicillin G) or aminopenicillins (e.g., ampicillin) for treatment of streptococcal infections

PRECAUTIONS/ CONTRAINDICATIONS

Precautions: Bacterial or fungal overgrowth may occur; indwelling lines/catheters ↑ risk. • May contribute to fluid overload/electrolyte imbalance, including hypernatremia, hypokalemia • May impair coagulation, cause abnormal bleeding
Use caution with: Hypersensitivity to cephalosporins, other drugs; risk of allergic reaction • Severe renal insufficiency; **P** lower dose/frequency • Children <12 yr: Safety not clearly established
B **Pregnancy category:** Safety not clearly established
Contraindications: Hypersensitivity to ticarcillin, any penicillin, clavulanate

ADVERSE EFFECTS

CNS: Headache, neuromuscular irritability/**seizures,** especially with high dose/renal insufficiency
GI: Nausea, vomiting, *diarrhea,* unpleasant taste, ↑ AST/ALT
GU: Hypokalemia, hypernatremia, increased BUN/creatinine
Hema: Eosinophilia, hemolytic anemia, other blood dyscrasias, coagulation disorders
Derm: *Rash,* urticaria, pruritus
Local: *Injection site pain,* thrombophlebitis
Misc: *Hypersensitivity,* **anaphylaxis,** serum sickness; *superinfection, colonization*

P pediatric   **G** geriatric   **V** Direct IV

TOXICITY/OVERDOSE

Symptoms: Neurotoxicity, including seizures, particularly with high-dose therapy, renal insufficiency • Acute allergic reaction, including anaphylaxis **Management:** Discontinue drug. Initiate symptomatic/supportive measures. For acute allergic reaction, see Appendix N. Hemodialysis effective in drug removal; minimal removal with peritoneal dialysis

INTERACTIONS

aminoglycosides (e.g., amikacin, gentamicin) Synergistic antibacterial activity
anticoagulants, PO Prolonged bleeding time
cephalosporins Unpredictable synergism/inactivation
chloramphenicol Inhibition of bactericidal activity
probenecid Higher/prolonged ticarcillin blood levels
tetracycline Inhibition of bactericidal activity

Y-SITE COMPATIBILITIES

Diltiazem, famotidine, fluconazole, insulin (regular), meperidine, morphine, ondansetron

Y-SITE INCOMPATIBILITIES

Aminoglycosides (e.g., amikacin, gentamicin, tobramycin), sodium bicarbonate

PATIENT CARE IMPLICATIONS

• Obtain specimens for culture and sensitivity before initiating antibiotic therapy. Initiate therapy before results received.
• Determine previous antibiotic use, including reactions to penicillins, cephalosporins. Cross-reactivity with cephalosporin allergies may occur; higher incidence of reactions reported with cystic fibrosis patients.
• Have epinephrine, antihistamine, resuscitation equipment readily available for use with severe allergic reaction.
• Do not discharge patient for at least 30 min after antibiotic administration.
• High sodium content may cause edema, electrolyte abnormalities, dysrhythmias and contribute to heart failure, particularly with high-dose therapy in susceptible patients.
• To avoid drug incompatibility/interaction, administer at separate site; stagger schedules when aminoglycosides (e.g., amikacin, gentamicin, tobramycin), tetracycline, chloramphenicol also prescribed.
• Reduce risk of suprainfection by limiting use of indwelling lines/catheters.
• Reduce risk of thrombophlebitis by using large veins, small catheters/needles, and rotating infusion sites.
Vital signs/hemodynamics: Monitor VS at beginning and throughout therapy. • Monitor I&O for imbalance.
Physical assessment: Assess for improvement in primary infection or symptoms of super/suprainfection: appearance of sputum, urine, stool, wound drainage; presence of fever, candidiasis, vaginitis. • Observe for symptoms of hypersensitivity: rash, pruritus, wheezing, laryngeal edema, hypotension. • Assess for unusual or occult bleeding, including ecchymosis, bleeding from gums/mucous membranes, excessive bleeding from venipuncture site/surgical incision. Note blood in urine,

T

other body fluids. Check emesis, stools for occult blood.
Laboratory tests: Monitor: CBC with differential; electrolytes, BUN, creatinine, liver enzymes, PT, PTT particularly important in patients with renal/cardiac impairment, elderly/debilitated patients • **Concurrent aminoglycoside therapy:** Closely monitor aminoglycoside levels, because aminoglycosides may be inactivated by ticarcillin. • **May cause:** Positive direct antiglobulin (Coombs') test

PATIENT/FAMILY TEACHING

Purpose of drug is to limit growth of infection-causing bacteria. • Immediately report rash, swelling, intense itching, difficulty breathing, other signs of allergic reaction. • Report diarrhea, fever, vaginal itching or discharge, furry growth on tongue. • Report unusual bruising, skin discoloration, bleeding from venipunctures, nose, mouth, urine, in stools/emesis.

AVAILABLE FORMS

Parenteral for IV use

---

tobramycin sulfate
(toe-bra-mye′sin)
Nebcin

Classification: Aminoglycoside antibiotic

USUAL DOSE

P **IV/IM, adults/children >1 mo:** 1-3 mg/kg/day in divided doses q6-8h • **Severe infections:** Up to 5 mg/kg/day in divided doses q6-8h; reduce to 3 mg/kg/day as soon as possible.

• **Extensive burns:** Altered pharmacokinetics result in ↓ serum levels; adjust to therapeutic levels. • **Renal insufficiency:** Reduce dose and/or frequency; adjust to therapeutic levels.

ADMINISTRATION

IM: Inject deep into large muscle mass (e.g., gluteus maximus, lateral thigh)
IV, intermit inf: Infuse prepared solution over 20-60 min.
• Toxicity possible with too-rapid infusion

PREPARATION

IV, intermit inf: Dilute single dose in 50-100 ml (less for children) compatible IV solution.
Compatible fluids: D_5W, 0.9% NaCl, LR, prepared combinations of these solutions above.
Stability: Reconstituted solution stable for 24 hr at room temperature. Stable for ≥8 hr when diluted in many peritoneal dialysis solutions, including those with 500 U/ml heparin.

ACTIONS

Bactericidal action; inhibits bacterial cell protein synthesis, causing cellular death • Active against many aerobic gram-negative bacteria, including *Pseudomonas aeruginosa, Escherichia coli, Enterobacter, Klebsiella, Proteus, Serratia* • Active against some aerobic gram-positive bacteria, including *Staphylococcus aureus* and *S. epidermidis*

P pediatric   **G** geriatric   **V** Direct IV

PHARMACOKINETICS

ROUTE	ONSET	PEAK	DURATION
IM	Rapid	30-90 min	Approx 6-8 hr
IV	Immed	End infusion	

DISTRIBUTION

Wide; low CSF levels

ELIMINATION

Filtered through glomeruli and excreted; half-life 2-3 hr, prolonged with renal impairment

Therapeutic levels: Peak levels, 4-10 µg/ml; trough levels, 1-2 µg/ml.

INDICATIONS

Treatment of serious, gram-negative bacterial infections, such as skin infections in burn patients; septicemia; bone, respiratory tract, postop intraabdominal infections • Useful with strains resistant to other antibiotics • Frequently combined with an extended-spectrum penicillin (e.g., piperacillin, ticarcillin) or other antibiotic for treatment of serious *Pseudomonas* infections, particularly in immunosuppressed patients • With penicillins for treatment of enterococcal endocarditis • Not indicated for gram-positive bacterial infections if other less toxic antibiotics could be used

PRECAUTIONS/ CONTRAINDICATIONS

Precautions: Bacterial or fungal overgrowth possible • Excessive serum levels associated with toxicity • Systemic absorption, toxicity possible when used in irrigating solutions or for intrapleural/peritoneal instillation • Some preparations contain sulfites, which can cause serious allergic reactions in susceptible individuals.

Use caution with: Renal impairment, advanced age, preexisting hearing disorder, high-dose/prolonged therapy, dehydration; ototoxicity, nephrotoxicity more likely • Preexisting neuromuscular disease, hypocalcemia, massive transfusions, general anesthesia, NMBAs; neurotoxicity more likely • Concurrent use of other ototoxic, neurotoxic, nephrotoxic agents

Pregnancy category: Risk of fetal damage; avoid pregnancy. Use only if safer alternative unavailable and risks explained to woman.

Contraindications: Hypersensitivity to tobramycin, possibly other aminoglycosides

ADVERSE EFFECTS

CNS: *Ototoxicity,* permanent hearing loss (rare), dizziness, peripheral numbness/twitching, weakness, neuromuscular blockade, **respiratory paralysis** (rare)
GI: Nausea, vomiting, ↑ liver enzymes
GU: *Nephrotoxicity,* ↑ BUN/creatinine, tubular necrosis, **renal failure**
Local: Irritation, pain
Misc: Hypersensitivity; superinfection, colonization

TOXICITY/OVERDOSE

Symptoms: Ototoxicity, nephrotoxicity • Neurotoxicity with neuromuscular blockade, seizures, possible respiratory paralysis
Management: Initiate symptomatic/supportive measures, including airway management/ventilation. • Hemodialysis or

peritoneal dialysis may be helpful.

INTERACTIONS

amphotericin B Nephrotoxicity
cephalosporins (e.g., cephalothin) Synergistic antibacterial activity; nephrotoxicity; possible chemical inactivation of aminoglycoside
cyclosporine Nephrotoxicity
ethacrynic acid Nephro/ototoxicity; extreme caution indicted
NMBAs Recent use increases risk of respiratory paralysis
NSAIDs ↑ Aminoglycoside levels
penicillins Synergistic antibacterial activity; chemical inactivation of aminoglycoside possible if given simultaneously

Y-SITE COMPATIBILITIES

Acyclovir, diltiazem, amiodarone, enalaprilat, esmolol, fluconazole, furosemide, hydromorphone, insulin, labetalol, magnesium sulfate, meperidine, morphine

Y-SITE INCOMPATIBILITIES

Cephalosporins, heparin, hetastarch, penicillins

PATIENT CARE IMPLICATIONS

• Obtain specimens for culture and sensitivity before initiating antibiotic therapy. Initiate therapy before results received.
• To avoid drug incompatibility/interaction, administer at separate site; stagger schedules when penicillins, cephalosporins also prescribed.
• IV route must be used for severe infections or when shock present.
Vital signs/hemodynamics: Monitor VS for indicators of infection, complications. • As available, monitor CVP, PCWP, central hemodynamics to optimize fluid volume balance.
Physical assessment: Assess for improvement in primary infection or symptoms of super/suprainfection: appearance of sputum, urine, stool, wound drainage; presence of fever, candidiasis, vaginitis. • Assess for evidence of neuromuscular blockade; numbness, tingling muscle twitching, weakness; possible progression to apnea; particular vigilance required for at-risk patients (see Precautions). • Assess hearing before initiating therapy. Monitor at intervals for symptoms of ototoxicity: tinnitus, roaring in ears, hearing loss, vertigo, nausea; **G** particularly important with advanced age, preexisting hearing disorder, renal impairment, high-dose/prolonged therapy. • Carefully monitor UO, evaluate I&O ratio. Keep patient well hydrated by PO or parenteral fluids of sufficient volume to produce adequate UO; older, debilitated, seriously ill, renal-impaired patients at greater risk for toxicity.
Laboratory tests: Peak/trough levels: Draw peak levels immediately after IV infusion complete or 30-60 min after IM injection. Draw trough levels just before next dose.
• Narrow therapeutic range requires close monitoring, particularly with advanced age, high-dose therapy, renal insufficiency. • **Monitor:** Electrolytes, liver enzymes, PT, PTT, CBC with differential • Urinalysis, BUN, creatinine, creatinine clearance before and regularly during therapy; follow closely **G** in older adults, renal impair-

---

ment, high-dose/prolonged therapy. Increase hydration if signs of renal irritation (e.g., casts, proteinuria); reduce dose or discontinue if renal dysfunction. • **Other:** Concurrent cephalosporin/penicillin therapy may cause inactivation of aminoglycoside levels; stagger schedules; avoid drawing aminoglycoside levels immediately after penicillin/cephalosporin administration.

PATIENT/FAMILY TEACHING

Purpose of drug is to limit growth of infection-causing bacteria. • Report rash, itching, diarrhea, fever, vaginal itching or discharge, dizziness, hearing difficulties. • Inform nurse or physician if you may be pregnant or are considering pregnancy.

AVAILABLE FORMS

Parenteral for IV/IM use • Premixed solution for IV infusion

---

tocainide HCl
(toe-kay'nide)
Tonocard

Classifications: Class IB antidysrhythmic, membrane stabilizer

USUAL DOSE

PO: Initially 400 mg q8h; increase gradually according to individual requirements. • Maintenance, 400-600 mg bid-tid; dosage rarely exceeds 2,400 mg/day. • May be given twice daily in well-controlled patients

ACTIONS

Membrane-stabilizing effects; decreases cardiac excitability by increasing threshold for electrical excitation • Does not prolong QRS complex, QT interval • Blocks fast sodium channels, increases effective refractory period, suppresses automaticity in His-Purkinje system • Peripheral vascular resistance may ↑ slightly, with resultant ↓ in CO. Electrophysiologic effects similar to lidocaine.

PHARMACOKINETICS

ROUTE	ONSET	PEAK	DURATION
PO	Rapid	30 min-2 hr	5 hr

DISTRIBUTION
Wide

ELIMINATION
Metabolized in liver; alkaline urine decreases renal excretion; half-life 15 hr

Therapeutic level: 3-10 µg/ml

INDICATIONS

Suppression/prevention of symptomatic ventricular dysrhythmias • Patients refractory to lidocaine usually refractory to tocainide; those successfully converted by lidocaine can generally be effectively managed with tocainide. • Ability to improve survival not well established.

PRECAUTIONS/CONTRAINDICATIONS

Precautions: May worsen frequent premature contractions, ventricular tachycardia • Has not been shown to prevent sudden death in patients with serious ventricular ectopy • May exacerbate heart failure, heart block • Bone marrow depression (i.e., leukopenia, anemia, thrombocytopenia), necessitating drug discontinuation is possible; monitor CBC closely, esp. during first 12 wks. Patients with

T

---

italic = common side effects   **bold** = life-threatening reactions

multisystem failure, polypharmacotherapy at greatest risk.
• Mild, transient neurologic/GI dysfunction may occur initially.

Use caution with: Renal/hepatic impairment; lower dose necessary

c Pregnancy category: Safety not established; use only if safer alternative unavailable.

Contraindications: Hypersensitivity to tocainide, other amide-type agents (e.g., lidocaine, novocaine) • 2nd/3rd degree heart block unless functional ventricular pacemaker in place or readily available

ADVERSE EFFECTS

CNS: *Dizziness, paresthesias, confusion, tremors, nervousness,* headache, mood alteration, **seizures** (rare)

EENT: Blurred vision, tinnitus, hearing loss

Resp: **Pulmonary edema,** dyspnea, cough, wheezing, pneumonia

CV: Hypotension, palpitations, **bradycardia, heart block,** tachycardia, ventricular dysrhythmias, **exacerbation of heart failure**

GI: *Nausea,* diarrhea, anorexia, vomiting

Derm: Rash, dermatitis, diaphoresis

Syst: Bone marrow depression with anemia, leukopenia, thrombocytopenia; positive ANA titer, Coombs' test; SLE-like syndrome

TOXICITY/OVERDOSE

Symptoms: Dizziness, vertigo, tremors, confusion, hallucinations, seizures • Heart block, heart failure, ventricular fibrillation • Severe nausea/vomiting, diarrhea • Severe dyspnea, respiratory depression, respiratory arrest

Management: After recent ingestion, implement guidelines for management of acute overdose (Appendix I). • **Heart failure:** Administer inotropic agents (e.g., dobutamine, dopamine) • **Hypotension:** Elevate legs, administer IV fluids; use vasopressors (e.g., norepinephrine, dopamine) for severe hypotension. • Manage symptomatic bradycardia, ventricular dysrhythmias according to ACLS guidelines (Appendix P). • Implement seizure precautions. Consider ET intubation to maintain airway/ventilation in unconscious/convulsing patients. Administer anticonvulsants if seizures continue after ventilation/O_2 therapy.

Toxic serum level: >10 µg/ml

INTERACTIONS

antidysrhythmics Additive/antagonistic effects
beta-blockers ↓ CO
lidocaine Additive effects; CNS toxicity

PATIENT CARE IMPLICATIONS

• Correct hypoxemia, hypercapnia, hypokalemia, other fluid/electrolyte imbalances before initiating therapy.
• High rate of adverse GI/CNS effects may necessitate discontinuation of therapy.

Vital signs/hemodynamics: Monitor BP, HR, RR frequently during initiation of therapy.
• Continuously monitor ECG for significant dysrhythmias until controlled.

Physical assessment: Assess for perfusion/oxygenation deficit: ↓ level of consciousness, chest pain, activity intolerance, hypotension, dizziness. • Assess for pulmonary insufficiency: dyspnea, cough, abnormal breath sounds.

Laboratory tests: Monitor: Electrolytes • CBC with differential • ANA titer • Plasma levels of tocainide; therapeutic level, 3-10 µg/ml • If positive ANA titer develops or SLE symptoms occur, consult physician, consider discontinuation of drug.

PATIENT/FAMILY TEACHING

Purpose of medication is to control abnormal heartbeats. • Nausea, vomiting, diarrhea, dizziness, lightheadedness, numbness, confusion, tremors, nervousness may occur. These symptoms usually improve after 1-2 wk of therapy. Immediately report prolonged or serious side effects. • Use caution when engaging in activities requiring mental alertness and coordination until individual effects established. • Immediately report chest pain, breathing difficulty, swelling of extremities, rapid weight gain, activity intolerance, persistent coughing, wheezing. • Report unusual bruising/bleeding, sore throat, other signs of infection.

AVAILABLE FORMS

Tablets

torsemide
(toor'si-mide)
Demadex

Classification: loop diuretic

USUAL DOSE

PO/IV, adults: PO/IV doses interchangeable. Initially, 5-10 mg once daily; for CHF, renal failure, use initial dose of 10-20 mg. Titrate by doubling dose each day until desired effect achieved. Maximum PO dose: 200 mg. Maximum IV dose: 200 mg. • **Cirrhosis, hepatic disease:** Must be given with spironolactone (Aldactone) or other potassium-sparing diuretic; maximal dose is 40 mg.

ADMINISTRATION

PO: May be given without regard to meals
▼ **Direct IV:** Inject each dose of 20 mg or less slowly over ≥2 min. Dilution not necessary. Too-rapid injection may cause ototoxicity.

ACTIONS

Diuretic that acts on loop of Henle to promote rapid diuresis • Action similar to other loop diuretics (e.g., furosemide, bumetanide) • Results in excretion of sodium, chloride, potassium, magnesium, water • Beneficial effects in CHF include reduced plasma volume, increased Hct, decreased peripheral resistance, increased CO • Reduced plasma volume results in hypotensive effects in some patients. • Affects glucose metabolism, may cause mild elevations of blood glucose

T

italic = common side effects   **bold** = life-threatening reactions

PHARMACOKINETICS

ROUTE	ONSET	PEAK	DURATION
PO	60 min	1-2 hr	6-8 hr
IV	10 min	1-2 hr	6-8 hr

DISTRIBUTION
99% Protein bound

ELIMINATION
Metabolized by liver. Half-life 3.5 hr

INDICATIONS

Edema associated with congestive heart failure, renal disorders, cirrhosis • Hypertension; used alone or with other agents • May be used with potassium-sparing diuretic, especially with liver disorders

PRECAUTIONS/CONTRAINDICATIONS

Precautions: May cause hypokalemia, metabolic alkalosis; use with spironolactone, other potassium-sparing diuretic reduces this risk. Hypokalemia more likely with cirrhosis; diminished oral intake of electrolytes; rapid diuresis; corticosteroid, adrenocorticotropic hormone therapy. Increased risk of hypokalemia-associated dysrhythmias in older adults, digitalize patients • Excessive diuresis may cause dehydration, hypovolemia, possible thromboembolism, especially in older adults. • Tinnitus, hearing loss possible with rapid IV injection, use of large doses.
Use caution with: Renal impairment; diuresis, reduced plasma volume may decrease GFR • Nephrotic syndrome; profound hypokalemia possible • Cirrhosis/hepatic failure; rapid changes in fluids/electrolytes can prompt hepatic coma; initiate torsemide diuresis in hospital • Digitalized patients; torsemide-related hypokalemia could promote dysrhythmias, toxicity • Children: Safety/efficacy not established
B Pregnancy category: Use only if clearly needed.
Contraindications: Hypersensitivity to torsemide, other sulfonylureas • Anuria • Untreated severe hepatic coma • Severe uncorrected electrolyte depletion

ADVERSE EFFECTS

CNS: *Headache, dizziness,* weakness
EENT: Tinnitus, hearing impairment
CV: Hypotension, hypovolemia
GI: Nausea, vomiting
GU: Excessive urination, thirst
Misc: Hypokalemia, hyperglycemia, hyperuricemia

TOXICITY/OVERDOSE

Symptoms: Dehydration, hypovolemia, hypotension, hyponatremia, hypokalemia, hypochloremic alkalosis, hemoconcentration
Management: After recent ingestion, implement guidelines for management of acute overdosage (Appendix I). • For hypotension, elevate legs, administer IV fluids (e.g., 0.9% NaCl). • Correct electrolyte imbalance.

INTERACTIONS

ACE inhibitors, beta-blockers, calcium channel blockers Hypotension
digoxin Hypokalemia, dysrhythmias, toxicity
indomethacin, possibly other NSAIDs ↓ Diuresis
probenecid ↓ Diuresis
salicylates Salicylate toxicity

PATIENT CARE IMPLICATIONS

• Correct electrolyte/acid-base imbalance before initiating therapy. Administration with potassium-sparing diuretic (e.g., spironolactone, amiloride) will help prevent hypokalemia.

• Adjust dose according to response to therapy. Consider diuresis, fluid balance, weight, electrolytes.

• If prerenal patients become progressively more oliguric or azotemic, discontinue use.

Vital signs/hemodynamics: Monitor BP, UO carefully, especially with initial, high-dose, or IV therapy. Consult physician for hypotension or oliguria.

• Monitor ECG, as available, especially with high-dose, IV therapy. Note presence of dysrhythmias, hypokalemic changes: PVCs, flattened ST, T wave inversion, U wave. If present, check potassium level, correct as necessary. Digitalized patients should be monitored for these and other dysrhythmias associated with digitalis toxicity.

• Hemodynamic monitoring recommended for patients with severe CHF, cardiogenic shock, hemodynamic instability. Monitor closely for overaggressive diuresis, excessive lowering of preload, resulting in reduced CO. • Monitor fluid balance; weigh daily.

Physical assessment: Assess for improvement in condition: resolution of ascites, diminished fatigue, unlabored breathing, stable BP. • Assess for electrolyte imbalance: dysrhythmias, confusion, dizziness, weakness, muscle cramps, fatigue, faintness, headache, paresthesias, anorexia, vomiting. • Assess for perfusion/oxygenation deficit cause by hypovolemia: chest discomfort, decreased level of consciousness, activity intolerance, hypotension, dizziness.

Laboratory tests: Monitor: Electrolytes, especially potassium • BUN, creatinine • Blood glucose, especially in patients with diabetes • Promptly correct imbalances. • **May cause:** Hypokalemia, hypomagnesemia, hyponatremia

PATIENT/FAMILY TEACHING

Purpose of medication is to eliminate excess body fluid.

• May cause dizziness, especially at first; use caution when changing positions, walking. IV: Call for assistance before getting out of bed. • Report symptoms of heart failure: breathing difficulty, palpitations, dizziness, activity intolerance, chest pain.

• Report symptoms of electrolyte imbalance: confusion, weakness, dizziness, fatigue, headache, numbness/tingling of hands, feet; loss of appetite, nausea, vomiting.

Outpatient: Take medicine in the morning. Do not stop taking medicine even if you feel better. Drug controls but does not cure condition. • Weigh twice/wk; report weight gain, edema. • Patients with diabetes: Blood glucose levels may increase. Insulin dose may need adjustment.

AVAILABLE FORMS

Tablets • Parenteral solution for IV use

T

---

italic = common side effects   **bold** = life-threatening reactions

tramadol
(tram′ah-dole)
Ultran

Classification: Non-opiate analgesic

USUAL DOSE

PO, adults: 50-100 mg q4-6h as needed for pain. Maximum dose: 400 mg/day or 300 mg/day if age >75 yrs • **Renal insufficiency:** 50-100 mg q12h. Maximum dose: 200 mg/day • **Hepatic insufficiency:** 50 mg q12h

ADMINISTRATION

PO: May be given without regard to meals

ACTIONS

Centrally acting synthetic analgesic; unrelated to opiates. Binds to *u*-opioid receptors; inhibits reuptake of norepinephrine, serotonin. Broken down in the liver to active metabolite, MI, which has high affinity for *u*-receptors. Like opioids may cause drowsiness, nausea, constipation; however, less likely to cause respiratory depression. Unlike morphine, does not cause histamine release. May cause vasodilation with orthostatic changes in some patients. Similar in analgesic efficacy to acetaminophen 300 mg with codeine 30 mg (Tylenol 3). Mild tolerance may develop, but withdrawal is less severe than with opioids.

PHARMACOKINETICS

ROUTE	ONSET	PEAK	DURATION
PO	1 hr	2-3 hr	6-8 hr

ELIMINATION

Metabolized by liver, excreted in urine. Half-life = 6-7 hr.

INDICATIONS

Relief of moderate to moderately severe pain

PRECAUTIONS/CONTRAINDICATIONS

Precautions: May cause seizures with: use of MAO inhibitors, neuroleptics; history of seizure disorders; other states, medications that lower seizure threshold. Naloxone increases seizure risk. • May cause respiratory depression when administered with other respiratory depressants or to high-risk patients • Not recommended for opioid-dependent patients; may precipitate withdrawal • May obscure clinical findings if used with acute abdominal conditions
Use caution with: CNS depressants, including alcohol, anesthesia, opioids, phenothiazines, tranquilizers, sedatives; respiratory depression possible; reduced dose indicated • COPD, asthma, respiratory disorders; may cause respiratory depression; use reduced dose. • CNS depression, head injury, craniotomy; may cause miosis, obscure clinical findings • Hepatic/renal insufficiency; use reduced dose. • MAO inhibitors
c Pregnancy category: Safe use not established
Contraindications: Hypersensitivity to tramadol • Acute intoxication with alcohol, opioids, **P** other CNS depressants • Children: Safe use not established

ADVERSE EFFECTS

CNS: *Sedation, dizziness, headache,* nervousness, anxiety, tremor, emotional lability, **seizures**

CV: Vasodilation, hypotension, tachycardia
GI: *Nausea, vomiting, constipation,* stomach upset
GU: Retention, urinary frequency
Misc: Dry mouth, diaphoresis, miosis, mild tolerance

TOXICITY/OVERDOSE

Symptoms: Sedation, seizures, respiratory depression
Management: Effects partially antagonized by naloxone, but use may not reverse all symptoms • Maintain airway, support ventilation, administer IV fluids if hypotensive. • Seizures: Administer benzodiazepines, barbiturates.

INTERACTIONS

alcohol, anesthetics, antihistamines, opioid analgesics, phenothiazines, sedatives, tranquilizers Additive CNS depression
carbamazepine ↑ Tramadol metabolism; higher doses of tramadol required
MAO inhibitors Tramadol interferes with detoxification mechanisms

PATIENT CARE IMPLICATIONS

• Administer prn doses before pain becomes severe. Regularly scheduled dosing is usually more effective than prn.
• Patients receiving tramadol for pain control do not develop psychologic dependence. Mild tolerance may develop, but withdrawal is less severe than with opioids.
Vital signs/hemodynamics: Assess VS according to patient condition. • Consider use of pulse oximetry in patients who are heavily sedated or who have pulmonary disease.
Physical assessment: Assess type, location, intensity of pain before and after administration.
• Evaluate adequacy of ventilation in patients who are heavily sedated or who have pulmonary disease. • Assess for signs of opioid withdrawal in patients with established opioid dependency: restlessness, sweating, abdominal cramps, vomiting, hypertension, elevated temperature.

PATIENT/FAMILY TEACHING

Purpose of drug is to relieve pain. • Request medication before pain becomes severe.
• Change position slowly to minimize dizziness. • Do not perform hazardous tasks requiring mental alertness or physical coordination until effects of drug are established. • Avoid concurrent use of alcohol or other sedatives when taking this medication.

AVAILABLE FORMS

Tablets

---

triamterene
(trye-am′ter-een)
Dyrenium
triamterene with hydrochlorothiazide
Dyazide, Maxzide

T

Classification: Potassium-sparing diuretic

USUAL DOSE

PO, adults: 100 mg bid after meals • Often given with other diuretics (e.g., furosemide, hydrochlorothiazide) • Maximum dose, 300 mg/day

---

italic = common side effects   **bold** = life-threatening reactions

P PO, children: 4 mg/kg/day bid after meals

PREPARATION

G-tube: Crush tablets, dissolve in water. Shake well before administration.
Stability: Stable for 1 month if refrigerated

ACTIONS

Acts directly on renal distal tubule to inhibit reabsorption of sodium/water, limit potassium/hydrogen excretion • Effects include excretion of sodium, calcium, magnesium, bicarbonate, water • Unlike thiazide/loop diuretics, does not cause potassium loss • Diuresis independent of aldosterone levels • With daily administration, GFR may be reduced. • When combined with non–potassium-sparing diuretics, diuresis increases, whereas potassium excretion caused by other agent decreases; when used alone, has little or no effect on BP.

PHARMACOKINETICS

ROUTE	ONSET	PEAK	DURATION
PO	2-4 hr	6-8 hr	12-16 hr

DISTRIBUTION
Wide: 50%-67% bound to plasma proteins
ELIMINATION
Metabolized by liver, eliminated in urine; half-life 3 hr

INDICATIONS

Edema associated with CHF, liver cirrhosis, nephrotic syndrome, steroid use, secondary hyperaldosteronism • Unlike loop/thiazide diuretics, conserves potassium; often used with other diuretics to prevent excessive potassium loss • With other agents in management of mild to moderate hypertension • Prophylaxis/treatment of hypokalemia • May be effective in patients with poor response to spironolactone

PRECAUTIONS/ CONTRAINDICATIONS

Precautions: Risk of hyperkalemia, especially with renal/
G hepatic impairment, older adults, patients with diabetes, with potassium supplements • May contribute to development of renal calculi; use caution with history of renal calculi • May deplete folate stores; use caution in pregnant/alcohol-dependent patients
Use caution with: Severely ill patients at risk for developing respiratory/metabolic acidosis, because sudden increases in serum potassium possible • Renal/hepatic impairment; may cause hyperkalemia
B Pregnancy category: Safety not clearly established; use only if safer alternative unavailable.
Contraindications: Hypersensitivity to triamterene • Rapidly deteriorating renal status; anu-
P ria; hyperkalemia • Children: Safety/efficacy not established

ADVERSE EFFECTS

CNS: Dizziness, headache, weakness, confusion, lethargy
Resp: Acidosis, compensatory hyperventilation
CV: Dysrhythmias due to electrolyte imbalance, intravascular fluid volume deficit, hypotension
GI: *Nausea,* vomiting, dry mouth, diarrhea, jaundice, ↑ liver enzymes
GU: ↑ BUN/creatinine, renal insufficiency, oliguria, renal stones

---

F&E: ↑ Potassium, chloride; ↓ sodium, magnesium, bicarbonate; hyperchloremic metabolic acidosis; dehydration

Hema: Megaloblastic anemia, thrombocytopenia

Derm: Rash, urticaria, photosensitivity

Misc: ↑ Uric acid, gout

TOXICITY/OVERDOSE

Symptoms: Hypotension • Hyperkalemia, hyponatremia, weakness, renal insufficiency, possible hyperchloremic acidosis • Nausea, vomiting, abdominal cramping

Management: After recent ingestion, implement guidelines for management of acute overdose (Appendix I). • Administer IV fluids, replace electrolytes based on laboratory results of serum levels. Closely monitor sodium, potassium balance. Treat hyperkalemia with dextrose, insulin. Additional measures for hyperkalemia include IV calcium, bicarbonate if acidotic, cation exchange resin.
• Hypotension: Elevate legs, administer IV fluids; if unresponsive to fluid replacement, use vasopressors (e.g., dopamine, epinephrine). • Hemodialysis may be moderately effective.

INTERACTIONS

angiotensin-converting enzyme inhibitors Hyperkalemia
beta-blockers Hypotension
calcium channel blockers Hypotension
digoxin Electrolyte disturbances; cardiac dysrhythmias
diuretics ↑ Diuretic effects
diuretics, potassium sparing Hyperkalemia

hypotensive agents Hypotension
NSAIDs ↓ Diuresis; NSAID-induced renal failure
potassium supplements Hyperkalemia

PATIENT CARE IMPLICATIONS

• Avoid use in severely ill patients at risk for developing respiratory/metabolic acidosis, because sudden increases in serum potassium may result. If use unavoidable, check electrolytes, acid-base balance frequently.
• Avoid use of $D_{50}W$ to test for hypoglycemia in comatose patients with diabetes receiving triamterene, because use could cause rapid, dangerous elevations in serum potassium.
• Evaluate response to therapy considering diuretic response, fluid balance, weight, electrolytes. Adjust dose accordingly.
• Avoid combination formulas with potential for profound hypotension when initiating therapy.
• If progressive oliguria or azotemia develops, discontinue drug.
Vital signs/hemodynamics: Monitor BP, HR, UO frequently, especially with parenteral therapy. Consult physician for hypotension, oliguria. • As available, continuously monitor ECG. Note presence of PVCs, dysrhythmias, hyperkalemic ECG changes (peaked T waves, PR prolongation, ST depression, widened QRS). If present, check potassium level, correct as necessary. Digitalized patients should be carefully monitored for these and other dysrhthmias associated with digitalis toxicity.

T

---

italic = common side effects   **bold** = life-threatening reactions

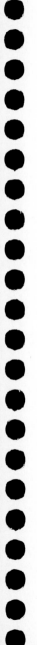

Physical assessment: Assess extremities, face, sacrum for improvement in edema. • Assess for signs/symptoms of electrolyte imbalance, including dysrhythmias, confusion, dizziness, weakness, muscle cramps, fatigue, faintness, headache, paresthesias, thirst, anorexia, vomiting. • Assess for perfusion/oxygenation deficit caused by hypovolemia: chest discomfort, ↓ level of consciousness, activity intolerance, hypotension, dizziness. • Weigh patient daily.
Laboratory tests: Monitor: Electrolytes, especially sodium, potassium • BUN, creatinine • Bilirubin, liver enzymes • CBC with differential • May interfere with laboratory tests for quinidine

PATIENT/FAMILY TEACHING

Purpose of drug is to eliminate excess body fluid, lower BP. • May cause dizziness, especially when starting therapy; use caution when changing positions, walking. • Report signs/symptoms of heart failure: breathing difficulty, palpitations, activity intolerance, chest pain. • Report signs/symptoms of electrolyte imbalance: confusion, weakness, dizziness, headache, numbness, tingling of legs, muscle cramps, persistent thirst, anorexia, nausea, vomiting. • Report unusual bleeding/bruising, persistent mouth sores, fever, sore throat.
Outpatient: Take medication in morning. Never double doses. • Continue taking medication as prescribed even if feeling better. Drug controls but does not cure condition. • Take with food to avoid nausea. • Avoid excessive ingestion of high-potassium foods, including salt substitutes. • Avoid alcohol, which could cause dizziness, fainting. • Do not take aspirin or other nonprescription drugs without consulting physician or pharmacist. • Use sunscreen, wear protective clothing to prevent photosensitivity reactions. • Weigh twice/wk; notify physician of weight gain, edema.

AVAILABLE FORMS

Tablets

trimethaphan camsylate
(trye-meth'a-fan)
Arfonad

Classifications: Antihypertensive, vasodilator

USUAL DOSE

Adjust dose carefully to individual response. Always use lowest effective dose.
IV, cont inf, adults: Initially 3-4 mg/min; increase by small increments to control BP. • Use lower dose range for older adults.
IV infusion, children: Initially 50-150 µg/kg/min; increase by small increments to control BP.

ADMINISTRATION

IV, cont inf: Increase by small increments q5-10min to control BP. • Use infusion pump. • Patient must be supine throughout therapy.

PREPARATION

DILUTION	CONCENTRATION
500 mg/500 ml	1 mg/ml
500 mg/250 ml	2 mg/ml

P pediatric   **G** geriatric   **V** Direct IV

Compatible fluids: D_5W (recommended), 0.9% NaCl, LR, Do not mix with any other drugs, solutions.

ACTIONS

Blocks sympathetic/parasympathetic ganglia of autonomic nervous system by competing with acetylcholine at receptor sites • Causes direct peripheral vasodilation, histamine release • Effects include vasodilation, peripheral pooling of blood, decreased BP • Additional BP lowering occurs with head-up position, because venous return/CO ↓ . • In heart failure, ↓ afterload/venous return may improve CO. • Bladder atony, GI hypomotility, dilated pupils, dry mouth may occur because of parasympathetic blockade. • Marked reduction in effectiveness develops within 24-72 hr.

PHARMACOKINETICS

ROUTE	ONSET	PEAK	DURATION
IV	Immed	5-10 min	10-30 min

DISTRIBUTION
Crosses placenta

ELIMINATION
Filtered, secreted by kidneys

INDICATIONS

Initial control of BP and rate of increasing left ventricular pressure in acute aortic dissection, usually with concurrent beta-blocker therapy • Management of pulmonary edema associated with systemic/pulmonary hypertension • To produce controlled hypotension, control small-vessel bleeding during head/neck surgery • Rapid reduction of BP in hypertensive crises, although other agents (e.g., sodium nitroprusside, diazoxide)

preferred because of adverse parasympatholytic effects of trimethaphan

PRECAUTIONS/CONTRAINDICATIONS

Precautions: Excessive doses result in prolonged action rather than ↑ hypotension. • *Large doses may cause apnea, respiratory arrest.* • Controlled hypotension during surgery may affect ventilation/perfusion ratio.
Use caution with: History of any allergy; drug causes histamine release • Arteriosclerosis, cardiac disease, cerebrovascular/degenerative CNS disease, diabetes mellitus, Addison's disease, corticosteroid therapy; risk of perfusion impairment • Older adults, debilitation, children: higher risk of complications
Pregnancy category: Risk of fetal damage; use in pregnancy only if benefits exceed risk and woman informed of possible fetal harm.
Contraindications: Hypersensitivity to trimethaphan camsylate • Anemia • Hypovolemia, shock • Asphyxia, persistent respiratory insufficiency • Glaucoma

ADVERSE EFFECTS

CNS: *Dizziness,* headache, weakness, confusion, restlessness, **CVA**
EENT: Dilate pupils
Resp: Tachypnea, shortness of breath, **apnea/respiratory arrest** (rare)
CV: *Hypotension,* **shock,** tachycardia, dysrhythmias, **angina, MI**
GI: *Nausea,* vomiting, dry mouth, constipation
GU: Urinary retention
Derm: Itching, urticaria

T

---

italic = common side effects   **bold** = life-threatening reactions

Misc: ↓ Potassium

TOXICITY/OVERDOSE

Symptoms: Profound hypotension, dizziness, angina, shock, loss of consciousness, vomiting • Apnea, respiratory arrest
Management: Support breathing as needed with O_2 and/or mechanical ventilation.
• Hypotension: Stop infusion, elevate feet, administer IV fluids; if prolonged, unresponsive to IV fluids, use vasopressors (e.g., dopamine, norepinephrine).

INTERACTIONS

anesthesia, general/spinal Profound hypotension
calcium channel blockers Additive hypotension
diuretics Hypotension
hypotensive agents Additive hypotension
NMBAs Prolonged neuromuscular blockade
procainamide Hypotension

Y-SITE COMPATIBILITIES

Heparin, hydrocortisone sodium succinate, potassium chloride

Y-SITE INCOMPATIBILITIES

Bromides, iodides, thiopental, tubocurarine chloride, strongly alkaline solutions

PATIENT CARE IMPLICATIONS

• Correct hypovolemia before administration.
• Patient must remain supine with appropriate safety precautions during administration.
• Have IV fluids, vasopressors immediately available.
• If progressing aortic aneurysm dissection, prepare patient for surgical intervention.

• Convert to PO/other antihypertensive therapy as soon as possible. Gradually reduce dose to avoid rebound hypertension.
Vital signs/hemodynamics: Initially, monitor BP continuously. Thereafter, monitor BP, HR frequently according to patient condition, titration schedule. For hypotension, reduce rate or stop infusion, elevate feet. Consult physician for hypotension not immediately responsive to positioning, rate adjustment. • Continuously monitor ECG, noting tachycardia, dysrhythmias, ECG changes. • Hemodynamic monitoring recommended with history of heart disease, CHF. Note filling pressures (e.g., CVP, PCWP), SVR; titrate agents to optimize CO/CI. • Consider continuous pulse oximetry, especially in patients with history of lung disease.
Physical assessment: Assess for perfusion/oxygenation deficit: chest discomfort, shortness of breath, ↓ level of consciousness, confusion, dizziness.
Laboratory tests: Evaluate renal, hepatic hematologic status before initiating therapy. In hypertensive crisis, immediately begin withdrawing sample while starting therapy. • Have typed, cross-matched blood immediately available when used for patients with acute aortic dissection.

PATIENT/FAMILY TEACHING

Purpose of drug is to lower BP.
• May cause dizziness, low BP; do not attempt to get out of bed. • Immediately report chest discomfort, breathing difficulty, dizziness, confusion.

AVAILABLE FORMS

Parenteral for IV infusion

trimethoprim/ sulfamethoxazole

(trye-meth'oh-prim sul-fa-meth-ox'ah-zole)
Bactrim, Cotrim, Cotrimoxazole, Roubac ♣, Septra, Sulfatrim, TMP-SMX, Uroplus

Classification: Sulfonamide antibiotic

USUAL DOSE

Dosage expressed as trimethoprim, which is present in commercial products in 1:5 fixed ratio with sulfamethoxazole
PO, adults: Urinary tract infection (UTI), enteritis, bronchitis: 160 mg q12h for 7-14 days • *Pneumocystis carinii* pneumonia: 20 mg/kg/24 hr in divided doses q6h • Renal impairment creatinine clearance [CrCl] 15-30 ml/min): Reduce dose by 50%.
℗PO, children >2 mo: Otitis media, enteritis: 8 mg/kg/24 hr in divided doses q12h for 5-14 days. • *P. carinii* pneumonia: 15-20 mg/kg/24 hr in divided doses q6h for 14-21 days
℗IV, intermit inf, adults/children: 8-10 mg/kg/24 hr in divided doses q6-12h for 5-14 days • *P. carinii* pneumonia: 15-20 mg/kg/24 hr in divided doses q6-8h for 14-21 days • Renal impairment (CrCl 15-30 ml/min): Reduce dose by 50%.

ADMINISTRATION

IV, intermit inf: Infuse prepared solution over 60-90 min. • Flush lines before and after. • Avoid rapid infusion or bolus injection. • Do not inject IM.

PREPARATION

IV: Dilute in 125 ml D_5W; infuse within 6 hr. • May dilute in 75 ml if fluid restriction necessary; use within 2 hr. • Do not refrigerate. • Discard cloudy or crystallized solutions.
Compatible fluids: D_5W, 0.9% NaCl, LR; solutions compatible up to 24 hr, concentrated solution compatible for at least 2 hr
Stability: Reconstituted solutions table for 2-6 hr at room temperature

ACTIONS

Broad-spectrum antibacterial/antiprotozoal activity against gram-positive, gram-negative organisms • Synergistic combination of trimethoprim/sulfamethoxazole prevents folic acid formation, reduces folates essential for growth of microorganisms

PHARMACOKINETICS

ROUTE	ONSET	PEAK	DURATION
PO	>1 hr	1-4 hr	
IV	Immed	60-90 min	To 10 hr

DISTRIBUTION
Widely distributed in all body tissue; highly protein bound

ELIMINATION
Metabolized in liver, excreted in urine; half-life 8-13 hr

INDICATIONS

UTI caused by *Escherichia coli, Proteus, Klebsiella, Enterobacter,* other organisms • Choice agent for treatment and preven-

T

tion of *P. carinii* pneumonia • Enteritis caused by *Shigella, E. coli,* other organisms • Ampicillin-resistant otitis media or when patient allergic to penicillin • Acute exacerbations of chronic bronchitis
Unlabeled/investigational: Empiric treatment of sepsis in granulocytopenic patients, *Nocardia* infections

PRECAUTIONS/ CONTRAINDICATIONS

Precautions: Not for IM use • Bacterial or fungal overgrowth may occur; indwelling lines/ catheters ↑ risk. • Commercial IV preparations contain sulfites, which may cause serious allergic reactions in susceptible individuals. • Inadequate hydration promotes crystalluria, stone formation. • Hematologic adverse effects more likely with folate [G] deficiency (e.g., advanced age, malnutrition, chronic alcohol ingestion, pregnancy, debilitation)
[G] **Use caution with:** Older adults • Severe allergies, bronchial asthma • Folate, glucose-6-phosphate (G6PD) deficiency • AIDS ↑ incidence of adverse effects • Renal/hepatic insufficiency; lower dose/frequency • Hypersensitivity to furosemide, thiazide diuretics, sulfonylureas
[C] **Pregnancy category:** Safe use not established; benefits must outweigh risk.
Contraindications: Hypersensitivity to trimethoprim, sulfonamides • Megaloblastic anemia caused by folate deficiency [P] • CrCl <15 ml/min • Infants <2 mo • Streptococcal pharyngitis; may be ineffective

ADVERSE EFFECTS

CNS: Headache, insomnia, depression, vertigo, fatigue, seizures, aseptic meningitis
GI: *Nausea, vomiting, anorexia,* **hepatitis** (rare)
GU: ↑ BUN/creatinine, crystalluria, stone formation
Hema: Bone marrow depression, agranulocytosis, aplastic anemia
Derm: *Rash, urticaria,* pruritus photosensitivity, **Stevens-Johnson syndrome**
Local: *Injection site pain,* irritation
Misc: *Superinfection, colonization;* hypersensitivity, **anaphylaxis;** serum sickness

TOXICITY/OVERDOSE

Symptoms: Major toxic or adverse reactions: rash, sore throat, fever, pallor, arthralgia, cough, shortness or breath, purpura, jaundice
Management: Discontinue drug for rash, bone marrow depression, major toxicity. • Initiate symptomatic/supportive measures. For acute allergic reaction, see Appendix N.

INTERACTIONS

cyclosporine Nephrotoxicity
digoxin ↑ Digoxin levels, espe-
[G]   cially in older adults
methotrexate ↑ Methotrexate levels
metronidazole Disulfiram (Antabuse)-like reaction caused by ethanol in IV preparation
phenytoin Folate deficiency
probenecid Potentiates bactericidal activity
warfarin Prolonged PT

COMPATIBILITIES

Acyclovir, atracurium, diltiazem, enalaprilat, esmolol, heparin, hydromorphone, labetalol, magnesium sulfate, meperidine, morphine sulfate, pancuronium, piperacillin-tazobactam, vecuronium, zidovudine

INCOMPATIBILITIES

Fluconazole, verapamil; no mixing in syringe or solution (manufacturer recommendation)

PATIENT CARE IMPLICATIONS

• Obtain specimens for culture and sensitivity before initiating antibiotic therapy. Initiate therapy before results received.
• Determine previous antibiotic use, including reactions to sulfonamides, sulfonamide derivatives (e.g., furosemide, thiazides, sulfonylureas).
• Have epinephrine, antihistamine, resuscitation equipment readily available for use with severe allergic reaction.
• Do not discharge patient for at least 30 min after IV antibiotic administration.
• Maintain adequate hydration (at least 2,000 ml/day) to prevent urinary crystallization, stone formation.
• Reduce risk of suprainfection by limiting use of indwelling lines/catheters.
• Reduce risk of thrombophlebitis by using large veins, small catheters/needles and rotating infusion sites.
Vital signs/hemodynamics: Monitor VS at beginning and throughout therapy. • Monitor I&O for imbalance.
Physical assessment: Assess for improvement in primary infection or symptoms of super/suprainfection: appearance of sputum, urine, stool, wound drainage; presence of fever, candidiasis, vaginitis. • Observe for symptoms of serious adverse reaction: rash, sore throat, fever, pallor, arthralgia, cough, shortness of breath, purpura, unusual bleeding, jaundice. If present, discontinue, consult physician.
Laboratory tests: Monitor: CBC with differential before and frequently throughout therapy; discontinue for any evidence of bone marrow suppression. • Blood glucose; may cause hypoglycemia • BUN, creatinine, urinalysis
May cause: ↑ Alkaline phosphatase, bilirubin, creatinine

PATIENT/FAMILY TEACHING

Purpose of drug is to limit growth of infection-causing bacteria. • Immediately report rash, swelling, intense itching, difficulty breathing, other signs of allergic reaction. • Report diarrhea, fever, vaginal itching or discharge, furry growth on tongue. • Report unusual bruising, skin discoloration, bleeding from venipunctures, nose, mouth, urine, in stools/emesis.
Outpatient: Take medication at least 1 hr before or 2 hr after meals. Take with full 8-oz glass of water. Drink plenty of water throughout the day. • Take at evenly spaced intervals over each 24-hr period. Take all of medication exactly as prescribed. Do not stop taking medicine even if you feel better. Failure to take all of antibiotic may result in recurrence or additional infection. Do not save or share unused medicine.
• Avoid sunlight, use sunscreen,

T

---

italic = common side effects   **bold** = life-threatening reactions

wear protective clothing to prevent burns.

AVAILABLE FORMS

Parenteral for IV use • Tablets • PO suspension

---

urokinase
(yoor-oh-kin'ase)
Abbokinase, Abbokinase
Open-Cath

Classification: Thrombolytic agent

USUAL DOSE

IV, acute pulmonary embolism, adults: Initially 4,400 IU/kg over 10 min; follow with continuous infusion of 4,400 IU/kg/hr for 12 hr.
Intracoronary, coronary artery thrombolysis, adults: Administer within 6 hr of onset of acute MI symptoms. • Initial bolus dose of heparin, 2,500-10,000 U IV • Then administer urokinase; average total dose 500,000 IU. Given at rate of 6,000 IU/min (e.g., 4 ml/min solution containing 1500 IU/ml), directly into coronary artery for up to 2 hr. • Angiography repeated q15min to determine response; therapy continued for 15-30 min after initial opening or up to 2hr. Other dosing regimens, including IV administration (investigational), used
IV, catheter occlusion, adults: 5,000 IU in 1 ml diluent; may repeat once if initial attempt unsuccessful

ADMINISTRATION

IV, acute pulmonary embolism: Measure thrombin time (TT) 3-4 hr after initiating therapy to ensure activation of fibrinolytic system. • Must use volumetric infusion pump or syringe infusion pump; reconstituted solution alters droplet size; inaccuracies result if other infusion devices used. • Use 0.45-μm IV filter; DO NOT USE STANDARD IN-LINE FILTER. • After infusion complete, flush catheter with 25-30 ml 0.9% NaCl to ensure delivery of entire dose. • Anticoagulant therapy initiated after infusion; heparin started after TT has decreased to < twice normal value
Intracoronary infusion: Must use volumetric infusion pump or syringe infusion pump; reconstituted solution alters droplet size; inaccuracies result if other infusion devices used. • Use 0.45-μm IV filter; DO NOT USE STANDARD IN-LINE FILTER.
IV catheter occlusion: Aseptically attach 1-ml TB syringe with urokinase solution to hub of catheter, without force slowly inject volume equal to internal volume of catheter. • Remove syringe, attach 5-ml syringe. • After 5 min attempt aspiration of urokinase solution, clot. If unsuccessful, repeat aspiration attempts q5min. • After 30 min of unsuccessful attempts, cap catheter for 30-60 min, then reattempt aspiration; 2nd urokinase injection may be necessary. • When patency restored, remove 4-5 ml blood, then gently flush with 10 ml 0.9% NaCl, reconnect. • When clearing central venous catheters, instruct patient to exhale, hold breath whenever catheter not connected to IV tubing/syringe • Avoid excessive pressure when inject-

---

℗ pediatric   **Ⓖ** geriatric   **▼** Direct IV

ing urokinase or attempting to clear catheter.

PREPARATION

Reconstitute each vial with sterile water for injection WITHOUT PRESERVATIVES; amount varies according to use (see following sections). • Add slowly, direct stream of diluent to sides of vial. • Roll and tilt gently to dissolve; do not shake. • Prepared solution is colorless to slightly straw colored and transparent. • Reconstitute immediately before use. • Do not use highly colored or cloudy solutions.

IV: Add 5 ml sterile water for injection to each vial of 250,000 IU. • Add reconstituted solution to D_5W or 0.9% NaCl. Do not exceed total volume of 200 ml.

Intracoronary: Add 5 ml sterile water for injection to each 250,000 IU. • Add contents of 3 reconstituted vials to 500 ml D_5W for solution containing 1,500 IU/ml.

IV catheter occlusion: When using Abbokinase Open-Cath, dilute 5,000 IU vial with 1 ml sterile water. • When using Abbokinase, reconstitute 250,000 vial with 5 ml sterile water. Remove 1 ml reconstituted solution, add to 9 ml of sterile water for solution containing 5,000 IU/ml.

ACTIONS

Enzyme produced by kidney that promotes thrombolysis (clot dissolution) by converting plasminogen to the proteolytic enzyme plasmin • Plasmin degrades fibrin clots, fibrinogen, other clotting factors, thus dissolving clots, improving blood flow through previously occluded arteries. • Decreases in circulating clotting factors present for 12-24 hr, may result in bleeding complications.

PHARMACOKINETICS

ROUTE	ONSET	PEAK	DURATION
IV	Rapid	1-2 hr	Fibrinolytic effect: 3 hr; anticoagulant effect: 12-24 hr

DISTRIBUTION
Throughout bloodstream
ELIMINATION
Excreted in bile, urine; half-life 10-20 min.

INDICATIONS

Lysis of clots, restoration of blood flow in various thromboembolic conditions • Limited availability, high cost, relative to streptokinase • Useful for patients with high concentrations of streptokinase antibodies • **Acute pulmonary emboli:** Initiate therapy as soon as possible, no later than 5 days after onset of symptoms; results in improved hemodynamic stability, ↓ pulmonary hypertension, reversal of right ventricular dysfunction; start anticoagulant therapy immediately after urokinase to minimize risk of reocclusion. • **Thrombolysis in evolving acute MI:** Used to restore coronary perfusion, limit infarct size, improve ventricular function, ↓ incidence of CHF, other complications; initiate therapy as soon as possible after onset of symptoms, preferably within 6 hr; concomitant therapy with anticoagulants (e.g., heparin, warfarin) and/or platelet-aggregation inhibitors (e.g., aspirin, dipyridamole) used to ↓ incidence of reocclusion. • **IV catheter occlusion:** Used to

U

---

italic = common side effects   **bold** = life-threatening reactions

clear occluded IV catheters obstructed by clotted blood, fibrin; not effective in clearing obstructions of substances other than blood (e.g., drug precipitates) *Unlabeled/investigational:* To lyse clot, restore perfusion in selected instances of peripherial arterial vascular occlusion

PRECAUTIONS/CONTRAINDICATIONS

Precautions: Bleeding, bruising, hematomas may occur, especially at vascular access sites, after invasive procedures, with IM injections. • Cerebral, other serious or fatal spontaneous bleeding may occur. • Atrial/ventricular dysrhythmias may occur during coronary reperfusion.

G **Use caution with:** Older adults; history of cerebrovascular disease, severe or uncontrolled hypertension; ↑ risk of cerebral hemorrhage

B **Pregnancy category:** Safety not well established; use only if safer alternative unavailable.

Minor relative contraindications: Recent (within 10 days) minor trauma, including CPR • History of cerebrovascular disease • Pregnancy • Likelihood of left-sided heart thrombus (e.g., atrial fibrillation, severe left ventricular dyskinesia) • Acute pericarditis • Subacute bacterial endocarditis • Hemostatic defects, including those associated with liver/renal dysfunction; anticoagulant therapy • Diabetic hemorrhagic retinopathy, other hemorrhagic ophthalmic conditions • Age >75 yr **G** • Septic thrombophlebitis, occluded AV cannula at seriously infected site • Any condition in which serious bleeding likely or would be difficult to control

Major relative contraindications: Recent (within 10 days) major surgery, serious trauma, obstetric delivery, organ biopsy/puncture of noncompressible vessels • GI/GU bleeding within 10 days • Hypertension (SBP >180 or DBP >110 mm Hg)

Absolute contraindications: Hypersensitivity to urokinase • Active internal bleeding • Recent CVA • Recent (within 2 mo) intracranial neoplasm, anteriovenous malformation/aneurysms • Recent (within 2 mos) intracranial/intraspinal surgery, trauma • Bleeding diathesis **P** • Severe, uncontrolled hypertension • Children: Safety not established

ADVERSE EFFECTS

CNS: **Cerebral hemorrhage**
EENT: Epistaxis, gingival bleeding, eye hemorrhage
Resp: Hemoptysis
CV: *Reperfusion dysrhythmias,* including accelerated idioventricular rhythm, PVCs, **ventricular tachycardia/fibrillation,** PACs, atrial fibrillation, junctional rhythm, sinus bradycardia; hypotension
GI: *Nausea, vomiting,* bleeding
GU: Hematuria
Hema: *Puncture site/soft tissue bleeding, bruising, ecchymosis/hematoma,* ↓ Hct
Misc: Fever, mild allergic reactions (rare)

TOXICITY/OVERDOSE

Symptoms: Bleeding, bruising, hematomas • Spontaneous bleeding from cerebral, retroperitoneal, GU, GI, soft tissue sources • Dose-dependent depletion of clotting proteins, production of fibrin degradation products.

Management: Stop infusion.
• Initiate local measures such as manual compression followed by pressure dressings. • Administer plasma volume expanders (avoid dextran), packed RBCs, fresh-frozen plasma, cryoprecipitate, as indicated by blood loss, clotting studies • Antifibrinolytics (e.g., aminocaproic acid) may be used in cases of life-threatening bleeding (e.g., intracranial hemorrhage).

INTERACTIONS

aminocaproic acid Inhibition of therapeutic effects
anticoagulants (e.g., heparin, warfarin) ↑ Bleeding risk
antiplatelet agents (e.g., abciximab, dipyridamole, NSAIDs, ticlodipine) ↑ Bleeding risk
cefamandol, cefoperazone, cefotetan, cephalosporins May ↓ prothrombin/ ↑ bleeding risk

INCOMPATIBILITIES

Do not mix, dilute, infuse with other agents.

PATIENT CARE IMPLICATIONS
Before starting therapy
• Obtain baseline 12-lead ECG.
• Review history for contraindications.
• Have emergency resuscitation equipment, including epinephrine, lidocaine, atropine, immediately available.
• Apply pressure dressings to unsuccessful venipuncture attempts.
• Start 2 or more 18-gauge or larger catheters for laboratory samples; medications, fluids, emergency use.

• See many precautions under Administration
During/immediately after therapy
• Avoid unnecessary venipuncture, invasive procedures, IM injections.
• If venipuncture necessary, hold manual pressure over site for 20 min or until bleeding stops, then apply pressure dressing. Inspect frequently for bleeding.
• If arterial puncture necessary, avoid femoral site, hold manual pressure over puncture site for 30 min or until bleeding stops. Apply pressure dressing, inspect frequently for bleeding.
• Avoid arterial/venous invasive procedures in areas inaccessible to manual compression (e.g., internal jugular, subclavian).
• Transient dysrhythmias, reduced chest pain, reduction of ST segment elevation suggest successful thrombolysis, coronary reperfusion.
• Notify physician of significant dysrhythmias, unusual or excessive bleeding, change in neurologic status, unrelieved or recurrent chest pain.
Vital signs/hemodynamics:
Initially, monitor BP, HR q5-15min; when stable progress to q30-60min during and for several hours after infusion. Hypotension may result from reperfusion dysrhythmias, hemorrhage, impaired myocardial contractility; carefully evaluate each case. • Immediately consult physician for severe or uncontrolled hypertension (SBP >180 or DBP >110 mm Hg). Prepare to initiate antihypertensive therapy. • Continuously monitor ECG for dysrhythmias, changes in ST segment eleva-

U

tion. Anticipate reperfusion dysrhythmias; if symptomatic, manage according to ACLS guidelines (Appendix P).
Physical assessment: Assess/document chest pain intensity, character, location, radiation, duration. Note any associated symptoms. • Monitor all vascular access sites, assess for bleeding at 15-min intervals during and immediately after infusion, then q4h for 24 hr. If bleeding occurs, apply pressure, continue to monitor closely. Infusion may need to be discontinued if bleeding becomes excessive. • Assess peripheral pulses for diminished intensity, especially those distal to arterial puncture or other invasive procedures. • Assess neurologic status before initiating therapy, frequently during, and immediately after infusion. Immediately consult physician for changes. • Assess for retroperitoneal bleeding (e.g., low back pain, flank ecchymosis). • Note blood in urine, other body fluids. Check emesis, stools for occult blood. • If used for peripheral arterial thrombolysis, perform q1-2h neurovascular checks
Laboratory tests: Monitor: CPK, CBC, PT, PTT, TT, fibrinogen before and after therapy • TT at frequent intervals during therapy • Cardiac enzymes for coronary thrombolysis • **May cause:** Unreliable results with coagulation studies; notify lab.

PATIENT/FAMILY TEACHING

Purpose of drug is to dissolve clots blocking blood flow. • Frequent monitoring is necessary because of many side effects. • Immediately report chest pain or discomfort, unusual bleeding (e.g., from venipunctures, nose, mouth, urine), breathing difficulty, itching. • Remain on bed rest throughout therapy. • Avoid potential trauma from shaving, toothbrushing, excessive activity for 24 hr after therapy.

AVAILABLE FORMS

Parenteral for IV injection/infusion

vancomycin
(van-koe-mye'sin)
Lyphocin, Vancocin, Vancoled, Vancor

Classification: Miscellaneous antibiotic

USUAL DOSE

NOT FOR IM USE
PO, adults: 500 mg-2 g/24 hr in divided doses q6-8h
P PO, children: 40 mg/kg/24 hr in divided doses q6-8h; do not exceed 2 g daily.
IV, adults: 500 mg q6h or 1 g q12h • **Renal insufficiency:** Initially 15 mg/kg; adjust subsequent doses to serum levels, creatinine clearance
P IV, children: 40 mg/kg/24 hr in divided doses q6h

ADMINISTRATION

IV, intermit inf: Infuse each dose over 60-90 min. Infusion rate of 10 mg/min results in fewer adverse reactions. "Red man's syndrome" (see Adverse Effects), hypotension may occur with too-rapid infusion • Rotate infusion sites. Use dilute solution, large vein, small catheter/needle to reduce risk of phlebitis.

PREPARATION

IV: Reconstitute 500-mg vial with 10 ml sterile water for injection; use 20 ml for 1-g vial; yields concentration of 50 mg/ml. • Further dilute each 500-mg dose with 100 ml compatible IV solution to yield concentration of 5 mg/ml.

Compatible fluids: D_5W, $D_{10}W$, 0.9% NaCl, LR • Peritoneal dialysis fluid, 1.5% or 4.25% dextrose, with and without heparin added to dialysis fluid; solution may precipitate if >6.9 g/L vancomycin used. • May not be compatible in alkaline solutions

Stability: Reconstituted IV solution stable for at least 24 hr at room temperature • Reconstituted PO solution stable for 14 days if refrigerated

ACTIONS

Bactericidal antibiotic that binds to bacterial cell wall, blocks bacterial synthesis/division • Active against most gram-positive bacteria, including staphylococci, methicillin-resistant staphylococci, group A beta-hemolytic streptococci, enterococci, *Streptococcus pneumoniae, Corynebacterium, clostridium* • Very active against *Enterococcus faecalis, Clostridium difficile* • Not active against gram-negative organisms • Oral forms not systemically absorbed; only effective against colitis caused by staphyloccal or *clostridium difficile* organisms

PHARMACOKINETICS

ROUTE	ONSET	PEAK	DURATION
IV	Immed	End infusion	Approx 6-12 hr

DISTRIBUTION
Widely distributed; CSF levels low

ELIMINATION
Eliminated in urine via glomerular filtration; half-life 4-6 hr

Therapeutic levels: Peak levels, 5-40 µg/ml; trough levels, 5-10 µg/ml.

INDICATIONS

Serious infections caused by gram-positive organisms when less toxic antibiotics such as penicillins, cephalosporins not effective • Choice agent for treatment of methicillin-resistant *Staphylococcus aureus* (MRSA), many other penicillin-resistant organisms • Alternate antibiotic for bacterial endocarditis prophylaxis • PO vancomycin choice agent for treatment of antibiotic-associated pseudomembranous colitis (AAPC) caused by *c. difficile*

PRECAUTIONS/ CONTRAINDICATIONS

Precautions: Bacterial or fungal overgrowth possible • Rapid IV infusion may cause "Red man's syndrome". • PO vancomycin not effective in treatment of systemic infections.

Use caution with: High-dose/prolonged therapy, concurrent use of other oto/nephrotoxic agents • Renal impairment, advanced age, preexisting hearing disorder, dehydration; oto/nephrotoxicity more likely. If use necessary, consider reduced dose/frequency. • Premature neonates, young infants

c Pregnancy category: Risk of fetal damage unknown; use only if safer alternative unavailable.

Contraindications: Hypersensitivity to vancomycin

ADVERSE EFFECTS

CNS: Headache, dizziness, insomnia/other sleep disorders, fatigue, **increased ICP (rare)**

EENT: *Ototoxicity,* including deafness, tinnitus, dizziness

CV: Hypotension

GI: Nausea, vomiting (PO), unpleasant taste (PO)

GU: ↑ Creatinine/BUN, renal insufficiency, vaginitis

Hema: Leukopenia, eosinophilia

Derm: Rash, pruritus

Local: *Pain, thrombophlebitis* (IV)

Misc: Superinfection, colonization; hypersensitivity, including **anaphylaxis, "Red man's syndrome"** (flushing and/or rash on face, neck, chest, upper extremities; hypotension; fever; chills; wheezing; seizures; cardiac arrest)

TOXICITY/OVERDOSE

Symptoms: Hypotension, "Red man's syndrome," other allergic reactions occur in up to 10% of patients with IV use.

Management: After recent ingestion, implement guidelines for management of acute overdose (Appendix I). • Optimize hydration with parenteral fluids. • For acute allergic reaction, see Appendix N. Premedication with antihistamine may prevent allergic reaction. • **Hypotension:** Elevate legs, administer IV fluids; use vasopressors if unresponsive to fluid replacement. • Hemodialysis or peritoneal dialysis not likely to be useful

INTERACTIONS

aminoglycosides, amphotericin B, bacitracin, cisplatin, polymyxin B Oto/nephrotoxicity

Y-SITE COMPATIBILITIES

Acyclovir, amiodarone, atracurium, diltiazem, enalaprilat, erythromycin, esmolol, fluconazole, hydromorphone, insulin, labetalol, magnesium sulfate, meperidine, morphine, ondansetron, pancuronium, potassium chloride, vecuronium, zidovudine

Y-SITE INCOMPATIBILITIES

Aminophylline, ceftazidime, cefotaxime, chloramphenicol, chlorothiazide, dexamethasone, methicillin, penicillin G, phenytoin, piperacillin-tazobactam, secobarbital

PATIENT CARE IMPLICATIONS

• Obtain specimens for culture and sensitivity before initiating antibiotic therapy. Initiate therapy before results received.

• Have epinephrine, antihistamine, resuscitation equipment readily available for use with severe allergic reaction.

• Do not discharge patient for at least 30 min after antibiotic administration.

• PO/NG routes not indicated for systemic infections; used only for enterocolitis or pseudomembranous colitis

IV injection/infusion

• Reduce risk of thrombophlebitis by using large veins, small catheters/needles; rotating infusion sites; using slow infusion rates.

• Assess hearing before and at **G** intervals during therapy in older

---

P pediatric   **G** geriatric   **V** Direct IV

adults, patients with preexisting hearing disorder/renal impairment. Early detection reduces risk of permanent deafness.
• Pretreatment with antihistamine may relieve symptoms of "Red man's syndrome" in patients who have previously experienced reaction.
Vital signs/hemodynamics: Monitor VS for indicators of infection, complications. • Monitor BP, HR closely during IV infusion, particularly during first few doses. • Carefully monitor UO, elevate I&O ratio. Decreasing volume, cloudy or pink urine may indicate nephrotoxicity. Keep patient well hydrated by oral or parenteral fluids of sufficient volume to produce adequate UO; Older, debilitated, seriously ill, renal-impaired patients at greater risk for toxicity.
Physical assessment: Assess for improvement in primary infection or symptoms of super/suprainfection: appearance of sputum, urine, stool, wound drainage; presence of fever, candidiasis, vaginitis. • Monitor all patients at intervals for symptoms of ototoxicity: hearing loss, dizziness, tinnitus. • Observe for symptoms of hypersensitivity: rash, pruritus, wheezing, laryngeal edema, hypotension
Laboratory tests: Monitor: Electrolytes, CBC with differential • Urinalysis, BUN, creatinine, creat. cl. before and regularly during therapy; follow closely in older adults, renal impairment, high-dose/prolonged therapy. • Serum vancomycin levels

PATIENT/FAMILY TEACHING

Purpose of drug is to limit growth of infection-causing bacteria. If used for MRSA, inform family members of appropriate transmission precautions. Immediately report flushing, rash, chills, difficulty breathing, other signs of allergic reaction. • Report diarrhea, blood in stool, fever, vaginal itching or discharge, furry growth on tongue, hearing difficulty, dizziness.
• Drink plenty of fluid. • Take all medication exactly as prescribed. Do not stop taking medicine even if you feel better. Failure to take all of antibiotic may result in recurrence or additional infection. Do not save or share unused medicine.

AVAILABLE FORMS

Parenteral for IV use • Capsules
• Powder for PO solution

---

vasopressin
(vay-soe-press'in)
Pitressin, Pressyn ✿

Classifications: Posterior pituitary hormone/antidiuretic, vasopressor

USUAL DOSE

SC/IM, adults: Central diabetes insipidus: 5-10 U 2-4 times daily; range, 5-60 U/day; adjust to patient response. • **Abdominal distention:** 5-10 U q3-4h
SC/IM, children: Central diabetes insipidus: 2.5-10 U 2-4 times daily; adjust to patient response.
Unlabeled/investigational:
IV, adults: Initially 20 U in 100 ml D_5W over 20 min • Im-

V

---

mediately follow with continuous infusion of 0.2-0.4 U/min; may increase up to 1 U/min.
• Use lowest effective dose.
• Other dosing regimens used
Intraarterial, adults: 0.1-1.5 U/min via angiographically placed arterial catheter

ADMINISTRATION

SC/IM: Administer with 1-2 glasses of water.
Unlabeled/investigational:
IV infusion: Initially 20 U dose over 20 min (1 U/min); follow with continuous infusion at 0.2 U. Adjust gradually q10-15min to control bleeding while minimizing adverse effects; do not exceed 1 U/min. • Infuse via central, antecubital, or other large vein. • Use infusion pump.
• Slow or stop for symptomatic bradycardia, serious dysrhythmias (e.g., multifocal PVCs, ventricular tachycardia), chest pain, ECG evidence of myocardial ischemia.
Intraarterial: Administer via angiographically placed catheter into superior mesenteric or other artery according to bleeding source. • Start at 0.1 U/min, adjust gradually q10-15min to control bleeding while minimizing adverse effects. • Use infusion pump or syringe delivery device (do not use low-pressure or drop-counting device).
• Slow or stop for symptomatic bradycardia, serious dysrhythmias (e.g., multifocal PVCs, ventricular tachycardia), chest pain, ECG evidence of myocardial ischemia.

PREPARATION

COMMON DILUTIONS	CONCENTRATION
20 U/100 ml (initial)	0.2 U/ml
200 U/500 ml (continuous)	0.4 U/ml

Compatible fluids: D_5W, 0.9% NaCl, prepared combinations of these solutions

ACTIONS

Antidiuretic hormone that causes increased reabsorption of water by renal tubules, resulting in more concentrated urine; urine osmolality increases, UO decreases. • Has potent vasopressor effect when large doses used • Causes smooth muscle contraction, resulting in vasoconstriction/increased peristalsis • CV/hemodynamics: Causes vasoconstriction, particularly of capillaries, small arterioles; cardiac effects include ↑ afterload; ↓ HR; ↓ coronary blood flow, contractility, CO; causes generalized reduction in blood flow, especially of splanchnic, portal systems • GI: Increases tone, peristaltic activity, especially of large bowel; ↓ splanchnic, portal, pancreatic, mesenteric blood flow; reduces ↑ portal venous pressure, decreases blood loss from acute variceal bleeding; may lead to bowel ischemia, necrosis

PHARMACOKINETICS

ROUTE	ONSET	PEAK	DURATION
SC/IM	10-15 min	1-2 hr	2-8 hr
IV	Immed	Rapid	15-20 min

DISTRIBUTION
Throughout extracellular fluid
ELIMINATION
Rapidly destroyed by liver, kidneys; half-life 10-20 min

INDICATIONS

Prevention/control of excessive UO, dehydration in patients with central diabetes inspidus • Reduction of postop abdominal distention • Treatment of other conditions associated with intestinal hypomotility, excessive gas, distention
Unlabeled/investigational:
Adjunct in treatment of acute massive upper GI bleeding, especially that associated with ruptured esophageal varices; IV route generally considered safer, as effective as intraarterial; may be given concomitantly with IV nitroglycerin to counteract cardiotoxic effects, enhance reduction of portal venous pressure

PRECAUTIONS/ CONTRAINDICATIONS

Precautions: Tissue necrosis, sloughing may result from extravasation during IV infusion.
Use caution with: Cardiac disease • Severe vascular disease • Seizure disorders, coma, migraine • Asthma • Renal disease
c Pregnancy category: Use in pregnancy only when clearly needed and benefits outweigh risk.
Contraindications: Hypersensitivity to beef/pork proteins • Chronic nephritis with ↑ BUN

ADVERSE EFFECTS

CNS: *Tremor, pounding in head, vertigo,* **cerebral hemorrhage**
Resp: **Respiratory arrest**
CV: *Peripheral/visceral vasoconstriction,* hypertension, **reflex bradycardia, dysrhythmias,** myocardial ischemia, angina, **acute MI,** ↓ CO

GI: *Nausea, vomiting, abdominal cramps, passage of gas, belching,* diarrhea, hypermotility, bowel ischemia/necrosis
GU: ↓ UO, ↑ urine specific gravity
Derm: *Circumoral pallor, sweating,* paleness, sloughing/ necrosis of skin at infusion site, cutaneous gangrene
Misc: Water intoxication, fever
Hypersensitivity: Urticaria, angioedema, bronchoconstriction, rash, wheezing, dyspnea, circulatory collapse, cardiac arrest, anaphylaxis

TOXICITY/OVERDOSE

Symptoms: Water intoxication, drowsiness, listlessness, headache, confusion, anuria, weight gain • Possible seizures, coma, death • **IV:** Cardiotoxicity manifested by coronary insufficiency, ↓ CO, myocardial ischemia, angina, dysrhythmias
Management: Water intoxication: Discontinue drug, restrict fluid intake; if severe, promote diuresis with furosemide osmotic diuretics (e.g., mannitol, hypertonic dextrose, urea) • **Cardiotoxicity:** Reduce or discontinue infusion. Use concomitant IV nitroglycerin to counter vasoconstriction. Treat dysrhythmias according to ACLS guidelines (Appendix P).

INTERACTIONS

alcohol ↓ Antidiuretic effects
carbamazepine ↑ Antidiuretic effects
epinephrine ↓ Antidiuretic effects
heparin ↓ Antidiuretic effects
lithium ↓ Antidiuretic effects
TCAs ↑ Antidiuretic effects

V

Y-SITE COMPATIBILITIES
Information not available

PATIENT CARE IMPLICATIONS
• Use lowest effective dose for shortest possible time.
• **SC/IM:** Unless contraindicated by patient condition, administer with 1-2 glasses of water to reduce adverse effects, improve drug efficacy.
• Many precautions necessary with IV use; see Administration.
Vital signs/hemodynamics: Obtain baseline 12-lead ECG before initiating therapy and periodically during IV/intra-arterial therapy. Check for evidence of ischemia/infarction. • **GI bleeding:** Monitor BP, pulse q15-30min. • Continuously monitor ECG for significant dysrhythmias, ischemic changes, including ST depression. Anticipate immediate lowering of HR with initiation of therapy. • Monitor CVP, central hemodynamics as available. Monitor fluid intake carefully to avoid water intoxication.
Physical assessment: Assess for water intoxication: drowsiness, listlessness, headache, confusion, anuria, weight gain.
• Weigh patient daily. • Monitor/measure I&O. • **Diabetes insipidus:** Evaluate response to therapy by assessing for dehydration (thirst, tachycardia, dry mucous membranes, poor skin turgor). Measure urine specific gravity regularly. • **GI bleeding:** Evaluate response to therapy by monitoring amount/frequency of bleeding, presence of abdominal distention, bowel sounds. Titrate as necessary to control bleeding while minimizing side effects. • Assess for perfusion/oxygenation deficit: ↓ level of consciousness, hypotension, chest discomfort, dizziness. • Assess for diminished peripheral perfusion: coolness, ↓ pulse intensity, paresthesias, delayed capillary refill. • Check infusion site frequently for signs of extravasation (e.g., blanching along vein pathway, coldness, hardness). If this occurs, change infusion site immediately, infiltrate affected area with 5-10 mg phentolamine mixed with 10 ml saline. • Monitor UO qh; consult physician if ≤5 ml/kg/hr or ≤30 ml/hr for 2 consecutive hr.
Laboratory tests: Monitor: Electrolytes • Urine osmolality, specific gravity • Hct/Hgb in patients with GI bleeding

PATIENT/FAMILY TEACHING
Explain drug action, need for frequent monitoring. • Immediately report chest pain or discomfort, palpitations, headache, pain at IV infusion site. • Inform patient of common side effects such as abdominal cramping, elimination of gas, sweating.

AVAILABLE FORMS
20 U/ml in 0.5- and 1-ml ampules

---

vecuronium bromide
(vek-yoo-roe′nee-um)
Norcuron

Classification: Nondepolarizing neuromuscular blocking agent

USUAL DOSE

Direct IV injection, adults/
❶ children: Initially 0.08-0.1
mg/kg (usually 5-7 mg for aver-
age-sized adult) • Maintenance,
0.008-0.015 mg/kg q12-40min
as needed for skeletal muscle
❶ relaxation • Children >10yr,
dose same as adults; children
1-9 yr may require slightly
higher dosage. • **Major burns:**
Resistance to neuromuscular
blocking effects usually occurs;
increased doses are necessary.
• **Renal insufficiency:** Initial
dose same; less frequent, lower
maintenance doses required
IV, cont inf, adults: 1 μg/kg/
min; adjust to maintain desired
neuromuscular blockade; usual
range, 0.8-1.2 μg/kg/min. • Decreased dose usually effective in
❶ older adults

ADMINISTRATION

▼ Direct IV: Inject each dose over
30-60 sec. • *Causes respiratory*
depression, paralysis; means for
airway management, and con-
tinuous artificial ventilation
must be in place or provided
immediately after injection.
IV, cont inf: Adjust infusion to
minimal dose required to maintain 90% suppression of twitch
response (using peripheral nerve
stimulator) or desired neuromuscular blockade.

PREPARATION

Dilute each 10 mg with 10 ml
sterile bacteriostatic water supplied by manufacturer. Concentration will be 1 mg/ml. • May
be further diluted in compatible
solution for ease in administration or continuous infusion

Compatible fluids: D_5W,
0.9% NaCl, LR, prepared combinations of these solutions

ACTIONS

Causes skeletal muscle paralysis
by interfering with transmission
of nerve impulses at neuromuscular junction • Competes with,
blocks activity of acetylcholine,
the neurotransmitter that normally produces electrical depolarization • First muscles, affected include eyes, face, neck;
followed by limbs, abdomen,
chest; diaphragm affected last.
Recovery usually occurs in reverse order, takes ≥60 min.
• Unlike other nondepolarizing
NMBAs, has minimal CV ef-
fects • More potent than pancuronium with shorter duration;
vecuronium less likely to stimulate histamine release • No analgesic, sedative effects

PHARMACOKINETICS

ROUTE	ONSET	PEAK	DURATION
IV	30 sec	3-5 min	25-60 min

DISTRIBUTION
Throughout extracellular fluid
ELIMINATION
Excreted in urine, feces; half-life 31-80
min

INDICATIONS

Adjunct to general anesthesia to
produce skeletal muscle relaxation during surgery • To facilitate ET intubation in nonemergency situations; succinylcholine preferred during emergencies because of rapid onset
of action • No effects on con-
sciousness/pain threshold; used
only after induction of general
anesthesia or with appropriate
analgesics/anxiolytics
• Particularly useful with critically ill/cardiac patients in

V

---

italic = common side effects   **bold** = life-threatening reactions

whom CV alterations caused by other NMBAs would be undesired • To provide skeletal muscle relaxation, increase lung compliance, during mechanical ventilation of critically ill patients.

PRECAUTIONS/ CONTRAINDICATIONS

Precautions: *Causes respiratory paralysis; must use with artificial airway, ventilatory support, O_2 administration* • Long-term use to facilitate mechanical ventilation associated with prolonged paralysis, skeletal muscle weakness • Does not cause tachycardia; will not counteract bradycardia caused by some anesthetics (e.g., fentanyl) • Burn patients may develop resistance to neuromuscular blocking effects, particularly if burn exceeds 25% body surface area; increased doses usually necessary.

Use caution with: Renal insufficiency; reduce dose for creatinine clearance <10 L/min • Hepatic dysfunction • Pulmonary impairment, respiratory depression • Advanced age • Debilitation • Myasthenia gravis; extreme caution indicated • Neonates • Electrolyte disturbances (i.e., hypermagnesemia, hypokalemia, hypocalcemia)

C **Pregnancy category:** Use only if safer alternative unavailable.

Contraindications: Hypersensitivity to vecuronium or bromides • Children <7: Safety/efficacy not established

ADVERSE EFFECTS

CNS: Muscle weakness, **paralysis**

Resp: **Respiratory depression, prolonged apnea**

Misc: Hypersensitivity reactions (rare)

TOXICITY/OVERDOSE

Symptoms: Prolonged effects • Hypersensitivity, anaphylaxis
Management: Provide airway/continuous artificial ventilation. • Neostigmine or pyridostigmine with atropine q5-30min to reverse neuromuscular blockade; may worsen severe overdose • For management of acute allergic reaction, see Appendix N.

INTERACTIONS

aminoglycosides, amphotericin B, beta-blockers, calcium channel blockers, corticosteroids, diuretics (potassium wasting), lidocaine, magnesium sulfate Prolonged neuromuscular blockade
opiate analgesics Respiratory depression

Y-SITE COMPATIBILITIES

Aminophylline, cefazolin, cefuroxime, cimetidine, dobutamine, dopamine, epinephrine, esmolol, fentanyl, gentamicin, heparin, isoproterenol, lorazepam, midazolam, morphine, nitroglycerin, nitroprusside, ranitidine, vancomycin

Y-SITE INCOMPATIBILITIES

Diazepam, any alkaline solution

PATIENT CARE IMPLICATIONS

• Drug has no effect on consciousness/pain threshold; patient will be fully awake and feel all sensations. USE ONLY WITH GENERAL ANESTHESIA OR ANALGESICS (e.g., MORPHINE)/ANXIOLYTICS

(e.g., DIAZEPAM, MIDAZO-LAM).
• Causes respiratory paralysis, apnea; use only for patients under direct observation and continuous mechanical ventilation.
• Prevent corneal drying by instillation of artificial tears, eye patching.
• Cholinesterase inhibitors such as neostigmine, pyridostigmine, used to reverse effects; multiple doses may be necessary.
• Long-term use with mechanical ventilation associated with prolonged paralysis, skeletal muscle weakness. Monitor closely; use lowest effective dose.
• Patients thought to have recovered from neuromuscular blockade may develop apnea when given certain drugs that potentiate vecuronium (see Interactions).
• Effects prolonged with acidosis, shortened with alkalosis.
Vital signs/hemodynamics: Monitor ECG continuously, observe for dysrhythmias. • Monitor BP, observing for hypotension, q3-5min during initiation of therapy and frequently thereafter. Be aware that ↑ HR, BP could indicate inadequate sedation or need for analgesics.
• Use continuous pulse oximetry to monitor oxygenation during and immediately after extubation.
Physical assessment: Closely monitor respiratory status: rate, depth, pattern of ventilation until fully recovered. • Use peripheral nerve stimulator to monitor effectiveness of NMBAs. Maintain 90% suppression of twitch response. Paralysis of muscle groups usually occurs in following order: eyelids, jaws, limbs,

abdomen, glottis, intercostals, diaphragm. Recovery occurs in reverse order. Assess frequently for residual muscle weakness, respiratory distress until fully recovered from effects. • Monitor I&O; Foley catheter required.
Laboratory tests: Monitor electrolytes closely, especially magnesium, potassium, calcium. Hypermagnesemia, hypokalemia, hypocalcemia may cause prolonged neuromuscular blockade.

PATIENT/FAMILY TEACHING

Purpose of medication is to paralyze body muscles temporarily to facilitate procedures, surgery. • When recovering from effects, it may be difficult to swallow, talk. These effects are temporary. • Drug does not affect consciousness; explain all procedures, provide information/emotional support, remind family to communicate with patient.

AVAILABLE FORMS

Parenteral for IV injection
Storage: Refrigerated storage recommended for optimal stability; stable for 6 mo at room temperature; do not store in plastic syringes.

verapamil HCl
(ver-ap'a-mill)
Apo Verap ✱, Calan, Calan SR, Isoptin, Isoptin SR, Nu-Verap ✱, Verelan

Classifications: Class IV antidysrhythmic, calcium channel blocker, antihypertensive, antianginal

USUAL DOSE

G PO, adult: Standard preparation, 80-120 mg q6-8h • Older adults, 40 mg q8h • Sustained-release preparation, 120-240 mg qAM • **Hepatic impairment:** Reduced dosage indicated

Direct IV, adults: 5-10 mg; may repeat in 15-20 min

IV, cont inf, adults: 5-10 mg/hr • Sometimes used for prophylaxis of SVT after initial conversion

P IV, children <1 yr: 0.1-0.2 mg/kg

P IV, children 1-15 yr: 0.1-0.3 mg/kg; may repeat in 30 min • Do not exceed 5 mg total dose in single injection.

ADMINISTRATION

V Direct IV, adults: Inject each dose of ≤10 mg SLOWLY over 2-3 min • Too-rapid injection may cause profound hypotension; monitor BP closely. • Continuously monitor ECG for dysrhythmias.

IV, cont inf, adults: Initiate at 5 mg/hr; may increase to 10 mg/hr as needed to control SVT. • Use infusion pump.

Compatible fluids: D_5W, 0.9% NaCl, prepared combinations of these solutions

ACTIONS

Inhibits movement of calcium ions across myocardium, vascular smooth muscle • Inhibits myocardial contractility, causes vasodilation • Slows AV conduction, prolongs AV node refractoriness; PR interval may be prolonged; no change in QT interval. • May cause 2nd/3rd degree heart block • Has little effect on antegrade, retrograde conduction in accessory pathways • Afterload reduction decreases myocardial O_2 requirements.

PHARMACOKINETICS

ROUTE	ONSET	PEAK	DURATION
IV	3-5 min	10-15 min	1-6 hr
PO, std	30 min	1-2 hr	6-8 hr

DISTRIBUTION

Wide; 83%-92% bound to plasma proteins

ELIMINATION

Metabolized in liver; eliminated by kidneys, in feces; half-life 2-8 hr

Therapeutic level: 80-300 ng/ml

INDICATIONS

Suppression/prevention of SVT • Management of vasospastic, chronic stable/unstable angina • Control of essential hypertension • Sustained-release preparations used exclusively for control of hypertension

PRECAUTIONS/ CONTRAINDICATIONS

Precautions: May cause transient hypotension when therapy initiated. IV dose may cause significant hypotension, especially with too-rapid administration. • Negative inotropic effects may exacerbate heart failure, particularly in patients with pre-existing heart disease. • Dysrhythmias possible after rhythm conversion

G Use caution with: Older adults, hepatic impairment; dosage reduction may be necessary.

C Pregnancy category: Use only if safer alternative unavailable.

Contraindications: Hypersensitivity to verapamil • Significant hypotension • Sick sinus syndrome; accessory conduction pathways or preexcitation syn-

---

drome (WPW, Lown-Ganong-Levine [LGL] syndrome) • Sinus bradycardia, 2nd/3rd degree heart block without functional ventricular pacemaker in place or readily available • Severe heart failure

ADVERSE EFFECTS

CNS: *Dizziness,* fatigue, headache, depression, blurred vision

Resp: Dyspnea, pulmonary edema

CV: *Hypotension,* bradycardia, peripheral edema, **exacerbation of heart block/failure;** rarely—**ventricular fibrillation, asystole**

GI: *Constipation,* nausea, ↑ of liver enzymes

GU: Polyuria, urinary retention

Derm: Rash, pruritus, sweating

Misc: Tachyphylaxis, worsening of symptoms of Duchenne's muscular dystrophy

TOXICITY/OVERDOSE

Symptoms: Profound hypotension • Dysrhythmias: bradycardia, 2nd/3rd degree heart block, junctional rhythm, ventricular fibrillation, asystole • Heart failure, generalized edema • Dizziness, drowsiness, confusion, slurred speech

Management: After recent ingestion, implement guidelines for management of acute overdose (Appendix H). • **Hypotension:** Elevate legs, administer IV fluids; beta-adrenergic agonists/IV calcium chloride, except in patients with hypertrophic cardiomyopathy; vasopressors (e.g., norepinephrine, dopamine) used if unresponsive to other measures. In patients with hypertrophic cardiomyopathy or IHSS, alpha-adrenergic agents (e.g., metaraminol, methoxamine, phenylephrine) used • **Symptomatic bradycardia, heart block:** Use IV atropine, calcium, epinephrine, possibly isoproterenol; consider temporary pacemaker. • **Other dysrhythmias:** Rapid ventricular response from antegrade conduction (e.g., WPW, LGL): direct-current cardioversion, IV lidocaine, or procainamide; asystole. Other dysrhythmias managed according to ACLS guidelines (Appendix P) • Calcium may be helpful in reversing adverse hemodynamic effects but may not always reverse electrophysiologic toxicity. • Hemodialysis cannot remove drug.

INTERACTIONS

angiotension-converting enzyme inhibitors Profound hypotension

antihypertensives Profound hypotension

beta-blockers Heart failure, profound hypotension, heart block

calcium ↓ Verapamil effectiveness

digoxin Heart block, ↑ digoxin levels

disopyramide Heart failure

diuretics Profound hypotension

fentanyl Profound hypotension

NMBAs Prolonged neuromuscular blockade

theophylline ↑ Theophylline levels/toxicity

vasodilators Profound hypotension

Y-SITE COMPATIBILITIES

Amrinone, ciprofloxacin, dobutamine, dopamine, famotidine, meperidine, methicillin, milrinone, penicillin G potassium, piperacillin, ticarcillin

V

---

italic = common side effects   **bold** = life-threatening reactions

Y-SITE INCOMPATIBILITIES
Alkaline solutions (pH >6), aminophylline, amphotericin B, ampicillin, nafcillin, oxacillin, sodium bicarbonate

PATIENT CARE IMPLICATIONS
G • Older adults may experience profound hypotension. Use lowest effective dose; monitor closely.
• Anticipate higher incidence of adverse effects in patients receiving multiple or high-dose therapy.
SVT
• Consider appropriate vagal maneuvers to convert rhythm before administration.
• Use synchronized cardioversion for immediate stabilization of unstable patients with SVT.
• Before drug administration, evaluate 12-lead ECG for short PR interval, delta waves, other evidence of preexcitation syndrome (i.e., WPW, LGL).
• Patient should remain in bed for at least 3 hr after last dose and will require assistance with initial ambulation.
Vital signs/hemodynamics: Monitor BP, HR. • For hypotension, symptomatic bradycardia, withhold therapy, consult with physician. • Monitor central hemodynamics, CO frequently as available. Be alert for ↑ PCWP, other evidence of left ventricular failure.
IV: Continuously monitor cardiac rhythm for return of sinus rhythm, dysrhythmias (atrial fibrillation with rapid ventricular response, extreme bradycardia, asystole). • Monitor BP q2-5min during and immediately after IV administration.

Physical assessment: Assess for evidence of pulmonary edema: bibasilar crackles, neck vein distention, S_3 gallop, breathing difficulty, especially in patients with CHF, cardiomyopathy. • Assess for perfusion/oxygenation deficit: ↓ level of consciousness, decreased BP, activity intolerance, chest discomfort. • Observe for signs of hepatic dysfunction (e.g., elevated liver enzymes, jaundice, abdominal discomfort) in patients receiving long-term therapy.

PATIENT/FAMILY TEACHING
Purpose of medication is to control high BP, relieve angina pain, or slow rapid heartbeat.
• May cause dizziness, especially during initiation of therapy; use caution, change positions slowly • Report breathing difficulty, chest pain, palpitations, activity intolerance, swelling of feet/ankles. • Sustained-release tablets should never be broken, chewed, or crushed.
• Sustained-release preparations should be taken with food. • IV: Remain in bed during and for several hours after last dose.

AVAILABLE FORMS
Parenteral for IV injection
• Standard tablets • Sustained-release tablets, capsules

---

warfarin sodium
(war'far-in)
Coumadin, Panwarfin, Sofarin

Classification: Anticoagulant

USUAL DOSE

PO, adults: Initially 10-15 mg once daily for 2-4 days, then individualized by serial PT, clinical condition • Maintenance range, 2-10 mg once daily; adjust dose to maintain INR of 2.0-3.0 (e.g., PT ratio of 1.2-1.5); maintain INR of 2.5-3.5 in patients with mechanical heart valves. • Older adults: Use lower end of dosage range.

ACTIONS

Promotes anticoagulation by altering synthesis of vitamin K–dependent coagulation factors (II, VII, IX, X) • Inhibits thrombus formation, may prevent extension of existing thrombi • Does not dissolve established clots • Maximal anticoagulation with antithrombogenic effects after 2-7 days of therapy

PHARMACOKINETICS

ROUTE	ONSET	PEAK	DURATION
PO	8-12 hr	0.5-3 days*	2-5 days

DISTRIBUTION
Up to 99% bound to plasma protein

ELIMINATION
Metabolized in liver, excreted in urine/feces; half-life 0.5-3 days

*Time to peak PT.

INDICATIONS

Prophylaxis/treatment of venous thrombosis and its extension, embolism related to atrial fibrillation or mitral valve disease, and pulmonary embolism • As adjunct in treatment of coronary occlusion • Heparin may be used for immediate anticoagulations; with concurrent warfarin therapy used for 5-10 days until full antithrombogenic effects

achieved. • Prevention of thromboembolism after prosthetic heart valve placement; often used with antiplatelet agents.

PRECAUTIONS/ CONTRAINDICATIONS

Precautions: May cause minor to major bleeding resulting in death; usual sites of massive hemorrhage are GI/GU tissues. • ↑ Risk of bleeding with recent trauma, surgery, uncontrolled hypertension, indwelling catheters • Diet, drugs, other factors affect response to warfarin therapy, may ↑ risk of hemorrhage or ↓ therapeutic effects. • Certain factors ↑ risk of hemorrhage: vitamin K deficiency, malabsorption, alterations in intestinal bacteria, some antibiotic therapy, malnutrition/cachexia, small body size, hepatic/renal impairment, hypermetabolic states (e.g., fever, sepsis, hyperthyroidism), infectious disease, carcinoma, CHF, diarrhea, advanced age. • Certain factors ↓ therapeutic effects: increased intake of vitamin K, diabetes mellitus, edema, hyperlipidemia, hypothyroidism, viceral carcinoma, hereditary resistance to coumarin derivatives.

✗ Pregnancy category: Do not use during pregnancy.
Contraindications: Hypersensitivity • Active bleeding • Tartrazine sensitivity (Panwarfin 7.5-mg tablets only) • Hemorrhagic blood disorders • Recent major surgery, CNS surgery, eye surgery, procedures with potential for uncontrollable bleeding • Open wounds or ulceration of the GI, respiratory, GU tracts • Cerebrovascular hemorrhage • Aneurysms (cerebral, aortic) • Pericarditis, peri-

W

cardial effusion • Bacterial endocarditis • Uncontrolled hypertension • Children: Safe use not established

ADVERSE EFFECTS

EENT: Mouth ulcers, gingival bleeding, epistaxis

GI: Nausea/vomiting, anorexia, abdominal cramps, diarrhea

GU: Hematuria

Endo: **Adrenal hemorrhage with acute adrenal insufficiency**

Hema: *Hemorrhage, bruising, ecchymosis, hematoma,* agranulocytosis, eosinophilia, leukopenia

Derm: Dermatitis; urticaria; alopecia; rarely—**skin necrosis, gangrene**

Misc: Fever, purple toe syndrome (bilateral discoloration of toes with pain but not necrosis)

TOXICITY/OVERDOSE

Symptoms: Excessive bleeding; bleeding from gums, other mucous membranes; oozing from nicks made by shaving • Hematuria, hematemesis, melena, petechiae, ecchymoses

Management: After recent ingestion, implement guidelines for management of acute overdose (Appendix I). • Administer vitamin K_1 (phytonadione), using lowest effect dose to minimize risk of hypercoagulable state. • Initiate local measures such as manual compression followed by pressure dressings. • If bleeding severe, administer fresh whole blood, fresh frozen plasma, and/or commercial factor IX complex concomitantly. • Packed RBCs may be used to replace significant blood loss.

INTERACTIONS

cephalosporins, dextran, dipyridamole, heparin, NSAIDs, penicillins, sulfonamides ↑ Anticoagulation

phenytoin, sucralfate, vitamin K ↓ Anticoagulation

PATIENT CARE IMPLICATIONS

• Inform all personnel caring for patient of bleeding precautions associated with anticoagulant therapy. Place highly visible, written notice in patient's room.

• Avoid unnecessary venipuncture, arterial punctures, invasive procedures, IM injections.

• If IM injections necessary, use upper extremity so that site can be easily observed and bleeding managed.

• Avoid arterial/venous invasive procedures in areas inaccessible to manual compression, such as internal jugular or subclavian venipunctures.

Physical assessment: Assess for unusual bleeding, including petechiae, ecchymosis, bleeding from gums/mucous membranes, excessive bleeding from superficial injury. • Assess for evidence of occult bleeding, including paralysis; headache; pain in chest, abdomen, joints; shortness of breath; unexplained swelling; unexplained hypotension/shock. • Note blood in urine, other body fluids. Check emesis, stools for occult blood. • Assess fatty tissues of abdomen, breasts, buttocks, thighs for warfarin-induced necrosis. Observe for painful, erythematous patches that progress rapidly to dark, hemorrhagic areas. Consult physician immediately.

• Assess for improvement or deterioration of thromboembolic condition.

Laboratory tests: Obtain baseline PT, monitor at prescribed intervals during therapy. Maintain INR of 2.0-3.0 (e.g., PT ratio of 1.2-1.5); in patients with mechanical heart valves, maintain INR of 2.5-3.5. Monitor CBC, hepatic enzymes at intervals throughout therapy.

PATIENT/FAMILY TEACHING

This medication prevents excessive blood clotting. • Strict compliance with dosing schedule, instructions for lab testing are necessary to prevent serious complications. • Take medicine at same time each day. If dose missed, take as soon as remembered. Do not take more than 1 dose each day. Notify prescriber of missed doses at time of checkup or lab tests. • Immediately report unusual bruising, skin discoloration, bleeding (e.g., from venipunctures, nose, mouth, urine, in stools or emesis), diarrhea. • Do not take any other medicine or discontinue any medicine except on advice of prescriber or pharmacist. • Avoid alcohol, aspirin, NSAIDs, (e.g., ibuprofen). • Be aware of foods high in vitamin K (e.g., asparagus, beans, broccoli, brussel sprouts, cabbage, fish, green leafy vegetables, milk products, pork, rice); do not drastically alter intake. • Inform dentist, surgeon, lab personnel, other health care workers of anticoagulant therapy. • Avoid activities that may cause injury (e.g., use soft toothbrush, electric razor). • May cause harmless redorange discoloration of urine

• Wear Medic-Alert bracelet stating use of anticoagulant therapy.

AVAILABLE FORMS

Tablets

W

---

italic = common side effects   **bold** = life-threatening reactions

References

Acute pain management: operative and medical procedures and trauma, clinical practice guideline, AHCPR Pub No 92-0032, Agency for Health Care Policy and Research, Public Health Service, Rockville, Md, 1992, US Department of Health and Human Services.

American Heart Association's Educational Task Force of the ACLS Subcommittee: *ACLS algorithms and drugs,* Dallas, 1993, American Heart Association.

Chameides L, editor: *Textbook of pediatric advanced life support,* Dallas, 1990, American Heart Association.

Chernow B, editor: *The pharmacologic approach to the critically ill patient,* ed 3, Baltimore, 1994, William & Wilkins.

Cummins R, editor: *Textbook of advanced cardiac life support,* Dallas, 1994, American Heart Association.

Denniston P: *Physicians GenRx 1995,* ed 5, Riverside, Conn, 1995, Denniston Publishing.

Drug Evaluation Monographs, Micromedix, Vol 74, 1993.

Estoup M: Medication delivery in patients with enteral feeding tubes, *Crit Care Nurse* 14(1):68-79.

Gahart B: *Intravenous medications,* ed 11, St Louis, 1995, Mosby.

Hansten P, editor: *Drug interactions and updates quarterly,* ed 4, Vancouver, Wash, 1993, Applied Therapeutics.

Heyneman CA: Histamine-2 antagonists in allergic disorders, *The Ann Pharmacother* 28(6):742-3.

Kahn MG: *Cardiac drug therapy,* ed 3, London, 1992, Saunders.

Katz SL: Hepatitis B: a comprehensive strategy for eliminating transmission in the United States through universal childhood vaccination, *MMWR* 40:(RR13):1-25, 1991.

Kinney M, Packa D, Dunbar S, editors: *AACN's Clinical Reference for Critical-Care Nursing,* ed 3, St Louis, 1993, Mosby.

Koda-Kimble MA, Young LY, editors: Applied therapeutics: *the clinical use of drugs,* ed 5, Vancouver, Wash, 1992, Applied Therapeutics.

Leff R, Roberts R: *Practical aspects of intravenous drug administration,* ed 2, Bethesda, Md, 1992, American Society of Hospital Pharmacists.

McEvoy G, editor: *Drug information,* Bethesda, Md, 1995, American Society of Hospital Pharmacists.

Miyagawa C: Drug-nutrient interactions in critically ill patients, *Crit Care Nurse* 13(5):69-90.

Olin BR et al: *Drug facts and comparisons,* St Louis, 1995, Facts and Comparisons.

Phelps S, Cochran E: *Guidelines for administration of intravenous medications to pediatric patients,* ed 4, Bethesda, Md, 1993, American Society of Hospital Pharmacists.

Swearingen P, Keen J, editors: *Manual of critical care,* ed 3, St Louis, 1995, Mosby.

Thelan LA et al: *Critical care nursing: diagnosis and management,* ed 2, St Louis, 1994, Mosby.

Trissel LA: *Handbook on injectable drugs,* ed 4, Bethesda, Md, 1994, American Society of Hospital Pharmacists.

Whipple J et al: Selected vasoactive drugs: a readily available chart reference, *Crit Care Nurse* 12(3):23-29, 1992.

APPENDIX A

Conversions and Calculations

CONVERSIONS

Volume
5 ml = 1 teaspoon (tsp)
15 ml = 1 tablespoon (T)
30 ml = 1 ounce (oz) = 2 T
500 ml = 1 pint (pt)
1000 ml = 1 quart (qt)

Length
2.5 centimeters (cm) = 1 inch

Pressure
1 mm Hg = 1.36 cm H_2O

Weight
1 kilogram (kg) = 2.2 pounds (lb)
1 gram (g) = 1000 milligrams (mg)
1 mg = 1000 micrograms (μg)
1 grain (gr) = 60 mg
$1/100$ gr = 0.6 mg
$1/150$ gr = 0.4 mg

Centigrade (C)/Fahrenheit (F)
$°C = (F - 32) \times 5/9$
$°F = (C \times 9/5) + 32$

CRITICAL CARE CALCULATIONS

Drug concentration
mg/ml = Drug in solution (mg)/Volume of solution (ml)
μg/ml = mg/ml $\times$ 1000

Delivery rate
ml/min = ml/hr $\div$ 60 min/hr

$$\mu g/kg/min = \frac{\mu g/ml \times ml/min}{\text{Weight (kg)}}$$

$$ml/hr = \frac{\mu g/kg/min \text{ prescribed} \times kg \times 60 \text{ min/hr}}{\mu g/ml \text{ of solution}}$$

Rule of 15

Use for drugs that are dosed in μg/kg/min.

Patient weight (kg) $\times$ 15 = mg of drug to add to 250 cc.

Set flow rate to deliver desired dose as follows:

1 μg/kg/min = 1 microgtt/min (1 ml/hr)
2 μg/kg/min = 2 microgtt/min (2 ml/hr)

APPENDIX B

Hemodynamic Formulas and Normal Values

Cardiac output (CO)	$\dfrac{O_2 \text{ consumption}}{\text{A-V}O_2 \text{ difference}}$	4-7 L/min
Cardiac index (CI)	$\dfrac{\text{CO}}{\text{Body surface area (BSA)}}$	2.5-4 L/min/m²
Stroke volume (SV)	$\dfrac{\text{CO}}{\text{HR}} \times 1{,}000$	55-100 ml/beat
Arterial oxygen content (Ca_{O_2})	$(\text{Hgb} \times 1.34) \times Sa_{O_2}$	18-20 ml/vol%
Venous oxygen content (Cv_{O_2})	$(\text{Hgb} \times 1.34) \times Sv_{O_2}$	15.5 ml/vol%
Oxygen delivery (Do_2)	$Ca_{O_2} \times \text{CO} \times 10$	800-1,000 ml/min
Arteriovenous oxygen content difference ($C[a\text{-}v]o_2$)	$Ca_{O_2} - Cv_{O_2}$	4-6 ml/vol%
Oxygen consumption ($\dot{V}o_2$)	$\text{CO} \times 10 \times C(a\text{-}v)o_2$	200-250 ml/min
Systemic vascular resistance (SVR)	$\dfrac{\text{MAP} - \text{RAP}}{\text{CO}} \times 80$	900-1,200 dynes/sec/cm⁻⁵
Pulmonary vascular resistance (PVR)	$\dfrac{\text{PAM} - \text{PAWP}}{\text{CO}} \times 80$	60-100 dynes/sec/cm⁻⁵
Left ventricular stroke work index (LVSWI)	$\text{SVI} \times (\text{MAP} - \text{PAWP}) \times 0.136$	40-75 g/m²beat
Mean arterial pressure (MAP)	$\dfrac{\text{Systolic BP} + 2(\text{Diastolic BP})}{3}$	70-105 mm Hg
Mean pulmonary artery pressure (MPAP, PAM)	$\dfrac{\text{PAS} + 2(\text{PAD})}{3}$	10-15 mm Hg
Mixed venous oxygen saturation (Sv_{O_2})	$(\text{CO} \times Ca_{O_2} \times 10) - \dot{V}o_2$	60%-80%
Central venous pressure (CVP)		2-6 mm Hg
Right atrial pressure (RAP)		4-6 mm Hg
Left atrial pressure (LAP)		8-12 mm Hg
Right ventricular pressure (RVP)		25/0-5 mm Hg
Pulmonary artery pressure (PAP)		20-30/8-15 mm Hg
Pulmonary artery wedge pressure (PAWP)		6-12 mm Hg

Specialized Administration Routes Used in Critical and Emergency Care

ROUTE

Endotracheal (ET)

When IV access not available, selected emergency medications (e.g., epinephrine, lidocaine, atropine) can be administered endotracheally; dose usually 2-2.5 times recommended IV dose.

MANAGEMENT

- For adults dilute drug in 10 ml 0.9% NaCl or sterile water. Use smaller volume (e.g., 1-2 ml) for children.
- Place sterile catheter just past tip of ET tube; quickly spray medication into tube.
- Follow with 3-4 rapid insufflations to aerosolize medication.

Intraosseous (IO)

During emergencies in children <6 yr, catheter may be placed into proximal tibia to administer drugs/fluids; blood products, isotonic fluids, medications may be administered IO; used for temporary access only.

- Using sterile technique, insert standard 16- to 18-gauge hypodermic, spinal, or bone marrow needle into anterior surface of tibia.
- Confirm placement by aspiration of bone marrow, freely flowing IV solution without evidence of infiltration.
- Secure firmly with sterile dressing; tape to prevent dislodgement.
- Monitor for extravasation, patency.
- Flush with dilute heparin or saline to prevent clotting.
- Dilute hypertonic/alkaline solutions before administration.

ROUTE	MANAGEMENT

Intraperitoneal (IP)

Medications, especially antibiotics, sometimes added to peritoneal dialysate or lavage; medications have local/systemic effects, depending on absorption; local instillation of antibiotics reduces intraperitoneal bacteria

- Use sterile technique when adding medications to fluid for peritoneal lavage/dialysis.
- Confirm compatibility before adding multiple medications.
- Systemic absorption of aminoglycoside antibiotics may depress respiration, especially if patient has recently received NMBAs.

Gastric feeding tube (G-tube)

Route used for patients with functioning GI tracts/swallowing impairment; G-tube usually placed previously for enteral feeding or gastric decompression

- Verify presence of GI activity (e.g., bowel sounds), tube placement before medication administration.
- Use commercial liquid preparations when possible. If liquid is not available, many standard tablets can be crushed and mixed with water for administration. NEVER CRUSH TIME-RELEASED, LIQUID-FILLED, OR ENTERIC COATED PREPARATIONS. When in doubt, consult pharmacist.
- Use only commercially prepared liquid preparations with small-bore feeding tubes. Suspensions of crushed tablets may obstruct tube.
- Flush tube thoroughly before and after medication administration.
- Hyperosmolar liquids such as KCl, sorbitol, may cause gastric irritation, diarrhea. Dilute with water before administration.
- Administer multiple medications separately, flushing after each, to avoid incompatibilities.
- If suction prescribed, do not reconnect for 1-2 hr after medication administration.
- Feedings may affect the absorption of some drugs (e.g., phenytoin, warfarin, carbamazepine). Avoid resuming feedings for 1-2 hrs if absorption could be affected.

U.S. Food and Drug Administration Pregnancy Risk Categories

All drugs should be avoided during pregnancy, if possible. Potential benefits of any drug used during pregnancy must be weighed against possible fetal harm.

CATEGORY A

Well-controlled studies in women do not demonstrate fetal risk, and risk of harm is minimal.

CATEGORY B

Animal studies do not show risk, but data from studies in pregnant women or animals are insufficient to show clear evidence of risk to fetus, or studies in women have failed to demonstrate fetal harm.

CATEGORY C

Animal studies show adverse effects, but there are no studies in women, or no data are available from animal or human studies. In some situations, benefits of use may outweigh possible risks.

CATEGORY D

Human fetal harm has been demonstrated. In life-threatening illness, benefits of use may outweigh risks.

CATEGORY X

Human fetal harm has been clearly demonstrated, and possible risks to fetus outweigh any possible benefit to pregnant woman. Do not use during pregnancy.

Controlled Substances Classification

Controlled substances are classified by the U.S. Drug Enforcement Administration (DEA). State laws often are more stringent than federal laws. Health care providers must comply with both federal and state laws.

DESCRIPTION OF CATEGORIES

DRUG EXAMPLES

Schedule I

No accepted medical use; high potential for abuse; drug may be used for research when approved by application to DEA.

- *Cannabinols:* marijuana, hashish, tetrahydrocannabinol
- *Hallucinogens:* LSD, MDA, DMT, peyote, mescaline, psilocybin

Schedule II

High abuse potential exists, with possibility of severe psychologic/physical dependence.

- *Narcotics:* morphine, opium, codeine, hydromorphone (Dilaudid), methadone (Dolophine), meperidine (Demerol), oxycodone (Percodan)
- *Stimulants:* cocaine, amphetamine, dextroamphetamine, methamphetamine, methylphenidate (Ritalin)
- *Depressants:* amobarbital, methaqualone, pentobarbital, phencyclidine, secobarbital

Schedule III

Abuse potential less than with schedule I/II drugs; misuse leads to psychologic/physical dependence.

- *Narcotics:* opiates in limited amounts and combined with other nonnarcotic drugs (e.g., acetaminophen with codeine), paregoric
- *Depressants:* barbiturates, except those listed under other schedules

Schedule IV

Abuse potential less than with schedule III drugs; misuse leads to psychologic/possible physical dependence.

- *Narcotics:* pentazocine, propoxyphene (Darvon)
- *Depressants:* benzodiazepines (e.g., alprazolam, chlordiazepoxide, diazepam, flurazepam, lorazepam, midazolam, oxazepam), chloral hydrate, paraldehyde, phenobarbital

Schedule V

Abuse potential less than with schedule IV drugs; contains limited amount of narcotics; includes preparations used for cough, diarrhea.

- buprenorphine, diphenoxylate/atropine (Lomotil), loperamide, antitussives containing codeine/dihydrocodeine

Equianalgesic Doses of Opioid Analgesics

Class/Name	Route	Equianalgesic Dose (Mg)*	Average Duration (Hr)
Morphinelike agonists			
codeine	IM, SC	75†	3
	PO	130†	3
hydromorphone (Dilaudid)	IM, SC	1.5	4
	PO	7.5	4
levorphanol (Levo-Dromoran)	IM, SC	2.0	6
	PO	4.0	6
morphine	IM, SC	10	4
	PO	30-60	
oxycodone (Percodan)	PO	30†	4
hydrocodone (Cortab, Vicodin)	PO	30†	4
oxymorphone (Numorphan)	IM, SC	1.0-1.5	4
	rectal	10	4
Meperidine-like agonists			
fentanyl (Sublimaze)	IV, IM, SC, TD	0.1-0.2	1‡
meperidine (Demerol)	IM, SC	100	3
	PO	300†	3
Methadone-like agonists			
methadone (Dolophine)	IM, SC	10	6
	PO	20	6
propoxyphene (Darvon)	PO	130-250†	4
Mixed agonist-antagonists§			
buprenorphine (Buprenex)	IM	0.3-0.4	4
butorphanol (Stadol)	IM, SC	2.0	3
nalbuphine (Nubain)	IM, SC	10	4
pentazocine (Talwin)	IM	60	3
	PO	150†	3

Adapted from Koda-Kimble MA et al: *Applied therapeutics: the clinical use of drugs, ed 5, Vancouver, Wash, 1992, Applied Therapeutics and Acute Pain Management: operative and medical procedures and trauma, clinical practice guideline,* AH CPR Pub No 92-0032, Agency for Health Care Policy and Research, Public Health Service, Rockville, Md, 1992, US Dept of Health and Human Services.

*Recommended starting dose; actual dose must be titrated to patient response.

†Starting doses lower (codeine 30 mg, oxycodone 5 mg, meperidine 50 mg, propoxyphene 65-130 mg, pentazocine 50 mg).

‡Respiratory depressant effects persist longer than analgesic effects.

§Mixed agonist/antagonist analgesics may precipitate withdrawal in opioid-dependent patients.

Modified Vaughan-Williams Classification of Antidysrhythmics

Class/Drugs	Electrophysiologic Effects	Indications
IA disopyramide moricizine* procainamide quinidine	Exhibit membrane-stabilizing effects; inhibit rapid sodium influx: "fast channel" blocking agents; may slightly prolong or shorten action potential duration, decrease myocardial irritability; QRS complex, QT interval increased	Atrial fibrillation, PACs, PVCs, ventricular tachycardia, WPW
IB lidocaine mexiletine phenytoin tocainide	Exhibit membrane-stabilizing effects (see IA); depending on specific agent, may slightly prolong or shorten action potential duration, decrease ventricular irritability; no change in QRS/QT	PVCs, ventricular tachycardia/fibrillation
IC encainide* flecainide* lorcainide propafenone	Exhibit membrane-stabilizing effects (see IA); minimal effects on action potential duration; increase QRS width without changes in QT	Severe ventricular dysrhythmias
II acebutolol atenolol esmolol metoprolol nadolol propranolol timolol	Exhibit beta-adrenergic blocking effects; inhibit sympathetic stimulation of cardiac electrical system, reduce HR, decrease myocardial irritability	Supraventricular/ventricular dysrhythmias, general myocardial depression
III amiodarone* bretylium sotalol*	Delay repolarization, prolong effective refractory period/action potential duration, thus decreasing myocardial irritability	Ventricular tachycardia/fibrillation
IV diltiazem verapamil	Exhibit calcium channel–blocking effects, inhibit "slow channel" calcium influx, decrease HR	SVT, atrial fibrillation/flutter
UNCLASSIFIED adenosine	Slows conduction time through AV node, interrupts reentry pathways to decrease HR	SVT

*Use limited to symptomatic, life-threatening ventricular dysrhythmias, such as sustained ventricular tachycardia.

Tetanus Prophylaxis in Routine Wound Management

History of Adsorbed Tetanus Toxoid (Doses)	Clean, Minor Wounds		All Other Wounds*	
	Td†	TIG	Td†	TIG
Unknown or < three	Yes	No	Yes	Yes
≥three‡	No§	No	No‖	No

Adapted from Centers for Disease Control: *MMW* 34(27):422, 1985.

*Such as, but not limited to, wounds resulting from missiles, crushing, burns, frostbite.

†For children <7 yr; DPT (DT, if pertussis vaccine contraindicated) preferred to tetanus toxoid alone. For persons ≥7 yr, Td preferred to tetanus toxoid alone

‡If only 3 doses of *fluid* toxoid received, 4th dose of toxoid, preferably adsorbed toxoid, should be given.

§Yes, if >10 yr since last dose.

‖Yes, if >5 yr since last dose. (More frequent boosters not needed, can accentuate side effects.)

Emergency Management of Poisonings and Overdoses

GENERAL GUIDELINES

- **ABCs:** Stabilize airway, breathing, circulatory status.
- **Initial assessment:** Obtain history of ingestion/exposure, past medical history, physical assessment.
- **ID:** Identify causative agent(s). When possible, verify history (e.g., obtain substance container).
- **Antidote:** Administer specific antidote as indicated.
- **Decontamination:** Remove causative agent from exposed area (eyes, skin, GI tract). Decontamination assumes higher priority depending on agent, body system involved.
- Provide symptomatic/supportive measures.

LABORATORY EXAMINATION

- **Toxicology screen:** Collect blood/urine for general screening if multiple or unknown substances ingested.
- **Screening for specific toxins:** Request tests for opiates, benzodiazepines, TCAs acetaminophen, other toxins based on history, presentation.
- **Management:** Do not withhold therapy while waiting for toxicology screen; essential to initiate therapy as soon as possible, especially with acetaminophen overdose. Negative screen does not rule out toxic ingestion.

GI ELIMINATION OF TOXINS

- **Ipecac:** Use only if ingestion recent; optimal effectiveness when given within 30 min of ingestion. Patient must be alert, have gag reflex present, not be at risk for aspiration. *Do not use if patient has ingested caustic agents, petroleum distillates or if ingested substance is known to cause coma, seizures, dysrhythmias.*

Ipecac administration

AGE	USUAL DOSE	COMMENTS
<6 mo	5-10 ml	Follow ipecac with 6-8 oz water for
6-12 mo	15 ml	adults, 4-8 oz for children; repeat
>1 yr	30 ml	dose in 30 min if no response.

- **Gastric lavage:** Insert large (30-40 French) orogastric tube; irrigate using 250-300 ml warm tap water for total of at least 1 L and until clear; used for patients with seizures, decreased level of consciousness, when induced vomiting poses a risk of aspiration.

- **Cathartics:** Promotes elimination of toxins from lower GI tract; encourages movement, elimination of activated charcoal when used

CATHARTIC	ADULT DOSE	PEDIATRIC DOSE
Magnesium sulfate	15-30 g	250 mg/kg
Magnesium citrate	6 oz	1-3 ml/kg
Sodium sulfate	15-30 g	250 mg/kg
Sorbitol	1 g/kg	1 g/kg

- **Activated charcoal:** Absorbs most toxins or poisons; typically given with sorbitol, which hastens elimination; to prevent intestinal obstruction from charcoal, administer 1 dose of sorbitol or saline q24h in patients receiving charcoal.

ELIMINATION OF ABSORBED TOXINS

- **Activated charcoal:** Helpful in absorbing toxins even after they have entered bloodstream.
- **Urinary alkalinization:** Sodium bicarbonate or acetazolamide used to increase pH of urine, encourage urinary excretion of phenobarbital, certain other toxins
- **Hemodialysis or hemoperfusion:** Certain drugs or toxins (e.g., aspirin, acetaminophen) can be successfully removed using dialysis techniques.

Specific Antidotes

Poison	Antidote	Dosage
acetaminophen	N-acetylcysteine (Mucomyst)	Initially 140 mg/kg PO, then 70 mg/kg PO q4h FOR 17 DOSES or for 72 hours
anticholinergics	physostigmine (Antilirium)	Adults: 2 mg IV (slowly) Children: 0.5 mg IV (slowly)
carbon monoxide	oxygen	100%
cholesterase inhibitors	atropine	Adults: 1-2 mg IV Children: 0.05 mg/kg IV NOTE: Repeat above until signs of atropinization.
benzodiazepines	flumazenil (Romazicon)	0.2 mg IV q30-60 sec until patient awakens or until total dose of 1 mg reached
cyanide	1st: amyl nitrite pearls	Inhale for 30 sec of every min
	2nd: sodium nitrite	10 ml 3% solution IV over 3 min (children: 0.33 ml/kg; not to exceed 10 ml)
	3rd: sodium thiosulfate	50 ml 25% solution IV over 10 min (children: 1.65 ml/kg (IV)
methanol/ethylene glycol	ethyl alcohol	1 ml/kg IV 95%-100% absolute ethyl alcohol in glucose solution over 20 min; maintain blood level of 100 mg/dl
narcotics	naloxone (Narcan)	Adults/children: 0.8-2 mg IV
TCAs	sodium bicarbonate	1 mEq/kg IV; repeat as necessary to keep serum pH physiologic, reverse cardiac conduction abnormalities.

Management of Extravasation

RISK FACTORS

- Inability to communicate pain sensation (e.g., infants, children, altered mental status, sensory impairment, general anesthesia, CPR)
- Frequent venipuncture attempts
- IV line on dorsum of hand or foot
- Presence of peripheral vascular disease
- Use of infusion pumps
- History of radiation to injection site

GENERAL TREATMENT

1. Stop infusion/injection if patient complains of pain, burning.
2. Assess for infiltration: redness, swelling, tenderness, inability to aspirate blood, resistance to injection.
3. Leave needle/catheter in place to aspirate fluid/drug, administer specific antidote when indicated (Appendix J). Remove cannula after any necessary therapy.
4. Elevate limb to minimize swelling.
5. During first 48-72 hr apply cool compresses for 20 min tid-qid. Cool compresses produce vasoconstriction, reduce cellular activity, which may limit tissue injury. Warm compresses may be preferred for specific drugs (e.g., *Vinca* alkaloids). They increase blood flow, enhance drug absorption.
6. Assess tissue perfusion locally and distal to injury.
7. Surgical debridement or other specialized therapy may be necessary for persistent pain, tissue necrosis.

Antidotes Used with IV Extravasations

Mechanism of Injury	Specifications	Treatment
	IV FLUIDS/ELECTROLYTES	
Osmotic	calcium salts ≥ 10% dextrose solutions mannitol parenteral nutrition solutions potassium salts sodium bicarbonate	Hyaluronidase 15 U/ml in normal saline (5 injections of 0.2 ml each)
	SYMPATHOMIMETIC AMINES	
Ischemic	dobutamine dopamine epinephrine metaraminol norepinephrine	Phentolamine 5-10 mg diluted in 10 ml normal saline injected with fine hypodermic needle around extravasation site
	MISCELLANEOUS	
Irritant	diazepam nafcillin phenytoin thiopental vasopressin	Hyaluronidase 15 U/ml in normal saline (5 injections of 0.2 ml each)

APPENDIX M

Using IV Filters

Filter use: Use of in-line filters varies according to unique requirements of population served by health care facility. Policies should be developed collaboratively with input from IV therapy, pharmacy, nursing.

Microporous membrane filters: Typically used in hospital setting to decrease incidence of phlebitis, reduce particulate contamination of IV solutions; in-line 0.22 μm filter is generally recommended. 0.45 μm filter generally used with TPN solutions. 0.8 μm filter often used with chemotherapy. 1.2 μm filter used with lipids.

Effectiveness: Microporous filters retain most bacteria, fungi, latexes, emulsified fats, blood cells, larger particles, including glass fragments from ampules. They may allow passage of viruses, polymers, proteins, pyrogens, low–molecular-weight solutes, antibiotics, amino acids, sugars, salts. Therapeutic effectiveness is impaired when certain agents filtered. List of agents that require specialized filter or that should NOT be filtered follows:

alteplase (tPA)	fat emulsions*
amphotericin B	ganciclovir
blood/blood products*	iron/dextran (Imferon)
cancer chemotherapeutic agents*	immune globulin
colony-stimulating factors	insulin
cyclosporine	interleukins
dextran	streptokinase
	urokinase

*Specialized filter may be required. 20-40 μm microaggregates filter often used for stored blood to remove particulates, platelets, leukocytes, fibrin. 170 μm standard blood filter will remove gross clots.

Acute Hypersensitivity (Allergic) Reactions

CLINICAL PRESENTATION

Symptoms generally start within 30 min of exposure, almost always within 2 hr; if not treated, may lead to death by asphyxia, CV collapse. "Late-phase" reactions may occur; patient appears to be recovered, but 6-8 hr later anaphylaxis recurs.

SYSTEM	MANIFESTATIONS
Derm	Pruritus, urticaria, erythema, angioedema
GI	Nausea, abdominal pain, vomiting, diarrhea
Resp	Chest tightness, stridor, bronchospasm
CV	Hypotension, tachycardia, dysrhythmias

MANAGEMENT

1. Discontinue suspected drug.
2. Airway: Establish/maintain patency.
3. O_2: Administer at 6-10 L/min or as indicated by clinical condition.
4. Epinephrine: Causes bronchodilation, increases BP; administer SC/IM adults: 1:1000, 0.3-0.5 mg; children: 1:1000, 0.01 ml/kg.
5. IV fluids: Establish IV access; administer crystalloids for hypotension; use vasopressors (e.g., norepinephrine) for hypotension unresponsive to fluid therapy.
6. Diphenhydramine: Blocks histamine-1 receptors; administer IV; IM route may be used if CV status stable; adults: 10-50 mg, may repeat; children: 1-2 mg/kg, may repeat. Combination therapy with H-2 antagonists (e.g., cimetimine) may benefit patients with allergic skin disorders who do not respond adequately to H-1 receptor blockade.
7. Hydrocortisone sodium succinate: Blocks late phase reaction; adults/children: $\geq$100 mg IV, up to 2 g; follow with 100 mg IV q2-4h; convert to PO therapy when possible, continue for 1-3 days.
8. Aminophylline: Sometimes used for severe or refractory bronchospasm.

Drugs Used in Pediatric Resuscitation

Drug	Dose	How Supplied*
epinephrine HCl	0.01 mg/kg 0.1 ml/kg	1:10,000 (0.1 mg/ml)
sodium bicarbonate	1 mEq/kg 1 ml/kg	1 mEq/ml (8.4% solution)
atropine sulfate	0.02 mg/kg 0.2 ml/kg	0.1 mg/ml
calcium chloride	20 mg/kg (0.2 ml/kg)	100 mg/ml (10% solution)
glucose	0.5-1 g/kg	0.5 g/ml $D_{50}W$
lidocaine HCl	1 mg/kg	10 mg/ml (1%) 20 mg/ml (2%)
bretylium tosylate	5 mg/kg	50 mg/ml $D_{50}W$

INFUSIONS

Drug	Dose	How Supplied*
epinephrine	0.1-1 µg/kg/min	1 mg/ml 1:1000
dopamine HCl	2-20 µg/kg/min	40 mg/ml
dobutamine	5-20 µg/kg/min	250 mg/vial lyophilized
isoproterenol	0.1-1.0 µg/kg/min	1 mg/5 ml
lidocaine	20-50 µg/kg/min	40 mg/ml (4%)

From Chameides L, editor: *Textbook of pediatric advanced life support,* Dallas, 1990, American Academy of Pediatrics, American Heart Association. Reproduced with permission. Textbook of Pediatric Advanced Life Support, 1988, 1990. Copyright American Heart Association.
*For IV push medications, preparation listed is form available in prefilled syringes.

Remarks
Most useful drug in cardiac arrest; 1:1000 must be diluted.

Infuse slowly and ONLY when ventilation adequate.

Minimum dose of 0.1 mg (1 ml); use for bradycardia after assessing ventilation.
Maximum dose, infants/children: 10 mg; adolescents: 2 mg
Use only for hypocalcemia, calcium blocker overdose, hyperkalemia, hypermagnesemia; give slowly.

Dilute 1:1 with water ($D_{25}W$); dose then 2-4 ml/kg.

Use for ventricular dysrhythmias only.

Use if lidocaine not effective; repeat dose with 10 mg/kg if first dose not effective.

Titrate to desired hemodynamic effect.
Titrate to desired hemodynamic response.
Titrate to desired hemodynamic response; may cause vasodilation.

Titrate to desired hemodynamic effect; may cause vasodilation.
Use lower infusion dose with shock, liver disease.

Advanced Cardiac Life Support Algorithms

Figure 1.
Universal Algorithm for Adult Emergency Cardiac Care

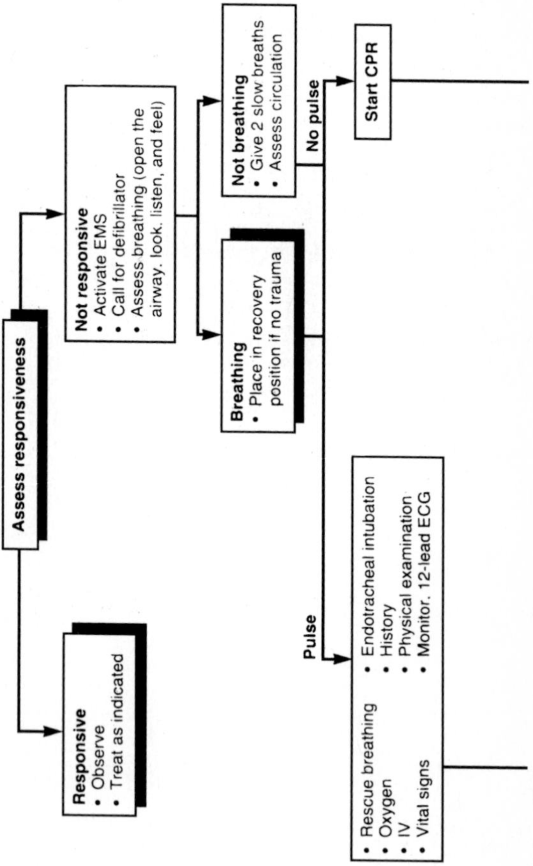

Assess responsiveness

Responsive
- Observe
- Treat as indicated

Not responsive
- Activate EMS
- Call for defibrillator
- Assess breathing (open the airway, look, listen, and feel)

Breathing
- Place in recovery position if no trauma

Not breathing
- Give 2 slow breaths
- Assess circulation

Pulse
- Rescue breathing
- Oxygen
- IV
- Vital signs
- Endotracheal intubation
- History
- Physical examination
- Monitor, 12-lead ECG

No pulse

Start CPR

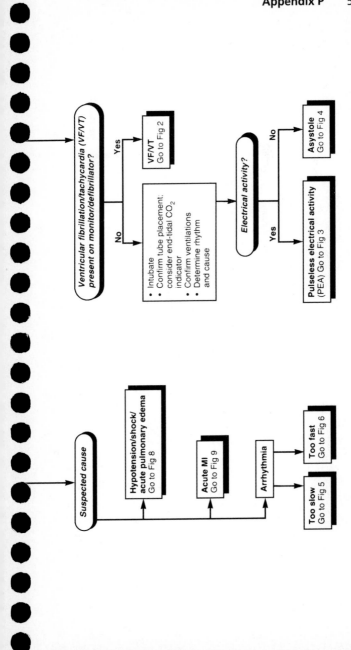

All algorithms in this appendix modified from Emergency Cardiac Care Committee and Subcommittees, American Heart Association: Guidelines for cardiopulmonary resuscitation and emergency cardiac care, *JAMA* 286(16): 2216, 2217, 2219, 2220, 2221, 2223, 2224, 2227, 2230.

Figure 2.
Algorithm for ventricular fibrillation and pulseless ventricular tachycardia (VF/VT)

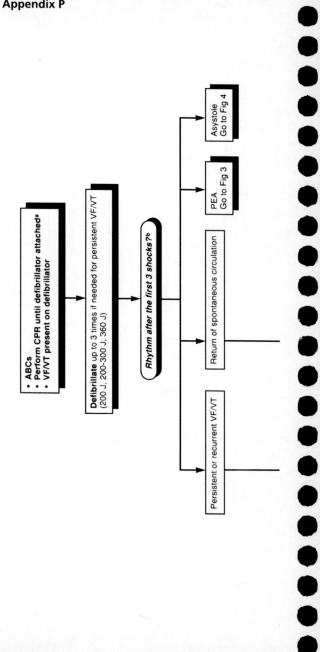

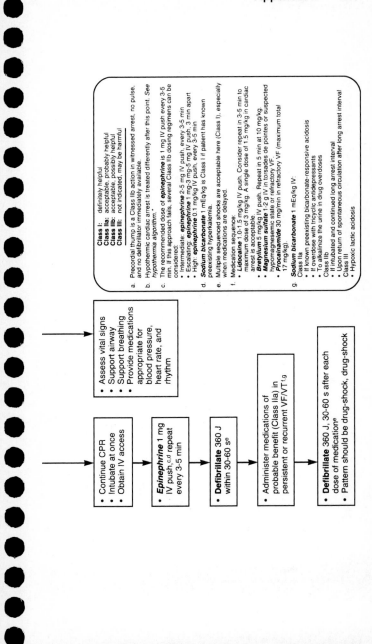

- Continue CPR
- Intubate at once
- Obtain IV access

- *Epinephrine* 1 mg IV push,[c,d] repeat every 3-5 min

- **Defibrillate** 360 J within 30-60 s[e]

- Administer medications of probable benefit (Class IIa) in persistent or recurrent VF/VT[f,g]

- **Defibrillate** 360 J, 30-60 s after each dose of medication[e]
- Pattern should be drug-shock, drug-shock

- Assess vital signs
- Support airway
- Support breathing
- Provide medications appropriate for blood pressure, heart rate, and rhythm

Class I: definitely helpful
Class IIa: acceptable, probably helpful
Class IIb: acceptable, possibly helpful
Class III: not indicated, may be harmful

a. Precordial thump is a Class IIb action in witnessed arrest, no pulse, and no defibrillator immediately available.

b. Hypothermic cardiac arrest is treated differently after this point. *See hypothermia algorithm.*

c. The recommended dose of *epinephrine* is 1 mg IV push, every 3-5 min. If this approach fails, several Class IIb dosing regimens can be considered:
 • Intermediate: *epinephrine* 2-5 mg IV push, every 3-5 min
 • Escalating: *epinephrine* 1 mg-3 mg-5 mg IV push; 3 min apart
 • High: *epinephrine* 0.1 mg/kg IV push, every 3-5 min

d. *Sodium bicarbonate* 1 mEq/kg is Class I if patient has known preexisting hyperkalemia.

e. Multiple sequenced shocks are acceptable here (Class I), especially when medications are delayed.

f. Medication sequence:
 • *Lidocaine* 1.0-1.5 mg/kg IV push. Consider repeat in 3-5 min to maximum dose of 3 mg/kg. A single dose of 1.5 mg/kg in cardiac arrest is acceptable.
 • *Bretylium* 5 mg/kg IV push. Repeat in 5 min at 10 mg/kg.
 • *Magnesium sulfate* 1-2 g IV in torsades de pointes or suspected hypomagnesemic state or refractory VF
 • *Procainamide* 30 mg/min in refractory VF (maximum total 17 mg/kg).

g. *Sodium bicarbonate* 1 mEq/kg IV:
 Class IIa
 • If known preexisting bicarbonate-responsive acidosis
 • If overdose with tricyclic antidepressants
 • To alkalinize the urine in drug overdoses
 Class IIb
 • If intubated and continued long arrest interval
 • Upon return of spontaneous circulation after long arrest interval
 Class III
 • Hypoxic lactic acidosis

Figure 3.
Algorithm for pulseless electrical activity (PEA) (electromechanical dissociation [EMD])

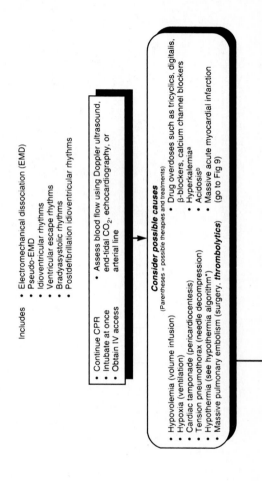

Includes
- Electromechanical dissociation (EMD)
- Pseudo-EMD
- Idioventricular rhythms
- Ventricular escape rhythms
- Bradyasystolic rhythms
- Postdefibrillation idioventricular rhythms

- Continue CPR
- Intubate at once
- Obtain IV access

- Assess blood flow using Doppler ultrasound, end-tidal CO_2, echocardiography, or arterial line

Consider possible causes
(Parentheses = possible therapies and treatments)

- Hypovolemia (volume infusion)
- Hypoxia (ventilation)
- Cardiac tamponade (pericardiocentesis)
- Tension pneumothorax (needle decompression)
- Hypothermia (see hypothermia algorithm*)
- Massive pulmonary embolism (surgery, *thrombolytics*)

- Drug overdoses such as tricyclics, digitalis, β-blockers, calcium channel blockers
- Hyperkalemia[a]
- Acidosis[b]
- Massive acute myocardial infarction (go to Fig 9)

- **Epinephrine** 1 mg IV push,[a,c] repeat every 3-5 min

- If absolute bradycardia (<60 BPM) or relative bradycardia, give **atropine** 1 mg IV
- Repeat every 3-5 min to a total of 0.03-0.04 mg/kg[d]

Class I: definitely helpful
Class IIa: acceptable, probably helpful
Class IIb: acceptable, possibly helpful
Class III: not indicate*: may be harmful

a. **Sodium bicarbonate** 1 mEq/kg is Class I if patient has known preexisting hyperkalemia.

b. **Sodium bicarbonate** 1 mEq/kg:
   Class IIa
   - If known preexisting bicarbonate-responsive acidosis
   - If overdose with tricyclic antidepressants
   - To alkalinize the urine in drug overdoses
   Class IIb
   - If intubated and continued long arrest interval
   - Upon return of spontaneous circulation after long arrest interval
   Class III
   - Hypoxic lactic acidosis

c. The recommended dose of **epinephrine** is 1 mg IV push every 3-5 min. If this approach fails, several Class IIb dosing regimens can be considered:
   - Intermediate: **epinephrine** 2-5 mg IV push, every 3-5 min
   - Escalating: **epinephrine** 1 mg-3 mg-5 mg IV push, 3 min apart
   - High: **epinephrine** 0.1 mg/kg IV push, every 3-5 min

d. The shorter **atropine** dosing interval (3 min) is possibly helpful in cardiac arrest (Class IIb).

Figure 4.
Asystole treatment algorithm

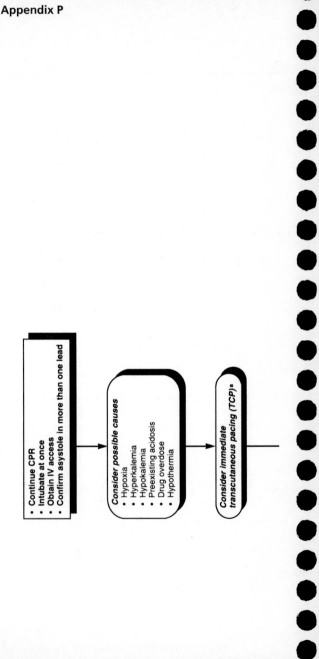

- Continue CPR
- Intubate at once
- Obtain IV access
- Confirm asystole in more than one lead

Consider possible causes
- Hypoxia
- Hyperkalemia
- Hypokalemia
- Preexisting acidosis
- Drug overdose
- Hypothermia

Consider immediate transcutaneous pacing (TCP) a

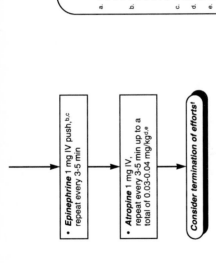

- *Epinephrine* 1 mg IV push, repeat every 3-5 min.[b,c]

- *Atropine* 1 mg IV, repeat every 3-5 min up to a total of 0.03-0.04 mg/kg[d,e]

Consider termination of efforts[f]

Class I: definitely helpful
Class IIa: acceptable, probably helpful
Class IIb: acceptable, possibly helpful
Class III: not indicated, may be harmful

a. TCP is a Class IIb intervention. Lack of success may be due to delays in pacing. To be effective TCP must be performed early, simultaneously with drugs. Evidence does not support routine use of TCP for asystole.

b. The recommended dose of *epinephrine* is 1 mg IV push every 3-5 min. If this approach fails, several Class IIb dosing regimens can be considered:
 • Intermediate: *epinephrine* 2-5 mg IV push, every 3-5 min
 • Escalating: *epinephrine* 1 mg-3 mg-5 mg IV push, 3 min apart
 • High: *epinephrine* 0.1 mg/kg IV push, every 3-5 min

c. *Sodium bicarbonate* 1 mEq/kg is Class I if patient has known preexisting hyperkalemia.

d. The shorter *atropine* dosing interval (3 min) is Class IIb in asystolic arrest.

e. *Sodium bicarbonate* 1 mEq/kg:
 Class IIa
 • If known preexisting bicarbonate-responsive acidosis
 • If overdose with tricyclic antidepressants
 • To alkalinize the urine in drug overdoses
 Class IIb
 • If intubated and continued long arrest interval
 • Upon return of spontaneous circulation after long arrest interval
 Class III
 • Hypoxic lactic acidosis

f. If patient remains in asystole or other agonal rhythm after successful intubation and initial medications and no reversible causes are identified, consider termination of resuscitative efforts by a physician. Consider interval since arrest.

Figure 5.
Bradycardia algorithm (patient not in cardiac arrest)

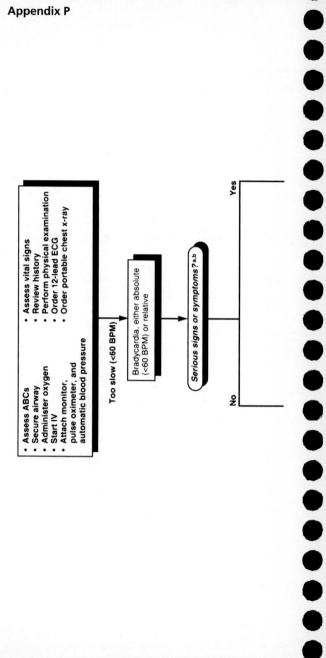

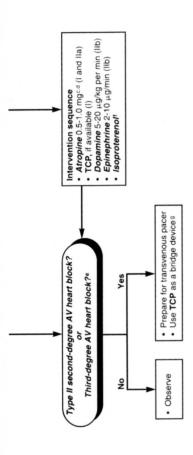

Intervention sequence
- *Atropine* 0.5-1.0 mg[c,d] (I and IIa)
- *TCP*, if available (I)
- *Dopamine* 5-20 μg/kg per min (IIb)
- *Epinephrine* 2-10 μg/min (IIb)
- *Isoproterenol[f]*

Type II second-degree AV heart block?
or
Third-degree AV heart block?[e]

No → • Observe

Yes → • Prepare for transvenous pacer
• Use **TCP** as a bridge device[g]

a. Serious signs or symptoms must be related to the slow rate. Clinical manifestations include
   - Symptoms (chest pain, shortness of breath, decreased level of consciousness)
   - Signs (low BP, shock, pulmonary congestion, CHF, acute MI)
b. Do not delay TCP while awaiting IV access or for *atropine* to take effect if patient is symptomatic.
c. Denervated transplanted hearts will not respond to *atropine*. Go at once to pacing, *catecholamine* infusion, or both.
d. *Atropine* should be given in repeat doses every 3-5 min up to total of 0.03-0.04 mg/kg. Use the shorter dosing interval (3 min) in severe clinical conditions. It has been suggested that *atropine* should be used with caution in atrioventricular (AV) block at the His-Purkinje level (type II AV block and new third-degree block with wide QRS complexes) (Class IIb).
e. Never treat third-degree heart block plus ventricular escape beats with *lidocaine.*
f. *Isoproterenol* should be used, if at all, with extreme caution. At low doses it is Class IIb (possibly helpful); at higher doses it is Class III (harmful).
g. Verify patient tolerance and mechanical capture. Use analgesia and sedation as needed.

Figure 6.
Tachycardia algorithm

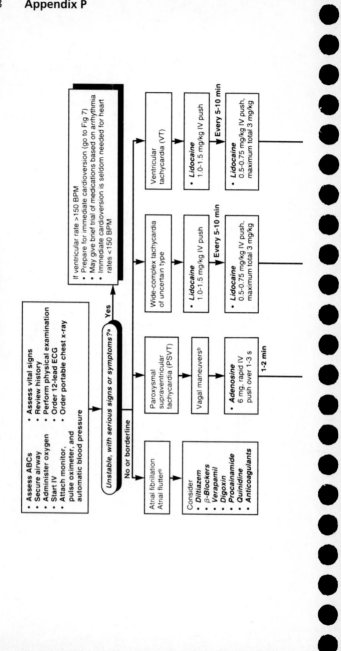

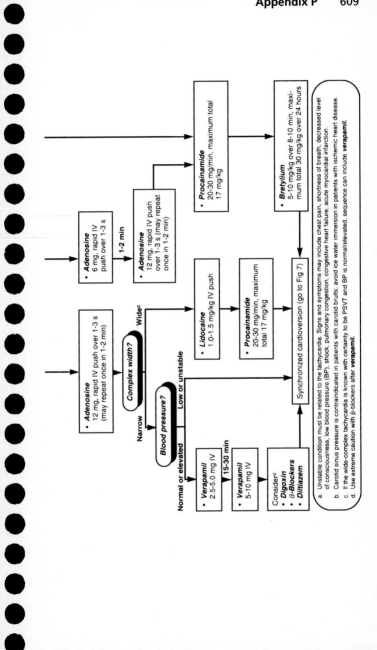

Figure 7.
Electrical cardioversion algorithm (patient not in cardiac arrest)

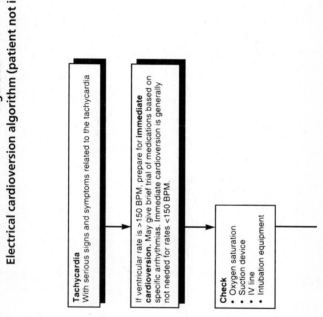

Tachycardia
With serious signs and symptoms related to the tachycardia

If ventricular rate is >150 BPM, prepare for **immediate cardioversion**. May give brief trial of medications based on specific arrhythmias. Immediate cardioversion is generally not needed for rates <150 BPM.

Check
• Oxygen saturation
• Suction device
• IV line
• Intubation equipment

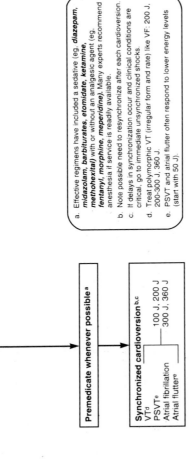

Premedicate whenever possible[a]

Synchronized cardioversion[b,c]

VT[d]	100 J, 200 J
PSVT[e]	300 J, 360 J
Atrial fibrillation	
Atrial flutter[e]	

a. Effective regimens have included a sedative (eg, *diazepam, midazolam, barbiturates, etomidate, ketamine, methohexital*) with or without an analgesic agent (eg, *fentanyl, morphine, meperidine*). Many experts recommend anesthesia if service is readily available.

b. Note possible need to resynchronize after each cardioversion.

c. If delays in synchronization occur and clinical conditions are critical, go to immediate unsynchronized shocks.

d. Treat polymorphic VT (irregular form and rate) like VF: 200 J, 200-300 J, 360 J.

e. PSVT and atrial flutter often respond to lower energy levels (start with 50 J).

Figure 8.
Algorithm for hypotension, shock, and acute pulmonary edema

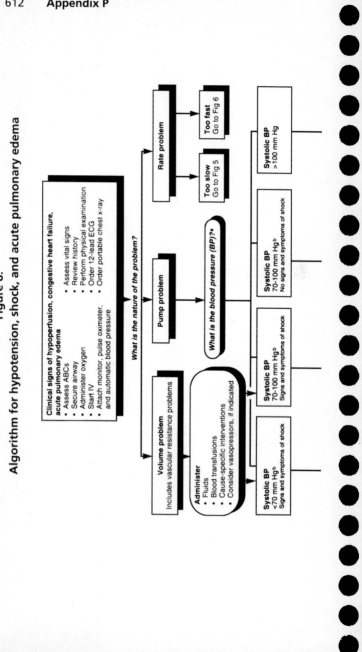

Clinical signs of hypoperfusion, congestive heart failure, acute pulmonary edema
- Assess ABCs
- Secure airway
- Administer oxygen
- Start IV
- Attach monitor, pulse oximeter, and automatic blood pressure
- Assess vital signs
- Review history
- Perform physical examination
- Order 12-lead ECG
- Order portable chest x-ray

What is the nature of the problem?

Volume problem
Includes vascular resistance problems

Pump problem

Rate problem

Too slow
Go to Fig 5

Too fast
Go to Fig 6

Administer
- Fluids
- Blood transfusions
- Cause-specific interventions
- Consider vasopressors, if indicated

*What is the blood pressure (BP)?*ᵃ

Systolic BP <70 mm Hgᵇ
Signs and symptoms of shock

Systolic BP 70-100 mm Hgᵇ
Signs and symptoms of shock

Systolic BP 70-100 mm Hgᵇ
No signs and symptoms of shock

Systolic BP >100 mm Hg

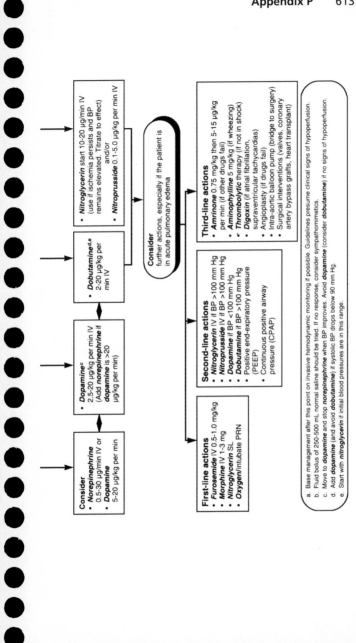

Consider
- *Norepinephrine* 0.5-30 µg/min IV or
- *Dopamine* 5-20 µg/kg per min

- *Dopamine*[c] 2.5-20 µg/kg per min IV (Add *norepinephrine* if *dopamine* is >20 µg/kg per min)

- *Dobutamine*[d,e] 2-20 µg/kg per min IV

- *Nitroglycerin* start 10-20 µg/min IV (use if ischemia persists and BP remains elevated. Titrate to effect)
  and/or
- *Nitroprusside* 0.1-5.0 µg/kg per min IV

Consider
further actions, especially if the patient is in acute pulmonary edema

First-line actions
- *Furosemide* IV 0.5-1.0 mg/kg
- *Morphine* IV 1-3 mg
- *Nitroglycerin* SL
- *Oxygen*/intubate PRN

Second-line actions
- *Nitroglycerin* IV if BP >100 mm Hg
- *Nitroprusside* IV if BP >100 mm Hg
- *Dopamine* if BP <100 mm Hg
- *Dobutamine* if BP >100 mm Hg
- Positive end-expiratory pressure (PEEP)
- Continuous positive airway pressure (CPAP)

Third-line actions
- *Amrinone* 0.75 mg/kg then 5-15 µg/kg per min (if other drugs fail)
- *Aminophylline* 5 mg/kg (if wheezing)
- *Thrombolytic* therapy (if not in shock)
- *Digoxin* (if atrial fibrillation, supraventricular tachycardias)
- Angioplasty (if drugs fail)
- Intra-aortic balloon pump (bridge to surgery)
- Surgical interventions (valves, coronary artery bypass grafts, heart transplant)

a. Base management after this point on invasive hemodynamic monitoring if possible. Guidelines presume clinical signs of hypoperfusion.
b. Fluid bolus of 250-500 mL normal saline should be tried. If no response, consider sympathomimetics.
c. Move to *dopamine* and stop *norepinephrine* when BP improves. Avoid *dopamine* (consider *dobutamine*) if no signs of hypoperfusion.
d. Add *dopamine* (and avoid *dobutamine*) if systolic BP drops below 90 mm Hg.
e. Start with *nitroglycerin* if initial blood pressures are in this range.

Figure 9.
Acute myocardial infarction (MI) algorithm

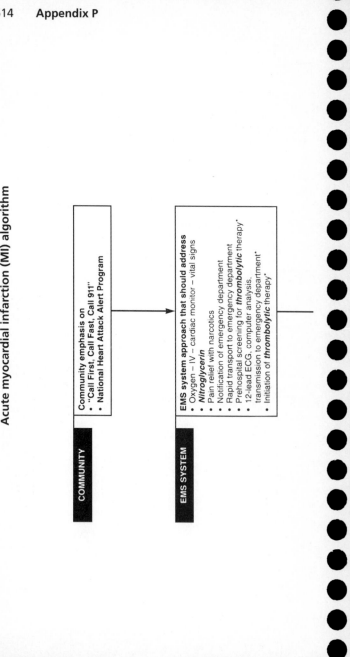

COMMUNITY

Community emphasis on
- "Call First, Call Fast, Call 911"
- National Heart Attack Alert Program

EMS SYSTEM

EMS system approach that should address
- Oxygen – IV – cardiac monitor – vital signs
- *Nitroglycerin*
- Pain relief with narcotics
- Notification of emergency department
- Rapid transport to emergency department
- Prehospital screening for *thrombolytic* therapy*
- 12-lead ECG, computer analysis,
  transmission to emergency department*
- Initiation of *thrombolytic* therapy*

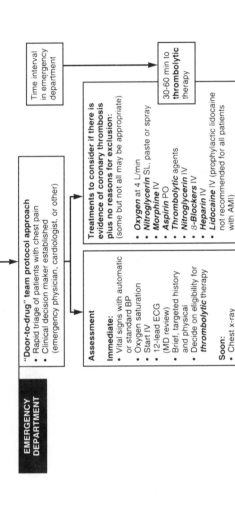

EMERGENCY DEPARTMENT

"Door-to-drug" team protocol approach
- Rapid triage of patients with chest pain
- Clinical decision maker established (emergency physician, cardiologist, or other)

Time interval in emergency department

Assessment

Immediate:
- Vital signs with automatic or standard BP
- Oxygen saturation
- Start IV
- 12-lead ECG (MD review)
- Brief, targeted history and physical
- Decide on eligibility for **thrombolytic** therapy

Soon:
- Chest x-ray
- Blood studies (electrolytes, enzymes, coagulation studies)
- Consult as needed

Treatments to consider if there is evidence of coronary thrombosis plus no reasons for exclusion:
(some but not all may be appropriate)

- ***Oxygen*** at 4 L/min
- ***Nitroglycerin*** SL, paste or spray
- ***Morphine*** IV
- ***Aspirin*** PO
- ***Thrombolytic*** agents
- ***Nitroglycerin*** IV
- ***β-Blockers*** IV
- ***Heparin*** IV
- ***Lidocaine*** IV (prophylactic lidocaine not recommended for all patients with AMI)
- ***Magnesium sulfate*** IV
- ***Coronary angiography/angioplasty***

30-60 min to **thrombolytic** therapy

*Optional guidelines

Figure 10.
Algorithm for treatment of hypothermia

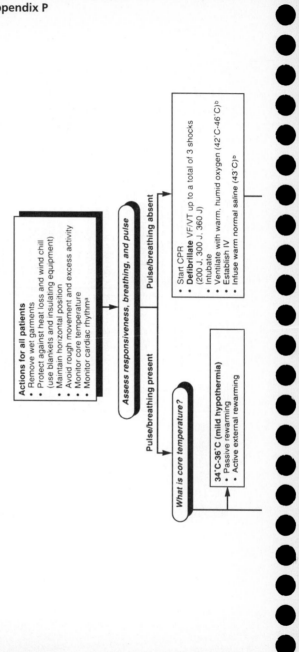

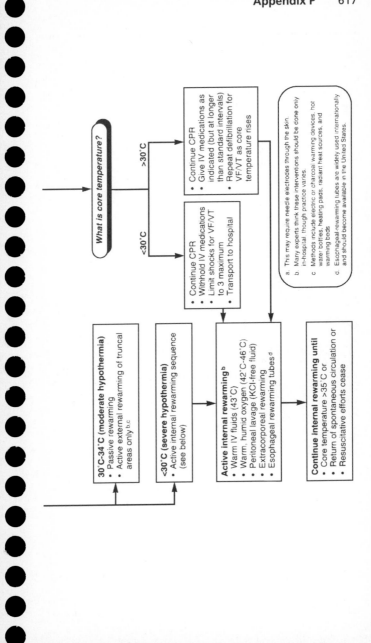

What is core temperature?

<30°C
- Continue CPR
- Withhold IV medications
- Limit shocks for VF/VT to 3 maximum
- Transport to hospital

>30°C
- Continue CPR
- Give IV medications as indicated (but at longer than standard intervals)
- Repeat defibrillation for VF/VT as core temperature rises

30°C-34°C (moderate hypothermia)
- Passive rewarming
- Active external rewarming of truncal areas only[b,c]

<30°C (severe hypothermia)
- Active internal rewarming sequence (see below)

Active internal rewarming[b]
- Warm IV fluids (43°C)
- Warm, humid oxygen (42°C-46°C)
- Peritoneal lavage (KCl-free fluid)
- Extracorporeal rewarming
- Esophageal rewarming tubes[d]

Continue internal rewarming until
- Core temperature >35°C or
- Return of spontaneous circulation or
- Resuscitative efforts cease

a. This may require needle electrodes through the skin.
b. Many experts think these interventions should be done only in-hospital, though practice varies.
c. Methods include electric or charcoal warming devices, hot water bottles, heating pads, radiant heat sources, and warming beds.
d. Esophageal-rewarming tubes are widely used internationally and should become available in the United States.

Infusion Rate Tables

Aminocaproic Acid
(Amicar)

USUAL DOSE

Initial: 4-5 g during first hour
Maintenance: 1-1.25 g/hr for 6-8 hrs
Maximal: 30 g in 24 hr

TITRATION

*Give priming dose over first hr
*Follow by continuous infusion of 1-1.25 g/hr for 6-8 hr or until hemorrhage is controlled

Aminocaproic Acid		
	Infusion Rate (ml/hr)	
Dose gm/hr	5000 mg/500 ml (10 mg/ml)	5000 mg/250 ml (20 mg/ml)
0.5	50	25
1	100	50
1.25	125	63
1.5	150	75
2	200	100
3	300	150
4	400	200
5	500	250

Aminophylline
(Aminophyllin)

USUAL DOSE

Loading: 6 mg/kg
Initial Infusion: 0.5-1 mg/kg/hr
Maintenance: 0.1-0.8 mg/kg/hr
Maximal: 3 mg/kg/hr

TITRATION

Loading dose over 20 min. Start infusion at 0.5 mg/kg/hr; titrate up until desired response

Aminophylline: 500 mg/250ml*

Concentration: 2 mg/ml

	Patient Weight in Kilograms								
	50	60	70	80	90	100	110	120	130
Loading Dose (6 mg/kg) →	280	336	392	448	504	560	616	672	728
Dose mg/kg/hr	*Infusion Rate (ml/hr)*								
0.1	3	3	4	4	5	5	6	6	7
0.2	5	6	7	8	9	10	11	12	13
0.3	8	9	11	12	14	15	17	18	20
0.4	10	12	14	16	18	20	22	24	26
0.5	13	15	18	20	23	25	28	30	33
0.6	15	18	21	24	27	30	33	36	39
0.7	18	21	25	28	32	35	39	42	46
0.8	20	24	28	32	36	40	44	48	52
0.9	23	27	32	36	41	45	50	54	59
1	25	30	35	40	45	50	55	60	65
2	50	60	70	80	90	100	110	120	130
3	75	90	105	120	135	150	165	180	195

*When infusion rates fall in the lightly shaded area, a more concentrated drip may be indicated.

Aminophylline: 1,000 mg/250 ml*

Concentration: 4 mg/ml

				Patient Weight in Kilograms					
	50	60	70	80	90	100	110	120	130
Loading Dose (6 mg/kg) →	280	336	392	448	504	560	616	672	728
Dose mg/kg/hr	Infusion Rate (ml/hr)								
0.1	1	2	2	2	2	3	3	3	3
0.2	3	3	4	4	5	5	6	6	7
0.3	4	5	5	6	7	8	8	9	10
0.4	5	6	7	8	9	10	11	12	13
0.5	6	8	9	10	11	13	14	15	16
0.6	8	9	11	12	14	15	17	18	20
0.7	9	11	12	14	16	18	19	21	23
0.8	10	12	14	16	18	20	22	24	26
0.9	11	14	16	18	20	23	25	27	29
1	13	15	18	20	23	25	28	30	33
2	25	30	35	40	45	50	55	60	65
3	38	45	53	60	68	75	83	90	98

*When infusion rates fall in the lightly shaded area, a more concentrated drip is indicated.

Aminophylline Pediatric Table

USUAL DOSE	TITRATION
Initial: 0.5-1 mg/kg/hr	Loading dose over 20 min. Start in-
Maintenance: 0.1-0.8 mg/kg/hr	fusion at 0.5 mg/kg/hr and titrate
Maximal: 3 mg/kg/hr	until desired response

Aminophylline: 500 mg/250 ml*
Concentration: 2 mg/ml

	Patient Weight in Kilograms								
	5	10	15	20	25	30	35	40	45
Loading Dose (6 mg/kg) →	28	56	84	112	140	168	196	224	252
Dose mg/kg/hr	*Infusion Rate (ml/hr)*								
0.1		1	1	1	1	2	2	2	2
0.2	1	1	2	2	3	3	4	4	5
0.3	1	2	2	3	4	5	5	6	7
0.4	1	2	3	4	5	6	7	8	9
0.5	1	3	4	5	6	8	9	10	11
0.6	2	3	5	6	8	9	11	12	14
0.7	2	4	5	7	9	11	12	14	16
0.8	2	4	6	8	10	12	14	16	18
0.9	2	5	7	9	11	14	16	18	20
1	3	5	8	10	13	15	18	20	23
2	5	10	15	20	25	30	35	40	45
3	8	15	23	30	38	45	53	60	68

*When infusion rates fall in the lightly shaded area, a more concentrated drip is indicated.

Amrinone
(Inocor)

USUAL DOSE

Loading: 0.75 mg/kg
Initial: 2.5-5 µg/kg/min
Maintenance: 5-10 µg/kg/min
Maximal: 20 µg/kg/min

TITRATION

Loading dose over 2-3 min. Start at 2.5-5 µg/kg/min; titrate q 10 min to optimize CO

Amrinone: 500 mg/250 ml*
Concentration: 2,000 µg/ml

	Patient Weight in Kilograms							
	50	60	70	80	90	100	110	120
Loading Dose (0.75 mg/kg)→	38	45	53	60	68	75	83	90
Dose µg/kg/min	Infusion Rate (ml/hr)							
5	8	9	11	12	14	15	17	18
6	9	11	13	14	16	18	20	22
7	11	13	15	17	19	21	23	25
8	12	14	17	19	22	24	26	29
9	14	16	19	22	24	27	30	32
10	15	18	21	24	27	30	33	36
11	17	20	23	26	30	33	36	40
12	18	22	25	29	32	36	40	43
13	20	23	27	31	35	39	43	47
14	21	25	29	34	38	42	46	50
15	23	27	32	36	41	45	50	54
20	30	36	42	48	54	60	66	72

*When infusion rates fall in the lightly shaded area, a more concentrated drip is indicated.

Amrinone: 1,000 mg/250 ml*

Concentration: 4,000 μg/ml

	Patient Weight in Kilograms							
	50	60	70	80	90	100	110	120
Loading Dose (0.75 μg/kg) →	38	45	53	60	68	75	83	90
Dose μg/kg/min	*Infusion Rate (ml/hr)*							
5	4	5	5	6	7	8	8	9
6	5	5	6	7	8	9	10	11
7	5	6	7	8	9	11	12	13
8	6	7	8	10	11	12	13	14
9	7	8	9	11	12	14	15	16
10	8	9	11	12	14	15	17	18
11	8	10	12	13	15	17	18	20
12	9	11	13	14	16	18	20	22
13	10	12	14	16	18	20	21	23
14	11	13	15	17	19	21	23	25
15	11	14	16	18	20	23	25	27
20	15	18	21	24	27	30	33	36

*When infusion rates fall in the lightly shaded area, a more concentrated drip is indicated.

Dobutamine
(Dobutren)

USUAL DOSE

Initial: 2.5 µg/kg/min
Maintenance: 2.5-10 µg/kg/min
Maximal: 40 µg/kg/min

TITRATION

Start at 2.5 mg/kg/min. Increase by
2.5 µg/kg/min increments every 10
minutes to optimize CO

Dobutamine: 250 mg/250 ml*
Concentration: 1,000 µg/ml

Dose µg/kg/min	Patient Weight in Kilograms								
	50	60	70	80	90	100	110	120	130
	Infusion Rate (ml/hr)								
2.5	8	9	11	12	14	15	17	18	20
5	15	18	21	24	27	30	33	36	39
7.5	23	27	32	36	41	45	50	54	59
10	30	36	42	48	54	60	66	72	78
12.5	38	45	53	60	68	75	83	90	98
15	45	54	63	72	81	90	99	108	117
17.5	53	63	74	84	95	105	116	126	137
20	60	72	84	96	108	120	132	144	156
22.5	68	81	95	108	122	135	149	162	176
25	75	90	105	120	135	150	165	180	195
27.5	83	99	116	132	149	165	182	198	215
30	90	108	126	144	162	180	198	216	234
32.5	98	117	137	156	176	195	215	234	254

*When infusion rates fall in the lightly shaded area, consider a more concentrated drip.

Dobutamine: 500 mg/250 ml*

Concentration: 2,000 µg/ml

Dose µg/kg/min	Patient Weight in Kilograms								
	50	60	70	80	90	100	110	120	130
	Infusion Rate (ml/hr)								
2.5	4	5	5	6	7	8	8	9	10
5	8	9	11	12	14	15	17	18	20
7.5	11	14	16	18	20	23	25	27	29
10	15	18	21	24	27	30	33	36	39
12.5	19	23	26	30	34	38	41	45	49
15	23	27	32	36	41	45	50	54	59
17.5	26	32	37	42	47	53	58	63	68
20	30	36	42	48	54	60	66	72	78
22.5	34	41	47	54	61	68	74	81	88
25	38	45	53	60	68	75	83	90	98
27.5	41	50	58	66	74	83	91	99	107
30	45	54	63	72	81	90	99	108	117
32.5	49	59	68	78	88	98	107	117	127

*When infusion rates fall in the lightly shaded area, consider a more concentrated drip.

Dopamine
(Dopastat, Intropin)

USUAL DOSE

Low: 0.5-2 µg/kg/min (dopaminergic effects)
Intermediate: 2-10 µg/kg/min (beta-1 adrenergic effects)
High > 10 µg/kg/min (alpha-adrenergic effects)
Maximal: 40 µg/kg/min

TITRATION

Increase by 1-4 µg/kg/min q 10-30 min until desired response

Dopamine: 200 mg/250 ml*
Concentration: 800 µg/ml

Dose µg/kg/min	Patient Weight in Kilograms							
	50	60	70	80	90	100	110	120
	Infusion Rate (ml/hr)							
2	8	9	11	12	14	15	17	18
4	15	18	21	24	27	30	33	36
6	23	27	32	36	41	45	50	54
8	30	36	42	48	54	60	66	72
10	38	45	53	60	68	75	83	90
12	45	54	63	72	81	90	99	108
14	53	63	74	84	95	105	116	126
16	60	72	84	96	108	120	132	144
18	68	81	95	108	122	135	149	162
20	75	90	105	120	135	150	165	180
25	94	113	131	150	169	188	206	225
30	113	135	158	180	203	225	248	270
40	150	180	210	240	270	300	330	360

*When infusion rates fall in the lightly shaded area, a more concentrated drip is indicated.

Dopamine: 400 mg/250 ml*

Concentration: 1,600 µg/ml

Dose µg/kg/min	Patient Weight in Kilograms							
	50	60	70	80	90	100	110	120
	Infusion Rate (ml/hr)							
2	4	5	5	6	7	8	8	9
4	8	9	11	12	14	15	17	18
6	11	14	16	18	20	23	25	27
8	15	18	21	24	27	30	33	36
10	19	23	26	30	34	38	41	45
12	23	27	32	36	41	45	50	54
14	26	32	37	42	47	53	58	63
16	30	36	42	48	54	60	66	72
18	34	41	47	54	61	68	74	81
20	38	45	53	60	68	75	83	90
25	47	56	66	75	84	94	103	113
30	56	68	79	90	101	113	124	135
40	75	90	105	120	135	150	165	180

*When infusion rates fall in the lightly shaded area, a more concentrated drip is indicated.

Epinephrine
(Adrenalin)

USUAL DOSE

Low: 1-4 µg/min
Moderate: 4-12 µg/min
Maximal: 40 µg/min

TITRATION

Start at 1 µg/min. Increase by 1
µg/min increments every 5 min until
desired response

Epinephrine*			
	Infusion Rate (ml/hr)		
Dose in µg/min	1 mg/250 ml (4 µg/ml)	3 mg/250 ml (12 µg/ml)	8 mg/250 ml (32 µg/ml)
1	15	5	2
2	30	10	4
3	45	15	6
4	60	20	8
5	75	25	9
6	90	30	11
7	105	35	13
8	120	40	15
9	135	45	17
10	150	50	19
15	225	75	28
20	300	100	38
25	375	125	47
30	450	150	56
35	525	175	66
40	600	200	75

*When infusion rates fall in the lightly shaded area, a more concentrated drip is indicated.

Esmolol
(Brevibloc)

USUAL DOSE

Initial: 50 μg/kg/min
Maintenance: 50-200 μg/kg/min
Maximal: < 300 μg/kg/min

TITRATION

Bolus LD of 500 μg/kg/min over 1 min, if no response repeat LD and increase infusion rate in increments of 50 μg/kg/min until desired response

---

Esmolol: 2,500 mg/250 ml

Concentration: 10 mg/ml

	Patient Weight in Kilograms								
	50	60	70	80	90	100	110	120	130
Loading Dose	*dose in ml/hr given for 1 min*								
	150	180	210	240	270	300	330	360	390
(500 μg/kg/)→	(25 mg)	(30 mg)	(35 mg)	(40 mg)	(45 mg)	(50 mg)	(55 mg)	(60 mg)	(65 mg)
Dose μg/kg/min	*Infusion Rate (ml/hr)*								
25	8	9	11	12	14	15	17	18	20
50	15	18	21	24	27	30	33	36	39
75	23	27	32	36	41	45	50	54	59
100	30	36	42	48	54	60	66	72	78
125	38	45	53	60	68	75	83	90	98
150	45	54	63	72	81	90	99	108	117
175	53	63	74	84	95	105	116	126	137
200	60	72	84	96	108	120	132	144	156

Esmolol: Infusion Rates in Milliliters per Hour
Concentration: 20 µg/ml

	Patient Weight in Kilograms							
	50 55	60	65	70 75	80	90	100 110	120
Loading Dose (500 µg/kg) →	dose in ml/hr given for 1 min							
	75 (25 mg)	90 (30 mg)	105 (35 mg)	120 (40 mg)	135 (45 mg)	150 (50 mg)	165 (55 mg)	170 (60 mg)
Dose µg/kg/min	Infusion Rate (µg/kg/min)							
2.5	4	5	5	6	7	8	8	9
5	8	9	11	12	14	15	17	18
7.5	11	14	16	18	20	23	25	27
10	15	18	21	24	27	30	33	36
12.5	19	23	26	30	34	38	41	45
15	23	27	32	36	41	45	50	54
17.5	26	32	37	42	47	53	58	63
20	30	36	42	48	54	60	66	72

Heparin Sodium

USUAL DOSE

Initial: loading dose of 5000 U
Maintenance: 20-40,000 U/24 hr or (800-1600 U/hr)

TITRATION

Rate adjusted according to desired response as measured by clotting tests

Heparin			
	Infusion Rate (ml/hr)		
Dose in U/hr	10,000 U/500 ml (20 U/ml)	20,000 U/500 ml (40 U/ml)	25,000 U/250 ml (100 U/ml)
500	25	13	5
750	38	19	8
1000	50	25	10
1250	63	31	13
1500	75	38	15
1750	88	44	18
2000	100	50	20

Isoproterenol
(Isuprel)

USUAL DOSE

Initial: 0.5 µg/min
Maintenance: lowest effective dose
Maximal: <10 µg/min

TITRATION

Titrate by 0.5-2 µg/min increments every 5-15 min until desired response

Isoproterenol*			
	Infusion Rate (ml/hr)		
Dose µg/min	1 mg/250 ml (4 µg/ml)	2 mg/250 ml (8 µg/ml)	4 mg/250 ml (16 µg/ml)
0.5	8	4	2
1	15	8	4
2	30	15	8
3	45	23	11
4	60	30	15
5	75	38	19
6	90	45	23
7	105	53	26
8	120	60	30
9	135	68	34
10	150	75	38
15	225	113	56
20	300	150	75
25	375	188	94
30	450	225	113

*When infusion rates fall in the lightly shaded area, a more concentrated drip is indicated.

Lidocaine HCl (Xylocaine), **Procainamide HCl** (Pronestyl), **Bretylium** (Bretylol)

USUAL DOSE

Initial: 1-2 mg/min
Maintenance: 1-4 mg/min

TITRATION

Start at 1-2 mg/min and titrate for
dysrhythmia control

Lidocaine/Procainamide HCl/Bretylium

Dose mg/min	*Infusion Rate (ml/hr)*			
	500 mg/500 ml (1 mg/ml)	500 mg/250 ml (2 mg/ml)	1000 mg/25 ml (4 mg/ml)	200 mg/250 ml (8 mg/ml)
1	60	30	15	8
2	120	60	30	15
3	180	90	45	23
4	240	120	60	30

Milrinone

USUAL DOSE

Initial: 0.25 µg/kg/min
Maintenance: 0.375-0.75 µg/kg/min
Maximal: 1.13 µg/kg/min

TITRATION

Loading dose over 10 min. Start at
0.4-0.8 µg/kg/min. Frequent titration
not necessary; adjust rate at 2-4 hr
intervals

Milrinone: 20 mg/100 ml
Concentration: 200 µg/ml

	Patient Weight in Kilograms							
	50	60	70	80	90	100	110	120
Loading Dose (50 µg/kg) →	3	3	4	4	5	5	6	6
Dose µg/kg/min	*Infusion Rate (ml/hr)*							
0.3	5	6	7	8	9	11	12	13
0.4	6	7	8	10	11	12	13	14
0.5	8	9	11	12	14	15	17	18
0.6	9	11	13	14	16	18	20	22
0.7	11	13	15	17	19	21	23	25
0.8	12	14	17	19	22	24	26	29
0.9	14	16	19	22	24	27	30	32
1	15	18	21	24	27	30	33	36

Nitroglycerin
(Tridil)

USUAL DOSE

Initial: 5-10 µg/min
Maintenance: use lowest effective
dose
Maximal: <200 µg/min

TITRATION

Titrate by 5-10 µg/min increments
q5-10 min until angina subsides

Nitroglycerin			
	Infusion Rate (ml/hr)		
Dose µg/min	25 mg/250 ml (100 µg/ml)	50 mg/250 ml (200 µg/ml)	100 mg/250 ml (400 µg/ml)
5	3	—	—
10	6	3	2
20	12	6	3
30	18	9	5
40	24	12	6
50	30	15	8
60	36	18	9
70	42	21	10
80	48	24	12
90	54	27	14
100	60	30	15
150	90	45	23
200	120	60	30
250	150	75	38
350	210	105	53

Nitroprusside
(Nipride, Nitropress)

USUAL DOSE

Initial: 0.3 µg/kg/min
Maintenance: 3-5 µg/kg/min
Maximal: 10 µg/kg/min

TITRATION

Start at 0.3 µg/kg/min. Increase in
small increments every 2-3 min until
BP controlled.

Nitroprusside: 50 mg/250 ml*

Concentration: 200 µg/ml

Dose µg/kg/min	Patient Weight in Kilograms							
	50	60	70	80	90	100	110	120
	Infusion Rate (ml/hr)							
0.3	5	5	6	7	8	9	10	11
0.5	8	9	11	12	14	15	17	18
1	15	18	21	24	27	30	33	36
2	30	36	42	48	54	60	66	72
3	45	54	63	72	81	90	99	108
4	60	72	84	96	108	120	132	144
5	75	90	105	120	135	150	165	180
6	90	108	126	144	162	180	198	216
7	105	126	147	168	189	210	231	252
8	120	144	168	192	216	240	264	288
9	135	162	189	216	243	270	297	324
10	150	180	210	240	270	300	330	360

*When infusion rates fall in the lightly shaded area, a more concentrated drip is indicated.

Nitroprusside: 100 mg/250 ml*

Concentration: 400 µg/ml

Dose µg/kg/min	Patient Weight in Kilograms							
	50	60	70	80	90	100	110	120
	Infusion Rate (ml/hr)							
0.3	2	3	3	4	4	5	5	5
0.5	4	5	5	6	7	8	8	9
1	8	9	11	12	14	15	17	18
2	15	18	21	24	27	30	33	36
3	23	27	32	36	41	45	50	54
4	30	36	42	48	54	60	66	72
5	38	45	53	60	68	75	83	90
6	45	54	63	72	81	90	99	108
7	53	63	74	84	95	105	116	126
8	60	72	84	96	108	120	132	144
9	68	81	95	108	122	135	149	162
10	75	90	105	120	135	150	165	180

*When infusion rates fall in the lightly shaded area, a more concentrated drip is indicated.

Norepinephrine
(Levophed)

USUAL DOSE

Initial: 8-12 µg/min
Maintenance: 2-4 µg/min
Maximum: 40 µg/min

TITRATION

Adjust every 2-3 min as necessary
to maintain desired systolic or
mean BP

Norepinephrine*			
	Infusion Rate (ml/hr)		
Dose µg/min	4 mg/500 ml (8 µg/ml)	8 mg/500 ml (16 µg/ml)	8 mg/250 ml (32 µg/ml)
2	15	8	4
4	30	15	8
6	45	23	11
8	60	30	15
10	75	38	19
12	90	45	23
14	105	53	26
16	120	60	30
18	135	68	34
20	150	75	38
25	188	94	47
30	225	113	56
35	263	131	66
40	300	150	75

*When infusion rates fall in the lightly shaded area, a more concentrated drip is indicated.

Phenylephrine
(Neo-Synephrine)

USUAL DOSE

Initial: 100-180 µg/min
Maintenance: 40-60 µg/min

TITRATION

Titrate to systolic or mean BP adjust
q10-15 min to maintain low normal
systolic BP

Phenylephrine			
	Infusion Rate (ml/hr)		
Dose µg/min	10 mg/500 ml (20 µg/ml)	10 mg/250 ml (40 µg/ml)	50 mg/500 ml (100 µg/ml)
20	60	30	12
40	120	60	24
60	180	90	36
80	240	120	48
100	300	150	60
120	360	180	72
140	420	210	84
160	480	240	96
180	540	270	108
200	600	300	120

Propofol
(Diprivan)

USUAL DOSE

Initial: 5 µg/kg/min
Maintenance: 5-50 µg/kg/min
Maximum: 150 µg/kg/min

TITRATION

Start at 5 µg/kg/min, increase by increments of 5 µg/kg/min q 5-10 min until desired level of sedation

Propofol: 500 mg/50 ml
Concentration: 10 mg/ml

Dose µg/kg/min	Patient Weight in Kilograms										
	50	55	60	65	70	75	80	90	100	110	120
	Infusion Rate (ml/hr)										
5	2	2	2	2	2	2	2	3	3	3	4
10	3	3	4	4	4	5	5	5	6	7	7
15	5	5	5	6	6	7	7	8	9	10	11
20	6	7	7	8	8	9	10	11	12	13	14
25	8	8	9	10	11	11	12	14	15	17	18
30	9	10	11	12	13	14	14	16	18	20	22
35	11	12	13	14	15	16	17	19	21	23	25
40	12	13	14	16	17	18	19	22	24	26	29
45	14	15	16	18	19	20	22	24	27	30	32
50	15	17	18	20	21	23	24	27	30	33	36
60	18	20	22	23	25	27	29	32	36	40	43
70	21	23	25	27	29	32	34	38	42	46	50
80	24	26	29	31	34	36	38	43	48	53	58
90	27	30	32	35	38	41	43	49	54	59	65
100	30	33	36	39	42	45	48	54	60	66	72

Propranolol HCl
(Inderal)

USUAL DOSE

Initial: 2 mg/hr
Maintenance: 2-3 mg/hr

TITRATION

Most patients well controlled on 2-3 mg/hr, if needed can give intermittent bolus doses of 1 mg

Propanolol		
	Infusion Rate (ml/hr)	
Dose mg/hr	15 mg/500 ml (30 µg/ml)	15 mg/250 ml (60 µg/ml)
1	33	17
2	67	33
3	100	50
4	133	67

Vasopressin
(Pitressin)

USUAL DOSE

Initial: 0.2 U/min
Maintenance: increase qh by 0.2
U/min until hemorrhage controlled

TITRATION

Start at 0.2 U/min
Increase in increments of 0.2 U/min
each hour until hemorrhage controlled
Maximum dose 1-2 U/min

Vasopressin			
Dose		Infusion Rate (ml/hr)	
U/min	U/hr	100 U/100 ml (1 U/ml)	200 U/250 ml (0.8 U/ml)
0.2	12	12	15
0.4	24	24	30
0.6	36	36	45
0.8	48	48	60
1	60	60	75
1.2	72	72	90
1.4	84	84	105
1.6	96	96	120
1.8	108	108	135
2	120	120	150

Abbreviations

ABGs	arterial blood gases
ACE	angiotension converting enzyme
ACLS	advanced cardiac life support
ACT	activated coagulation time
AIDS	acquired immunodeficiency syndrome
ALT (SGPT)	alanine aminotransferase (serum glutamic pyruvate transaminase)
ANA	antinuclear antibody
approx	approximately
APTT	activated partial thromboplastin time
ARDS	adult respiratory distress syndrome
AST (SGOT)	aspartate aminotransaminase (serum glutamic-oxaloacetic transaminase)
AV	atrioventricular
bid	two times daily
BP	blood pressure
BPH	benign prostatic hypertrophy
bpm	beats per minute
BSA	body surface area
BUN	blood urea nitrogen
CAD	coronary artery disease
caps	capsules
CBC	complete blood count
CDC	Centers for Disease Control
CHF	congestive heart failure
CI	cardiac index
CNS	central nervous system
CO	cardiac output
CO$_2$	carbon dioxide
COPD	chronic obstructive pulmonary disease
CPK	creatine phosphokinase
CPR	cardiopulmonary resuscitation
creat cl	creatinine clearance
C & S	culture and sensitivity
CTZ	chemoreceptor trigger zone
CV	cardiovascular
CVA	cerebrovascular accident
CVP	central venous pressure
D$_5$W	5% dextrose in water
DBP	diastolic blood pressure
Derm	dermatologic
DIC	disseminated intravascular coagulation
dl	deciliter
DNA	deoxyribonucleic acid
ECG	electrocardiogram
EEG	electroencephalogram
EENT	eye, ear, nose, and throat
EMS	emergency medical services
Endo	endocrine
ERP	effective refractory period
ET	endotracheal
ETT	endotracheal tube
ext rls	extended release
F&E	fluid and electrolyte
FD&C	food, drugs, and cosmetics
g	gram
g-tube	gastric tube
GFR	glomerular filtration rate
GGT	gamma-glutamyltransferase
GI	gastrointestinal
GU	genitourinary
HCl	hydrochloride
Hct	hematocrit
Hema	hematologic
Hgb	hemoglobin
HIV	human immunodeficiency virus
HR	heart rate
hr	hour
hs	before sleep (at bedtime)
ICP	intracranial pressure
ID	identification
Ig	immunoglobulin
IHSS	idiopathic hypertropic subaortic stenosis

643

IM	intramuscular	**PAP**	pulmonary artery pressure(s)
immed	immediate	**PAS**	pulmonary artery systolic (pressure)
inhal	inhalation	**PAT**	paroxysmal atrial tachycardia
I&O	intake and output	**PCA**	patient-controlled analgesia
IPPB	intermittent positive-pressure breathing	**PCWP**	pulmonary capillary wedge pressure(s)
IU	international units	**pH**	hydrogen ion concentration
IV	intravenous	**PID**	pelvic inflammatory disease
kg	kilogram	**PO**	*per os*, by mouth
L	liter	**postop**	postoperative
lb	pounds	**preop**	preoperative
LDH	lactate dehydrogenase	**prn**	as needed
LR	lactated Ringer's solution	**PT**	prothrombin time
LVEDP	left ventricular end-diastolic pressure	**PTCA**	percutaneous tranluminal coronary angioplasty/atherectomy
m	meter	**PTT**	partial thromboplastin time
MAO	monoamine oxidase	**PVC**	premature ventricular contraction
MAP	mean arterial pressure	**PVR**	pulmonary vascular resistance
mEq	milliequivalent	**q**	every
mg	milligram	**qd**	once every day
MI	myocardial infarction	**qid**	four times daily
min	minute(s)	**RBC**	red blood cell
misc	miscellaneous	**RE**	reticuloendothelial
ml	milliliter	**Resp**	respiratory
mm Hg	millimeters mercury (pressure)	**RR**	respiratory rate
mo	month(s)	**SA**	sinoatrial
MRSA	methacillin resistant staphylococcus aureus	**SBP**	systolic blood pressure
MS	musculoskeletal	**SC**	subcutaneous
NaCl	sodium chloride	**sec**	second(s)
ND	not determined	**SIADH**	syndrome of inappropriate secretion of antidiuretic hormone
Neuro	neurologic	**SL**	sublingual
ng	nanogram	**SLE**	systemic lupus erythematosus
NG	nasogastric	**std**	standard
NMBA	neuromuscular blocking agent	**sus rls**	sustained release
nmol	nanomole	**susp**	suspension
NPO	nothing by mouth	**SV**	stroke volume
NSAID	nonsteroidal antiinflammatory drug	**SVR**	systemic vascular resistance
O₂	oxygen	**SVT**	supraventricular tachycardia
Ophth	ophthalmic	**Syst**	systemic
oz	ounces	**TCA**	tricyclic antidepressant
PAC	premature atrial contraction	**TD**	transdermal
PAD	pulmonary artery diastolic (pressure)	**temp**	temperature
PAM	pulmonary artery mean		

TEN	toxic epidermal necrolysis	**WBC**	white blood cell (count)
TIA	transient ischemic attack	**wk**	week
tid	three times daily	**WPW**	Wolff-Parkinson-White syndrome
TPN	total parenteral nutrition	**yr**	year(s)
tsp	teaspoon	μ	micron
U	units	μg	microgram
UO	urine output	>	greater than
var	variable	<	less than
vs	versus	≥	greater than/equal
VS	vital signs	≤	less than/equal

Index

Entries can be identified as follows: Trade Name; generic; DRUG CATEGORY.

Entries can be identified as follows: Trade Name; generic; DRUG CATEGORY.

Entries can be identified as follows: Trade Name; generic; DRUG CATEGORY.

Entries can be identified as follows: Trade Name; generic; DRUG CATEGORY.

Entries can be identified as follows: Trade Name; generic; DRUG CATEGORY.

Entries can be identified as follows: Trade Name; generic; DRUG CATEGORY.

Entries can be identified as follows: Trade Name; generic; DRUG CATEGORY.

Entries can be identified as follows: Trade Name; generic; DRUG CATEGORY.

Entries can be identified as follows: Trade Name; generic; DRUG CATEGORY.

Entries can be identified as follows: Trade Name; generic; DRUG CATEGORY.

Entries can be identified as follows: Trade Name; generic; DRUG CATEGORY.

Entries can be identified as follows: Trade Name; generic; DRUG CATEGORY.

Entries can be identified as follows: Trade Name; generic; DRUG CATEGORY.

Entries can be identified as follows: Trade Name; generic; DRUG CATEGORY.

Entries can be identified as follows: Trade Name; generic; DRUG CATEGORY.

Entries can be identified as follows: Trade Name; generic; DRUG CATEGORY.

Entries can be identified as follows: Trade Name; generic; DRUG CATEGORY.

Entries can be identified as follows: Trade Name; generic; DRUG CATEGORY.

Entries can be identified as follows: Trade Name; generic; DRUG CATEGORY.

Y-Site and Solution Compatibility

AGENT	Aminophylline	Amrinone	Amphotericin	Atracurium	Bretylium	Diltiazem	Dobutamine	Dopamine	Epinephrine	Esmolol	Fentanyl	Furosemide	Heparin	Insulin, reg	Isoproterenol	Labetalol
Aminophylline		C		C		I	I		I	C			C		I	C
Amrinone	C				C		C	C	C			I	C		C	
Amphotericin						C										
Atracurium	C						C	C	C	C	C		C		C	
Bretylium		C				C	C								C	
Diltiazem	I		C		C		C	C	C	C			I	I	I	
Dobutamine	I	C		C	C	C		C					I	C		
Dopamine		C		C		C	C			C			I			C
Epinephrine		C		C		C							C			
Esmolol	C			C		C		C			C	I	C			
Fentanyl				C						C			C			C
Furosemide						I	I	I		I			C			
Heparin	C			C		I	I	I	I	C	C	C		C	C	C
Insulin, reg						I	C					C	C			
Isoproterenol	I	C		C	C								C			
Labetalol	C							C			C	I	C			
Lidocaine		C	I			C	C	C	I			C			I	C
Magnesium							C			C		C	C			C
Midazolam				C												
Milrinone												I				
Morphine	C			C		C		C				I	C	C	C	
Nitroglycerin		C		C		C	C	C					C			
Nitroprusside		C		C		C	C						C			
Norepinephrine	I	C				C							C			
Pancuronium	C						C	C	C	C	C		C		C	
Phenylephrine		C														
Potassium chl	C	C				C	C	C	C	C	C	C		C	C	C
Procainamide		I				C							C			
Propranolol		C											C			
Sodium bicarb		I				I	I	I	I				C	C		
Vancomycin	I			C						C			C		C	C
Vecuronium	C						C	C	C	C	C		C		C	
Verapamil		C					C	C								

D5W = Dextrose 5%
NS = Sodium Chloride 0.9%
RL = Ringer's injection, Lactated
C = Y-site compatibility at typical concentrations
I = One or more sources reported incompatibility
☐ = Compatibility unknown or conflicting reports in literature
This chart is not an exhaustive review. The clinician is encouraged to consult the full text as well as specialized literature in order to compare specific test conditions with actual clinical situations.